# Recent Advances in

# Obstetrics and Gynaecology 28

# Recent Advances in

# Obstetrics and Gynaecology 28

**Mausumi Das** MD MRCOG MPH
Consultant Gynaecologist
Department of Gynaecology and
Reproductive Medicine
Imperial College Healthcare NHS Trust and
Chelsea and Westminster Hospitals NHS Foundation Trust
London, UK

**Togas Tulandi** MD MHCM FRCSC FACOG FCAHS
Professor and Chair
Department of Obstetrics & Gynecology and
Milton Leong Chair in Reproductive Medicine
McGill University
Chief of Department of Obstetrics and Gynecology
McGill University Health Center
Montreal, Canada

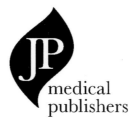

JP
medical
publishers

London • New Delhi

© 2023 Jaypee Brothers Medical Publishers

Published by Jaypee Brothers Medical Publishers,
4838/24 Ansari Road, New Delhi, India

Tel: +91 (011) 43574357          Fax: +91 (011)43574390

Email: info@jpmedpub.com, jaypee@jaypeebrothers.com
Web: www.jpmedpub.com, www.jaypeebrothers.com

JPM is the imprint of Jaypee Brothers Medical Publishers.

The rights of Mausumi Das and Togas Tulandi to be identified as the editors of this work have been asserted by them in accordance with the Copyright, Designs and Patents Act 1988.

**ISBN: 978-1-78779-173-2**

**British Library Cataloguing in Publication Data**
A catalogue record for this book is available from the British Library

**Library of Congress Cataloging in Publication Data**
A catalog record for this book is available from the Library of Congress

Development Editor:     Nikita Chauhan
Editorial Assistant:     Keshav Kumar
Cover Design:     Seema Dogra

Printed at: Printed in India

# Preface

This latest volume of *Recent Advances in Obstetrics and Gynaecology* features an outstanding collection of comprehensive reviews of the latest advances in Obstetrics and Gynaecology. It brings together seventeen chapters written by renowned experts from around the world and it is with great appreciation that we thank them for their immense contribution to this volume.

The field of Obstetrics and Gynaecology is expanding rapidly, driven by the need to provide safe and effective treatment options for patients. Each chapter provides an authoritative review of current knowledge and highlights the latest developments of relevance to clinical practice. The chapters are presented in an accessible and easy to read format, making this latest volume an invaluable resource for both busy clinicians and trainees preparing for postgraduate examinations.

**Mausumi Das**
**Togas Tulandi**
June, 2022

# Contents

# Chapter 1

# Non-invasive prenatal testing: An update

*María Mar Gil, Kypros Herodotos Nicolaides*

## INTRODUCTION

The most frequent indication for invasive prenatal diagnosis is the detection of chromosomal aneuploidies, major causes of perinatal death and childhood handicap. However, these tests are only recommended in high-risk pregnancies since both, amniocentesis and chorionic villous sampling, are associated with an increased risk of subsequent pregnancy loss [1].

During the past decade, several externally blinded validation and implementation studies have been carried out, showing that, using analysis of cell-free (cf) DNA in maternal blood, it is possible to detect a high proportion of fetuses affected by trisomies 21, 18 and 13 at a much lower false positive rate (FPR) than by all other existing screening methods [2]. There is also some recent evidence that cfDNA testing can detect other autosomal trisomies, sex chromosome aneuploidies, and even sequence the complete fetal genome which has led some laboratories to offer screening for fetal chromosomal aberrations of >3 megabases on any chromosome [2–5].

However, and despite the advances in the technique, neither sensitivity nor specificity of cfDNA testing for detecting any condition is 100%. Therefore, it should not be considered a diagnostic test to replace invasive testing, but a screening test capable of identifying high-risk pregnancies that will require further investigation by invasive testing.

This chapter aims to review both, technical and clinical considerations for the implementation of cfDNA testing in current routine practice.

## SCREENING FOR ANEUPLOIDIES

### Current methods of screening

In the 1970s, maternal age was the only method of screening for trisomy 21 but 10 years later, maternal serum biochemistry and detailed ultrasonographic examination performed

**María Mar Gil** MD PhD, Obstetrics and Gynaecology Department, Hospital Universitario de Torrejón, Torrejón de Ardoz, Madrid, School of Medicine, Universidad Francisco de Vitoria (UFV), Pozuelo de Alarcón, Madrid, Spain, Fetal Medicine Research Institute, King's College Hospital, London, UK
Email: mariadelmar.gil@ufv.es

**Kypros Herodotos Nicolaides** MD, Fetal Medicine Research Institute, King's College Hospital, London, UK
Email: kypros@fetalmedicine.com

in the second trimester of the pregnancy were incorporated. In the 1990s, the first-trimester combined test was developed and the introduction of the measurement of the fetal nuchal translucency (NT) thickness by ultrasound and maternal serum β-human chorionic gonadotropin (β-hCG) and pregnancy-associated plasma protein A (PAPP-A), together with maternal age, shifted the time of screening from the second to the first trimester. Using this method of screening, the detection rate (DR) of trisomy 21 increased to 90% at the same FPR of 5% [6]. This is the method of screening currently implemented as first-line screening in many countries, like the UK, where there is a national screening programme for trisomy 21. Essentially, women who receive a risk estimation above a certain threshold are offered the possibility of an invasive test. However, most countries lack national screening guidelines and a variety of first and/or second-trimester screening methods are offered by individual practitioners or institutions, generally driven by the rules of supply/demand or market forces. Consequently, this individual criterion leads to a high invasive testing rate, ranging from 20 to 40% in some countries before cfDNA testing was implemented. However, the use of cfDNA testing for screening of the major aneuploidies has widely spread all over the world from 2012, not only in the private sector but also in many public systems, followed by a significant decrease in the invasive testing rate. Nonetheless, a national policy for offering the cfDNA test has only been established by a few countries and different strategies and approaches have been adopted by those which have, from universal first-line screening to contingent screening following another method, generally the first-trimester combined test.

## Genetic abnormalities included in the screening

Traditionally, trisomy 21 has been the main target of the prenatal aneuploidy screening. However, while performing invasive testing in screened positive cases for trisomy 21, some common patterns in the expression of the biophysical and biochemical markers were observed with some other aneuploidies, like trisomies, 18 and 13, triploidy, and Turner syndrome [6–9]. As a consequence, many of these conditions are secondarily diagnosed when performing an invasive test because of a high risk for trisomy 21 from the first-trimester combined test, without a significant increase in the FPR. However, this is not applicable for cfDNA testing because every condition which is included in the analysis, adds it's related FPR; e.g. the FPR is only 0.04% when trisomy 21 is tested alone, but it goes up to 0.12% when trisomies 18 and 13 are incorporated in the analysis [2]. Although, it may still seem extremely low, a continuous increase is expected with every single new condition analysed. Moreover, the diagnosis of any genetic condition potentially associated to fetal malformations still requires invasive testing for deep analysis, which cannot be replaced by any method of screening.

Moreover, including other conditions such as sex chromosome aneuploidies, rare autosomal trisomies (RATs) or subchromosomal anomalies in routine cfDNA screening may be a challenge in parental counselling since there is a wide spectrum in their clinical manifestation, low understanding of the disease, and insufficient scientific evidence. However, for the last few years, cfDNA testing has being offered to all pregnant women, as an alternative to the first-trimester combined test in Belgium and the Netherlands. In these countries, as an alternative to the first-trimester combined test, genome-wide analysis rather than confined screening for the three major trisomies is offered to all pregnant women in an attempt to also diagnose RATs and other rare additional segmental imbalances (SIs). The results from the first 56,818 women that had the test during the first year of implementation of such strategy in the Netherlands (TRIDENT-2 study) showed that 0.4% (207) of the population screened positive for RATs ($n = 95$) or SIs ($n = 101$) [10]. Only 6 of the 95 cases testing positive for RATs were confirmed and, among those, only one case was associated with an abnormal phenotype. On the other hand, 29 of the 101 cases which tested positive for SIs were confirmed but it was not defined how many of those presented any abnormality which was not discoverable through ultrasound. Additionally, there were seven cases reporting results consistent with maternal malignancies or pre-malignancies, but the benefit of such discovery was not demonstrated. Since an abnormal test result inevitably leads to anxiety and in some cases termination of pregnancy or further maternal and fetal testing, clear management protocols must be developed before routine genome-wide analysis can be implemented. Finally, several concerns also arise from mosaicisms detected prenatally. First, it is impossible to predict the clinical outcome when a true fetal mosaicism is found following a high-risk result for RATs and, second, there is evidence that, in an unselected population, the incidence of adverse pregnancy outcomes in the presence of a confined placental mosaicism (CPM) is not different from that in pregnancies with normal karyotype (except CPM for trisomy 16) [11].

For all the reasons above and even if technically possible, no other condition apart from trisomies 21, 18, and 13 is currently recommended to be analysed by cfDNA testing in maternal blood [12,13].

## SCREENING FOR ANEUPLOIDIES BY CELL-FREE DNA ANALYSIS OF MATERNAL BLOOD

### Performance of the test in screening for trisomies 21, 18, and 13

A meta-analysis summarising the results from 1,963 cases of trisomy 21, 563 cases of trisomy 18, 119 cases of trisomy 13, and over 200,000 unaffected singleton pregnancies reported that the weighted pooled DR was 99.7% (95% CI 99.1–99.9%) for trisomy 21, 97.9% (95% CI 94.9–99.1%) for trisomy 18 and 99.0% (95% CI 65.8–100%) for trisomy 13 and the weighted pooled FPR were 0.04% (95% CI 0.02–0.07%), 0.04% (95% CI 0.03–0.07%) and 0.04% (95% CI 0.02–0.07%) for trisomies 21, 18, and 13, respectively [2].

Similarly, a recent meta-analysis in twin pregnancies reported that in a combined total of 56 trisomy 21, 18 cases of trisomy 18 and over 3,000 unaffected twin pregnancies, the weighted pooled DR was 98.2% (95% CI 83.2–99.8%) for trisomy 21 and 88.9% (95% CI 64.8–97.2%) for trisomy 18 and the weighted pooled FPR were 0.05% (95% CI 0.01–0.26%) and 0.03% (95% CI 0.00–0.33%) for trisomies 21 and 18, respectively [14]. The number of twin pregnancies affected by trisomy 13 ($n = 3$) was insufficient to accurately assess the DR, but the average FPR of 0.19% found for trisomy 13 seems higher than that reported for singleton pregnancies.

These results show that cfDNA testing is the best available method for screening of these conditions in singleton pregnancies and the best method for screening of trisomy 21 in twin pregnancies.

### Performance of the test in screening for other aneuploidies

A smaller number of cases have been analysed to demonstrate the ability of cfDNA analysis in maternal blood to detect sex chromosome aneuploidies, RATs, triploidy, microdeletion, and microduplication syndromes and even monogenic disorders [5,10,15–18]. Nonetheless, further investigation is required to determine the exact performance and clinical utility of the test.

## Laboratory methods for analysis

Millions of nucleotide sequences can be amplified and sequenced by parallel sequencing of the numerous cfDNA fragments that are present in the maternal circulation. This results in a large amount of data subsequently analysed by bioinformatics and normally, a comparison with a genome of reference is carried out for interpretation. Two main approaches have been used for analysis in the main clinical studies assessing the performance of cfDNA testing: (1) massively parallel shotgun sequencing (MPSS) and (2) targeted chromosome analysis. While the MPSS method sequences and normally analyses the entire genome, in the targeted approach the analysis is limited only to the chromosomes of interest either by next-generation sequencing, custom microarray or single nucleotide polymorphisms (SNPs) analysis, among others.

## Massively parallel shotgun sequencing

This method consists on the sequencing of millions of cfDNA fragments from the maternal plasma, belonging to both, the mother and the fetus, whose origin and chromosome of origin are possible to identify. This makes it possible to quantify the number of fragments that comes from each one of the studied chromosomes. Since trisomies consist of the presence of an additional chromosome in a certain pair, the amount of fragments derived from that chromosome in these cases is higher (usually, chromosome 3 is used as a reference) [19,20]. A large number of sequences (depth of sequencing or "coverage") and a great biomathematical effort are needed to examine these numerical differences, which are sometimes minute.

Since all DNA fragments coming from the entire genome are analysed, this method is potentially able to identify all aneuploidies as well as many other genetic conditions. However, chromosome 21 represents only 1–2% of the human genome, therefore, many millions of molecules from the whole genome need to be sequenced to ensure a minimum amount of chromosome 21 which allows to differentiate between pregnancies affected by trisomy 21 and euploids.

This method has shown a high performance in the screening for the three major trisomies and a low no-result rate (<1%).

## Chromosome selective sequencing

The basic principle of chromosome selective sequencing (CSS) is the same as that of MPSS, sequencing DNA from maternal plasma. However, in CSS, the selective assay is directed specifically towards chromosomes 21, 18, and 13 (plus or minus chromosomes X and Y) before sequencing. Since the number of regions to be sequenced is much less than the entire genome, the process may be simplified. In addition, the CSS is capable of estimating the fetal fraction by evaluating the SNPs in other chromosomes [21]. This method has shown a high performance in the screening for the three major trisomies; however, although a recent meta-analysis did not show significant differences, the no-result rate may be higher (up to 2%) by CSS than by MPSS [2].

## Microarray analysis

Microarray analysis was developed to substitute CSS and, by this method, a custom microarray is used as a counting method instead of next-generation sequencing [22]. The results obtained by this approach are comparable to those obtained by CSS, but with a shorter turnaround time and more cost-effective results [22,23].

## Single nucleotide polymorphisms analysis

SNPs are small differences in the DNA that are unique for each individual. A SNP represents a variation in one single base (a nucleotide) from a certain DNA sequence, which is identical between individuals for everything else. This method is based on the principle that the mother and the fetus have different SNPs. To perform the test, the maternal plasma, which contains both fetal and maternal DNA, and the buffy coat, which contains only maternal DNA, are analysed. Then, >13,000 polymorphic loci are quantified simultaneously on chromosomes 21, 18, 13, X, and Y using a multiplex polymerase chain reaction (PCR). Finally, the small differences in the SNPs pattern between the mother and the fetus throughout the genome are used to estimate if the fetal distribution is consistent with disomy, trisomy, or monosomy [17]. It could be expected that, even at lower fetal fractions, this method would be the most accurate. However, the performance for the detection of the three major trisomies reported in published studies is similar to that of MPSS or CSS, but the no-result rate is higher (up to 3–5%) [2].

## Other methods

Many research groups were simultaneously working on the development of a cfDNA test for screening of aneuploidies based on PCR, such as real-time PCR or digital PCR, even before the spread of next-generation sequencing [24]. This method is already offered by several laboratories and, despite similar performance was shown in the validation studies, there is yet no large-scale prospective study reporting results in the general population. More recently, a method based on highly specific chromosomal fluorescent labelling, called the rolling-circle method, has been developed [25].

## Limitations of the cfDNA test

CfDNA testing has two important disadvantages which may make its implementation as a method of screening for aneuploidies more difficult. The first one is its cost, similar to the cost of an invasive test but considerably higher than the cost of other methods for screening of aneuploidies, such as the first-trimester combined test. The second disadvantage is the no-result rate or the proportion of cases where a result cannot be provided after analysis. A low fetal fraction is the most important cause for not getting a result from cfDNA testing and the two main reasons for the fetal fraction to be low are first, maternal obesity and second, a small placental mass [26,27].

# CLINICAL IMPLEMENTATION OF CELL-FREE DNA TESTING FOR SCREENING OF FETAL ANEUPLOIDIES

In the last 40 years performing prenatal screening techniques, we have learnt that pregnant women are capable of making scientifically and ethically reasoned decisions about invasive testing when they have the appropriate information about these tests [28,29]. Screening techniques have contributed to a worldwide marked reduction in the number of invasive tests, and an exponential increase in the rate of invasive tests has been observed as the risk predicted by these systems increases [28,29]. Despite this, there is still a small fraction of women who, despite obtaining a low-risk screening result, wish to undergo an invasive test. Similarly, there is a percentage of women who prefer not to undergo an invasive test even after obtaining a high-risk result. In these cases, the cfDNA test is especially beneficial, since it reinforces the screening result, which has a positive impact on patient care and pregnancy monitoring.

Although many studies on the efficacy of the cfDNA test have been performed in women at high-risk of aneuploidies, an increasing number of studies performed in routine population have shown that this method is equally effective in both, high-risk and low-risk patients. This, added to the fact that reliable results are obtained from week 10, has led to worldwide recommendation of cfDNA testing in routine, average-risk, populations in the first trimester. Since, by this approach, the result is obtained in the first trimester, most of the parents receiving a low-risk result will be early reassured that the fetus is unlikely to have the aneuploidy while those parents receiving a high-risk result will have the possibility of an earlier and safer termination of the pregnancy. Having assessed the risk of fetal aneuploidies, efforts can then focus into early screening for other pregnancy complications, such as pre-eclampsia [30].

## CfDNA as primary method of screening

Essentially, there are two options for performing cfDNA testing universally, as a primary method of screening: the first one is to take the blood sample at 10 weeks of gestation and, the second is to take it at 11–13 weeks, during the first-trimester ultrasound. The main advantage of the 10 weeks' sampling is that the results will be available at the 12–13 weeks' first-trimester scan, which allows the chance to perform a rescue first-trimester combined test if no results are obtained from the cfDNA test [31]. The disadvantage of this approach is that several unnecessary tests will be performed, as some of the pregnant women will suffer an spontaneous miscarriage before 12–13 weeks' and there will also be some cases in which a high NT or a major fetal defect will be diagnosed, therefore, requiring an invasive test irrespective of the result from the cfDNA test. On the other hand, the option of taking the blood sample at 12 weeks' gestation, would avoid doing the test on such cases, but it would not be possible to perform a rescue first-trimester combined test in cases without a result, likely falling outside the 11–13 weeks window [32].

## CfDNA offered contingently

When universal screening by cfDNA testing is not a feasible option, the cfDNA test can be alternatively offered as a contingent screening on the basis of the results obtained by another method performed as first-line screening, preferably the first-trimester combined test. If the main objective of such policy is to reduce the invasive testing rate, the cfDNA test can be limited to the high-risk group, as an alternative to invasive testing; however, if the objective is not only that, but also to increase the DR of fetal aneuploidies, the offering of cfDNA testing can be expanded to the intermediate-risk group [33]. However, the recommended cut-offs which define the high-risk or intermediate-risk groups will inevitably depend on the economic cost of cfDNA testing that will define the proportion of pregnant women who can benefit from the test [34].

## Interpretation of results from cfDNA testing: Special situations

### High-risk results

If the cfDNA report shows a high-risk result for any aneuploidy, it does not mean that the fetus is definitely affected and, therefore, it is important to perform an invasive procedure for genetic diagnosis, which confirms or refutes the result. Since the cfDNA analysed is actually not fetal but placental in origin, many authors recommend amniocentesis as the preferred invasive test for confirmation. However, the cfDNA test can be performed as early as the 10th week of gestation and the amniocentesis should not be performed before the 15th week; therefore, performing an amniocentesis would require a long waiting time for the parents. Recent studies have analysed the results of over 2,000 chorionic villus samplings and concluded that, even in the absence of fetal defects, in 97% of the cases, mesenchyme culture of placental villi would be informative and only 3% would require a subsequent amniocentesis to exclude CPM [35,36]. CPM occurs most frequently in those cases where the cfDNA test shows a high risk for trisomy 13 or monosomy X, therefore, only these two results would necessitate an amniocentesis for confirmation, if the ultrasound scan shows no compatible fetal malformations [35].

### Low-risk results

On the other hand, if the cfDNA test result shows a low risk, the parents can be reassured that it is highly unlikely that the fetus is affected by any of the three major aneuploidies. However, as for high-risk results, low-risk reports should also be interpreted together with a detailed ultrasound examination to exclude major fetal defects or increased NT. In such cases, the parents should be offered invasive testing for microarray analysis irrespective of the results from the cfDNA test, since other chromosomal and subchromosomal conditions need to be excluded in addition to the three main trisomies.

### No results or failed results

An individual management is needed for those cases where the cfDNA test does not provide a result. It was previously explained that the main reason for not getting a result after cfDNA analysis is an insufficient proportion of fetal DNA in the maternal blood sample. The main determinants of a low fetal fraction are maternal obesity and a small placental mass; therefore, fetal aneuploidies presenting with a smaller placenta, such as trisomies 18, 13, and triploidy but not trisomy 21, usually show a lower fetal fraction and a higher no-result rate than unaffected pregnancies [37]. Consequently, those pregnancies where the cfDNA test does not provide a result due to a low fetal fraction should be considered at a higher risk for trisomies 18, 13, and triploidy (but not for trisomy 21) and a detailed ultrasound examination looking for specific features of such conditions should be performed. If there are fetal defects concordant with the suspected aneuploidy, an invasive test should be recommended [37]. However, if the scan is normal, results from other screening methods, if available, should be evaluated. For example, if there was a previous screening that had already shown a low-risk result, repeating the test is the most sensible option since there is >60% chance to obtain a result in the second attempt [31]. Conversely, in those cases where a previous screening had already shown a high-risk result but the fetal ultrasound is normal, invasive testing or repeat testing is a reasonable option to consider. Finally, if the test fails a second time, the options of invasive testing or expectant management should be discussed with the parents.

Another important source of failed results from cfDNA testing is the presence of a vanishing twin. The cfDNA fetal fraction of the deceased fetus increases in maternal blood after the demise, peaking about 7–9 weeks later, to decrease gradually over gestation to almost become undetectable [38]. cfDNA analysis detects the presence of DNA material from the vanished twin up to 15–16 weeks after demise [38–40]. This persisting material from the vanished twin in the maternal circulation may reduce DR and increase false positive and no-result rates but actual performance of screening by cfDNA testing in the presence of a vanishing twin is unknown. For all this reasons, cfDNA testing should not be performed in vanishing-twin pregnancies unless new scientific evidence emerges. An alternative to cfDNA testing in these cases is the first-trimester combined test. Although it was generally recommended not to use serum biomarkers when there is a measurable fetal pole [41], it has been recently reported that, unlike PAPP-A levels which are always increased in vanishing-twin pregnancies even if only an empty sac is visible, free β-hCG levels are not significantly different from those in normal singleton pregnancies, regardless of the time the fetal demise occurred [42]. This knowledge may allow performing first-trimester screening by combining maternal age, fetal NT thickness, and free β-hCG in these pregnancies, increasing DR from 80 to 85% as compared to screening by maternal age and NT alone, both at 5% FPR [41].

## CONCLUSION

- cfDNA testing is the most accurate screening method for trisomy 21 both in singleton and twin pregnancies
- Inclusion of other genetic conditions in the cfDNA panel besides the three common trisomies is still controversial and therefore, not recommended
- Different technologies for cfDNA testing have been developed with similar results.
- High-risk results from cfDNA testing necessitate confirmation by invasive testing, preferably by first-trimester chorionic villus sampling. Only those cases testing positive for trisomy 13 or monosomy X and without any fetal defects detected by a detailed ultrasound examination would require a second-trimester amniocentesis due to a higher chance of encountering a CPM
- Low-risk results must always be interpreted in the context of a normal ultrasound examination which has excluded major fetal defects and an increased NT
- An individual management is needed for those cases where the cfDNA test does not provide a result: ultrasound and clinical findings must guide the decision on whether an invasive test is required or not
- The presence of a vanishing twin is currently a contraindication for performing cfDNA testing since the accuracy of the test in such cases is unknown

## REFERENCES

1. Gil MM, Molina FS, Rodriguez-Fernandez M, et al. New approach for estimating risk of miscarriage after chorionic villus sampling. Ultrasound Obstet Gynecol 2020; 56:656–663.
2. Gil MM, Accurti V, Santacruz B, et al. Analysis of cell-free DNA in maternal blood in screening for aneuploidies: updated meta-analysis. Ultrasound Obstet Gynecol 2017; 50:302–314.
3. Christina Fan H, Gu W, Wang J, et al. Non-invasive prenatal measurement of the fetal genome. Nature 2012; 487:320-324.
4. Kitzman JO, Snyder MW, Ventura M, et al. Noninvasive whole-genome sequencing of a human fetus. Sci Transl Med 2012; 4:137ra76.

5. Rabinowitz M, Savage M, Pettersen B, et al. Noninvasive Cell-Free DNA-Based Prenatal Detection of Microdeletions Using Single Nucleotide Polymorphism-Targeted Sequencing. Obs Gynecol 2014; 123:167S.

6. Wright D, Syngelaki A, Bradbury I, et al. First-trimester screening for trisomies 21, 18 and 13 by ultrasound and biochemical testing. Fetal Diagn Ther 2014; 35:118–126.

7. Sebire NJ, Snijders RJ, Brown R, et al. Detection of sex chromosome abnormalities by nuchal translucency screening at 10-14 weeks. Prenat Diagn. 1998; 18:581–584.

8. Spencer K, Tul N, Nicolaides KH. Maternal serum free beta-hCG and PAPP-A in fetal sex chromosome defects in the first trimester. Prenat Diagn. 2000; 20:390–394.

9. Kagan KO, Anderson JM, Anwandter G, et al. Screening for triploidy by the risk algorithms for trisomies 21, 18 and 13 at 11 weeks to 13 weeks and 6 days of gestation. Prenat Diagn. 2008; 28:1209–1213.

10. van der Meij KRM, Sistermans EA, Macville MVE et al. TRIDENT-2: National Implementation of Genome-Wide Non-Invasive Prenatal Testing as a First-Tier Screening Test in the Netherlands. Am J Hum Genet. 2019; 105:1091–1101.

11. Grati FR, Ferreira J, Benn P, et al. Outcomes in pregnancies with a confined placental mosaicism and implications for prenatal screening using cell-free DNA. Genet Med. 2020; 22:309–316.

12. Dondorp W, De Wert G, Bombard Y, et al. Non-invasive prenatal testing for aneuploidy and beyond: Challenges of responsible innovation in prenatal screening. Eur J Hum Genet. 2015; 23:1438–1450.

13. Committee Opinion No. 640. Cell-free DNA screening for fetal aneuploidy. Obstet Gynecol. 2015; 126:e31–37.

14. Gil MM, Galeva S, Jani J, et al. Screening for trisomies by cfDNA testing of maternal blood in twin pregnancy: update of The Fetal Medicine Foundation results and meta-analysis. Ultrasound Obstet Gynecol. 2021; 58:178–189.

15. Nicolaides KH, Musci TJ, Struble CA, et al. Assessment of fetal sex chromosome aneuploidy using directed cell-free DNA analysis. Fetal Diagn Ther. 2014; 35:1–6.

16. Nicolaides KH, Syngelaki A, Gil MM, et al. Prenatal Detection of Fetal Triploidy from Cell-Free DNA Testing in Maternal Blood. Fetal Diagn Ther. 2014; 35:212–217.

17. Nicolaides KH, Syngelaki A, Gil M, et al. Validation of targeted sequencing of single-nucleotide polymorphisms for non-invasive prenatal detection of aneuploidy of chromosomes 13, 18, 21, X, and Y. Prenat Diagn. 2013; 33:575–579.

18. Chitty LS, Mason S, Barrett AN, et al. Non-invasive prenatal diagnosis of achondroplasia and thanatophoric dysplasia: next-generation sequencing allows for a safer, more accurate, and comprehensive approach. Prenat Diagn. 2015; 35:656–662.

19. Chiu RWK, Chan KCA, Gao Y, et al. Noninvasive prenatal diagnosis of fetal chromosomal aneuploidy by massively parallel genomic sequencing of DNA in maternal plasma. Proc Natl Acad Sci. 2008; 105:20458–20463.

20. Fan HC, Blumenfeld YJ, Chitkara U, et al. Noninvasive diagnosis of fetal aneuploidy by shotgun sequencing DNA from maternal blood. Proc Natl Acad Sci. 2008; 105:16266–16271.

21. Sparks AB, Wang ET, Struble CA, et al. Selective analysis of cell-free DNA in maternal blood for evaluation of fetal trisomy. Prenat Diagn. 2012; 32:3–9.

22. Juneau K, Bogard PE, Huang S, et al. Microarray-based cell-free DNA analysis improves noninvasive prenatal testing. Fetal Diagn Ther. 2014; 36:282–286.

23. Stokowski R, Wang E, White K, et al. Clinical performance of non-invasive prenatal testing (NIPT) using targeted cell-free DNA analysis in maternal plasma with microarrays or next generation sequencing (NGS) is consistent across multiple controlled clinical studies. Prenat Diagn. 2015; 35:1243–1246.

24. Patsalis PC. A new method for non-invasive prenatal diagnosis of Down syndrome using MeDIP real time qPCR. Appl Trans Genom. 2012; 1:3–8.

25. Dahl F, Ericsson O, Karlberg O, et al. Imaging single DNA molecules for high precision NIPT. Sci Rep. 2018; 8:4549.

26. Ashoor G, Poon L, Syngelaki A, et al. Fetal fraction in maternal plasma cell-free DNA at 11–13 weeks' gestation: Effect of maternal and fetal factors. Fetal Diagn Ther. 2012; 31:237–243.

27. Poon LCY, Musci T, Song K, et al. Maternal plasma cell-free fetal and maternal DNA at 11–13 weeks' gestation: Relation to fetal and maternal characteristics and pregnancy outcomes. Fetal Diagn Ther. 2013; 33:215–223.

28. Nicolaides KH, Chervenak FA, McCullough LB, et al. Evidence-based obstetric ethics and informed decision-making by pregnant women about invasive diagnosis after first-trimester assessment of risk for trisomy 21. Am J Obstet Gynecol. 2005; 193:322–326.

29. Gil MM, Giunta G, Macalli EA, et al. UK NHS pilot study on cell-free DNA testing in screening for fetal trisomies: factors affecting uptake. Ultrasound Obstet Gynecol. 2015; 45:67–73.

30. Nicolaides KH. A model for a new pyramid of prenatal care based on the 11 to 13 weeks' assessment. Prenat Diagn. 2011; 31:3–6.

31. Gil MM, Quezada MS, Bregant B, et al. Implementation of maternal blood cell-free DNA testing in early screening for aneuploidies. Ultrasound Obstet Gynecol. 2013; 42:34–40.

32. Kagan KO, Wright D, Nicolaides KH. First-trimester contingent screening for trisomies 21, 18 and 13 by fetal nuchal translucency and ductus venosus flow and maternal blood cell-free DNA testing. Ultrasound Obstet Gynecol. 2015; 45:42–47.

33. Gil MM, Revello R, Poon LC, et al. Clinical implementation of routine screening for fetal trisomies in the UK NHS: cell-free DNA test contingent on results from first-trimester combined test. Ultrasound Obstet Gynecol. 2016; 47:45–52.

34. Nicolaides KH, Syngelaki A, Poon LC, et al. First-trimester contingent screening for trisomies 21, 18 and 13 by biomarkers and maternal blood cell-free DNA testing. Fetal Diagn Ther. 2014; 35:185–192.

35. Grati FR, Bajaj K, Malvestiti F, et al. The type of feto-placental aneuploidy detected by cfDNA testing may influence the choice of confirmatory diagnostic procedure. Prenat Diagn. 2015; 35:994–998.

36. Van Opstal D, Srebniak MI. Cytogenetic confirmation of a positive NIPT result: evidence-based choice between chorionic villus sampling and amniocentesis depending on chromosome aberration. Expert Rev Mol Diagn. 2016; 16:513–550.

37. Revello R, Sarno L, Ispas A, et al. Screening for trisomies by cell-free DNA testing of maternal blood: Consequences of a failed result. Ultrasound Obstet Gynecol. 2016; 47:698–704.

38. Chen M, Su F, Wang J, et al. Temporal persistence of residual fetal cell-free DNA from a deceased cotwin after selective fetal reduction in dichorionic diamniotic twin pregnancies. Prenat Diagn 2021; 41:1602–1610.

39. Niles KM, Murji A, Chitayat D. Prolonged duration of persistent cell-free fetal DNA from vanishing twin. Ultrasound Obstet Gynecol. 2018; 52:547–548.

40. Zou Y, Cui L, Xue M, et al. Applications of noninvasive prenatal testing in vanishing twin syndrome pregnancies after treatment of assisted reproductive technology in a single center. Prenat Diagn. 2021; 41:226–233.

41. Khalil A, Rodgers M, Baschat A, et al. ISUOG Practice Guidelines: role of ultrasound in twin pregnancy. Ultrasound Obstet Gynecol. 2016; 47:247–263.

42. Chaveeva P, Wright A, Syngelaki A, et al. First-trimester screening for trisomies in pregnancies with vanishing twin. Ultrasound Obstet Gynecol. 2020; 55:326–331.

# Chapter 2

# Pre-eclampsia: Pathophysiology, prediction, and management

*Angela B Lu, Ben W Mol, Daniel L Rolnik*

## INTRODUCTION

Pre-eclampsia is a multi-system disorder of pregnancy characterised by hypertension arising after 20 weeks' gestation with proteinuria, other signs of end-organ injury or uteroplacental dysfunction [1]. Eclampsia, a rare but serious complication featuring seizures, can also occur with pre-eclampsia. Pre-eclampsia affects 3–5% of all pregnancies and is associated with significant maternal and perinatal morbidity and mortality, particularly in early-onset disease and in low- and middle-income countries. Globally, 76,000 women and 500,000 babies die each year from pre-eclampsia [2]. Recent evidence also suggests that the disease, particularly when early-onset [3,4], is associated with increased risks for vascular disease including chronic hypertension, future cardiovascular disease, and stroke[3,5,6]; metabolic syndrome [4]; cognitive impairment [7]; and chronic end-stage renal disease [8–10]. Pre-eclampsia may also be associated with poorer outcomes for the offspring of pregnancies affected by the condition, including increased cardiovascular risk factors [11] and neurodevelopmental disorders [12].

Although a significant amount of research has been dedicated to investigating pre-eclampsia and interventions to improve outcomes for mothers and babies, the incidence of the disease has been relatively unchanged in the last decades [13]. Pre-eclampsia also continues to be a significant burden on healthcare systems, with the cost of the disease within the first 12 months of delivery estimated at $2.2 billion in the United States and largely driven by prematurity [14]. This review will focus on the emerging evidence about the pathophysiology of pre-eclampsia, and the implications of this in the prediction and management of the disease.

**Angela B Lu** MBBS FRANZCOG, Department of Obstetrics and Gynaecology, Monash Health, Victoria, Australia
Email: angela.lu@monashhealth.org

**Ben W Mol** MD PhD FRANZCOG, Department of Obstetrics and Gynaecology, Monash University, Victoria, Australia and Aberdeen Centre for Women's Health Research, Institute of Applied Health Sciences, School of Medicine, Medical Sciences and Nutrition, University of Aberdeen, Aberdeen, UK
Email: ben.mol@monash.edu

**Daniel L Rolnik** MSc MD PhD Diploma in Fetal Medicine (Fetal Medicine Foundation, UK), FRANZCOG, Department of Obstetrics and Gynaecology, Monash Health, Victoria, Australia
Email: daniel.rolnik@monash.edu

# PATHOPHYSIOLOGY

A century after pre-eclampsia and eclampsia were first described as a "disease of theories" [15,16], our understanding of the complex pathophysiology underlying this disease is still evolving. The term "toxaemia" was first used in the late 19th century to describe a syndrome in pregnancy of seizures, oedema, proteinuria, and hypertension thought to be driven by toxins such as urea [17]. It was only in the 1960's and 1970's that our current understanding of pre-eclampsia began to develop with Brosens et al observations of abnormal placentation and uteroplacental spiral artery remodelling in pre-eclampsia [18,19]. Roberts and Redman then proposed the broadly adopted two-stage model of pre-eclampsia in the early 1990's, with abnormal placentation and uteroplacental hypoperfusion (stage one) driving the clinical manifestations of pre-eclampsia (stage two) including hypertension and proteinuria [20]. However, new concepts regarding the pathophysiology of pre-eclampsia continue to be identified and challenge our traditional understanding of the disease.

## Disease processes in pre-eclampsia

It is widely understood that abnormalities in the development of placental vasculature drive the disease processes of pre-eclampsia. Placental tissue is necessary for the development of pre-eclampsia but the presence of a fetus is not, as seen in molar pregnancies. Conversely, delivery of the placenta is seen as a curative measure with pre-eclampsia features subsequently resolving in the days to weeks post-partum. There is likely a complex interplay between maternal, fetal, and placental factors driving pre-eclampsia although this is yet to be fully elucidated.

In normal pregnancy, the physiological changes of placentation occur early in gestation and are likely completed by 18–20 weeks of pregnancy. Cytotrophoblast cells of the developing placenta migrate through the decidua and the inner third of the myometrium to invade the endothelium and highly muscular tunica media of the maternal spiral arteries. These terminal branches of the uterine artery undergo transformation from small muscular arterioles into large capacity vessels with low resistance flow. This facilitates greater blood flow to the placenta compared to other areas of the uterus, to maximise efficient maternal-fetal nutrient exchange.

## Abnormal placentation promoting uteroplacental hypoperfusion, hypoxia, and ischaemia

In pregnancies affected by pre-eclampsia, cytotrophoblast cells infiltrate the decidual portion of the spiral arteries but fail to penetrate the myometrial segment [18,19]. This failure in spiral artery remodelling results in these vessels remaining narrow, resulting in placental hypoperfusion and ischaemia. Defective placentation has been associated with several adverse pregnancy outcomes, including second trimester fetal death in utero, placental abruption, pre-eclampsia, and fetal growth restriction.

As gestation increases, hypoperfusion becomes more pronounced since abnormal uterine vasculature is unable to manage the normal physiological increase in blood flow to the fetus and placenta. Ischaemic changes in the placenta may occur including placental infarction, decidual arteriopathy, and accelerated villous maturation, and can be more pronounced in severe or early-onset pre-eclampsia compared to mild and later-onset disease [21,22]. The hypoperfused placenta also progressively secretes elevated amounts of anti-angiogenic factors that cause vascular inflammation, endothelial dysfunction, and maternal vascular injury [18,20]. The net result of this altered angiogenic profile is the clinical manifestation of hypertension and injury to maternal organs.

## Endothelial dysfunction causing clinical features of pre-eclampsia

All of the clinical features of pre-eclampsia can be explained as clinical responses to generalised endothelial dysfunction. Hypertension results from disturbed endothelial control of vascular tone, proteinuria, and oedema are caused by increased vascular permeability, and coagulopathy occurs due to abnormal endothelial expression of procoagulants. Headache, seizures, visual symptoms, epigastric pain, and fetal growth restriction are the consequences of endothelial dysfunction in the vasculature of target organs including the brain, liver, kidney, and placenta. This is supported by laboratory evidence in pre-eclamptic women including increased production of vasoconstrictors such as endothelins and thromboxanes, decreased production of endothelial-derived vasodilators such as nitric oxide and prostacyclin, and enhanced vascular reactivity to angiotensin II [23].

## Angiogenic and anti-angiogenic factors

Placentation requires extensive angiogenesis to establish a suitable vascular network to effectively supply oxygen and nutrients to the fetus. A balance between pro-angiogenic and anti-angiogenic factors is important for normal placental development. In pre-eclampsia, increased production of anti-angiogenic factors disturbs this balance, resulting in systemic endothelial dysfunction. The pre-eclamptic placenta secretes many factors that could contribute to endothelial dysfunction: Pro-inflammatory cytokines, exosomes [24], extracellular vesicles [25], and anti-angiogenic molecules such as soluble fms-like tyrosine kinase-1 (sFlt-1) [26] and soluble endoglin (sEng) [27]. These placenta-derived factors can act on the maternal vascular endothelium to incite local endothelial release of other factors that worsen endothelial dysfunction such as thromboxane, proinflammatory cytokines, and possibly sFlt-1 itself. This is combined with suppression of the release of the pro-angiogenic placental growth factor (PlGF) and vascular endothelial growth factor (VEGF) [26].

sFlt-1 is an anti-angiogenic protein which antagonises the pro-angiogenic VEGF and PlGF by binding to and preventing their interaction with their endothelial receptors [26]. Although binding of sFlt-1 to VEGF is not the primary pathogenic event triggering pre-eclampsia, sFlt-1 has many features that implicate it as a major driver of disease in pre-eclampsia. Elevated concentrations of sFlt-1 are seen weeks before the clinical onset of pre-eclampsia and during pre-eclampsia [26-28], with women who went on to develop pre-eclampsia seen to have an increase in sFlt-1 levels earlier in gestation than normotensive controls (at 21–24 weeks, vs. 33–36 weeks), and to reach higher sFlt-1 levels overall [26]. As sFlt-1 is anti-angiogenic, it is biologically plausible that it plays a pathogenic role in pre-eclampsia and this is supported by animal models in which administration of sFlt-1 generates phenotypes of clinical disease [29].

Soluble endoglin is another placenta-derived anti-angiogenic protein which has been implicated in pre-eclampsia. In vivo, sEng increased vascular permeability and induced hypertension, and appeared to potentiate the vascular effects of sFlt-1 in pregnant rats to induce a severe pre-eclampsia-like state [30]. Levine et al demonstrated that sEng is elevated in the sera of pre-eclamptic women 2–3 months prior to the onset of clinical signs of pre-eclampsia regardless of gestation at onset of disease, and falls after delivery [27]. Increased levels of sEng were also usually accompanied by an increased sFlt-1:PlGF ratio, and if present together was most predictive of developing pre-eclampsia [27].

## Complement dysregulation

The maternal complement system has also been recently implicated in the development of pre-eclampsia. The complement system has a central role in the human body for host defence against foreign pathogens, and innate immunity. To achieve normal pregnancy, the complement system must reach a homeostasis of clearing normal (effectively semi-allogeneic) placental apoptotic debris from the maternal circulation [31], with appropriate regulation to allow immunological tolerance to the fetus and placenta [32]. Placental expression of complement regulatory proteins appears to help protect the fetus, by inhibiting complement activation at different steps along the complement activation cascade.

In placenta-mediated disorders such as pre-eclampsia, there is an increase in apoptotic and necrotic placental debris, leading to an excess inflammatory response [33]. There is a shift towards increased complement activation and decreased complement regulation. The terminal effector of the complement pathway, C5b-9, has been found at higher levels in placentas of women with pre-eclampsia, and its lytic and sublytic inflammatory effects may contribute to placental injury in these pregnancies by stimulating trophoblasts to secrete sFlt-1 [32]. Severe pre-eclampsia has also been associated with marked elevations in urinary C5b-9 relative to subjects with chronic hypertension and healthy controls, with urinary C5b-9 detected in 96% of women with severe pre-eclampsia in a small American case-control study [34].

## Potential factors influencing the development of pre-eclampsia

The sentinel upstream event that triggers the cascade of events leading to poor placental implantation and subsequent maternal vascular hypoperfusion has not been completely identified. This remains an area of on-going research, with the anticipation of future treatments for pre-eclampsia coming from these findings.

## Immunological factors

Hypotheses around immunological factors contributing to abnormal placentation are based on the observations that prior exposure to paternal or fetal antigens appears to protect against pre-eclampsia. Nulliparous women [35] and women who change partners between pregnancies, have long interpregnancy intervals, use barrier contraception, or conceive via intracytoplasmic sperm injection have less exposure to paternal antigens and higher risks of developing pre-eclampsia in some studies. In addition, meta-analyses show that women who conceive through oocyte donation, a situation in which all the embryonic genetic material is allogeneic, have a more than two-fold higher rate of pre-eclampsia than women who conceive via other assisted reproductive techniques and a four-fold higher rate of pre-eclampsia than women who have a natural conception, which also supports the hypothesis that immunologic intolerance between the mother and fetus may play a role in the pathogenesis of pre-eclampsia.

Other immunological abnormalities involving human leucocyte antigen (HLA) antigens in extravillous trophoblastic cells and interaction with natural killer cells have also been suggested to underlie pre-eclampsia. However, a systemic review found no clear evidence that one or several specific HLA alleles were involved in the pathogenesis of pre-eclampsia [36].

# Genetic factors

Most cases of pre-eclampsia are sporadic; however, genetic factors are thought to play a role in disease susceptibility. Family history of pre-eclampsia is widely acknowledged as a risk factor for the development of pre-eclampsia [2,37,38], with daughters or sisters of women with a history of pre-eclampsia three to four times more likely to develop pre-eclampsia than women without a family history [2,39]. Despite this, genome-wide association studies have not identified reproducible maternal sequence variants [2,40], suggesting that inheritance is likely complex and multi-factorial. There also appears to be some influence from paternal genes, with men who were the product of a pregnancy complicated by pre-eclampsia more likely to father a pregnancy complicated by pre-eclampsia [39].

Pathogenic mutations or deletions in complement regulatory genes have been detected in women with pre-eclampsia. These variants are not causative in isolation, but may predispose affected women to increased complement activation in combination with other risk factors. In the PROMISSE cohort of 250 pregnant patients with systemic lupus erythematosus and/or antiphospholipid antibodies, autoimmune conditions driven by complement-mediated injury, and associated with increased risks of pre-eclampsia, variants in complementary regulatory proteins were identified in women with pre-eclampsia, both with and without pre-existing autoimmune disease [41].

Fetal genomes have also been examined for gene variants that may contribute to the development of pre-eclampsia. A genome-wide association study found that the only gene variant across the entire fetal genome that was significantly associated with pre-eclampsia was a locus on chromosome 13 near the gene encoding Fms-like tyrosine kinase 1 (FLT1), an isoform of sFlt-1 [40]. Interestingly, in pregnancies affected by trisomy 13, the incidence of pre-eclampsia is increased above other trisomies and non-trisomic pregnancies, and an increased ratio of circulating sFlt-1:PlGF has been noted [42].

# Environmental factors

### Low calcium intake

Epidemiological studies have identified low dietary intake of calcium as a risk factor for pre-eclampsia, leading to the hypothesis that an increase in calcium intake during pregnancy may reduce the incidence of hypertensive disorders in pregnancy. It is unclear how this may occur but may be related to reduction in smooth muscle contractility. Nonetheless, recent data suggests that calcium supplementation has improved uteroplacental blood flow with lowered resistance indexes in the uterine and umbilical arteries [43].

### Behavioural factors

Some epidemiological studies have suggested that cigarette smoking is a protective factor against the development of pre-eclampsia [44,45]. However, this paradoxical association seems to be spuriously caused by inappropriate confounding control and by collider-stratification bias [46].

### High body mass index

Increased maternal body mass index is widely recognised as a risk factor for the development of pre-eclampsia [35,37], with a linear relationship between increasing body mass index and increasing pre-eclampsia risk. It is suggested that maternal obesity increases susceptibility to pre-eclampsia by inducing chronic inflammation and endothelial dysfunction, with lower levels of sFlt-1 and PlGF seen in pregnant women with higher maternal BMI, with and without clinically evident placental dysfunction [47].

## Vascular factors

Pre-existing vascular disease and associated endothelial cell damage are thought to increase susceptibility to developing pre-eclampsia [48]. Risk factors for pre-eclampsia such as maternal age older than 40 years, obesity, pre-existing diabetes, or chronic hypertension suggest an association with pre-existing endothelial dysfunction. It may also explain why women who develop pre-eclampsia are also at increased risk of developing cardiovascular disease [3,5,6] and end-stage renal disease later [8–10] in life.

It has recently been hypothesised that pre-eclampsia is a primary cardiovascular disorder that influences placental perfusion and function, rather than the other way around. Two clinically recognisable phenotypes result, reflecting an imbalance of supply-demand on the maternal cardiovascular system—women with pre-existing poor cardiovascular reserve who are at risk of preterm pre-eclampsia as detected on first-trimester screening, and women who are at risk of late pre-eclampsia due to the inability of their cardiovascular system to cope with the excessive cardiovascular demands of advancing gestation.

Defendants of the placental hypothesis suggest that significant placental histological findings, imbalances between angiogenic and anti-angiogenic factors and the anti-inflammatory effects of aspirin strongly support the theory of a primary placental origin. Conversely, defendants of the cardiovascular theory argue that fetal growth restriction and significant placental histological findings are common in early-onset pre-eclampsia but often absent in late-onset pre-eclampsia that pre-eclampsia is an early manifestation of cardiovascular disease triggered by pregnancy (in much the same way that gestational diabetes increases the risk of type 2 diabetes mellitus in the future), and that aspirin is often used as a strategy to prevent cardiovascular events. The cardiovascular theory also does not explain why pre-eclampsia is more common in young nulliparous women than in subsequent pregnancies. It is possible that both mechanisms result in placental hypoperfusion, leading to the common final cascade characterised by imbalances between angiogenic and anti-angiogenic factors and the clinical features of pre-eclampsia, with varying contribution according to gestational age at disease onset.

## PREDICTION

Accurate predictive models for pre-eclampsia are highly sought after, in order to identify those in early pregnancy who are at increased risk of developing pre-eclampsia so that preventative measures can be commenced promptly. Ideally, such a model should be safe and acceptable to women, non-invasive, inexpensive, reproducible, and able to be applied as a point of care test in the first trimester. Many predictive factors for pre-eclampsia have been reported in primary research studies, with a 2019 umbrella review identifying 90 predictors and 52 prediction models; however, risk factors associated with pre-eclampsia do not necessarily translate into clinically useful prediction, and many prediction models lack independent and external validation [49].

## Maternal risk factors

Multiple maternal risk factors for the development of pre-eclampsia have been described in international guidelines (**Table 2.1**) [1,37,38]. A large systematic review and meta-analysis of 92 studies, including over 25 million pregnancies, evaluated the association between clinical risk factors identified before 16 weeks' and the risk of pre-eclampsia [35]. The most significant risk factors for pre-eclampsia were personal history of pre-eclampsia and chronic hypertension, with other risk factors including nulliparity, maternal age >35 years, conception by assisted reproductive technology, pre-pregnancy BMI >30 kg/m$^2$, and pre-gestational diabetes mellitus [35].

Guidelines internationally such as those by the American College of Obstetricians and Gynecologists (ACOG) [38] and the National Institute for Health and Care Excellence (NICE) [37] have proposed screening for pre-eclampsia based on maternal risk factors alone, with each risk factor simply seen as a separate screening test with additive detection rate (DR) and screen-positive rate. However, this approach fails to appreciate the relative weighting of various risk factors and does not account for protective factors such as

| Table 2.1  Clinical risk factors to identify women at risk of pre-eclampsia, from international guidelines | | | | |
|---|---|---|---|---|
| | **ACOG [38,88]** | **NICE [37]** | **ISSHP [1]** | **FIGO [2]** |
| Chronic hypertension | High | High | High | Included |
| Type 1 or type 2 diabetes mellitus | High | High | High | Included |
| Renal disease | High | High | High | Included |
| Autoimmune disease (SLE and APLS) | High | High | High | Included |
| History of pre-eclampsia | High | High | High | Included |
| Multifetal pregnancy | High | Moderate | High | Included |
| History of other pregnancy hypertensive disorder | Moderate | High | Not included | Included |
| Use of assisted reproductive technology | Not included | Not included | High | Included |
| High BMI | Moderate (>30 kg/m$^2$) | Moderate (≥35 kg/m$^2$) | High (>30 kg/m$^2$) | Included |
| Nulliparity | Moderate | Moderate | Not included | Included |
| Family history of pre-eclampsia (mother and sister) | Moderate | Moderate | Not included | Included |
| More than 10 year pregnancy interval | Moderate | Moderate | Not included | Included |
| Maternal age | Moderate (>35 years old) | Moderate (≥40 years old) | Not included | Included |
| Maternal height | Not included | Not included | Not included | Included |
| Obstetric history (low birthweight, small for gestational age, or previous adverse pregnancy outcome) | Moderate | Moderate | Not included | Included |
| Sociodemographic characteristics (black, low socioeconomic status) | Moderate | Not included | Not included | Included |

Adapted for use from Chappell et al. [183]
APLS, antiphospholipid syndrome; SLE, systemic lupus erythematosus.

previous normotensive pregnancies. It also has suboptimal performance, with the NICE recommendation only achieving DRs of 40.8% and 30.4% for preterm and all pre-eclampsia respectively, at a 10% false positive rate [50]. Likewise, the ACOG approach from 2013, only achieved DRs of 5% and 2% for preterm and term pre-eclampsia respectively, with a 0.2% false-positive rate [51]. The expanded list of clinical risk factors included in the United States Preventive Services Task Force (USPSTF) recommendation from 2014 led to considerably improved DRs of 90% [95% confidence interval (CI) 79–96] and 89% (95% CI 84–94) for preterm and term pre-eclampsia, respectively; however, the false positive rate also increased to as high as 64% [52].

## Biophysical markers

### Blood pressure in the first trimester

All women, as part of routine antenatal care, should have their blood pressure recorded at each antenatal visit. The International Federation of Gynaecology and Obstetrics (FIGO) recommends that blood pressure should be taken with the woman in a sitting position after 5 minutes of rest, with their arm well supported at the level of the heart and using a validated automated or semiautomated device and appropriately sized blood pressure cuff for the woman's mid-arm circumference [2]. Blood pressure should be measured in both arms simultaneously with two sets of recordings taken at 1-minute intervals, and the four sets of systolic and diastolic blood pressures used to calculate a final mean arterial pressure (MAP) [2]; for practicality, two blood pressure recordings in one arm 1-minute apart is also accepted [2,53].

The FIGO recommends that MAP should be measured as part of the risk assessment for pre-eclampsia [2]. MAP is calculated from the systolic and diastolic blood pressure, using the average of the two or four separate blood pressure measurements. Further conversion of the MAP into a multiple of median (MoM) allows for adjustment for gestational age and other maternal characteristics that can affect MAP, including maternal weight, height, Afro-Caribbean racial origin, cigarette smoking, family history of pulmonary embolism (PE), history of PE in the previous pregnancy, interpregnancy interval, chronic hypertension, and diabetes mellitus [2,54]. Use of MAP has been proposed as part of a standardised protocol at 11–13 weeks of gestation for the prediction of pre-eclampsia, with DRs of 38% improving to 63% in combination with maternal history at a 10% false-positive rate [55].

## Ultrasound indices

### Uterine artery Doppler

As pregnancy progresses, impedance to flow in the uterine arteries normally decreases, reflecting the previously mentioned process of trophoblastic invasion, specifically defective invasion of spiral arteries, and failure of these vessels to transform into low resistance vessels. Increased impedance for gestational age on first trimester Doppler ultrasound is associated with the development of pre-eclampsia [56], particularly early-onset disease as it correlates well with disease severity as given by gestational age at birth with pre-eclampsia. Assessment of the uterine artery resistance therefore provides a useful non-invasive method to assess the uteroplacental circulation.

Analysis of the uterine artery Doppler flow waveform ratios (e.g. high resistance index or pulsatility index, systolic/diastolic ratio) and/or presence or absence of diastolic notching in the uterine arcuate vessels may help to identify women at risk of disorders related to impaired placentation such as pre-eclampsia. A 2008 systematic review found that uterine artery Doppler ultrasound best predicted the overall risk of pre-eclampsia in the presence of second-trimester elevation of the pulsatility index with the presence of uterine artery notching (sensitivity 19%, specificity 99%, positive likelihood ratio 21, and negative likelihood ratio 0.82) and that severe pre-eclampsia was best predicted by second-trimester elevated resistance index (sensitivity 80%, specificity 78%, positive likelihood ratio 3.7, and negative likelihood ratio 0.26) [57]. However, studies of uterine artery Doppler measurements for the prediction of pre-eclampsia are difficult to compare due to differences in Doppler sampling techniques, definitions of abnormal flow velocity waveform, populations, gestational ages at examination, and criteria for diagnosis of pre-eclampsia. As with MAP, the first mean uterine artery pulsatility index (UTPI) should be converted into MoM adjusting for maternal characteristics and medical history. In isolation, UTPI performs poorly; however, FIGO recommends that where feasible, UTPI should be measured at 11–13 weeks of gestation as part of first-trimester combined pre-eclampsia risk assessment in singleton pregnancies [2].

### Ophthalmic artery Doppler

The ophthalmic artery is the first branch of the internal carotid artery, and is an easily accessible vessel for Doppler assessment that provides information on the less accessible intracranial circulation. In the 1990s, cross-sectional studies reported that in women with pre-eclampsia, compared with normotensive pregnant women, there is a decrease in impedance to flow and an increase in the flow velocity in the ophthalmic arteries. This observation is more likely related to maternal haemodynamic changes unlike the uterine artery which is directly impacted by the effects of trophoblast invasion. A meta-analysis incorporating 1,119 pregnancies across three studies suggested that some ophthalmic artery Doppler indices measured either in the first or second trimester had a significant association with the subsequent development of early-onset pre-eclampsia [58]. Although it is a safe, non-invasive point-of-care test, it is also limited by availability of suitably credentialled obstetric providers and so may have little clinical utility as a standalone predictive test for pre-eclampsia.

## Biochemical markers

Traditionally, maternal blood tests have played a role in the management of pre-eclampsia through analysis of end-organ (renal, hepatic, and haematological) dysfunction. However, there is an emerging role for the use of serum maternal analytes in the prediction of pre-eclampsia, such as the angiogenic (VEGF and PlGF) and anti-angiogenic (sFlt-1 and sEng) proteins implicated in the endothelial dysfunction of pre-eclampsia. These tests are potentially useful as predictive biomarkers due to the alterations in their levels preceding the onset of clinical pre-eclampsia by weeks to months, their correlation with disease severity, and their normalisation post-partum [26,28]. To date, the overall test performance of first trimester analytes indicates that when used alone, they are likely of low predictive value for screening [59-61].

Placental growth factor is recognised by FIGO as the best biochemical marker for pre-eclampsia first-trimester screening [2]. PlGF alone has a DR of 55% and 33% respectively, for the identification of early- and late-onset pre-eclampsia, at a 10% false positive rate [62]. A systematic review and meta-analysis demonstrated that PlGF was superior to other biomarkers for predicting pre-eclampsia, with a DR of 56% at 9% false positive rate for the prediction of early-onset disease [61]. In contrast, sFlt-1 levels are comparable between control groups and women who go on to develop clinical pre-eclampsia until about 20 weeks' gestation [26] and in keeping with this the sFlt-1:PlGF ratio has not been shown to be useful in early pregnancy [63].

Pregnancy associated plasma protein A (PAPP-A) is a metalloproteinase insulin-like growth factor binding protein secreted by the syncytiotrophoblast, that plays an important role in placental growth and development. Low circulating levels of PAPP-A have been associated with pre-eclampsia, presumably due to reduced availability of unbound PAPP-A in the maternal circulation. It is already a well-established biochemical marker in serum screening for fetal trisomies 21, 18, and 13, and therefore relatively widely available. A PAPP-A level below the 5th percentile has been found to be significantly associated with pre-eclampsia [64,65]; however, this is only present in 8–23% of women with pre-eclampsia and therefore as a single marker it is not an accurate predictive test for pre-eclampsia [2].

## Risk prediction models

All aforementioned biophysical and biochemical markers used in the prediction of pre-eclampsia perform poorly in isolation. In an effort to increase sensitivity of screening, investigators have used variables such as those listed above to create predictive tools to predict an individual woman's risk of developing pre-eclampsia whilst still early in pregnancy. The predictive performance of maternal risk factors as suggested by ACOG or NICE is modest, and fails to account for protective factors such as previous normotensive pregnancy, and does not distinguish between early-onset and term pre-eclampsia, which have different risk profiles and recurrence rates. Recently developed algorithms are mathematical equations that incorporate maternal characteristics, medical history, and various combinations of biophysical and biochemical markers (such as MAP, UTPI, PAPP-A, and PlGF) to improve DR. Such algorithms, usually based on logistic regression models or on Bayesian probabilistic competing risks models, attribute the right weight to different predictors and achieve an DRs of 82% for preterm pre-eclampsia, as compared to 41% with the NICE guidelines [50] and increasing sensitivity for overall pre-eclampsia by 18% (95% CI 0–56) [66].

The Fetal Medicine Foundation (FMF) combined first trimester prediction model, or triple test, has been identified by FIGO as one of the most predictive models available for preterm pre-eclampsia currently [2]. Using a Bayesian competing risks model derived from large datasets, it calculates a patient-specific risk for preterm pre-eclampsia using maternal factors, MAP, UTPI, and serum PlGF and/or PAPP-A, in line with the concept of personalised medicine. A high-risk result in this model has often been considered when the risk of preterm pre-eclampsia is ≥1 in 100 [2,67], however, can be influenced by local disease prevalence, and resources available for screening and treatment. It has undergone successful internal and external validation in large populations, with DRs of 90% and 75% for the prediction of early and preterm pre-eclampsia respectively, at a 10% false-positive rate.

- A large European multicentre, prospective, non-intervention study conducted in 2017 validated the FMF first trimester combined test in 8,775 pregnant women, including 2.7% with pre-eclampsia [51]. DRs for very early (100%), preterm (75%), and term (43%) pre-eclampsia at a 10% false positive rate were similar to the screening performance of previous data from the development set [56]
- The screening program for pre-eclampsia (SPREE) study from 2018 was a British prospective multicentre cohort study of 16,747 singleton pregnancies at 11–13 weeks of

gestation, screened for pre-eclampsia using the FMF algorithm. 2.8% developed pre-eclampsia. In comparison to clinical risk factors alone as defined by NICE (DR 30.4%; 95% CI 26.3–34.6), this algorithm had a higher DR for all pre-eclampsia (DR 42.5%; 95% CI 38.0–46.9). In preterm pre-eclampsia, the FMF algorithm also outperformed the NICE method with DRs of 82% and 41% respectively (difference in DR 41.6%; 95% CI 33.2–49.9) [50]. A further UK retrospective study in the public healthcare system, with a modified FMF algorithm using PAPP-A instead of PlGF and used a risk cut-off of 1 in 50, also demonstrated a doubling of pre-eclampsia detection [68]

- A large multicentre study in Asia in 2019 of 10,935 women with 0.67% developing preterm pre-eclampsia, further validated the FMF triple test and in a population completely different than that used for the original development of the model. It demonstrated a DR of 64.0% at 10% false positive rate for preterm pre-eclampsia, superior to the risk factors-based approaches recommended by ACOG and NICE [52]
- An Australian retrospective study of prospectively collected data compared 29,618 women with singleton pregnancies who underwent screening with the FMF algorithm at 11–14 weeks with 301,566 unscreened pregnancies (unpublished data) [69]. Compared to the women who received standard care, women identified as high-risk through the FMF screening were more likely to develop preterm pre-eclampsia [2.1% vs. 0.7%; relative risk (RR) 3.04; 95% CI 2.46–3.77], while low-risk women had significantly lower rates of preterm pre-eclampsia (0.2% vs. 0.7%; RR 0.26; 95% CI 0.19–0.35) and other pregnancy complications. Screening with the FMF algorithm detected 65.2% (95% CI 56.4–73.2%) of women who would go on to develop preterm pre-eclampsia, at a false positive rate of 13.4% (95% CI 13.1–13.8)

This first trimester screen and treat approach is already endorsed in international guidelines [1,2]. However, use of these algorithms with maternal biomarkers and ultrasound indices may not be achievable in resource-limited settings. Nonetheless, pre-eclampsia individual risk prediction using a simpler combination of maternal risk factors and MAP should be used rather than maternal risk factors alone, to optimise detection [2]. A contingent screening approach whereby serum biomarkers and ultrasound markers can be then reserved for a subgroup of the population identified by maternal risk factors and MAP may also be considered in these resource-limited settings. A prospective screening study evaluating this two-stage strategy with 30% of the population undergoing PlGF and UTPI demonstrated a DR of 71% at a fixed screen-positive rate of 10% [70].

# PREVENTION

Given the significant burden of pre-eclampsia on mothers, babies, and healthcare systems, measures to prevent pre-eclampsia continue to be an intense area of research. As there is no curative treatment for pre-eclampsia other than delivery, an intervention that could successfully prevent pre-eclampsia would have a significant impact on maternal and infant health worldwide. Although many approaches have been investigated, few have been successful reflecting the complexities of the underlying pathophysiology of pre-eclampsia.

## Risk factor modification

Most risk factors for pre-eclampsia are non-modifiable. One exception to this is maternal obesity and excessive gestational weight gain. Overweight and obese women should be recommended to optimise their weight pre-pregnancy, for a variety of reproductive, pregnancy, and overall health benefits. A cohort study of women with previous pre-eclampsia found that weight loss between pregnancies, regardless of their BMI, reduced the risk of recurrent pre-eclampsia in their subsequent pregnancy [71]. Therefore, women at risk of pre-eclampsia should be counselled about weight management peri-conception as well as the gestational weight gain recommendations as established by the Institute of Medicine [72].

## Aspirin

Aspirin (acetylsalicylic acid) is the only drug treatment for pre-eclampsia prevention that is supported by strong randomised evidence. As a non-steroidal anti-inflammatory drug, it inhibits two cyclooxygenase (COX) isoenzymes, COX-1 and COX-2, which are essential for prostaglandin synthesis in a dose-dependent fashion. At lower doses (60–300 mg daily) aspirin irreversibly acetylates COX-1 resulting in decreased biosynthesis of thromboxane A2, a potent vasoconstrictor and promotor of platelet aggregation, without affecting levels of vascular prostacyclin, which acts as a vasodilator and inhibitor of platelet aggregation. This process is irreversible in platelets, where COX is inhibited for the platelet's entire lifespan, whereas prostacyclin production is re-established relatively quickly. Although the resulting alteration in the ratio of prostacyclin to thromboxane A2 in the placenta is suggested to play a role in preventing or delaying the onset of pre-eclampsia, aspirin's mechanism of action in pre-eclampsia prevention remains unclear with alternative hypotheses including improved placentation, reduced inflammation, stabilisation of the endometrium, and increased PlGF production.

Aspirin has been investigated as a potential prevention for pre-eclampsia since the 1970s, when it was first demonstrated in observational studies that nulliparous women who had taken aspirin more than once a fortnight antenatally had a lower risk of pre-eclampsia compared to those who had no reported history of aspirin intake [73]. However, until recently, there were only several small randomised trials conducted with conflicting results about aspirin's benefits, and Askie et al individual patient-data meta-analysis in 2007 [74] suggested only a 10% reduction in pre-eclampsia although the studies included largely gave aspirin at <100 mg daily dosing commencing after 16 weeks' gestation. Several large landmark trials have occurred to examine the benefit of aspirin for pre-eclampsia prevention, with the most notable benefits in the risk reduction of preterm pre-eclampsia:
- Beaufils et al published the first randomised trial of aspirin for the prevention of placental-mediated complications in 1985 [75]. Almost 102 pregnant women with a history of risk factors for pre-eclampsia and fetal growth restriction were randomised to treatment with 150 mg aspirin and 300 mg dipyridamole daily from 12 weeks' gestation or standard care. A significant reduction in the risk of pre-eclampsia, fetal growth restriction, and stillbirth was seen, with none of these events occurring in the treatment arm
- The Collaborative Low-dose Aspirin Study in Pregnancy (CLASP) [76] was a double-blinded, placebo-controlled trial examined the use of aspirin 60 mg daily in 9,356 women at high-risk of pre-eclampsia according to maternal characteristics and medical history or with established pre-eclampsia, and suggested a 12% non-statistically significant risk reduction in pre-eclampsia with aspirin. However, this study lacked statistical power for this effect, and used an aspirin dose which is now thought to be less effective for pre-eclampsia prevention
- The Combined Multimarker Screening and Randomised Patient Treatment with Aspirin for Evidence-Based Prevention (ASPRE) trial [67] was a multicentre, double-blind, placebo-controlled trial where women deemed high risk of pre-eclampsia by the FMF triple test received aspirin 150 mg nightly from 11 to 14 weeks until 36 weeks' gestation.

A total of 26,941 women underwent screening in 13 sites across six European countries, and although there was no significant reduction in the rate of delivery with term pre-eclampsia [odds ratio (OR) 0.95 in the aspirin group; 95% CI 0.57–1.57], there was a significant reduction in the primary outcome of delivery with preterm pre-eclampsia with aspirin use [adjusted OR (aOR) 0.38 in the aspirin group; 95% CI 0.20–0.74; number needed to treat (NNT) to avoid one primary outcome 38]. In addition, aspirin was considered safe as there were no significant differences between the groups in adverse events including vaginal bleeding and upper gastrointestinal symptoms. A secondary analysis of ASPRE [77] also identified a 68% reduction in the total length of stay in neonatal intensive care for neonates whose mothers were in the aspirin group, in keeping with a reduction in preterm births due to effective prevention of preterm pre-eclampsia

- The Aspirin Supplementation for Pregnancy Indicated Risk Reduction in Nulliparas (ASPIRIN) trial [78] was a randomised, international, double-masked, placebo-controlled trial examining the effect of universal low-dose (81 mg daily) aspirin commenced in the first trimester on preterm birth rates. There was an 11% reduction in the primary outcome of preterm birth (RR 0.89; 95% CI 0.81–0.98; $p = 0.012$). The incidence of women who delivered before 34 weeks' gestation with hypertensive disorders of pregnancy was significantly reduced in the low-dose aspirin (RR 0.38; 95% CI 0.17–0.85; $p = 0.015$). However, this was not the primary outcome of the study, and the overall incidence of hypertensive disorders of pregnancy was no different between the treatment and placebo groups

A 2019 Cochrane review also confirmed that there is high-quality evidence that low-dose aspirin taken daily from the first trimester until 36 weeks' gestation reduces the risk of developing pre-eclampsia by approximately 18% (RR 0.82; 95% CI 0.77–0.82; NNT 61) [79], with a much stronger effect on early-onset disease. Subgroup analysis of ASPRE found no difference on the effect of aspirin between subgroups according to maternal characteristics and medical history, although benefit was not seen in women with chronic hypertension [80]. Although a policy of universal prophylaxis with aspirin has been suggested [81], such a strategy for the prevention of pre-eclampsia has not been properly assessed in randomised trials, and is likely to be associated with poor adherence to treatment, lower effectiveness, and an increase in rates of side-effects. A recent population-wide observational study suggested an increase in haemorrhagic complications in women who used aspirin during pregnancy [82]. Cost-effectiveness studies demonstrate that both a screen-and-treat policy with the use of biomarkers and universal prophylaxis are more cost-effective than no screening or risk factor-based screening [83–86], but make the unrealistic assumption that compliance and effectiveness would be the same with universal prophylaxis as seen with a screen-and-treat approach [87].

In clinical practice, international guidelines (**Table 2.2**) reflect that there is still uncertainty about some aspects of the use of aspirin in pregnancy for the prevention of pre-eclampsia:

- *Timing of commencement*: Early commencement of low-dose aspirin is likely important since the underlying disease processes involving placental development occur early in pregnancy, weeks before clinical disease is apparent. International guidelines generally recommend optimal timing of commencement between approximately 11 and 16 weeks' gestation [1,2,37,88,89], with this timing supported in ASPRE [67] and ASPIRIN [78]. Systematic reviews and meta-analyses also suggest that aspirin commencing before 16 weeks' gestation is associated with a significant reduction for the prevention

**Table 2.2 Recommendations for aspirin prophylaxis, from international guidelines**

| | ACOG [38,88] | NICE [37] | ISSHP [1] | FIGO [2] |
|---|---|---|---|---|
| When to offer aspirin | Any high-risk factor, or two moderate-risk factors | Any high-risk factor, or two moderate-risk factors | Any high-risk factor. No recommendation to take aspirin in the presence of moderate-risk factors | High-risk on the Fetal Medicine Foundation first trimester combined test |
| Universal first trimester screening | Does not recommend | Does not recommend | Supports its use when integrated into the local health system, but does not specifically recommend it | Supports universal first trimester screening |
| Recommended daily dose of aspirin | 81 mg Initiated between 12 and 28 weeks' gestation, ideally <16 weeks' gestation | 75–150 mg Initiated from 12 weeks' gestation | 75–162 mg Initiated ideally <16 weeks' gestation, but definitely before 20 weeks' gestation | 150 mg at night Initiated between 11 and 14 weeks' gestation |
| When to cease aspirin | Continue until delivery | Continue until delivery | No recommendation | Continue until 36 weeks' gestation, delivery or when pre-eclampsia is diagnosed |

Adapted for use from Chappell et al. [183]

of pre-eclampsia [90,91], particularly in preterm [90] and severe [91] disease, although no benefit is seen in term pre-eclampsia [90,91]. Commencement of aspirin prior to 11 weeks' gestation did not significantly decrease pre-eclampsia in women at increased risk of the disease [92]. Starting low-dose aspirin after 16 weeks (but before symptoms develop) may also still have a smaller benefit in pre-eclampsia prevention [91,93], although has been suggested to not reduce the risk of severe pre-eclampsia or fetal growth restriction [91]. However, there is no evidence to suggest benefit in women who have already developed pre-eclampsia nor does aspirin appear to prevent progression to more severe disease

- *Dose*: There is no consensus regarding this, with recommended dosing varying from 81 to 150 mg daily [1,37,88,89], influenced by local availability. A study by Caron et al suggested that approximately 30% of high-risk pregnant women showed a lack of platelet function response at a daily dose of 81 mg, and this proportion was below 5% when the dose was doubled to 162 mg [94]. The optimal aspirin dose for pre-eclampsia prevention is largely based on systematic reviews and meta-analyses comparing <100 mg and >100 mg doses. A 2017 meta-analysis suggested a dose-response effect for the prevention of pre-eclampsia and severe pre-eclampsia, with higher doses associated with greater risk reduction and suggesting that doses below 100 mg are likely to be ineffective [91]. A further meta-analysis from the same group in 2018, which included subgroup analyses of preterm and term pre-eclampsia, found that aspirin reduced the risk of preterm pre-eclampsia, but not term pre-eclampsia, and only when it was initiated at ≤16 weeks' gestation at a daily dose of ≥100 mg [90]. The 2019 Cochrane review suggested that trials using doses >75 mg appeared to show a greater risk reduction for pre-eclampsia than trials using doses <75 mg, but that the overall data was not conclusive [79]. FIGO suggests the minimum dosage of aspirin for prevention in women at high risk of pre-eclampsia should be 100 mg daily [2]

- *Timing of cessation*: There is no consensus about this, although international guidelines commonly recommend continuation until delivery [1,2,37,88]. Alternatively, aspirin could be discontinued at 36 weeks' gestation [2] to minimise haemorrhage during delivery

The short-term safety of low-dose aspirin in the second and third trimesters is well established [79], although there is conflicting data available. A 2019 Cochrane review did not identify any clear increases in the risk of placental abruption (RR 1.21; 95% CI 0.95–1.54), neonatal intraventricular haemorrhage (RR 0.99; 95% CI 0.72–1.36), or other neonatal bleeding (RR 0.90; 95% CI 0.75–1.08), in keeping with these outcomes in ASPRE [67] and ASPIRIN [78]. Interestingly, a 2018 meta-analysis suggested a significant difference in placental abruption and antepartum haemorrhage dependant on timing of aspirin commencement, with those starting before 16 weeks' gestation trending toward less risk of these outcomes (RR 0.62; 95% CI 0.31–1.26) compared to an increased risk in those who initiated aspirin after 16 weeks' gestation (RR 2.08; 95% CI 0.86–5.06); however, neither result was significant on its own [95]. Aspirin has, however, been associated with a probable slight increase in post-partum haemorrhage > 500 mL (RR 1.06; 95% CI 1.00–1.12) representing nine more post-partum haemorrhages > 500 mL/1,000 patients on aspirin compared to those not on aspirin [79]; this was also demonstrated in Hastie et al large Swedish population-based cohort study where a higher incidence of post-partum haemorrhage (10.2% vs. 7.8%; aOR 1.23; 95% CI 1.08–1.39) and post-partum haematoma (0.4% vs. 0.1%; aOR 2.21; 95% CI 1.13–4.34) was seen with aspirin treatment [82]. Longer-term safety data is limited to date, although there has not appeared to be any increase in adverse childhood outcomes such as neuromotor deficit or developmental delay at 18 months [96] or 5-year [97] follow-up.

## Calcium

Oral supplementation with calcium may prevent pre-eclampsia, especially when dietary intake of calcium is low (<800 mg daily). Low dietary calcium intake is known to be associated with hypertension in the general population. A 2018 meta-analysis of over 18,000 women, including two-thirds who lived in geographic areas where calcium rich foods were not commonly available or consumed, concluded that high dose calcium (≥1 g daily) reduced rates of pre-eclampsia (RR 0.45; 95% CI 0.31–0.65), with the most benefit seen in women with a low dietary calcium intake (RR 0.36; 95% CI 0.2–0.65) compared to those with adequate dietary calcium intake (RR 0.62; 95% CI 0.32–1.2) [98]. Although calcium supplementation may also reduce the composite outcome of maternal death or serious morbidity (RR 0.80; 95% CI 0.66–0.98) and preterm birth (RR 0.76; 95% CI 0.6–0.92), these effects may be overestimated due to small-study effects or publication bias [98]. Although lower doses of calcium may also show a trend towards reduction in pre-eclampsia, hypertension, and admission to neonatal high care, this evidence is limited to date [98]. A subsequent multicentre randomised trial assigned over 1,300 women with previous pre-eclampsia or eclampsia and a likely calcium deficient diet to low-dose calcium supplementation (500 mg) or placebo from pre-pregnancy until 20 weeks' gestation, after which all participants were prescribed 1.5 g calcium daily. The addition of early supplementation did not significantly reduce the risk of recurrent pre-eclampsia (23% vs. 29%; RR 0.80; 95% CI 0.61–1.06), although subgroup analysis suggested that women with >80% compliance with their calcium supplements had a statistically significant reduction in pre-eclampsia (RR 0.66; 95% CI 0.44–0.98) [99].

The World Health Organization and FIGO support daily calcium supplementation (1.5–2.0 g oral elemental calcium) for pregnant women in populations with low dietary calcium intake for pre-eclampsia prevention [2,89,100]. There is no clear evidence on the best timing to commence calcium supplementation but it has been suggested to commence at the first antenatal care contact [100].

## Investigational preventative therapies

### Low molecular weight heparin

As thrombosis is frequently seen in the uteroplacental circulation of pregnancies affected by severe and/or early-onset forms of placental-mediated complications, anticoagulation with low molecular weight heparin (LMWH) has been suggested as a method of improving placental perfusion. It has also been suggested that treatment with LMWH promotes a pro-angiogenic state, with significantly increased levels of PlGF seen in the third trimester in a small prospective cohort study of women on LMWH in pregnancy [101].

However, evidence to date has not supported the use of LMWH in pre-eclampsia prevention, and is limited by low quality studies with significant clinical and statistical heterogeneity. A 2016 meta-analysis of individual patient data from eight randomised controlled trials of LMWH versus no LMWH in pregnancy for women with any prior placental-mediated pregnancy complications (including term or preterm pre-eclampsia) did not demonstrate a significant reduction in the primary composite outcome which included early-onset or severe pre-eclampsia (RR 0.64; 95% CI 0.36–1.11), nor in the secondary outcomes of pre-eclampsia, severe pre-eclampsia, early-onset pre-eclampsia, and severe or early-onset pre-eclampsia [102]. Likewise, in a randomised controlled trial of women with prior severe pre-eclampsia diagnosed before 34 weeks' gestation where the women were allocated to either enoxaparin and aspirin, or aspirin alone prior to 14 weeks' gestation, there was no difference in the primary composite outcome (RR 0.84; 95% CI 0.61–1.16) which included pre-eclampsia [103]. A subsequent 2017 open-label randomised controlled trial of 149 women at high risk of pre-eclampsia and/or small for gestational age children based on their obstetric history demonstrated that the addition of enoxaparin to standard high-risk care had no effect on the rate of pre-eclampsia [104]; however, there were small numbers of women with a history of pre-eclampsia included in this study. Although a recent systematic review concluded that LMWH was associated with a significant reduction in the risk of pre-eclampsia and other placental-mediated complications when started before 16 weeks' gestation in women at high risk, the authors acknowledged that the meta-analysis was limited by the poor methodological quality of studies included, substantial heterogeneity identified in the analyses, wide CIs suggesting imprecision in results and possible publication bias relating to single-centre trials [105].

### Metformin

Small molecule inhibitors of hypoxic inducible factor $1\alpha$ have been found to reduce sFlt-1 and sEng secretion. Metformin is also reported to inhibit hypoxic inducible factor $1\alpha$ by reducing mitochondrial electron transport chain activity, and is known to be safe in pregnancy [106]. Although initial trials suggested reduction in the risk of pre-eclampsia with metformin [107] and certain trials of metformin in women with gestational diabetes or obesity found a reduced risk of pre-eclampsia as a secondary outcome [107], a 2018 Cochrane review suggested metformin makes little or no difference in the risk of women developing pre-eclampsia (RR 0.74; 95% CI 0.09–6.28) based on low-quality evidence [108].

## Statins

Pre-eclampsia and cardiovascular disease share the key components of endothelial dysfunction and inflammation. Therefore, statins, which are effective in primary and secondary prevention of cardiovascular disease, have been hypothesised to also reduce the risk of pre-eclampsia. This is supported by data from animal studies [109,110] and small clinical studies [111]. However, the recent STATIN multicentre, double-blind, placebo-controlled trial where women at high-risk of term pre-eclampsia identified in the third trimester were randomised to pravastatin or placebo from 35 to 37 weeks until delivery or 41 weeks failed to show any significant differences in the incidence of term pre-eclampsia (statin 14.6% vs. placebo 13.6%; hazard ratio 1.08; 95% CI 0.78–1.49, $p = 0.65$), any of the secondary outcomes studied or levels of maternal serum PlGF or sFlt-1 after randomisation [112].

## Ineffective preventative therapies

In the search for an effective intervention to prevent pre-eclampsia, several treatments have been demonstrated to have no significant benefit, including:

- *Anti-oxidants*: Vitamins C and E did not confer a reduction in the risk of pre-eclampsia in multiple large, randomised, multicentre trials including women at both high and low risk of developing pre-eclampsia [113–116]. Meta-analysis of such trials encompassing almost 20,000 women confirmed this finding (pre-eclampsia 9.6% vs. placebo 9.6%; RR 1.00; 95% CI 0.92–1.09) and also suggested an increased risk of gestational hypertension (RR 1.11; 95% CI 1.05–1.17) and premature rupture of membranes (RR 1.73; 95% CI 1.34–2.23) [117]
- *Nitric oxide donors*: Pre-eclamptic women have been suggested to be deficient in nitric oxide, which mediates vasodilatation and inhibits platelet aggregation. A small randomised controlled trial of supplementation with L-arginine (a nitric oxide precursor) and anti-oxidants supplementation in women with a history of pre-eclampsia suggested a significant reduction in pre-eclampsia compared with placebo (absolute RR 0.17; 95% CI 0.12–0.21) and anti-oxidants alone (absolute RR 0.09; 95% CI 0.05–0.14; $p = 0.004$); however, there were no significant differences in clinical outcomes such as gestational age at delivery, mean infant birth weight, small for gestational age infants, or placental abruption [118]. A subsequent Cochrane review also concluded that there was insufficient evidence to support the use of nitric oxide donors (e.g. glyceryl trinitrate) or pre-cursors (e.g. L-arginine) for the prevention of pre-eclampsia [119]
- *Vitamin D*: It has been hypothesised that vitamin D may prevent pre-eclampsia by modulating pro-inflammatory responses, decreasing oxidative stress, and promoting angiogenesis; however, a systematic review of clinical trials did not support vitamin D supplementation in preventing pre-eclampsia [120]. A 2019 Cochrane review suggested that, compared with placebo, the risk of pre-eclampsia was probably reduced with vitamin D alone (RR 0.48; 95% CI 0.30–0.79) as well as with vitamin D combined with calcium (RR 0.50; 95% CI 0.32–0.78), but recognised that the studies included were of very low to moderate quality and limited by study design, imprecision, and indirectness [121].

# DIAGNOSIS

Prompt diagnosis of pre-eclampsia aims to improve maternal and perinatal outcomes by ensuring appropriate management including treatment of severe hypertension, magnesium sulphate to prevent seizures when appropriate, antenatal corticosteroids for fetal lung maturation, and timely delivery.

Historically, there has been no clear consensus regarding the diagnostic criteria for pre-eclampsia, with various international statements creating uncertainty around best practice. Pre-eclampsia has traditionally been defined by the presence of both hypertension and proteinuria, as reflected in guidelines released by the International Society for the Study of Hypertension in Pregnancy (ISSHP) [122] and ACOG [123] in the early 2000s. However, in 2013 and 2014, ISSHP (Box 2.1) [1] and ACOG [124] revised these diagnostic criteria, stating that pre-eclampsia could be diagnosed in the absence of proteinuria if other evidence of maternal end-organ dysfunction was present. Although this principle has been reaffirmed in updated guidelines from both ISSHP in 2018 [125] and ACOG in 2020 [38], there remains subtle variations between them including the inclusion of uteroplacental dysfunction as a form of maternal end-organ dysfunction by ISSHP but not ACOG; 'severe' pre-eclampsia being defined by ACOG but not ISSHP; and differing thresholds for thrombocytopenia (platelet count in ISSHP < 150,000/μL, in ACOG <100,000 μL). Nonetheless, guidelines from both societies are accepted internationally with the ISSHP guidelines endorsed by FIGO [2,126] and NICE [37].

## Clinical assessment

In addition to routine antenatal care, women who are at increased risk of developing should have accurate pregnancy dating, baseline blood pressure, and baseline biochemistry (including platelet count, creatinine, liver function tests, and urinary protein: Creatinine ratio) recorded in early pregnancy. This is helpful later in gestation in distinguishing from underlying disorders which may be associated with similar clinical and laboratory findings.

---

**Box 2.1  The revised (2014) ISSHP definition of pre-eclampsia**

Gestational hypertension (systolic blood pressure ≥140 mmHg, or diastolic blood pressure ≥90 mmHg, or both) together with one or more of the following new-onset conditions at or after 20 weeks' gestation:

- Proteinuria, e.g. protein to creatinine ratio of ≥30 mg/mmol (0.3 mg/mg)
- Other maternal organ dysfunction, including:
  - *Acute kidney injury*: Creatinine ≥ 90 μmol/L (1 mg/dL)
  - *Liver involvement*: Elevated alanine aminotransferase or aspartate aminotransferase > 40 IU/L, with or without right upper quadrant or epigastric abdominal pain
  - Neurological complications, e.g. eclampsia, altered mental state, blindness, stroke, clonus, severe headaches, or persistent visual scotomata
  - Haematological complications, e.g. platelet count < 150,000 platelets per μL, disseminated intravascular coagulation, or haemolysis
- Uteroplacental dysfunction, e.g. fetal growth restriction, abnormal umbilical artery Doppler wave form analysis, or stillbirth

It is also prudent to educate higher-risk patients about the signs and symptoms of pre-eclampsia, and to monitor them more closely through more frequent antenatal appointments [126].

## Maternal serum biomarkers

Maternal serum biomarkers can be used in the diagnosis of suspected pre-eclampsia to help clarify the likelihood of pre-eclampsia where there is clinical uncertainty. Numerous biomarkers have been described [127] but most require further validation and evaluation in larger studies. The utility of PlGF alone, and the sFlt-1:PlGF ratio, in the diagnosis of pre-eclampsia is the most studied maternal serum analytes to date, and is particularly useful in the prediction of pre-eclampsia as findings of low PlGF and elevated sFlt-1 concentrations predate the clinical manifestations of pre-eclampsia by some weeks [26].

Placental growth factor is a pro-angiogenic protein secreted by the placenta that, in healthy pregnancies, increases in the maternal circulation with increasing gestation before decreasing towards term. In pregnancies affected by pre-eclampsia, however, PlGF concentrations are decreased, with this change predating clinical symptoms of pre-eclampsia by weeks [26]. Low PlGF has high sensitivity (96%; 95% CI 89–99%) and negative predictive value (98%; 95% CI 93.0–99.5) for a diagnosis of pre-eclampsia within 14 days, with improved predictive value compared to traditionally used investigations such as blood pressure measurement and serum biochemistry assessing for maternal end-organ dysfunction [128]. The PARROT trial, a multicentre pragmatic stepped-wedge cluster-randomised controlled trial in the UK, examined the use of PlGF in women with suspected pre-eclampsia, with revealed PlGF testing and subsequent targeted enhanced surveillance reducing the time to diagnosis of pre-eclampsia compared to usual care with additional concealed PlGF testing (1.9 days vs. 4.1 days; time rate 0.36; 95% CI 0.15–0.87; $p = 0.027$) [129]. This approach also was associated with a reduction in severe maternal outcomes as defined by the full pre-eclampsia integrated estimate of risk (fullPIERS) consensus (revealed testing 4% vs. concealed testing 5%, aOR 0.32; 95% CI 0.11–0.96; $p = 0.043$), with no difference in adverse perinatal outcomes (15% vs. 14%, aOR 1.45; 95% CI 0.73–2.90) [129]. Further analysis of the same cohort demonstrated that incorporating PlGF testing into clinical care costs less than current standard care (£149 saved per patient tested) after accounting for the local costs of testing [130]. UK guidelines have recently been updated to reflect this evidence, with NICE recommending PlGF-based testing for women with suspected pre-eclampsia before 35 weeks' gestation to help rule out the disease [37].

A ratio of sFlt-1:PlGF has also been reviewed for its role in the diagnosis of pre-eclampsia. In pregnancies complicated by pre-eclampsia, PlGF concentrations are decreased with sFlt-1 levels elevated compared to pregnancies not affected by the disease; therefore women with pre-eclampsia have significantly increased sFlt-1:PlGF ratio compared with women who are normotensive or have chronic hypertension [28,131–133]. Regardless of gestational age, in women with suspected pre-eclampsia, a sFlt-1:PlGF of ≤38 indicates a reasonable sensitivity (80.0%; 95% CI 51.9–95.7) and high negative predictive value (99.3%; 95% CI 97.9–99.9) for the diagnosis of pre-eclampsia in the subsequent week [28] and 4 weeks [131] thereafter. Because of the high negative predictive value of sFlt-1:PlGF ratio, it is most useful as a point of care test to rule out pre-eclampsia in women with clinical suspicion of the disease, potentially decreasing unnecessary interventions such as hospital admission, the costs associated with increased antenatal surveillance and unwarranted anxiety for women. Conversely, women with sFlt-1:PlGf levels that are in high or intermediate ranges for gestation are at increased risk of pre-eclampsia or another form of placental dysfunction within the next 4 weeks and justify closer surveillance. The single-centre INSPIRE prospective parallel-group randomised controlled trial in the UK found that sFlt-1:PlGF testing improved the clinical identification of women who developed pre-eclampsia within 7 days (100% in revealed testing group vs. 83% in non-revealed testing group; $p = 0.038$) without changing the primary outcome of overall maternal admission rate or altering gestational age at birth, birthweight, or neonatal unit admission [134].

## Prognostic models

As there is no single test that is able to predict pre-eclampsia with sufficient accuracy for clinical use and, most importantly, adverse outcomes in women with suspected or confirmed pre-eclampsia, multivariable models have been proposed that involve clinical and laboratory predictors. These risk prediction models, such as the fullPIERS and PREP-S models recommended in the NICE guidelines [37], have successfully undergone internal and external validation, and assist clinicians in risk stratifying women with pre-eclampsia to guide decisions about the most appropriate place of care (which may indicate need for in utero transfer) and thresholds for intervention. FullPIERS is intended for use at any time in pregnancy, while PREP-S is intended only for up to 34 weeks' gestation [37], and neither model predicts outcomes for infants.

The fullPIERS multivariable model predicts composite adverse maternal outcome within 48 hours in women admitted to hospital for pre-eclampsia [area under the receiver-operating characteristics curve (AUROC) 0.88; 95% CI 0.84–0.92], and can be used at any gestational age. Up to 7 days after eligibility, there was good performance of the model (AUROC > 0.7) with >99% negative predictive value [135]. Significant predictors of adverse maternal outcomes (maternal mortality or one or more of serious neurological, cardiorespiratory, hepatic, or renal or haematological morbidity) in the model were gestational age at eligibility, platelet count, chest pain or dyspnoea, oxygen saturation, serum creatinine concentration, and aspartate transaminase concentration [135]. Blood pressure was not identified as a predictor of maternal complications, possibly because this is one feature of pre-eclampsia for which effective intervention can be implemented. External validation of the fullPIERS model in an independent dataset (miniPIERS, developing for low- and middle-income countries) demonstrated reasonable discrimination [AUROC 0.768 (95% CI 0.735–0.80)] but poor calibration [136,137].

The PREP models can also be used to obtain predictions of adverse maternal outcome risk in women with confirmed early-onset pre-eclampsia, by 48 hours (PREP-S) and by discharge (PREP-L) [138]. The primary outcome of these models, similar to fullPIERS, was a composite of maternal complications including maternal death and organ dysfunction (neurological, hepatic, cardiorespiratory, renal, and haematological) but also included delivery before 34 weeks as a surrogate of iatrogenic delivery to avoid maternal and fetal complications as per national guidelines; exclusion of this as an adverse outcome would potentially underestimate the true incidence of adverse outcomes and lead to prognostic models that yield too low risk predictions of actually developing an adverse outcome.

# MANAGEMENT

Once pre-eclampsia has been diagnosed, it is typically a progressive condition with deterioration of maternal organ function over time. No intervention to date has been shown to reliably influence disease progression, and the only effective curative treatment is delivery of the fetus and placenta. Current approaches to improving clinical outcomes of pre-eclampsia include prompt diagnosis and appropriate stratification of antenatal care, with the ideal goal of prolonging pregnancy to term gestation with close surveillance if safe to do so.

## Maternal management

Admission to hospital for pre-eclampsia may be warranted in several circumstances, such as at initial diagnosis [1] or in the presence of higher-risk features such as severe hypertension, clinical concerns regarding mother or fetus, or increased risk of adverse events based on prognostic models [37,38]. This may involve transfer to facilities with maternal high dependency or intensive care unit capacity if they have features potentially reflecting severe pre-eclampsia (on-going or recurring severe headaches, visual scotomata, nausea/vomiting, epigastric pain, oliguria, severe hypertension, progressively worsening biochemical markers, and abnormal fetal Doppler measurements) [1]. If hypertension is controlled, and maternal and fetal wellbeing is confirmed, outpatient specialist management with increased surveillance may be appropriate [38].

Maternal blood tests, including haemoglobin, platelet count, liver enzymes, electrolytes, creatinine, and uric acid, should be performed at diagnosis as well as at least twice weekly in most women with pre-eclampsia [1,37]. Although the utility of uric acid has been challenged, evidence suggested that amongst hypertensive pregnant women, elevated corrected uric acid may still be valuable as an indicator for the possibility of fetal growth restriction [1].

## Blood pressure management

Most women with pre-eclampsia will require antihypertensive therapy, with the goal of reducing the risk of severe hypertension and other maternal complications. Although there is no clear consensus as to when regular anti-hypertensive treatment should be commenced, NICE suggests pharmacological management if a woman's blood pressure persistently remains ≥140/90 mmHg [37]. International guidelines generally recommend a target blood pressure of 135/85 mmHg or less [37]; less tight blood pressure control (diastolic blood pressure ≥ 100 mmHg) has been associated with increased risk of severe hypertensive episodes [139]. It is also recommended to not lower blood pressure below recommended limits as this may be associated with poor placental perfusion [1].

Agents commonly used for regular blood pressure control in pregnancy include oral labetalol, nifedipine, and methyldopa [1,37,38], which can be used in combination and all have favourable safety profiles. A Cochrane meta-analysis regarding antihypertensive treatment for mild-to-moderate hypertension in pregnancy concluded that β-blockers such as labetalol, and calcium-channel blockers such as nifedipine, were more effective that other antihypertensives in preventing severe hypertension [140]. Angiotensin-converting enzyme inhibitors and angiotensin receptor blockers should not be used in pregnancy because of potential adverse safety profiles for the fetus.

Acute antihypertensive management should be instituted at sustained blood pressures ≥160–170/110 mmHg, as these blood pressures are thought to be surrogate markers for an increased risk of stroke and placental abruption, as well as reflecting increased severity of pre-eclampsia [1]. Intravenous agents such as labetalol or hydralazine can be used for severe hypertension, but should be done with caution due to the risk of acute maternal hypotension and reduced placental perfusion. Oral agents, such as nifedipine, can also be used and may be more accessible than intravenous agents in some settings.

## Magnesium sulphate

Magnesium sulphate is widely recommended for seizure prophylaxis in women at acute risk of, or already with, eclampsia [1,37,38,89,126]. Although magnesium sulphate is not typically regarded as an anticonvulsant, it is the drug of choice for seizure prophylaxis in eclampsia as it is better than traditional anticonvulsants such as diazepam [141], phenytoin [142], or lytic cocktail [143]. Its mode of action in preventing eclamptic seizures is not clearly understood, but may include vasodilatation by antagonism of calcium channels in vascular smooth muscle, a reduction in peripheral resistance and vasoconstriction, protective effects on the blood-brain barrier and decreased cerebral oedema, and central anticonvulsant actions through inhibition of N-methyl-D-aspartate (NMDA) receptors [144]. Despite being a calcium antagonist, there is no evidence that it lowers systemic blood pressure [145] or is an effective antihypertensive drug [140].

Predicting who is at risk of eclampsia is difficult, as only around 1–2% of those with even severe pre-eclampsia will have a seizure [146]. Although neurological symptoms such as severe intractable headache, visual scotoma, or hyperreflexia may prompt commencement of magnesium sulphate treatment due to suggested higher risks of eclamptic seizures, no symptoms are accurate predictors of eclampsia [147].

There is no consensus on what the optimal magnesium sulphate regimen is, in regards to dosing, length of treatment or route of administration. The Collaborative Eclampsia Trial [148] regimen is commonly recommended [37,126], of a 4 g loading dose intravenously over 5–15 minutes, followed by a maintenance infusion of 1 g/h and a further 2–4 g load in the event of recurrent seizures. In this regimen, magnesium sulphate is recommended for a minimum of 24 hours, and extended to 24 hours after the last seizure if recurrent fits occur [148]. Alternative regimens include intramuscular dosing, which may offer lower risk of side effects due to more stable magnesium, therefore being of more use in low- and middle-income countries where dosing serum magnesium levels may be challenging.

Side effects include flushing, muscle weakness, and nausea. Serious adverse effects such as respiratory and cardiac arrest are rare, but if they do occur, are potentially life threatening. Caution must be exercised in women with renal insufficiency, as magnesium sulphate is excreted by the kidneys and may increase the risk of toxicity in these women. A reduction in maintenance dosing or monitoring with serum magnesium levels may assist in appropriate dosing.

In women with pre-eclampsia, magnesium sulphate more than halved the risk of eclampsia (RR 0.41; 95% CI 0.29–0.58; NNT for an additional beneficial outcome 100; 95% CI 50–100) compared to placebo or no anticonvulsant [145,146]. Treatment with magnesium sulphate also demonstrated a reduction in placental abruption (RR 0.64; 95% CI 0.50–0.83), although the risk of caesarean section was increased (RR 1.05; 95% CI 1.01–1.10) [146]. Maternal outcomes including a non-statistically significant reduction in maternal death (RR 0.54; 95% CI 0.26–1.1), and increased side effects such as flushing (24% vs. 5%; RR 5.26; 95% CI 4.59–6.03; number needed to harm 6; 95% CI 5–6) [146]. There was no clear difference in stillbirth or neonatal death (RR 1.04; 95% CI 0.93–1.15) [146].

There are also additional benefits in neonatal outcome when magnesium sulphate is given to women at risk of preterm birth. Antenatal magnesium sulphate treatment significantly reduced the risk of cerebral palsy (RR 0.68; 95% CI 0.54–0.87) and substantial gross motor dysfunction (RR 0.61; 95% CI 0.44–0.85) in the child without statistically significant effects on paediatric mortality (RR 1.04; 95% CI 0.92–1.17) [149]. The number of women needed to be treated to benefit one baby by avoiding cerebral palsy is 63 (95% CI 43–155) [149].

## Fetal management

Fetal surveillance should be increased in pregnancies affected by pre-eclampsia due to the risk of fetal growth restriction associated with uteroplacental dysfunction. In addition to fetal heart rate auscultation at every antenatal encounter, an ultrasound assessment of the fetal biometry should be undertaken at the time of pre-eclampsia diagnosis and repeated every 2 weeks to assess serial growth.

Cardiotocography (CTG) monitoring is indicated as per usual clinical indications. Notably, this includes severe maternal hypertension requiring urgent management, as there is a risk of acute maternal hypotension and subsequent placental hypoperfusion with intravenous antihypertensive treatment.

## Antenatal corticosteroids

Antenatal corticosteroids to accelerate fetal lung maturation should be administered if birth is to be expedited before 34 weeks' gestation and likely within 7 days [37,150], regardless of indication for delivery. If immediately indicated, however, birth should not be delayed for antenatal corticosteroid administration.

High certainty evidence demonstrates that a single course of antenatal corticosteroids reduces the risk of perinatal death (RR 0.85; 95% CI 0.77–0.93), neonatal death (RR 0.78; 95% CI 0.70–0.87), respiratory distress syndrome (RR 0.71; 95% CI 0.65–0.78) and probably intraventricular haemorrhage (RR 0.58; 95% CI 0.45–0.75) [150]. There is probably little or no difference in maternal outcomes including maternal death, chorioamnionitis, and endometritis, although all these outcomes had wide CIs.

## Birth

### Timing

Birth should be expedited irrespective of gestation if there is evidence of severe maternal end organ dysfunction, eclamptic seizure, pulmonary oedema, or placental abruption [37,126]. Delivery should also be considered if biochemistry demonstrates worsening parameters of thrombocytopaenia, haemolysis, coagulopathy, or renal or liver dysfunction [37,126]. Serum uric acid [1] and proteinuria [151,152] should not be used for indications for delivery, as they are poor predictors of maternal and fetal complications.

Before 34 weeks' gestation, a Cochrane review of six trials concluded that expectant management of severe early-onset pre-eclampsia may be associated with decreased morbidity for the child [153]. Therefore, continuation of the pregnancy until a more advanced gestation is achieved is recommended at this gestation if safe to do so. International guidelines support that women with pre-eclampsia before 34 weeks' gestation should be managed conservatively at a centre with maternal and fetal medicine expertise, with triggers for delivery such as uncontrolled maternal hypertension despite appropriate anti-hypertensive therapy; maternal pulse oximetry < 90%; progressive biochemical deterioration in liver, renal, and haematological parameters; neurological symptoms or eclampsia; placental abruption; or fetal indications including reversed end-diastolic flow in the umbilical artery, non-reassuring CTG, or stillbirth[1,37,38,89].

Between 34 and 37 weeks' gestation, timing of birth is a trade-off between maternal and fetal risks and so decision making should be individualised and shared with the woman.[89] The open-label randomised controlled trial HYPITAT-II randomised 703 women with non-severe hypertensive disorders of pregnancy to either immediate delivery within 24 hours, or expectant monitoring with the aim of prolonging pregnancy until 37 weeks' gestation [154]. This trial found that although immediate delivery may reduce the already small risks of adverse maternal outcomes, it significantly increased the risk of neonatal respiratory distress syndrome (RR 3.3; 95% CI 1.4–8.2; $p = 0.005$) and therefore recommended against routine immediate delivery at these late preterm gestations [154]. The PHOENIX trial in 2019 likewise compared planned early delivery with expectant management in women with late preterm pre-eclampsia between 34 and 37 weeks' gestation with a reduction in the risk of a composite of adverse maternal outcomes (RR 0.86; 95% CI 0.79–0.94) but with increased admission rates to the neonatal unit (RR 1.26; 95% CI 1.08–1.47)[155]. Those managed expectantly in the PHOENIX trial delivered a median of 6 days after diagnosis, with 55% of the expectant group requiring expedited delivery before 37 weeks' gestation due to clinical concerns[155].

At 37 weeks' gestation or beyond, delivery is warranted[1,37,38,126] because continuing expectant management will increase the likelihood of adverse maternal outcomes with little or no fetal gain[156]. This should be initiated within 24–48 hours[37,126].

## Mode of delivery

Mode of delivery should be individualised for each woman, based on the woman's clinical status, her preferences, and routine obstetric indications[37,38]. Should the woman proceed with labour, the following considerations should be made:

- Continue regular antenatal antihypertensive treatment during labour [37]
- During labour, measure blood pressure hourly in women with hypertension, increasing to every 15–30 minutes until blood pressure is <160/110 mmHg in women with severe hypertension [37]
- Continuous intrapartum fetal monitoring is indicated
- Judicious fluid management, including no intravenous fluid preloading in women with severe pre-eclampsia before establishing low-dose epidural analgesia or combined spinal-epidural analgesia
- Do not routinely limit the duration of second stage of labour if hypertension in appropriately controlled [37]
- Operative or assisted birth in second stage labour should be considered for women with severe hypertension, where hypertension has not responded to initial treatment [37]

## Investigational treatments

The search for new therapies for the treatment of pre-eclampsia is the subject of intensive research, given the significant global burden of maternal and fetal morbidity and mortality. However, as knowledge regarding the pathophysiology underlying pre-eclampsia increases, research around therapies specifically targeted at these mechanisms gains momentum.

## Antithrombin

Antithrombin is a complex glycoprotein which affects coagulation through inhibition of thrombin and factor Xa, and inflammation by inducing prostacyclin endothelial release [157]. Decreased antithrombin levels have been described in pre-eclampsia [158] However, the Pharmacokinetics, Safety and Efficacy of Recombinant Antithrombin Versus Placebo in Preterm Preeclampsia (PRESERVE-1) double-blind randomised placebo-controlled trial examining the use of intravenous recombinant human antithrombin versus placebo for women with early-onset pre-eclampsia from 23 to 30 weeks' gestation did not demonstrate any differences in pregnancy prolongation, maternal, or fetal outcomes [159].

## Metformin

Metformin is a commonly used oral hypoglycaemic agent that has been demonstrated as safe in pregnancy through its use as treatment for gestational diabetes mellitus. In addition to its hypoglycaemic effects, it has been demonstrated to block hypoxic inducible factor $1\alpha$, which is upregulated with ischaemia and facilitates sFlt-1 secretion. In functional experiments using primary human tissues, metformin has reduced sFLt-1 and sEng secretion and therefore endothelial dysfunction, as well as inducing angiogenesis and enhancing vasodilatation [106]. The PI2 trial, a double-blind randomised placebo-controlled trial, has shown that metformin as a treatment has shown to increase duration of pregnancy with 1 week [160]. Metformin has also been proposed in combination with other drugs such as esomeprazole [161] and sulfasalazine [162].

## Proton pump inhibitors

Proton pump inhibitors (PPI) are commonly used in pregnancy to treat gastroesophageal reflux, with extensive safety data available including in early pregnancy [163]. Pre-clinical evidence suggests PPIs decrease anti-angiogenic factor expression and secretion from the placenta and endothelial cells, mitigate markers of endothelial dysfunction and decrease secretion of pro-inflammatory molecules [164]. A secondary analysis of a prospective cohort study of women with confirmed or suspected pre-eclampsia also suggested that PPI use was associated with lower sFlt-1, sEng, and endothelin-1 levels [165]. However, a randomised placebo-controlled trial in South Africa of 40 mg esomeprazole daily in women diagnosed with preterm pre-eclampsia at 26–32 weeks' gestation did not demonstrate a statistically significant prolongation of pregnancy or a reduction in anti-angiogenic factors [166], although the authors suggest that the study may have been underpowered and may have better efficacy with higher dosing or alternative administration route. Nonetheless, on-going investigation into PPIs in combination with other therapeutics such as metformin [161] continue.

## Statins

Stains, or 3-hydroxy-methylglutaryl coenzyme A (HMG-CoA) reductase inhibitors, are primarily used in the treatment of cardiovascular disease and for lowering cholesterol, but have also been demonstrated to improve endothelial function. Pravastatin has been shown to reduce circulating sFlt-1 levels in mouse models of pre-eclampsia [167] and in vitro reduced secretion of sFlt-1 from human endothelial cells, trophoblast cells, and placental explants from women with preterm pre-eclampsia [168]. Although pravastatin has long been classed by the United States Food and Drug Administration as Category X, indicating that it is contraindicated in pregnancy, recent small pilot trials have confirmed the safety of pravastatin in pregnancy at 10–20 mg doses [111,169]. The Statins to Ameliorate Pre-Eclampsia (STaMP) double-blind, randomised, multicentre trial showed no evidence that 40 mg pravastatin lowered maternal plasma sFlt-1 levels once early-onset pre-eclampsia had developed [170]; however, the trial was limited by small sample size, non-compliance with study medication, and was underpowered for maternal and fetal outcomes.

## Other emerging treatments

There are also several emerging treatments that have been reported in case studies or small case series.

- *Therapies to modify the imbalance between angiogenic and anti-angiogenic factors*: Treatments traditionally used in the thrombotic microangiopathies of haemolytic-uremic syndrome (HUS), paroxysmal nocturnal haemoglobinuria, and thrombotic thrombocytopenic purpura (TTP) such as therapeutic plasma exchange (apheresis) [171–173] and complement inhibition with eculizumab, a targeted inhibitor of complement protein C5 [174,175] have been associated with prolongation of pregnancy in preterm pre-eclampsia in isolated reports
- *Sildenafil*: A phosphodiesterase type 5 inhibitor, sildenafil is thought to potentially increase in uteroplacental and fetoplacental blood flow and has been associated with prolongation of pregnancy [176] as well as reduced serum sFlt-1 and sEng secretion and increased PlGF secretion in preterm pre-eclampsia [177]; however, an increase in neonatal pulmonary hypertension in the Sildenafil Therapy in Dismal Prognosis Early-Onset Fetal Growth Restriction (STRIDER) trial has raised safety concerns about the drug in pregnancy [178]
- *Melatonin*: A potent anti-oxidant, melatonin was suggested in a phase I trial to prolong the time between diagnosis of pre-eclampsia and delivery [179], but a potential beneficial effect is yet to be confirmed in larger double-blind randomised controlled trials

There are also several novel therapies that have been demonstrated in animal models such as treatment with recombinant VEGF [180] and PlGF [181], and RNA interference with short interfering RNA therapeutics to suppress sFlt-1 overexpression.[182]

# CONCLUSION

Pre-eclampsia and eclampsia are a significant cause of maternal and perinatal morbidity and mortality, and continue to be a burden on healthcare systems globally. Despite pre-eclampsia first being recognised over a century ago, our understanding of its underlying pathophysiology continues to expand and evolve, challenging traditional thinking around treatment of the disease. Major advances have also occurred in the search for effective screening and prevention of pre-eclampsia over the last two decades. On-going research to refine, validate, and implement effective interventions for screening, prevention, and treatment of pre-eclampsia continues with the goal of improving maternal and perinatal outcomes.

# REFERENCES

1.  Tranquilli AL, Dekker G, Magee L, et al. The classification, diagnosis and management of the hypertensive disorders of pregnancy: A revised statement from the ISSHP. Pregnancy Hypertens 2014; 4:97–104.
2.  Poon LC, Shennan A, Hyett JA, et al. The International Federation of Gynecology and Obstetrics (FIGO) initiative on pre-eclampsia: A pragmatic guide for first-trimester screening and prevention. Int J Gynaecol Obstet 2019; 145:1–33.
3.  Dall'Asta A, D'Antonio F, Saccone G, et al. Cardiovascular events following pregnancy complicated by pre-eclampsia with emphasis on comparison between early- and late-onset forms: systematic review and meta-analysis. Ultrasound Obstet Gynecol 2021; 57:698–709.
4.  Stekkinger E, Zandstra M, Peeters LLH, Spaanderman MEA. Early-onset preeclampsia and the prevalence of postpartum metabolic syndrome. Obstet Gynecol 2009; 114:1076–1084.
5.  Bellamy L, Casas JP, Hingorani AD, et al. Pre-eclampsia and risk of cardiovascular disease and cancer in later life: systematic review and meta-analysis. BMJ 2007; 335:974.
6.  Staff AC. Long-term cardiovascular health after stopping pre-eclampsia. Lancet 2019; 394:1120–1121.
7.  Fields JA, Garovic VD, Mielke MM, et al. Preeclampsia and cognitive impairment later in life. Am J Obstet Gynecol 2017; 217:74.e1–e11.
8.  Kristensen JH, Basit S, Wohlfahrt J, et al. Pre-eclampsia and risk of later kidney disease: nationwide cohort study. BMJ 2019; 365:11516.
9.  Khashan AS, Evans M, Kublickas M, et al. Preeclampsia and risk of end stage kidney disease: A Swedish nationwide cohort study. PLOS Medicine 2019; 16:e1002875.
10. Vikse BE, Irgens LM, Leivestad T, et al. Preeclampsia and the Risk of End-Stage Renal Disease. N Eng J Med 2008; 359:800–9.
11. Andraweera PH, Lassi ZS. Cardiovascular Risk Factors in Offspring of Preeclamptic Pregnancies—Systematic Review and Meta-Analysis. J Pediatr 2019; 208:104–113.e6.
12. Sun BZ, Moster D, Harmon QE, et al. Association of Preeclampsia in Term Births With Neurodevelopmental Disorders in Offspring. JAMA Psychiat 2020; 77:823.
13. Ananth CV, Keyes KM, Wapner RJ. Pre-eclampsia rates in the United States, 1980-2010: age-period-cohort analysis. BMJ 2013; 347:f6564.
14. Stevens W, Shih T, Incerti D, et al. Short-term costs of preeclampsia to the United States health care system. Am J Obstet Gynecol 2017; 217:237–248.e16.
15. Broughton Pipkin F, Rubin PC. Pre-eclampsia—the 'disease of theories'. Br Med Bull 1994; 50:381–396.
16. Higgins JR, Brennecke SP. Pre-eclampsia--still a disease of theories? Curr Opin Obstet Gynecol 1998; 10:129–133.
17. Chesley LC. History and epidemiology of preeclampsia-eclampsia. Clin Obstet Gynecol 1984; 27:801–820.
18. Brosens IA, Robertson WB, Dixon HG. The role of the spiral arteries in the pathogenesis of preeclampsia. Obstet Gynecol Annu 1972; 1:177–191.
19. Robertson WB, Brosens I, Dixon HG. The pathological response of the vessels of the placental bed to hypertensive pregnancy. J Pathol Bacteriol 1967; 93:581–592.
20. Roberts JM, Redman CW. Pre-eclampsia: more than pregnancy-induced hypertension. Lancet 1993; 341:1447–1451.
21. Vinnars MT, Nasiell J, Ghazi S, et al. The severity of clinical manifestations in preeclampsia correlates with the amount of placental infarction. Acta Obstetricia et Gynecologica Scandinavica 2011; 90:19–25
22. Fillion A, Guerby P, Menzies D, et al. Pathological investigation of placentas in preeclampsia (the PEARL study). Hypertens Pregnancy 2021; 40:56–62.
23. Granger J. Pathophysiology of pregnancy-induced hypertension. Am J Hypertension 2001; 14:S178–S85.
24. Chang X, Yao J, He Q, et al. Exosomes From Women With Preeclampsia Induced Vascular Dysfunction by Delivering sFlt (Soluble Fms-Like Tyrosine Kinase)-1 and sEng (Soluble Endoglin) to Endothelial Cells. Hypertension 2018; 72:1381–1390.
25. Gill M, Motta-Mejia C, Kandzija N, et al. Placental Syncytiotrophoblast-Derived Extracellular Vesicles Carry Active NEP (Neprilysin) and Are Increased in Preeclampsia. Hypertension 2019; 73:1112–1119.
26. Levine RJ, Maynard SE, Qian C, et al. Circulating Angiogenic Factors and the Risk of Preeclampsia. N Eng J Med 2004; 350:672–683.
27. Levine RJ, Lam C, Qian C, et al. Soluble Endoglin and Other Circulating Antiangiogenic Factors in Preeclampsia. N Eng J Med 2006; 355:992–1005.

28. Zeisler H, Llurba E, Chantraine F, et al. Predictive Value of the sFlt-1:PlGF Ratio in Women with Suspected Preeclampsia. N Eng J Med 2016; 374:13–22.
29. Gatford KL, Andraweera PH, Roberts CT, et al. Animal Models of Preeclampsia. Hypertension 2020; 75:1363–1381.
30. Venkatesha S, Toporsian M, Lam C, et al. Soluble endoglin contributes to the pathogenesis of preeclampsia. Nat Med 2006; 12:642–649.
31. Huppertz B, Kingdom J, Caniggia I, et al. Hypoxia Favours Necrotic Versus Apoptotic Shedding of Placental Syncytiotrophoblast into the Maternal Circulation. Placenta 2003; 24:181–190.
32. Burwick RM, Feinberg BB. Complement activation and regulation in preeclampsia and hemolysis, elevated liver enzymes, and low platelet count syndrome. Am J Obstet Gynecol 2020; 226:S1059–S1070.
33. Redman CWG, Sargent IL. Placental Debris, Oxidative Stress and Pre-eclampsia. Placenta 2000; 21:597–602.
34. Burwick RM, Fichorova RN, Dawood HY, et al. Urinary Excretion of C5b-9 in Severe Preeclampsia. Hypertension 2013; 62:1040–1045.
35. Bartsch E, Medcalf KE, Park AL, et al. Clinical risk factors for pre-eclampsia determined in early pregnancy: systematic review and meta-analysis of large cohort studies. BMJ 2016; 353:i1753.
36. Saftlas AF, Beydoun H, Triche E. Immunogenetic determinants of preeclampsia and related pregnancy disorders: a systematic review. Obstet Gynecol 2005; 106:162–172.
37. National Institute for Health and Care Excellence. Hypertension in pregnancy: diagnosis and management. London: National Institute for Health and Care Excellence: Clinical Guidelines; 2019.
38. American College of Obstetricians and Gynaecologists. Gestational Hypertension and Preeclampsia: ACOG Practice Bulletin Summary, Number 222. Obstet Gynecol 2020; 135:1492–1495.
39. Esplin MS, Fausett MB, Fraser A, et al. Paternal and Maternal Components of the Predisposition to Preeclampsia. N Eng J Med 2001; 344:867–872.
40. McGinnis R, Steinthorsdottir V, Williams NO, et al. Variants in the fetal genome near FLT1 are associated with risk of preeclampsia. Nat Genet 2017; 49:1255–1260.
41. Salmon JE, Heuser C, Triebwasser M, et al. Mutations in Complement Regulatory Proteins Predispose to Preeclampsia: A Genetic Analysis of the PROMISSE Cohort. PLoS Med 2011; 8:e1001013.
42. Bdolah Y, Palomaki GE, Yaron Y, et al. Circulating angiogenic proteins in trisomy 13. Am J Obstet Gynaecol 2006; 194:239–245.
43. Carroli G, Merialdi M, Wojdyla D, et al. Effects of calcium supplementation on uteroplacental and fetoplacental blood flow in low-calcium-intake mothers: a randomized controlled trial. Am J Obstet Gynecol 2010; 202:45 e1–9.
44. Marcoux S, Brisson J, Fabia J. The effect of cigarette smoking on the risk of preeclampsia and gestational hypertension. Am J Epidemiol 1989; 130:950–957.
45. Conde-Agudelo A, Althabe F, Belizan JM, et al. Cigarette smoking during pregnancy and risk of preeclampsia: a systematic review. Am J Obstet Gynecol 1999; 181:1026–1035.
46. Luque-Fernandez MA, Zoega H, Valdimarsdottir U, et al. Deconstructing the smoking-preeclampsia paradox through a counterfactual framework. Eur J Epidemiol 2016; 31:613–623.
47. Zera CA, Seely EW, Wilkins-Haug LE, et al. The association of body mass index with serum angiogenic markers in normal and abnormal pregnancies. Am J Obstet Gynecol 2014; 211:247 e1–7.
48. Levine RJ, Qian C, Maynard SE, et al. Serum sFlt1 concentration during preeclampsia and mid trimester blood pressure in healthy nulliparous women. Am J Obstet Gynaecol 2006; 194:1034–1041.
49. Townsend R, Khalil A, Premakumar Y, et al. Prediction of pre-eclampsia: review of reviews. Ultrasound Obstet Gynecol 2019; 54:16–27.
50. Tan MY, Wright D, Syngelaki A, et al. Comparison of diagnostic accuracy of early screening for pre-eclampsia by NICE guidelines and a method combining maternal factors and biomarkers: results of SPREE. Ultrasound Obstet Gynecol 2018; 51:743–750.
51. O'Gorman N, Wright D, Poon LC, et al. Multicenter screening for pre-eclampsia by maternal factors and biomarkers at 11-13 weeks' gestation: comparison with NICE guidelines and ACOG recommendations. Ultrasound Obstet Gynecol 2017; 49:756–760.
52. Chaemsaithong P, Pooh RK, Zheng M, et al. Prospective evaluation of screening performance of first-trimester prediction models for preterm preeclampsia in an Asian population. Am J Obstet Gynecol 2019; 221:650 e1–e16.
53. Poon LCY, Zymeri NA, Zamprakou A, et al. Protocol for Measurement of Mean Arterial Pressure at 11-13 Weeks' Gestation. Fetal Diagn Ther 2012; 31:42–48.
54. Wright A, Wright D, Ispas CA, et al. Mean arterial pressure in the three trimesters of pregnancy: effects of maternal characteristics and medical history. Ultrasound Obstet Gynecol 2015; 45:698–706.

55. Poon LCY, Kametas NA, Pandeva I, et al. Mean Arterial Pressure at 11 +0 to 13 +6 Weeks in the Prediction of Preeclampsia. Hypertension 2008; 51:1027–1033.

56. O'Gorman N, Wright D, Syngelaki A, et al. Competing risks model in screening for preeclampsia by maternal factors and biomarkers at 11–13 weeks' gestation Am J Obstet Gynecol 2016; 214:103.e1–.e12.

57. Cnossen JS, Morris RK, Ter Riet G, et al. Use of uterine artery Doppler ultrasonography to predict pre-eclampsia and intrauterine growth restriction: a systematic review and bivariable meta-analysis. Can Med Assoc J 2008; 178:701–711.

58. Kalafat E, Laoreti A, Khalil A, et al. Ophthalmic artery Doppler for prediction of pre-eclampsia: systematic review and meta-analysis. Ultrasound Obstet Gynecol 2018; 51:731–737.

59. Widmer M, Cuesta C, Khan KS, et al. Accuracy of angiogenic biomarkers at 20 weeks' gestation in predicting the risk of pre-eclampsia: A WHO multicentre study. Pregnancy Hypertens 2015; 5:330–338.

60. Kleinrouweler C, Wiegerinck M, Ris-Stalpers C, et al. Accuracy of circulating placental growth factor, vascular endothelial growth factor, soluble fms-like tyrosine kinase 1 and soluble endoglin in the prediction of pre-eclampsia: a systematic review and meta-analysis. BJOG 2012; 119:778–787.

61. Zhong Y, Zhu F, Ding Y. Serum screening in first trimester to predict pre-eclampsia, small for gestational age and preterm delivery: systematic review and meta-analysis. BMC Pregnancy Childbirth 2015; 15:191.

62. Akolekar R, Zaragoza E, Poon LCY, et al. Maternal serum placental growth factor at 11 + 0 to 13 + 6 weeks of gestation in the prediction of pre-eclampsia. Ultrasound Obstet Gynecol 2008; 32:732–739.

63. Agrawal S, Cerdeira AS, Redman C, et al. Meta-Analysis and Systematic Review to Assess the Role of Soluble FMS-Like Tyrosine Kinase-1 and Placenta Growth Factor Ratio in Prediction of Preeclampsia. Hypertension 2018; 71:306–316.

64. Morris RK, Bilagi A, Devani P, Kilby MD. Association of serum PAPP-A levels in first trimester with small for gestational age and adverse pregnancy outcomes: systematic review and meta-analysis. Prenat Diagn 2017; 37:253–265.

65. Dugoff L, Hobbins JC, Malone FD, et al. First-trimester maternal serum PAPP-A and free-beta subunit human chorionic gonadotropin concentrations and nuchal translucency are associated with obstetric complications: A population-based screening study (The FASTER Trial). Am J Obstet Gynecol 2004; 191:1446–1451.

66. Al-Rubaie Z, Askie L, Ray J, et al. The performance of risk prediction models for pre-eclampsia using routinely collected maternal characteristics and comparison with models that include specialised tests and with clinical guideline decision rules: a systematic review. BJOG 2016; 123:1441–1452.

67. Rolnik DL, Wright D, Poon LC, et al. Aspirin versus Placebo in Pregnancies at High Risk for Preterm Preeclampsia. N Eng J Med 2017; 377:613–622.

68. Guy G, Leslie K, Diaz Gomez D, et al. Implementation of routine first trimester combined screening for pre-eclampsia: a clinical effectiveness study. BJOG 2021; 128:149–156.

69. Rolnik DL, Selvaratnam RJ, Wertaschnigg D, et al. Routine first trimester combined screening for preterm preeclampsia in Australia: A multicenter clinical implementation cohort study. Int J Gynaecol Obstet 2021.

70. Wright D, Gallo DM, Gil Pugliese S, et al. Contingent screening for preterm pre-eclampsia. Ultrasound Obstet Gynecol 2016; 47:554–559.

71. Mostello D, Jen Chang J, Allen J, et al. Recurrent preeclampsia: the effect of weight change between pregnancies. Obstet Gynecol 2010; 116:667–672.

72. Institute of Medicine, National Research Council. In: Rasmussen KM, Yaktine AL, editors. Weight Gain During Pregnancy: Reexamining the Guidelines. Washington (DC): The National Academies Collection: Reports funded by National Institutes of Health; 2009.

73. Crandon AJ, Isherwood DM. Effect of aspirin on incidence of pre-eclampsia. Lancet 1979; 1:1356.

74. Askie LM, Duley L, Henderson-Smart DJ, et al. Antiplatelet agents for prevention of pre-eclampsia: a meta-analysis of individual patient data. Lancet 2007; 369:1791–1798.

75. Beaufils M, Uzan S, Donsimoni R, et al. Prevention of pre-eclampsia by early antiplatelet therapy. Lancet 1985; 1:840–842.

76. CLASP (Collaborative Low-dose Aspirin Study in Pregnancy) Collaborative Group. CLASP: a randomised trial of low-dose aspirin for the prevention and treatment of pre-eclampsia among 9364 pregnant women. Lancet 1994; 343:619–629.

77. Wright D, Rolnik DL, Syngelaki A, et al. Aspirin for Evidence-Based Preeclampsia Prevention trial: effect of aspirin on length of stay in the neonatal intensive care unit. Am J Obstet Gynecol 2018; 218:612.e1–e6.

78. Hoffman MK, Goudar SS, Kodkany BS, et al. Low-dose aspirin for the prevention of preterm delivery in nulliparous women with a singleton pregnancy (ASPIRIN): a randomised, double-blind, placebo-controlled trial. Lancet 2020; 395:285–293.

79. Duley L, Meher S, Hunter KE, et al. Antiplatelet agents for preventing pre-eclampsia and its complications. Cochrane Database Syst Rev 2019; 10:CD004659.
80. Poon LC, Wright D, Rolnik DL, et al. Aspirin for Evidence-Based Preeclampsia Prevention trial: effect of aspirin in prevention of preterm preeclampsia in subgroups of women according to their characteristics and medical and obstetrical history. Am J Obstet Gynecol 2017; 217:585.e1–e5.
81. Mone F, Mulcahy C, McParland P, et al. Should we recommend universal aspirin for all pregnant women? Am J Obstet Gynecol 2017; 216:141.e1– e5.
82. Hastie R, Tong S, Wikstrom AK, et al. Aspirin use during pregnancy and the risk of bleeding complications: a Swedish population-based cohort study. Am J Obstet Gynecol 2021; 224:95.e1–e12.
83. Park F, Deeming S, Bennett N, et al. Cost effectiveness analysis of a model of first trimester prediction and prevention for preterm preeclampsia against usual care. Ultrasound Obstet Gynecol 2021; 58:688–697.
84. Mallampati D, Grobman W, Rouse DJ, et al. Strategies for Prescribing Aspirin to Prevent Preeclampsia. Obstet Gynecol 2019; 134:537–544.
85. Dubon Garcia A, Devlieger R, Redekop K, et al. Cost-utility of a first-trimester screening strategy versus the standard of care for nulliparous women to prevent pre-term pre-eclampsia in Belgium. Pregnancy Hypertens 2021; 25:219–224.
86. Ortved D, Hawkins TLA, Johnson JA, et al. Cost-effectiveness of first-trimester screening with early preventative use of aspirin in women at high risk of early-onset pre-eclampsia. Ultrasound Obstetr Gynecol 2019; 53:239–244.
87. Cuckle H. Strategies for Prescribing Aspirin to Prevent Preeclampsia: A Cost-Effectiveness Analysis. Obstet Gynecol 2020; 135:217.
88. American College of Obstetricians and Gynecologists. ACOG Committee Opinion No. 743: Low-Dose Aspirin Use During Pregnancy. Obstet Gynecol 2018; 132:e44–e52.
89. World Health Organization. WHO Recommendations for Prevention and Treatment of Pre-Eclampsia and Eclampsia. Geneva: WHO Guidelines Approved by the Guidelines Review Committee; 2011.
90. Roberge S, Bujold E, Nicolaides KH. Aspirin for the prevention of preterm and term preeclampsia: systematic review and metaanalysis. Am J Obstet Gynecol 2018; 218:287–293.
91. Roberge S, Nicolaides K, Demers S, et al. The role of aspirin dose on the prevention of preeclampsia and fetal growth restriction: systematic review and meta-analysis. Am J Obstet Gynecol 2017; 216:110–120.
92. Chaemsaithong P, Cuenca-Gomez D, Plana MN, et al. Does low-dose aspirin initiated before 11 weeks' gestation reduce the rate of preeclampsia? Am J Obstet Gynecol 2020; 222:437–450.
93. Meher S, Duley L, Hunter K, Askie L. Antiplatelet therapy before or after 16 weeks' gestation for preventing preeclampsia: an individual participant data meta-analysis. Am J Obstet Gynecol 2017; 216:121–128.
94. Caron N, Rivard GE, Michon N, et al. Low-dose ASA response using the PFA-100 in women with high-risk pregnancy. J Obstet Gynaecol Can 2009; 31:1022–1027.
95. Roberge S, Bujold E, Nicolaides KH. Meta-analysis on the effect of aspirin use for prevention of preeclampsia on placental abruption and antepartum hemorrhage. Am Jf Obst Gynecol 2018; 218:483-489.
96. CLASP (Collaborative Low-dose Aspirin Study in Pregnancy) Collaborative Group. Low dose aspirin in pregnancy and early childhood development: follow up of the collaborative low dose aspirin study in pregnancy. BJOG 1995; 102:861–868.
97. Marret S, Marchand L, Kaminski M, et al. Prenatal Low-Dose Aspirin and Neurobehavioral Outcomes of Children Born Very Preterm. Pediatrics 2010; 125:e29–e34.
98. Hofmeyr GJ, Lawrie TA, Atallah AN, et al. Calcium supplementation during pregnancy for preventing hypertensive disorders and related problems. Cochrane Database Syst Rev 2018; 10:CD001059.
99. Hofmeyr GJ, Betrán AP, Singata-Madliki M, et al. Prepregnancy and early pregnancy calcium supplementation among women at high risk of pre-eclampsia: a multicentre, double-blind, randomised, placebo-controlled trial. Lancet 2019; 393:330–339.
100. World Health Organization. WHO recommendation: Calcium supplementation during pregnancy for the prevention of pre-eclampsia and its complications. Geneva: WHO Guidelines Approved by the Guidelines Review Committee; 2018.
101. Yinon Y, Ben Meir E, Margolis L, et al. Low molecular weight heparin therapy during pregnancy is associated with elevated circulatory levels of placental growth factor. Placenta 2015; 36:121–124.
102. Rodger MA, Gris JC, De Vries JIP, et al. Low-molecular-weight heparin and recurrent placenta-mediated pregnancy complications: a meta-analysis of individual patient data from randomised controlled trials. Lancet 2016; 388:2629–2641.
103. Haddad B, Winer N, Chitrit Y, et al. Enoxaparin and Aspirin Compared With Aspirin Alone to Prevent Placenta-Mediated Pregnancy Complications: A Randomized Controlled Trial. Obstet Gynecol 2016; 128:1053–1063.

104. Groom KM, McCowan LM, Mackay LK, et al. Enoxaparin for the prevention of preeclampsia and intrauterine growth restriction in women with a history: a randomized trial. Am J Obstet Gynecol 2017; 216:296.e1–e14.

105. Cruz-Lemini M, Vázquez JC, Ullmo J, et al. Low-molecular-weight heparin for prevention of preeclampsia and other placenta-mediated complications: a systematic review and meta-analysis. Am J Obstet Gynecol 2021; 226:S1126–S1144.

106. Brownfoot FC, Hastie R, Hannan NJ, et al. Metformin as a prevention and treatment for preeclampsia: effects on soluble fms-like tyrosine kinase 1 and soluble endoglin secretion and endothelial dysfunction. Am J Obstet Gynecol 2016; 214:356.e1–e15.

107. Syngelaki A, Nicolaides KH, Balani J, et al. Metformin versus Placebo in Obese Pregnant Women without Diabetes Mellitus. N Engl J Med 2016; 374:434–443.

108. Dodd JM, Grivell RM, Deussen AR, et al. Metformin for women who are overweight or obese during pregnancy for improving maternal and infant outcomes. Cochrane Database Syst Rev 2018; 7:CD010564.

109. Fox KA, Longo M, Tamayo E, et al. Effects of pravastatin on mediators of vascular function in a mouse model of soluble Fms-like tyrosine kinase-1-induced preeclampsia. Am J Obstet Gynecol 2011; 205:366 e1–e5.

110. Bauer AJ, Banek CT, Needham K, et al. Pravastatin attenuates hypertension, oxidative stress, and angiogenic imbalance in rat model of placental ischemia-induced hypertension. Hypertension 2013; 61:1103–1110.

111. Costantine MM, Cleary K, Hebert MF, et al. Safety and pharmacokinetics of pravastatin used for the prevention of preeclampsia in high-risk pregnant women: a pilot randomized controlled trial. American J Obstet Gynecol 2016; 214:720.e1–e17.

112. Dobert M, Varouxaki AN, Mu AC, et al. Pravastatin versus Placebo in Pregnancies at High Risk of Term Preeclampsia. Circulation 2021; 144:670–679.

113. Roberts JM, Myatt L, Spong CY, et al. Vitamins C and E to Prevent Complications of Pregnancy-Associated Hypertension. N Eng J Med 2010; 362:1282–1291.

114. Poston L, Briley A, Seed P, et al. Vitamin C and vitamin E in pregnant women at risk for pre-eclampsia (VIP trial): randomised placebo-controlled trial. Lancet 2006; 367:1145–1154.

115. Villar J, Purwar M, Merialdi M, et al. World Health Organisation multicentre randomised trial of supplementation with vitamins C and E among pregnant women at high risk for pre-eclampsia in populations of low nutritional status from developing countries. BJOG 2009; 116:780–788.

116. Xu H, Perez-Cuevas R, Xiong X, et al. An international trial of antioxidants in the prevention of preeclampsia (INTAPP). Am J Obstet Gynecol 2010; 202:239.e1–e10.

117. Conde-Agudelo A, Romero R, Kusanovic JP, et al. Supplementation with vitamins C and E during pregnancy for the prevention of preeclampsia and other adverse maternal and perinatal outcomes: a systematic review and metaanalysis. Am J Obstet Gynecol 2011; 204:503.e1–12.

118. Vadillo-Ortega F, Perichart-Perera O, Espino S, et al. Effect of supplementation during pregnancy with L-arginine and antioxidant vitamins in medical food on pre-eclampsia in high risk population: randomised controlled trial. BMJ 2011; 342:d2901.

119. Meher S, Duley L. Nitric oxide for preventing pre-eclampsia and its complications. Cochrane Database Syst Rev 2007; 2:CD006490.

120. Purswani JM, Gala P, Dwarkanath P, et al. The role of vitamin D in pre-eclampsia: a systematic review. BMC Pregnancy Childbirth 2017; 17:231.

121. Palacios C, Kostiuk LK, Pena-Rosas JP. Vitamin D supplementation for women during pregnancy. Cochrane Database Syst Rev 2019; 7:CD008873.

122. Brown MA, Lindheimer MD, de Swiet M, et al. The classification and diagnosis of the hypertensive disorders of pregnancy: statement from the International Society for the Study of Hypertension in Pregnancy (ISSHP). Hypertens Pregnancy 2001; 20:IX–XIV.

123. American College of Obstetricians and Gynecologists. Diagnosis and management of preeclampsia and eclampsia. Int J Gynecol Obstet 2002; 77:67–75.

124. American College of Obstetricians and Gynecologists. Hypertension in pregnancy. Report of the American College of Obstetricians and Gynecologists' Task Force on Hypertension in Pregnancy. Obstet Gynecol 2013; 122:1122–1131.

125. Brown MA, Magee LA, Kenny LC, et al. Hypertensive Disorders of Pregnancy. Hypertension 2018; 72:24–43.

126. Poon LC, Magee LA, Verlohren S, et al. A literature review and best practice advice for second and third trimester risk stratification, monitoring, and management of pre-eclampsia. Int J Gynecol Obstet 2021; 154:3–31.

127. McCarthy FP, Ryan RM, Chappell LC. Prospective biomarkers in preterm preeclampsia: A review. Pregnancy Hypertension 2018; 14:72–78.
128. Chappell LC, Duckworth S, Seed PT, et al. Diagnostic Accuracy of Placental Growth Factor in Women With Suspected Preeclampsia. Circulation 2013; 128:2121–2131.
129. Duhig KE, Myers J, Seed PT, et al. Placental growth factor testing to assess women with suspected pre-eclampsia: a multicentre, pragmatic, stepped-wedge cluster-randomised controlled trial. Lancet 2019; 393:1807–1818.
130. Duhig K, Seed P, Myers J, et al. Placental growth factor testing for suspected pre-eclampsia: a cost-effectiveness analysis. BJOG 2019; 126:1390–1398.
131. Zeisler H, Llurba E, Chantraine FJ, et al. Soluble fms-like tyrosine kinase-1 to placental growth factor ratio: ruling out pre-eclampsia for up to 4 weeks and value of retesting. Ultrasound Obstet Gynecol 2019; 53:367–375.
132. Stubert J, Ullmann S, Bolz M, et al. Prediction of preeclampsia and induced delivery at <34 weeks' gestation by sFLT-1 and PlGF in patients with abnormal midtrimester uterine Doppler velocimetry: a prospective cohort analysis. BMC Pregnancy Childbirth 2014; 14:292.
133. Verlohren S, Herraiz I, Lapaire O, et al. The sFlt-1/PlGF ratio in different types of hypertensive pregnancy disorders and its prognostic potential in preeclamptic patients. Am J Obstet Gynecol 2012; 206:58.e1–e8.
134. Cerdeira AS, O'Sullivan J, Ohuma EO, et al. Randomized Interventional Study on Prediction of Preeclampsia/Eclampsia in Women With Suspected Preeclampsia. Hypertension 2019; 74:983–990.
135. Von Dadelszen P, Payne B, Li J, et al. Prediction of adverse maternal outcomes in pre-eclampsia: development and validation of the fullPIERS model. Lancet 2011; 377:219–227.
136. Payne BA, Hutcheon JA, Ansermino JM, et al. A Risk Prediction Model for the Assessment and Triage of Women with Hypertensive Disorders of Pregnancy in Low-Resourced Settings: The miniPIERS (Pre-eclampsia Integrated Estimate of RiSk) Multi-country Prospective Cohort Study. PLoS Med 2014; 11:e1001589.
137. Ukah UV, Payne B, Lee T, et al. External Validation of the fullPIERS Model for Predicting Adverse Maternal Outcomes in Pregnancy Hypertension in Low- and Middle-Income Countries. Hypertension 2017; 69:705–711.
138. Thangaratinam S, Allotey J, Marlin N, et al. Prediction of complications in early-onset pre-eclampsia (PREP): development and external multinational validation of prognostic models. BMC Med 2017; 15:68.
139. Magee LA, Von Dadelszen P, Rey E, et al. Less-Tight versus Tight Control of Hypertension in Pregnancy. N Eng J Med 2015; 372:407–417.
140. Abalos E, Duley L, Steyn DW, et al. Antihypertensive drug therapy for mild to moderate hypertension during pregnancy. Cochrane Database Syst Rev 2018; 10:CD002252.
141. Duley L, Henderson-Smart DJ, Walker GJ, et al. Magnesium sulphate versus diazepam for eclampsia. Cochrane Database Syst Rev 2010; CD000127.
142. Duley L, Henderson-Smart DJ, Chou D. Magnesium sulphate versus phenytoin for eclampsia. Cochrane Database Syst Rev 2010;CD000128.
143. Duley L, Gülmezoglu AM, Chou D. Magnesium sulphate versus lytic cocktail for eclampsia. Cochrane Database Syst Rev 2010; 2010:CD002960.
144. Euser AG, Cipolla MJ. Magnesium Sulfate for the Treatment of Eclampsia. Stroke 2009; 40:1169–1175.
145. Altman D, Carroli G, Duley L, et al. Do women with pre-eclampsia, and their babies, benefit from magnesium sulphate? The Magpie Trial: a randomised placebo-controlled trial. Lancet 2002; 359:1877–1890.
146. Duley L, Gulmezoglu AM, Henderson-Smart DJ, et al. Magnesium sulphate and other anticonvulsants for women with pre-eclampsia. Cochrane Database Syst Rev 2010;CD000025.
147. Hastie R, Brownfoot FC, Cluver CA, et al. Predictive Value of the Signs and Symptoms Preceding Eclampsia: A Systematic Review. Obstet Gynecol 2019; 134:677–684.
148. The Eclampsia Trial Collaborative Group. Which anticonvulsant for women with eclampsia? Evidence from the Collaborative Eclampsia Trial. Lancet 1995; 345:1455–1463.
149. Doyle LW, Crowther CA, Middleton P, et al. Magnesium sulphate for women at risk of preterm birth for neuroprotection of the fetus. Cochrane Database Syst Rev 2009; CD004661.
150. McGoldrick E, Stewart F, Parker R, Dalziel SR. Antenatal corticosteroids for accelerating fetal lung maturation for women at risk of preterm birth. Cochrane Database Syst Rev 2020; 12:CD004454.
151. Thangaratinam S, Coomarasamy A, O'Mahony F, et al. Estimation of proteinuria as a predictor of complications of pre-eclampsia: a systematic review. BMC Med 2009; 7:10.
152. Payne B, Magee LA, Côté A-M, et al. PIERS Proteinuria: Relationship With Adverse Maternal and Perinatal Outcome. J Obstet Gynaecol Can 2011; 33:588–597.

153. Churchill D, Duley L, Thornton JG, et al. Interventionist versus expectant care for severe pre-eclampsia between 24 and 34 weeks' gestation. Cochrane Database Syst Rev 2018; 10:CD003106.
154. Broekhuijsen K, Van Baaren GJ, Van Pampus MG, et al. Immediate delivery versus expectant monitoring for hypertensive disorders of pregnancy between 34 and 37 weeks of gestation (HYPITAT-II): an open-label, randomised controlled trial. Lancet 2015; 385:249–501.
155. Chappell LC, Brocklehurst P, Green ME, et al. Planned early delivery or expectant management for late preterm pre-eclampsia (PHOENIX): a randomised controlled trial. Lancet 2019; 394:1181–1190.
156. Koopmans CM, Bijlenga D, Groen H, et al. Induction of labour versus expectant monitoring for gestational hypertension or mild pre-eclampsia after 36 weeks' gestation (HYPITAT): a multicentre, open-label randomised controlled trial. Lancet 2009; 374:979–988.
157. Ornaghi S, Paidas MJ. Upcoming drugs for the treatment of preeclampsia in pregnant women. Expert Rev Clin Pharmacol 2014; 7:599–603.
158. Weiner CP, Kwaan HC, Xu C, et al. Antithrombin III activity in women with hypertension during pregnancy. Obstet Gynecol 1985; 65:301–306.
159. Paidas MJ, Tita ATN, Macones GA, et al. Prospective, randomized, double-blind, placebo-controlled evaluation of the Pharmacokinetics, Safety and Efficacy of Recombinant Antithrombin Versus Placebo in Preterm Preeclampsia. Am J Obstet Gynecol 2020; 223:739.e1–e13.
160. Cluver CA, Hiscock R, Decloedt EH, et al. 27 Metformin to treat Preterm Pre-eclampsia (PI-2): A randomised, double blind, placebo-controlled trial. Am J Obstet Gynecol 2021; 224:S20.
161. Kaitu'U-Lino TUJ, Brownfoot FC, Beard S, et al. Combining metformin and esomeprazole is additive in reducing sFlt-1 secretion and decreasing endothelial dysfunction – implications for treating preeclampsia. PLOS ONE 2018; 13:e0188845.
162. Brownfoot FC, Hastie R, Hannan NJ, et al. Combining metformin and sulfasalazine additively reduces the secretion of antiangiogenic factors from the placenta: Implications for the treatment of preeclampsia. Placenta 2020; 95:78–83.
163. Pasternak B, Hviid A. Use of Proton-Pump Inhibitors in Early Pregnancy and the Risk of Birth Defects. New Eng J Med 2010; 363:2114–2123.
164. Onda K, Tong S, Beard S, et al. Proton Pump Inhibitors Decrease Soluble fms-Like Tyrosine Kinase-1 and Soluble Endoglin Secretion, Decrease Hypertension, and Rescue Endothelial Dysfunction. Hypertension 2017; 69:457–468.
165. Saleh L, Samantar R, Garrelds IM, et al. Low Soluble Fms-Like Tyrosine Kinase-1, Endoglin, and Endothelin-1 Levels in Women With Confirmed or Suspected Preeclampsia Using Proton Pump Inhibitors. Hypertension 2017; 70:594–600.
166. Cluver CA, Hannan NJ, van Papendorp E, et al. Esomeprazole to treat women with preterm preeclampsia: a randomized placebo controlled trial. Am J Obstet Gynecol 2018; 219:388.e1–e17.
167. Costantine MM, Tamayo E, Lu F, et al. Using pravastatin to improve the vascular reactivity in a mouse model of soluble fms-like tyrosine kinase-1-induced preeclampsia. Obstet Gynecol 2010; 116:114–120.
168. Brownfoot FC, Tong S, Hannan NJ, et al. Effects of simvastatin, rosuvastatin and pravastatin on soluble fms-like tyrosine kinase 1 (sFlt-1) and soluble endoglin (sENG) secretion from human umbilical vein endothelial cells, primary trophoblast cells and placenta. BMC Pregnancy Childbirth 2016; 16:117.
169. Costantine MM, West H, Wisner KL, et al. A randomized pilot clinical trial of pravastatin versus placebo in pregnant patients at high risk of preeclampsia. Am J Obstet Gynecol 2021; 25:666.
170. Ahmed A, Williams D, Cheed V, et al. Pravastatin for early-onset pre-eclampsia: a randomised, blinded, placebo-controlled trial. BJOG 2020; 127:478–488.
171. Wind M, Gaasbeek AGA, Oosten LEM, et al. Therapeutic plasma exchange in pregnancy: A literature review. EuroJ Obstet Gynecol Reprod Biol 2021; 260:29–36.
172. Thadhani R, Hagmann H, Schaarschmidt W, et al. Removal of Soluble Fms-Like Tyrosine Kinase-1 by Dextran Sulfate Apheresis in Preeclampsia. J Am Soc Nephrol 2016; 27:903–913.
173. Nakakita B, Mogami H, Kondoh E, et al. Case of soluble fms-like tyrosine kinase 1 apheresis in severe pre-eclampsia developed at 15 weeks' gestation. J Obstet Gynaecol Res 2015; 41:1661–1663.
174. Lu AB, Lazarus B, Rolnik DL, et al. Pregnancy Prolongation After Eculizumab Use in Early-Onset Preeclampsia. Obstet Gynecol 2019; 134:1215–1218.
175. Burwick RM, Feinberg BB. Eculizumab for the treatment of preeclampsia/HELLP syndrome. Placenta 2013; 34:201–203.
176. Trapani A, Jr., Goncalves LF, Trapani TF, et al. Perinatal and Hemodynamic Evaluation of Sildenafil Citrate for Preeclampsia Treatment: A Randomized Controlled Trial. Obstet Gynecol 2016; 128:253–259.

177. Brownfoot FC, Tong S, Hannan NJ, et al. Effect of sildenafil citrate on circulating levels of sFlt-1 in preeclampsia. Pregnancy Hypertens 2018; 13:1–6.
178. Pels A, Derks J, Elvan-Taspinar A, et al. Maternal Sildenafil vs Placebo in Pregnant Women With Severe Early-Onset Fetal Growth Restriction. JAMA Network Open 2020; 3:e205323.
179. Hobson SR, Gurusinghe S, Lim R, et al. Melatonin improves endothelial function in vitro and prolongs pregnancy in women with early-onset preeclampsia. J Pineal Res 2018; 65:e12508.
180. Li Z, Zhang Y, Ying Ma J, et al. Recombinant Vascular Endothelial Growth Factor 121 Attenuates Hypertension and Improves Kidney Damage in a Rat Model of Preeclampsia. Hypertension 2007; 50:686–692.
181. Spradley FT, Tan AY, Joo WS, et al. Placental Growth Factor Administration Abolishes Placental Ischemia-Induced Hypertension. Hypertension 2016; 67:740–747.
182. Turanov AA, Lo A, Hassler MR, et al. RNAi modulation of placental sFLT1 for the treatment of preeclampsia. Nat Biotechnol 2018; 10.
183. Chappell LC, Cluver CA, Kingdom J, Tong S. Pre-eclampsia. Lancet 2021; 398:341–354.

# Chapter 3

# Infections in pregnancy: An update

Smriti Prasad, Asma Khalil

## INTRODUCTION

Infections during pregnancy continue to remain an important cause of maternal and perinatal morbidity and mortality. The causative organisms could be bacterial, viral, or parasitic. An infection is termed 'primary' if the host (the pregnant woman) acquires it for the first time, whereas a 'non-primary' or secondary infection is caused by either reactivation of a latent agent or infection with a different strain in a host who has been infected in the past. As a general rule, the fetus is less susceptible to damage following a secondary infection as it is readily protected by the passive immunity imparted by the placental transfer of immunoglobulin G (IgG) antibodies, whereas in primary infection, the slow maternal immune response is characterised by production of immunoglobulin M (IgM) antibodies which do not cross the placenta.

Infections in pregnancy can occur at any gestation with varying effects and the routes of transmission include vertical (transplacental passage) or perinatal transmission (by direct contact between mother and fetus during delivery). The likelihood of transmission of infection from mother to fetus depends on the gestational age at infection, type of infection (primary or non-primary), and maternal immune response, whereas fetal affection depends on virulence of the infectious agent and the immune response mounted by the fetus. Depending upon the interaction between the infectious agent and the fetus, the manifestations may vary from asymptomatic infections, structural abnormalities, or miscarriage/stillbirth. The infectious agents may have different implications for the mother and fetus – pregnant women themselves are minimally affected by Zika virus (ZIKV) infection which may cause significantly detrimental fetal effects. On the other hand, pregnant women have been reported to be more susceptible to severe illness secondary to viral diseases like H1N1 influenza and SARS-CoV-2, which cause minimal direct fetal effects.

**Smriti Prasad** MBBS MD MRCOG, Fetal Medicine Unit, St George's Hospital, St George's University of London, UK
Email: smriti.prasad@stgeorges.nhs.uk

**Asma Khalil** FRCOG MD MSc (Epi) DFSRH Dip (GUM), Fetal Medicine Unit, St George's Hospital, St George's University of London; Vascular Biology Research Centre, Molecular and Clinical Sciences Research Institute, St George's University of London; Fetal Medicine Unit, Liverpool Women's Hospital. University of Liverpool, UK
Email: akhalil@sgul.ac.uk

# CYTOMEGALOVIRUS

Cytomegalovirus (CMV), a double stranded DNA virus of the Herpesviridae family, is the most common cause of non-genetic sensorineural hearing loss and also accounts for most cases of infection-related congenital malformations in the high-income nations with a prevalence of 0.2–1% depending on country and seroprevalence [1]. Around 15% of newborns with congenital CMV may be symptomatic at birth, while another 25% may exhibit long-term sequelae. CMV infection in pregnancy can be primary or secondary (**Figure 3.1**).

## Screening for CMV in pregnancy

Routine antenatal serological screening of pregnant women is not recommended in most countries with conflicting opinions from scientific societies as the approach did not appear to fulfil the criteria of a good screening test [2]. Therefore, currently screening is only offered to pregnant women who have suggestive symptoms or there are signs of fetal CMV on antenatal ultrasound. However, there are arguments in favour of moving towards population-based universal serological screening in view of emerging evidence from prospective studies [3]. In a meta-analysis conducted by Chatzakis et al [4], the pooled rates of vertical transmission (10 studies, 2,942 fetuses) at the preconception period, periconception period, first trimester, second trimester, and third trimester were 5.5%, 21.0%, 36.8%, 40.3%, and 66.2%, respectively. For fetal affection in case of transmission (10 studies, 796 fetuses), the pooled rates were 28.8% (95% CI 2.4–55.1), 19.3% (95% CI 12.2–26.4), 0.9% (95% CI 0–2.4%), and 0.4% (95% CI 0–1.5), for maternal infection at the periconceptional period, first trimester, second trimester, and third trimester, respectively. The authors reported similar trends for sensorineural hearing loss following maternal infection at the first, second, and third trimester which were 22.8% (95% CI 15.4–30.2), 0.1% (95% CI 0–0.8), and 0% (95% CI 0–0.1), respectively. Recent evidence from a prospectively followed French cohort of 260 affected fetuses with a median follow up of 24 months report that the proportion of early/late auditory/neurological sequelae was around 30% following

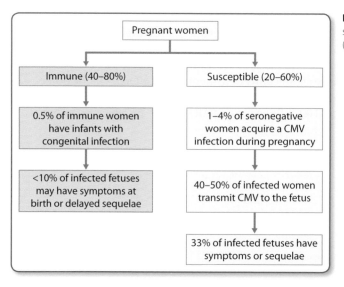

**Figure 3.1** Epidemiology and seroprevalence of cytomegalovirus (CMV) infection in pregnancy.

periconception and first trimester maternal CMV primary infections whereas there were no sequelae in fetuses of mothers with second or third trimester infections [5]. This implies that maternal CMV infection causes fetopathy only in periconceptional period and therefore there is a narrow time period when effective and targeted serological screening can be employed. Proponents of population-based serological screening also advocate a shift to universal approach as maternal valacyclovir therapy is increasingly being shown to be effective for prevention of fetal infection following maternal primary infection in early pregnancy [6,7]. However, a population-based screening also incurs increased costs. In a cost effectiveness study from the perspective of French National Health Insurance System comprising of a hypothetical cohort of 1,000,000 pregnant women, a population-based approach for targeting fetal CMV infections was associated with high organisational costs, albeit with an increased detection rates from 15 to 94% [3]. In the same cohort, secondary prevention with maternal valacyclovir resulted in a 58% decrease of severely infected newborns for 3.5% additional total costs. More evidence is needed regarding feasibility, acceptability, and cost effectiveness before implementation of population-based screening for CMV in routine obstetric practice.

## Diagnosis of maternal infection

Maternal infection may remain asymptomatic (90% cases) or manifest as a 'mononucleosis' like viral illness. A prototype of primary maternal infection is a young white pregnant woman with a child younger than 3 years [8]. Reactivation of a latent primary infection or infection by a different strain in an immune mother generally does not cause any maternal symptoms.

The diagnosis of maternal infection may be following occurrence of symptoms or during investigation of suspicious ultrasound features like ventriculomegaly, intracranial calcifications, microcephaly, sub-ependymal cysts, fetal growth restriction, hyperechogenic bowel, hepatomegaly, liver calcifications and pericardial effusion, etc. (**Figures 3.2** and **3.3**). The diagnosis can be established by either demonstration of seroconversion (IgG positivity in a previously seronegative woman) or presence of IgM antibody with a low avidity IgG test. IgG avidity <30% is strongly suggestive of a primary infection within the last 3 months whereas IgG avidity >60% is indicative of an infection which occurred >3 months previously. CMV IgM antibody as a standalone diagnostic test is not recommended as it is non-specific and shows cross-reactivity with other viruses like Epstein–Barr virus, may persist for months, and may be present during a non-primary infection.

Non-primary maternal CMV infection, which may account for about 50% of maternal infections in countries with higher seroprevalence, cannot be accurately predicted by serological tests, hence is not amenable to screening. The only way to confirm maternal infection is by demonstration of CMV DNA in the amniotic fluid.

## Diagnosis of fetal infection

The risk of vertical transmission varies according to the gestational age at which primary infection occurs, increasing from around 30% in the first trimester to 47% in the third trimester (**Table 3.1**). While the risk of viral transmission is lower in early pregnancy, the proportion of cases with a prenatal diagnosis of severe fetal infection is higher when infection occurs in the first compared to the third trimester of pregnancy. Nevertheless, fetuses with late infections should be monitored for growth restriction.

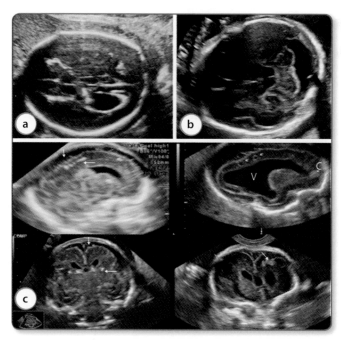

**Figure 3.2** Ultrasonographic cranial features of fetal cytomegalovirus (CMV) infection are variable, and include (a) ventriculomegaly, (b) mega cisterna magna, (c) intracranial calcifications and periventricular pseudocysts.

Detection of CMV DNA in the amniotic fluid/cord blood is diagnostic of fetal infection. However, negative polymerase chain reaction (PCR) does not completely rule out the possibility of congenital infection as late trans-placental passage has been reported. Infected fetuses excrete CMV virus in urine. In order to avoid false negative tests, amniocentesis should be delayed by at least 6–8 weeks after the suspected maternal infection or beyond 20 weeks (when fetal urination becomes established).

## Management of CMV infected fetuses

Following a diagnosis of fetal infection, the prognosis for the fetus depends on the timing of infection and presence or absence of cerebral/extracerebral findings on antenatal ultrasound. Ultrasound features of congenital infection might evolve as late as 12 weeks after maternal infection, therefore, serial ultrasound for the remainder of pregnancy is warranted. A normal ultrasound is reassuring and associated with low risk of infant disability; however, it is not predictive of sensorineural hearing loss. The main sonographic prognostic predictor of CMV-mediated damage is the presence of cranial lesions. In a CMV infected fetus, ultrasound and magnetic resonance imaging (MRI) are considered as complimentary imaging modality with a sensitivity of around 95% for detection of CMV-related brain lesions. Markers like amniotic fluid viral load, cord blood platelet count, or beta-2 microglobulin are of uncertain prognosis with scarce evidence exploring their utility.

Infected fetuses are classified into asymptomatic, mild or moderate symptomatic, and severely symptomatic fetuses [9]. Maternal valacyclovir is suggested in mild to moderately symptomatic fetuses. Maternal administration of high dose valacyclovir (8 g/day) initiated after confirmed fetal infection was associated with a significant increase in proportion of asymptomatic fetuses (82%) compared with a historical cohort (43%) and was well tolerated without increase in maternal adverse outcomes [7]. A recent randomised

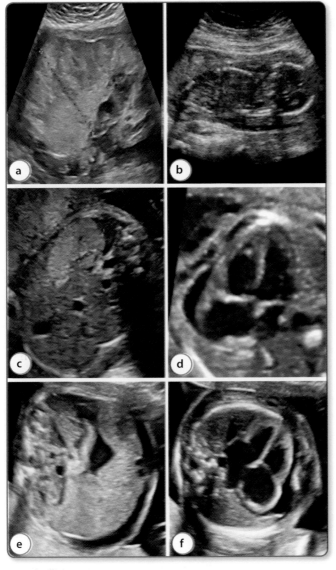

**Figure 3.3** Ultrasonographic extracranial features of fetal cytomegalovirus (CMV) infection, including (a) placentomegaly, (b) hyperechogenic bowel, (c) splenomegaly, (d and f) cardiomegaly, (e) ascites/pleural effusion/hydrops, (d and f) and pericardial effusion.

controlled trial (RCT) has reported that valacyclovir is effective in reducing (71%) the rate of fetal infection after maternal primary infection acquired in early pregnancy [6]. Valacyclovir appears to be promising in prevention of fetal CMV infection, although more evidence from large series is needed. Initially, there were reports from observational studies [10–12] suggesting effectiveness of CMV-specific hyper-immune globulin in reducing vertical transmission as well rates of fetal congenital defects. However, these results have not been confirmed in two RCTs by Hughes et al. [13] and Revello et al. [14] CMV-specific hyperimmune globulin did not significantly modify the course of primary CMV infection during pregnancy, nor was it effective in lowering composite adverse outcomes compared to placebo. Hence, it is not recommended outside of research setting for the treatment

| Table 3.1 Risk of vertical transmission, congenital infection, or fetal defects according to the gestational age at maternal infection/seroconversion | | |
|---|---|---|
| Cytomegalovirus[#] | Likelihood of vertical transmission after maternal primary infection | Likelihood of severe symptoms at birth in an infected fetus after maternal primary infection |
| Preconception | 0–10% | Negligible |
| Periconception | 25–45% | 70% |
| First trimester | 25–45% | 20% |
| Second trimester | 45% | 5% |
| Third trimester | 47–78% | Negligible |
| Toxoplasma GA at maternal seroconversion (weeks) | Risk of congenital infection % (95% CI) | Development of clinical signs in infected offspring % (95% CI) |
| 13 | 6 (3–9) | 61 (34–85) |
| 26 | 40 (33–47) | 25 (18–33) |
| 36 | 72 (60–81) | 9 (4–17) |
| Varicella[$] (weeks) | Risk of fetal varicella syndrome | |
| <13 | 0.5% | |
| 13–20 | 2% | |
| >20–36 | Negligible | |
| Rubella[µ] (weeks) | Vertical transmission | Risk of developing congenital defects |
| ≤12 | 90% | 97% |
| 12–16 | 55% | 20% |
| ≥16 | 45% | Minimal risk of deafness |

[#]For CMV secondary infection, the risk of congenital infection is low (1–2%).
[$]Maternal infection after 36 weeks is associated with a 50% fetal infection rate and a 25% clinical varicella rate in the neonate.
[µ]Beyond 20 weeks, very small risk of even deafness.
*Source:* Adapted from Khalil A, Sotiriadis A, Chaoui R, et al. ISUOG Practice Guidelines: role of ultrasound in congenital infection. Ultrasound Obstet Gynecol 2020; 56:128–151.

of primary CMV infection. Till date, there is no licensed vaccine for primary prevention against CMV; however, antenatal education about hygiene measures and avoidance of contact with urine/saliva of small children have been shown to be effective in reducing the risk of CMV infection.

After birth, the diagnosis of neonatal CMV must be confirmed by saliva swab/urine sample taken within 3 weeks of birth to confirm in-utero CMV infection.

## TOXOPLASMOSIS

Toxoplasmosis is a protozoal infection caused by obligate intracellular parasite *Toxoplasma gondii*. The parasite is transmitted through consumption of infected undercooked meat or raw vegetables and fruits contaminated with oocytes or contact with cat faeces. Like CMV, the majority of infected women remain asymptomatic or experience nonspecific symptoms like malaise, myalgia, and fever. Previous infection confers lifelong immunity. The overall risk of congenital toxoplasmosis following maternal infection ranges from 20 to 50% without treatment. Congenital toxoplasma infection typically involves the brain and eyes and results in intracranial calcifications, ventriculomegaly, microcephaly, and chorioretinitis. Other organ systems are also known to be affected like hepatosplenomegaly, anaemia, and jaundice. In up to 90% of the infected infants, some of the sequelae such as developmental delay, epilepsy, and blindness are evident only later in life. Diagnosis of maternal infection is based on demonstration of toxoplasma-specific IgM and IgG antibodies in maternal serum. In case of negative or equivocal IgM/IgG results, a repeat sample should be obtained in 2 weeks. Interpreting antibody levels can be challenging as toxoplasma serological assays are not standardised and hence, an experienced reference laboratory should be used. A high IgG avidity within first 16 weeks of pregnancy is reassuring and rules out maternal infection during pregnancy.

Diagnosis of congenital toxoplasmosis is confirmed by testing the amniotic fluid for toxoplasma DNA, at least after 4 weeks following maternal infection. Amniocentesis has a high rate of false negative result due to the low titres of viral DNA in amniotic fluid; however, these cases with less viral load generally have a favourable prognosis. Data from observational studies indicate that the presence of ventriculomegaly with intracranial calcifications is associated with poorer outcomes and long-term sequelae compared to cases with normal dilatation of the brain ventricles [15,16].

As soon as maternal infection is confirmed, spiramycin (1 g thrice daily orally) should be initiated as a measure to prevent vertical transmission and continued till amniocentesis at 18–20 weeks. If amniocentesis confirms fetal infection, a combination of pyrimethamine (50 mg daily orally) with sulphadiazine (1 g thrice daily orally), and folinic acid (50 mg weekly orally) should be commenced with the aim to attenuate fetal damage. This regiment should be continued throughout pregnancy and the infant should be treated till one year of age. On the other hand, if fetal infection is excluded by a negative amniocentesis, spiramycin therapy should be continued till delivery. Recently, the combination of pyrimethamine, sulfadiazine plus folinic acid was compared with spiramycin in the first RCT in the context of prevention of vertical transmission [17]. It was found that the transmission rate was 18.5% in the combined pyrimethamine + sulfadiazine + folinic acid group versus 30% in the spiramycin group, suggesting an overall trend of lower transmission rates with combination therapy although the results could not achieve statistical significance as enrolment was discontinued. There were no prenatal cerebral signs of congenital toxoplasmosis after prophylactic treatment with pyrimethamine combination therapy. Nonetheless, these promising results need to be supported by more evidence before application in clinical practice. G6PD deficiency testing should be done before starting sulphadiazine class of drugs. Fetuses with congenital toxoplasmosis should be followed up with 4 weekly ultrasound assessments for brain, eyes, and growth. Women should be counselled about the 30% risk of postnatal sequelae including vision loss, even if antenatal imaging was normal.

## GROUP B STREPTOCOCCUS

Group B streptococcus (GBS; *Streptococcus agalactiae*) is a gram-positive coccus that frequently colonises the human genital and gastrointestinal tracts, and less frequently, the upper respiratory tract of children and adults. GBS is the most common cause of severe early onset (<7 days) sepsis in neonates. It can also cause maternal chorioamnionitis, endometritis, wound infection, and puerperal sepsis. The incidence of early-onset GBS (EOGBS) disease in the UK and Ireland in 2015 was 0.57/1,000 births [18]. Apart from maternal colonisation, other risk factors for EOGBS is gestational age <37 weeks, prolonged rupture of membranes, young maternal age, and history of EOGBS in a previous neonate and black ethnicity. Intrapartum antibiotic prophylaxis (IAP) is shown to have an efficacy >80% in reducing the rates of EOGBS. The choice of antibiotic is intravenous penicillin or clindamycin/vancomycin (known cases of penicillin allergy). It is recommended that obstetric interventions, if indicated, should not be delayed in order to provide 4 hours of IAP.

## Variation in IAP strategies

There is significant variation in national policies surrounding routine GBS screening in pregnancy. Le Doare et al [19] performed a systematic review of the screening policies and IAP implementation worldwide. Out of 195 countries, they received policy information from nearly half the countries surveyed [95/195 (49%)]. Of these, 63% (60/95) had an IAP policy; 58% (35/60) used microbiological screening while the rest (25/60) used risk factors to guide IAP. Microbiological screening was associated with higher coverage (80%) compared with risk-factor-based IAP (29%). The authors concluded that there was considerable heterogeneity in IAP screening policies and coverage worldwide and emphasised the need of alternative approaches like maternal vaccination to reduce the global burden of disease.

Nonetheless, there are no RCTs which have compared efficacy of the two approaches – universal screening versus risk factors-based provision of IAP.

The American College of Obstetricians and Gynecologists (ACOG) recommends performing routine universal screening for GBS colonisation between 36 0/7 and 37 6/7 weeks of gestation [20]. All women whose vagino–rectal cultures at 36 0/7–37 6/7 weeks of gestation are positive for GBS should receive appropriate IAP unless a pre-labour caesarean birth is performed in the setting of intact membranes. The criticisms of universal screening include high rates of false positive results leading to overtreatment, increased medicalisation of labour, altered neonatal gut microbiome, increased antibiotic resistance, reports of maternal anaphylaxis, and uncertain effectiveness of this approach [21].

On the other hand, in the UK, the National Screening Committee in 2017 recommended to continue with risk factors-based screening for pregnant women when they present in labour. This approach is deemed inappropriate and imperfect as evidence suggests that around 65% of cases of EOGBS occur in neonates of pregnant women who did not have any clinical risk factors, whereas around 70% of women who are offered IAP based on presence of risk factors were shown to be non-colonisers. A meta-analysis by Hasperhoven et al [22] in 2020 has concluded that screening was associated with a reduced risk for EOGBS disease compared either with risk-based protocols (10 studies, RR 0.43; 95% CI 0.32–0.56) or with no policy (four studies, RR 0.31; 95% CI 0.11–0.84), without overexposing women to antibiotics. Currently, the National Institute for Health and Care Research (NIHR) funded trial GBS3 is recruiting pregnant women across 80 sites in the UK to study the clinical and cost effectiveness of two tests (antenatal extended culture medium testing and intra-partum rapid testing) to identify GBS in late pregnancy or labour compared with the current UK approach based on risk factors [23].

## Development of GBS vaccines

Although all 10 GBS serotypes have been found to cause disease, six serotypes (Ia, Ib, II, III, IV, and V) have been found to cause over 85% of the disease globally and 98% in South Africa. A GBS vaccine appears to be very promising in reducing the GBS disease given the drawbacks of current approach towards the disease – deficiencies of IAP strategies, rapid progression of the disease, and limitations associated with coverage [24,25]. A candidate vaccine will also have the potential to reduce the late-onset GBS disease against which IAP has no proven benefit. Till date, the development of a GBS vaccine was fraught with challenges due to the weak immunogenicity elicited by the earlier versions of polysaccharide vaccines. A recent trial has reported robust immune response at all doses following a hexavalent conjugate polysaccharide vaccine (GBS6) in a non-pregnant healthy population [26]. Currently, in the UK and South Africa, a phase 1/2, randomised, placebo-controlled, observer-blinded study is recruiting pregnant women for evaluation of safety, tolerability, and immunogenicity of various dose formulations of the investigational GBS6 vaccine [27].

# VARICELLA-ZOSTER VIRUS

Varicella-zoster virus (VZV) is one of eight herpes viruses, can cause maternal, fetal, and neonatal varicella syndrome as well as cause shingles (reactivation of the dormant virus in the ganglia). Routine antenatal serological screening for varicella is not recommended; however, around 90% of women in the UK are seropositive for VZV IgG antibody. The primary mode of transmission is through respiratory droplets. The incidence of primary VZV infection in pregnant women is about 3/1,000. For primary prevention, varicella vaccination is recommended in the pre-pregnancy or post-partum periods for seronegative women. Pregnant women who have significant contact with a known case of varicella and are found to be non-immune (absence of reliable history of previous chicken pox or seronegative for VZV IgG) should be offered VZV IgG within 10 days of the contact. Observational data indicate that administration of VZV IgG can attenuate development of maternal varicella as well as reduce the chance of fetal varicella syndrome in pregnant women. Most pregnant women with varicella infection present with a classical pruritic vesicular rash; however, a small proportion may develop systemic complications like pneumonia, encephalitis, and hepatitis and require hospitalisation. Oral acyclovir (800 mg five times a day for 7 days) should be offered to pregnant women with chickenpox if they present within 24 hours of the onset of the rash. Intravenous acyclovir should be considered for severe complications in pregnancy (oral forms have poor bioavailability).

# FETAL VARICELLA SYNDROME

Fetal varicella syndrome is characterised by any of the following features: limb and skin scarring, polyhydramnios, and central nervous system (CNS) defects like microcephaly, cortical atrophy, and ophthalmic lesions like microphthalmia and cataract. Maternal shingles does not pose any significant detrimental risk to the fetus.

Following a maternal infection before 13 weeks, the risk of fetal varicella is approximately 0.5% while the risk is 2% if maternal infection occurs between 13 and 20 weeks of gestation

(**Table 3.1**). The risk of spontaneous miscarriage does not appear to be increased if chickenpox occurs in the first trimester. Maternal infection between 20 and 36 weeks of gestation is not associated with the risk of fetal varicella syndrome.

Fetal infection can be confirmed by demonstration of VZV DNA in the amniotic fluid. Absence of viral DNA does not eliminate the possibility of an infected fetus; similarly, positive VZV DNA in the amniotic fluid does not imply fetal affection.

Following maternal varicella infection before 20 weeks, serial ultrasound assessment is warranted after 5 weeks from maternal infection or 16 weeks of gestation; whichever is earlier. Ultrasound features of fetal varicella are associated with severely infected fetus and termination of pregnancy should be offered as an option. A normal ultrasound is generally reassuring with low risk of neonatal sequelae. Maternal infection after 36 weeks is associated with a 50% fetal infection rate and around 25% of neonates would exhibit clinical varicella. It is imperative to avoid planned delivery for at least 7 days after the onset of the maternal rash to allow for the passive transfer of antibodies to the neonate.

## RUBELLA VIRUS

Rubella virus is a single stranded RNA virus of the Matonaviridae family which causes a self-limited infection or may remain asymptomatic in most hosts. However, it can result in catastrophic consequences in the fetus. Primary infection results in life-long immunity. In countries with robust immunisation programs, the incidence of congenital rubella syndrome (CRS) has drastically reduced and is rare. In most countries, serological screening for rubella antibodies is part of routine antenatal booking investigations to document immunity. Inadvertent vaccination during pregnancy is not an indication for termination of pregnancy [28].

The diagnosis of maternal infection is based on demonstration of positive rubella IgM on the background of exposure to a known case or typical rash or previous infection/vaccination status. Rubella IgM should not be used alone to diagnose infection because of the high false positive rates (15–50%) due to persistence/cross reactivity with other viruses. IgG avidity testing could be used to determine the timing of infection.

Following maternal infection, the rate of vertical transmission and fetal defects varies according to the gestational age at the time of infection (**Table 3.1**). The rate of miscarriage after first trimester infection is about 20%. Occasional reinfections have been reported without any fetal defects. There is no evidence that administration of rubella hyper-immune globulin to women reduces the rate of vertical transmission or attenuates fetal defects.

The main features of CRS are heart defects (patent ductus arteriosus and conotruncal anomalies), eye defects (cataract, microphthalmia, and retinopathy), sensorineural deafness, haematological abnormalities, neurodevelopmental delays, psychomotor retardation, and hepatosplenomegaly. Notably, some of these features like neurological deficits, hearing loss, endocrinopathies may not be apparent on prenatal ultrasound and may present only later in life.

As there is a significantly high chance of devastating effects of CRS following first trimester infection, it may be reasonable to offer termination without further invasive testing, if appropriate. Amniocentesis for rubella viral nucleic acid using PCR should be offered in cases of maternal infection for diagnosis of fetal infection, at least 6 weeks after maternal infection to reduce the chance of a false negative result.

# PARVOVIRUS B19

Parvovirus B19 is a single stranded DNA virus causing fifth disease (erythema infectiosum) and is common in children. Up to 50% of pregnant women who are seronegative are at risk of parvovirus B19 infection and the incidence of acute parvovirus B19 in pregnancy is about 1–2%. Parvovirus B19 is the most common cause of non-immune non-genetic cause of fetal hydrops. Most women remain asymptomatic and exhibit prodromal symptoms while few present with the characteristic 'slapped cheek' rash. Testing for parvovirus B19 infection in pregnancy is generally mandated after discovery of fetal hydrops on prenatal ultrasound or after recent exposure to a known case. Parvovirus B19-specific IgM and IgG antibodies should be tested in suspected cases while molecular methods like PCR and invasive testing for viral DNA in the amniotic fluid should be used as complimentary modalities where the IgM is negative. The ultrasound features of fetal parvovirus infection include hydrops, cardiomegaly, placentomegaly, and hepatosplenomegaly. The pathophysiologic mechanism of fetal infection is destruction of erythroid precursors, leading to aplastic crisis, and resultant profound anaemia. Fetal parvovirus B19 in itself is not associated with teratogenic effects or long-term disability/sequelae. However, these long-term sequelae are more likely to occur in cases complicated by fetal hydrops.

Following maternal infection, the risk of vertical transmission is around 30%. The manifestations of fetal infection like hydrops are apparent approximately after 3 weeks of maternal infection, but can present up to 8 weeks. Therefore, serial ultrasound monitoring for fetal anaemia from 4 weeks after infection or seroconversion is warranted and should be continued till 12 weeks. Although, the overall risk of fetal hydrops is low (4–13%), but, when it occurs, it carries a 50% risk of intrauterine fetal death. Spontaneous resolution of fetal anaemia has also been reported in few cases. Cordocentesis and intrauterine fetal blood transfusion are recommended in cases of fetal anaemia [middle cerebral artery peak systolic velocity (MCA PSV) >1.5 multiples of median (MoM)] and hydrops. Overall, the risk of perinatal death is 30% for fetuses presenting with hydrops versus 6% for non-hydropic fetuses.

No specific antiviral therapy or vaccine is presently available for parvovirus B19 infection but two vaccine candidates are being studied in preclinical setting.

# ZIKA VIRUS

The ZIKV is an arthropod-borne *Flavivirus* transmitted predominantly by *Aedes* mosquitoes, but also by sexual contact, vertical transmission from mother to fetus and by transfusion of blood products. The true rate of asymptomatic ZIKV infection is unknown; however, up to 20% of infected individuals exhibit symptoms like fever, myalgia and arthralgia, etc. Symptoms appear 3–14 days after infection and may last up to 1 week. Although sporadic outbreaks of ZIKV have been reported, it was only in October, 2015 epidemic that probable association of ZIKV infection in pregnancy and microcephaly was reported from Brazil. There is epidemiological, clinical, and laboratory evidence that prenatal transmission of ZIKV causes a spectrum of anomalies referred to as congenital Zika syndrome (CZS) [29]. CZS comprises a non-exhaustive pattern of anomalies, resulting from neurological damage and loss of intracranial volume, including microcephaly (fetal head circumference more than three SD below the mean), craniofacial disproportion, malformations of cortical development, ocular anomalies, congenital contractures, and fetal growth restriction. Microcephaly and other features of CZV are also seen with other congenital infections like CMV, VZV, and Rubella but organ involvement like hepatomegaly, rash, and hematologic abnormalities have not been reported in relation to CZS and could help in the differential diagnosis. Diagnosis of maternal ZIKV infection can be made by RTPCR of serum/urine for ZIKV. If ZIKV antibodies are not detected in a serum sample collected 4 or more weeks after the last possible travel-associated or sexual exposure, then recent ZIKV infection can be excluded. Additionally, all pregnant women with suggestive symptoms should be enquired about their travel history/sexual contact with a partner returning from affected areas and offered testing for ZIKV.

For couples considering/planning conception, consistent use of effective contraception is advised after travel to the endemic countries for at least 3 months.

Following a potential maternal exposure to ZIKV, a detailed assessment of fetal anatomy and growth should be undertaken. If there are any features of CZS, women should be referred to maternal fetal specialists for close surveillance and follow-up. In case, the initial assessment is normal and there are no features of CZS, a repeat assessment is warranted in the third trimester for fetal growth and extracerebral abnormalities. Ultrasound is the mainstay for diagnosis of CZS; however, MRI of the fetal brain may be employed in doubtful cases.

Amniocentesis for ZIKV should not be performed before 20 weeks of gestation due to high chance of false negative results. The correlation of ZIKV PCR in the amniotic fluid with fetal abnormalities is still to be elucidated and hence an expert virology opinion should be sought. In the UK, RIPL (Rare and Imported Pathogen Laboratory) is a specialist centre for advice and diagnosis for a wide range of unusual viral and bacterial infections including ZIKV. There is no vaccine against ZIKV infection or treatment for preventing fetal infection or reducing the risk of congenital defects once maternal infection is confirmed. Women with CZS should be followed up in multidisciplinary care settings with serial monitoring; their infants should be followed postnatally up to 1 year of age. Termination of pregnancy should be discussed where appropriate in cases of severe CZS. While counselling women, the limited and still-evolving knowledge surrounding ZIKV in pregnancy and CZS should be acknowledged.

# SARS-COV-2

The World Health Organization (WHO) declared a global pandemic of COVID-19 caused by SARS-CoV-2 in March 2020. SARS-CoV-2 is a single-stranded RNA-enveloped virus which predominantly affects the respiratory tract via the angiotensin-converting enzyme 2 (ACE2) expressed on type II alveolar cells of the lung. Pregnant women with COVID-19 do not appear to be at an increased risk of being affected with COVID-19; however, if symptomatic, they are twice as likely to be admitted to an intensive care unit (ICU) and to require extracorporeal membranous oxygenation (ECMO), and this risk appeared to be even higher during the period of Delta variant dominance [30]. Furthermore, pregnant women who had SARS-CoV-2 infection are at higher risk of preterm birth, stillbirth, preeclampsia, and cesarean birth.

The risk factors for severe disease appear to be similar to those in non-pregnant individuals: black ethnicity, increased body mass index, co-existing comorbidities, and socio-economic deprivation. Pregnant women in their third trimester are more susceptible to severe disease, which may be partly mediated through the physical burden on the lungs towards the end of pregnancy. Pregnant women with COVID-19 are at 50% increased risk of preterm birth, the majority of which are iatrogenic rather than spontaneous. According to a report by the Centers for Disease Control and Prevention (CDC), the risk of stillbirth is increased even further during the period when the delta strain was the predominant variant (July-September 2021) [31].

Vertical transmission of COVID-19 is rare, which might be due to low level of maternal viraemia and maternal COVID-19 infection is not shown to be associated with increased risk for congenital anomalies.

COVID-19 in pregnancy has been associated with preeclampsia; however, it is still unclear if COVID-19 causes preeclampsia or both the conditions share similar antecedents. There is evidence that COVID-19 infection may alter the vasoactive mediator balance which is critical for development of preeclampsia. A recent systematic review and meta-analysis by Conde–Agudelo and Romero of SARS-COV-2 infection during pregnancy and the risk of preeclampsia, which included 28 studies and 790,954 pregnant women, of whom 15,524 were diagnosed with SARS-CoV-2 infection, those with SARS-CoV-2 exhibited a significant increase in the odds of preeclampsia (pooled OR 1.58, 95% CI 1.39–1.80; 11 studies) [32].

There is limited evidence regarding the treatment of COVID-19 infection in pregnancy as most of the trials excluded pregnant women. A few treatment options might improve the outcomes. These include steroids, antiviral agents like remdesivir, monoclonal neutralizing antibody cocktails, heparin, Janus kinase inhibitors, and interleukin-6 inhibitors.

Following initial period of controversial guidance, COVID-19 vaccination is now recommended to pregnant people in parallel with their non-pregnant peers. COVID-19 vaccination has been shown to be as high as 96% effective in preventing the infection in pregnant population. Robust and consistent evidence continues to accrue from large population-based registries and observational studies about the safety of COVID-19 vaccination in pregnancy without causing any adverse pregnancy outcomes. Despite this, vaccination uptake amongst pregnant people continues to remain low. In the UK, the Royal College of Obstetricians and Gynaecologists (RCOG) has strongly encouraged to have the vaccine including the third booster dose (3 months after the second dose). Currently, there are three types of COVID-19 vaccines; mRNA, viral vector, and protein subunit (in phases of development) vaccines. In the UK, pregnant women are being offered the Pfizer-BioNTech or Moderna mRNA vaccines, where available; however, women who have already had one dose of AstraZeneca (before they became pregnant or earlier on in pregnancy), are advised to complete vaccination with a second dose of AstraZeneca (viral vector) vaccines. In the US pregnant or lactating women can opt for any one of the vaccines licensed by the FDA, namely, two mRNA vaccines (Pfizer-BioNTech and Moderna) and one viral vector vaccine (Johnson & Johnson-Janssen). Unlike the mRNA vaccines, the viral vector vaccines do not require stringent transport and storage conditions, therefore are of particular importance in resource limited nations. As of December 14, 2021, the WHO SAGE (Strategic Advisory Group of Experts) has classified the Bharat Biotech Covaxin (BBV152 A, BBV152 B, and BBV152 C), Sinopharm BIBP-CorV (Hayat-Vax), and Sinovac (Coronavac) (SARS-CoV-2 inactivated vaccine) vaccines to be 'permitted' for pregnant women, which imply that all pregnant persons can receive or choose to receive these vaccines. COVID-19 vaccination uptake amongst pregnant women continues to remain worryingly low and concerted efforts are required to promote vaccination.

# CONCLUSION

There is a constant risk of emergence and rapid spread of novel as well as endemic infectious diseases due to globalisation and increased population mobility, most recently reports of Monkey pox. However, it is heartening that recent advances in technology have drastically improved isolation, genetic sequencing and surveillance of these infectious pathogens with an aim to prevent/contain them. Concerted efforts are needed to continue collaborative research, education and awareness of health care providers such that optimal care can be provided to pregnant women and their babies.

# SUGGESTED READINGS

1. Khalil A, Sotiriadis A, Chaoui R, et al. ISUOG Practice Guidelines: role of ultrasound in congenital infection. Ultrasound Obstet Gynecol 2020; 56:128–151.
2. Royal College of Obstetricians & Gynaecologists. (2017). Group B Streptococcal Disease, Early-onset (Green-top Guideline No. 36). [online] Available from: https://www.rcog.org.uk/en/guidelines-research-services/guidelines/gtg36/ [Last accessed May, 2022].
3. Royal College of Obstetricians & Gynaecologists. (2015). Chickenpox in Pregnancy (Green-top Guideline No. 13). [online] Available from: https://www.rcog.org.uk/en/guidelines-research-services/guidelines/gtg13/ [Last accessed May, 2022].
4. Royal College of Obstetricians & Gynaecologists. (2021). COVID-19 vaccines, pregnancy and breastfeeding. [online] Available from: https://www.rcog.org.uk/en/guidelines-research-services/coronavirus-covid-19-pregnancy-and-womens-health/covid-19-vaccines-and-pregnancy/covid-19-vaccines-pregnancy-and-breastfeeding/ [Last accessed May, 2022].

# REFERENCES

1. Letamendia-Richard E, Périllaud-Dubois C, de La Guillonnière L, et al. Universal newborn screening for congenital cytomegalovirus infection: feasibility and relevance in a French type-III maternity cohort. BJOG 2022; 129:291–299.
2. Herman C. What Makes a Screening Exam "Good"? AMA J Ethics 2006; 8:34–37.
3. Seror V, Leruez-Ville M, Özek A, et al. Leaning towards Cytomegalovirus serological screening in pregnancy to prevent congenital infection: a cost-effectiveness perspective. BJOG 2022; 129:301–312.
4. Chatzakis C, Ville Y, Makrydimas G, et al. Timing of primary maternal cytomegalovirus infection and rates of vertical transmission and fetal consequences. Am J Obstet Gynecol 2020; 223:870–883.
5. Faure-Bardon V, Magny JF, Parodi M, et al. Sequelae of Congenital Cytomegalovirus Following Maternal Primary Infections Are Limited to Those Acquired in the First Trimester of Pregnancy. Clin Infect Dis 2019; 69:1526–1532.
6. Shahar-Nissan K, Pardo J, Peled O, et al. Valaciclovir to prevent vertical transmission of cytomegalovirus after maternal primary infection during pregnancy: a randomised, double-blind, placebo-controlled trial. Lancet 2020; 396:779–785.
7. Faure-Bardon V, Fourgeaud J, Stirnemann J, et al. Secondary prevention of congenital cytomegalovirus infection with valacyclovir following maternal primary infection in early pregnancy. Ultrasound Obstet Gynecol 2021; 58:576–581.
8. Leruez-Ville M, Foulon I, Pass R, et al. Cytomegalovirus infection during pregnancy: state of the science. Am J Obstet Gynecol 2020; 223:330–349.
9. Leruez-Ville M, Ghout I, Bussières L, et al. In utero treatment of congenital cytomegalovirus infection with valacyclovir in a multicenter, open-label, phase II study. Am J Obstet Gynecol 2016; 215:462.
10. Nigro G, Adler SP, La Torre R, et al. Passive immunization during pregnancy for congenital cytomegalovirus infection. N Engl J Med 2005; 353:1350–1362.
11. Nigro G, La Torre R, Pentimalli H, et al. Regression of fetal cerebral abnormalities by primary cytomegalovirus infection following hyperimmunoglobulin therapy. Prenat Diagn 2008; 28:512–517.
12. La Torre R, Nigro G, Mazzocco M, et al. Placental enlargement in women with primary maternal cytomegalovirus infection is associated with fetal and neonatal disease. Clin Infect Dis 2006; 43:994–1000.

13. Hughes BL, Clifton RG, Rouse DJ, et al. A Trial of Hyperimmune Globulin to Prevent Congenital Cytomegalovirus Infection. N Eng J Med 2021; 385:436–444.
14. Revello MG, Lazzarotto T, Guerra B, et al. A Randomized Trial of Hyperimmune Globulin to Prevent Congenital Cytomegalovirus. N Eng J Med. 2014; 370:1316–1326.
15. Malinger G, Werner H, Rodriguez Leonel JC, et al. Prenatal brain imaging in congenital toxoplasmosis. Prenat Diagn 2011; 31:881–886.
16. Dhombres F, Friszer S, Maurice P, et al. Prognosis of Fetal Parenchymal Cerebral Lesions without Ventriculomegaly in Congenital Toxoplasmosis Infection. Fetal Diagn Ther 2017; 41:8–14.
17. Mandelbrot L, Kieffer F, Sitta R, et al. Prenatal therapy with pyrimethamine + sulfadiazine vs spiramycin to reduce placental transmission of toxoplasmosis: a multicenter, randomized trial. Am J Obstet Gynecol 2018; 219:386.
18. Royal College of Obstetricians & Gynaecologists. (2017). Prevention of Early-onset Group B Streptococcal Disease (Green-top Guideline No. 36). [online] Available from: https://www.rcog.org.uk/en/guidelines-research-services/guidelines/gtg36/ [Last accessed May, 2022].
19. Le Doare, K, O'Driscoll, M, Turner, K, et al. Intrapartum antibiotic chemoprophylaxis policies for the prevention of group B streptococcal disease worldwide: systematic review. Clin Infect Dis 2017; 65:S143–S151.
20. ACOG. (2019). Prevention of Group B Streptococcal Early-Onset Disease in Newborns. [online] Available from: https://www.acog.org/en/clinical/clinical-guidance/committee-opinion/articles/2020/02/prevention-of-group-b-streptococcal-early-onset-disease-in-newborns [Last accessed May, 2022].
21. Seedat F, Geppert J, Stinton C, et al. Universal antenatal screening for group B streptococcus may cause more harm than good. BMJ 2019; 364:l463.
22. Hasperhoven G, Al-Nasiry S, Bekker V, et al. Universal screening versus risk-based protocols for antibiotic prophylaxis during childbirth to prevent early-onset group B streptococcal disease: a systematic review and meta-analysis. BJOG 2020; 127:680–691.
23. NIHR. (2019). New screening trial aims to improve detection and treatment for Group B Strep in pregnant women. [online] Available from: https://www.nihr.ac.uk/news/new-screening-trial-aims-to-improve-detection-and-treatment-for-group-b-strep-in-pregnant-women/20283 [Last accessed May, 2022].
24. Heath PT. Status of vaccine research and development of vaccines for GBS. Vaccine 2016; 34:2876–2879.
25. Lamagni T, Wloch C, Broughton K, et al. Assessing the added value of group B Streptococcus maternal immunisation in preventing maternal infection and fetal harm: population surveillance study. BJOG 2022; 129:233–240.
26. Absalon J, Segall N, Block SL, et al. Safety and immunogenicity of a novel hexavalent group B streptococcus conjugate vaccine in healthy, non-pregnant adults: a phase 1/2, randomised, placebo-controlled, observer-blinded, dose-escalation trial. Lancet Infect Dis 2021; 21:263–274.
27. NIH. (2022). Pfizer. A phase 1/2, randomized, placebo-controlled, observer-blinded trial to evaluate the safety, tolerability, and immunogenicity of a multivalent group b streptococcus vaccine in healthy nonpregnant women and pregnant women 18 to 40 years of age and their infants. [online] Available from https://clinicaltrials.gov/ct2/show/NCT03765073 [Last accessed May, 2022].
28. Mangtani P, Evans SJW, Lange B, et al. Safety profile of rubella vaccine administered to pregnant women: A systematic review of pregnancy related adverse events following immunisation, including congenital rubella syndrome and congenital rubella infection in the foetus or infant. Vaccine 2020; 38:963–978.
29. Moore CA, Staples JE, Dobyns WB, et al. Characterizing the Pattern of Anomalies in Congenital Zika Syndrome for Pediatric Clinicians. JAMA Pediatr 2017; 171:288–295.
30. Knight M, Bunch K, Vousden N, et al. Characteristics and outcomes of pregnant women admitted to hospital with confirmed SARS-CoV-2 infection in UK: National population based cohort study. BMJ 2020; 369:m2107.
31. DeSisto CL. (2021). Risk for Stillbirth Among Women With and Without COVID-19 at Delivery Hospitalization — United States, March 2020–September 2021. MMWR Morb Mortal Wkly Rep. [online] Available from: https://www.cdc.gov/mmwr/volumes/70/wr/mm7047e1.html [Last accessed May, 2022].
32. Conde-Agudelo A, Romero R. SARS-COV-2 infection during pregnancy and risk of preeclampsia: a systematic review and meta-analysis. Am J Obstet Gynecol 2022; 226:68–89.

# Chapter 4

# Pregnancy and heart disease

*Shrilla Banerjee*

## INTRODUCTION

The normal heart is put under pressure by the effects of pregnancy, so if the heart is already compromised, pregnancy may result in a suboptimal outcome for both fetus and mother. Cardiac disease is the leading cause of maternal death and accounts for 23% of the causes of maternal death in the UK [1]. Therefore, pregnancy must be planned and anticipated in a patient with an existing heart condition, pre-conception.

Cardiac disease as a first presentation in pregnancy or acquired in pregnancy is associated with poor outcomes. Acquired cardiac disease is more common with increasing maternal age [2], smoking [3,4], diabetes [5], hypertension [6], and obesity [7,8].

The cardiac causes of maternal death include those shown in **Figure 4.1** [1].

All patients with existing heart disease should be assessed before conception. The assessment should include a full history (including exercise capacity, history of heart failure or arrhythmia), an exercise test and echocardiogram [looking at pulmonary pressures, valve dysfunction, and left ventricular (LV) dimensions and function].

The patient should be assessed during each of the trimesters and at any time a change of symptoms occurs.

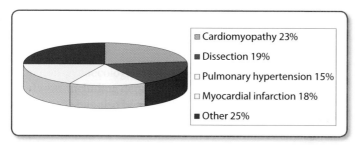

**Figure 4.1** The cardiac causes of maternal death.

- Cardiomyopathy 23%
- Dissection 19%
- Pulmonary hypertension 15%
- Myocardial infarction 18%
- Other 25%

**Shrilla Banerjee** MBChB MD FRCP, Consultant Cardiologist at NHS, UK
Email: Shrilla.Banerjee@nhs.net

# PHYSIOLOGICAL CHANGES ASSOCIATED WITH PREGNANCY

The changes in the cardiovascular system occur to meet the increased demands of the mother and fetus. The clinical signs and symptoms of a normal pregnancy are shown in **Box 4.1**. The total blood volume increases by 45% on average, and cardiac output increases by up to 50%, peaking in the second trimester [9,10].

## Cardiac output

*Stroke volume × heart rate = cardiac output*

Stroke volume, heart rate, and cardiac output increase in pregnancy [11,12]. Cardiac output increases rapidly by about 30–50% in the first two trimesters and remains elevated and peaks until 30 weeks, but then may decrease slightly because of the enlarging uterus on the vena cava [12–15]. There is some debate whether the cardiac output increases, reduces, or stays the same in later pregnancy. During labour, cardiac output increases by a further 30% due to the auto-transfusion of blood from the utero-placental circulation to the maternal systemic circulation [9,13]. Following delivery, the cardiac output falls to about 15–25% above normal levels and gradually declines until normal levels are reached at about 6 weeks post-partum [13].

## Systemic vascular resistance

The systemic vascular resistance (SVR) falls by 30–50% in the first 8 weeks and there is a further drop to 40% at 20–26 weeks which contributes to the hyper-dynamic circulation of pregnancy. The drop in SVR, triggers the renin–angiotensin–aldosterone system to retain sodium and water, manifests by peripheral oedema seen in pregnancy [16]. The drop in SVR corresponds to a reduction in mean arterial pressure, which starts to recover to normal pre-pregnancy levels from 26 to 28 weeks [13].

## Heart rate

The rise in cardiac output is mirrored by the rise in heart rate and is triggered by the lower systemic blood pressure (BP) and the reduction in afterload. The heart rate rises between 15 and 25% during pregnancy [11,12].

---

### Box 4.1 Clinical signs and symptoms in a normal pregnancy

- Shortness of breath and dyspnoea caused by hyperventilation
- Visible, elevated jugular venous pressure
- Displaced cardiac apex, palpable right ventricular apex
- Loud first heart sound, split second sound
- Ejection systolic murmur
- Pallor due to anaemia
- Weight gain

## Blood pressure

Both systolic and diastolic BPs drop by about 10 mmHg reaching trough levels at about 20 weeks. However, by term, BP levels return to pre-pregnancy levels.

## Left ventricular dimensions

The heart itself is displaced to the left and upwards, by the enlarging uterus. This results in apparent cardiomegaly on chest radiography. However, there is also a true increase in LV cavity size, caused by the increase in preload and contractility of the left ventricle secondary to increased catecholamine release results. These changes are accompanied by a degree of functional mitral valvular regurgitation and an increase in left atrial diameter.

## Electrocardiogram changes

Non-specific ST-segment, Q-wave (II, III, and aVF) and T-wave (inverted/flattened T-waves leads III, $V_1$-$V_3$) changes can be seen in pregnancy, along with a resting sinus tachycardia. The cardiac axis may be slightly left-deviated due to the displacement effects of the uterus on the heart [17].

# HYPERTENSION IN PREGNANCY

Hypertension complicates 10–15% of pregnancies and is responsible for up to 25% of all antenatal admissions [18]. There are recognised varieties of hypertension in pregnancy:
- Chronic hypertension
- Pregnancy-induced hypertension
- Pre-eclampsia

Risk factors for gestational hypertension include nulliparity, multiple pregnancy, previous pre-eclampsia, chronic hypertension, diabetes, obesity, and maternal age over 35 years [18].

The end effects of each of these varieties of hypertension are similar, in that they contribute significantly to maternal and fetal mortality and morbidity.

## Chronic or pre-existing hypertension

If hypertension is diagnosed in the first trimester, it is likely to have been a pre-existing disorder. However, this can only be confirmed 3–6 months post-partum if the baseline BP fails to return to normal. It is defined as a systolic BP of 140 mmHg or greater and/or a diastolic BP of 90 mmHg or more.

As with all new diagnoses of hypertension, no assumption of primary or essential hypertension should be made without the exclusion of important causes of secondary hypertension, such as renal or cardiac disease, coarctation, Cushing's syndrome, Conn's syndrome, or phaeochromocytoma [19].

Examination findings to look for include radio-femoral delay (coarctation) and renal bruits (renal artery stenosis). Investigations should include urine dipstick, urea and electrolytes, renal ultrasound scan, and urinary catecholamines.

If a patient with pre-existing hypertension becomes pregnant, it is imperative to review medications [20,21].

## First-line therapy – methyldopa

This is a superb drug for BP control and is known to be safe for the fetus. It can cause depression, so should be changed immediately post-partum (within 2 days of delivery). Other effects include sedation (that eventually patients become tolerant to) and postural hypotension, liver function abnormalities, and haemolytic anaemia.

## Second-line therapy – calcium antagonists

Used in conjunction with methyldopa, calcium antagonists (e.g., slow release nifedipine) and oral hydralazine are often helpful in those in whom monotherapy with methyldopa has failed. Alpha-receptor blockers (doxazosin) are also useful in conjunction with methyldopa.

## Third-line therapy – beta-blockers

Beta-blockers are generally well tolerated by pregnant women in addition to being effective anti-hypertensive agents. However, beta-blockers are known to cause intra-uterine growth retardation and hence patients need regular scans to assess for fetal growth. It is advisable to avoid atenolol in pregnancy. Labetalol in both tablet and parenteral form is a favoured formulation, preferably given in the second or third trimester. Also consider bisoprolol but with careful fetal growth monitoring.

- *Angiotensin-converting enzyme (ACE) inhibitors* can cause significant fetal abnormalities including oligohydramnios, renal failure, and hypotension. Patients on ACE inhibitors should be changed to a different type of medication immediately as ACE inhibitors are associated with congenital kidney abnormalities
- If a patient on ACE inhibitors becomes pregnant this is not an indication for termination, as the structural malformations caused are not related to the first trimester. The patient should be promptly converted to methyldopa. Methyldopa must be changed within 2 days of delivery due to increased risk of post-natal depression. Post-partum, ACE inhibitors can be restarted as their use in breastfeeding mothers is safe
- *Angiotensin receptor blockers* similar to ACE inhibitors. Suggest avoid in pregnancy
- *Diuretics* – not the drugs of choice in this physiological state, unless there is evidence of fluid overload, for instance in conditions such as heart failure, pulmonary oedema, or idiopathic intracranial hypertension

## Management of hypertension in pregnancy

Blood pressure should be taken with the patient seated or semi-reclining but not recumbent. Tight BP control is key. Target levels lower than 150/100 mmHg, but ideally <140/90 mmHg.

- *Urine testing* for proteinuria regularly, if more than 1+ of protein, then arrange a spot urinary protein:creatinine ratio to quantify proteinuria. If >30 mg/mmol, treat as per pre-eclampsia. Consider placental growth factor (PIGF)-based testing to help rule out pre-eclampsia
- *Fetal ultrasound* at 28–30 weeks and 32–34 weeks to assess fetal growth and amniotic fluid levels

## Pregnancy-induced hypertension

This usually appears in the second half of pregnancy and resolves within 6 weeks of delivery. It can persist for up to 3 months post-partum. It is a complication seen in about 5–10% of pregnancies.

Pregnancy-induced hypertension is defined as hypertension without proteinuria or other features of pre-eclampsia. The main difference between the two conditions is that the outcome is much worse with pre-eclampsia. The later the presentation in the pregnancy, the less likely the progression to pre-eclampsia (40% before 30 weeks vs. 7% after 38 weeks). Management is similar to that of hypertension in pregnancy [19].

## Pre-eclampsia

Pre-eclampsia is defined as pregnancy-induced hypertension and proteinuria and/or fetal growth restriction and/or biochemical and haematological abnormalities. The risks of developing pre-eclampsia are shown in **Box 4.2**. It is a multi-system disorder, due to diffuse vascular endothelial dysfunction. The first abnormalities occur in the first weeks of pregnancy, with abnormal placenta formation due to remodelling of the uterine spiral arteries, resulting in reduced vascular resistance, and leading to systemic endothelial dysfunction, hypertension, and renal impairment [22].

Women may present with headache, visual disturbance, epigastric or right upper quadrant pain, nausea, vomiting, or rapidly progressive oedema. The most common cause of death is cerebral haemorrhage and adult respiratory distress syndrome [23]. Fetal effects are intra-uterine growth retardation, placental abruption, and intra-uterine death [22].

## Management

The aim should be to manage the patient supportively, with delivery at or after 34 weeks' gestation, if at all possible. Recommended investigations are shown in **Table 4.1**. BP control has to be a balance between reduction of maternal BP, whilst protecting the utero-placental

### Box 4.2 Risks of developing pre-eclampsia

- First pregnancy
- Age 40 years or more
- Body Mass Index (BMI) of 35 or more at presentation
- Family history of pre-eclampsia (mother or sister)
- Multiple pregnancy
- 10 years or more since last pregnancy

| Table 4.1 Investigations in pre-eclampsia | |
|---|---|
| Urinalysis | Microscopy and culture |
| Bloods | FBC (HELLP syndrome – platelets < 100 × 10$^9$)<br>U + Es<br>LFTs (ALT or AST > 70 IU/L) |
| Clotting studies | |
| 24-hour urine collection | Quantify protein loss |
| Fetal ultrasound | Fetal growth and assessment of amniotic fluid volumes |
| Cerebral imaging | Only if focal neurology, to exclude haemorrhage or prolonged coma |

ALT, alanine transaminase; AST, aspartate transaminase; FBC, full blood count; HELLP, haemolysis, elevated liver enzymes and low platelet syndrome; LFT, liver function test.

> ## Box 4.3 Management of hypertension in pre-eclampsia
>
> - Mild hypertension: 140–149/90–99 mmHg
>   - Monitor BP four times daily
>   - Check bloods for FBC, renal function, and LFTs twice weekly
> - Moderate hypertension: 150–159/100–109 mmHg
>   - Monitor BP four times daily
>   - Start anti-hypertensives (labetalol/methyldopa/nifedipine)
>   - Target BP < 150/80–90 mmHg
>   - Check bloods for FBC, renal function, and LFTs three times weekly
> - Severe hypertension: >160/110 mmHg
>   - Monitor BP four times daily
>   - Check bloods for FBC, renal function, and LFTs three times weekly
>   - Fetal ultrasound
>   - Cardiotocography to assess fetal movements
>
> BP, blood pressure; FBC, full blood count; LFT, liver function test.

circulation and maintaining fetal blood flow. BP levels over 140/90 mmHg should provoke consideration of treatment. It is mandatory for BPs over 170/110 mmHg to be treated. Headache and epigastric pain should be assessed for at every BP assessment. Management depends on severity of BP – mild, moderate, or severe, as shown in **Box 4.3**.

## Management of acute severe pre-eclampsia

Delivery of the fetus is the ultimate resolution of the situation. This has to be balanced against extending the gestational period to be beyond 34 weeks if possible.
*Blood pressure management* includes the use of:
- Hydralazine (intermittent intravenous bolus)
- Labetalol (oral continuous intravenous infusion)
- Nifedipine tablets (oral only – never use sublingually)

If using hydralazine or nifedipine as second-line agents, the concomitant use of methyldopa reduces the side effects of headache and tachycardia.

### Seizure management

Magnesium sulphate is the drug of choice to prevent and control seizures in pre-eclampsia [24]. However, when used in conjunction with nifedipine, profound hypotension may ensue.

### Fluid balance

Fluid restriction is advised to reduce the risk of overload and pulmonary oedema. Pulmonary oedema is a significant contributor to maternal death.

### Post-partum

- Careful BP monitoring is essential to time change/reduction of medications
- Stop methyldopa (risk of post-partum depression)

- Blood tests – monitor full blood count (FBC), liver function tests (LFTs) and creatinine 72 hours post-partum
- Offer ACE inhibitor/angiotensin II receptor blocker (ARB) medication to manage BP, even if breastfeeding
- Black (African-Caribbean) women are better managed with nifedipine or amlodipine

## Prognosis

- Recurrence rate of 15% in women who had pre-eclampsia in first pregnancy [25]
- Increased risk of hypertension and heart disease [26]
- Maternal mortality rate of eclampsia is 1.8% [27]
- Low-dose aspirin (from 12 weeks' gestation) has been shown to reduce risk in those at high-risk of pre-eclampsia [28–30]

# PALPITATIONS AND ARRHYTHMIA

Palpitations are a common complaint and can occur in up to 50–60% of the pregnant population [31]. Holter data for pregnant women were analysed in one study, which showed that 76% of those experiencing palpitation were found to be in sinus tachycardia alone. Only 24% of the Holter tests demonstrated any arrhythmia, most of which were benign [32]. The physical and hormonal changes associated with pregnancy may produce a pro-arrhythmic state. Increasing cardiac output results in myocardial stretch and increases left ventricular end-diastolic (LVED) pressure volumes. These changes can promote arrhythmogenesis. Arrhythmia is the most common pregnancy-related cardiac complication. The increased circulating volume in pregnancy, can contribute to increased atrial and ventricular stretch, and combined with autonomic and hormonal factors, makes pregnancy a time of increased arrhythmogenesis [31,32].

Most palpitations experienced will be due to isolated atrial and ventricular ectopic beats. In **Box 4.4** the features that may warrant further investigation are shown. Treatment includes reassurance and avoidance of precipitants. Episodes of tachycardia are more symptomatic in pregnancy and can occur in any of the trimesters.

## Investigations

A thorough history, baseline 12-lead electrocardiogram (ECG), ambulatory ECG monitoring, and echocardiogram should be considered.

---

### Box 4.4 Areas in history that suggest further investigation is necessary

- Fast and irregular palpitation
- Palpitations waking from sleep
- Pre-syncope in association with palpitations
- Pre-existing cardiac condition
- Family history of cardiac disease
- Worsening symptoms with exertion
- Associated chest pain, shortness of breath, and syncope

## Sinus tachycardia

This is common in normal pregnancy. However, if the tachycardia is over 25% greater than the normal pre-pregnant heart rate, then consider hyperthyroidism, or other causes such as anaemia, hypovolaemia, sepsis, or respiratory or cardiac pathology. Cardio-respiratory causes include pulmonary embolism, phaeochromocytoma, and postural orthostatic tachycardia syndrome (POTS).

## Atrial and ventricular ectopic beats

Again, it is very common in pregnancy. It is found in about 50% of pregnant women on ambulatory monitoring [32]. At low burdens (<7.5% of total beats) are considered benign and rarely require treatment.

## Supraventricular tachycardia

Paroxysmal supraventricular tachycardia (SVT) is the most common non-benign arrhythmia encountered in pregnancy. A pregnant patient has a risk of developing new SVT 34% higher than at other times in her life [33]. Most are caused by atrioventricular nodal re-entrant tachycardia (AVNRT) [34]. SVT classically has an abrupt symptomatic onset and cessation. Management of an AVNRT is similar in pregnant and non-pregnant patients. Vagal manoeuvres should be the first choice. If successful in terminating the arrhythmia, no further treatment is necessary. However, if vagal manoeuvres fail, then it is worth considering intravenous adenosine that is safe in these circumstances, but whilst the women is monitored [35]. Subsequent strategies can include intravenous adenosine, propranolol, or metoprolol that are also safe to use in pregnancy. Some suggest that adenosine use in late pregnancy should be used with fetal heart rate monitoring. Flecainide and amiodarone are best avoided. Both carry the risks of teratogenesis.

If the arrhythmia is resistant to all therapies suggested, direct current (DC) cardioversion is safe, especially if performed within 48 hours of onset obviating the need for anticoagulation [36,37].

Beta-blockers are helpful agents for prophylaxis of paroxysmal SVT.

Curative catheter ablation is also possible in pregnancy, preferably in the second trimester with radiation shields placed over the abdomen. Pulsed fluoroscopy should help to limit radiation exposure. In patients with pre-existing tachycardia, a catheter ablation should be planned prior to conception if possible.

## Atrial fibrillation and flutter

Atrial fibrillation (AF) and atrial flutter are rarely seen in isolation in pregnancy. These rhythms are often seen in conjunction with congenital heart disease (Ebstein's anomaly), rheumatic heart disease (mitral stenosis), or hyperthyroidism [37,38].

In patients with permanent AF, adding beta-blockers (not atenolol) and digoxin can optimise rate control. AF increases the risk of systemic thromboembolism. Anticoagulation should be considered in those at high risk of stroke such as women with permanent AF, structural heart disease, rheumatic mitral valve disease, and those with previous emboli. Heparin is safe in early pregnancy (before 12 weeks) and this can be replaced with warfarin in the second and third trimesters. It is imperative that there is collaborative planning of the delivery between cardiologists, haematologists, and obstetricians [39].

## Ventricular tachycardia

A broad complex rapidly conducted heart rhythm with haemodynamic compromise should be treated as ventricular tachycardia (VT), until otherwise proven. VT is often associated with structural heart disease [hypertrophic cardiomyopathy (HCM), peri-partum cardiomyopathy (PPCM), arrhythmogenic right ventricular cardiomyopathy (ARVC)] or a primary electrical problem [long QT syndrome (LQTS)] [40].

Right ventricular outflow tract (RVOT) tachycardia is the most likely source of VT seen in pregnancy. RVOT tachycardia is known to occur in patients without recognised structural heart disease. Most episodes are related to stress and are probably catecholamine driven, given that they respond to beta-blocker therapy. One study showed that in 11 women with VT in pregnancy, 73% had monomorphic VT originating from the right ventricle [i.e. left bundle branch block (LBBB) morphology], with an inferior axis [41]. The tachycardia resolves post-delivery and the prognosis for mother and baby is good.

An echocardiogram and ECG are necessary to determine if there is any evidence of structural heart disease. The antiarrhythmic of choice for VT in pregnancy is lidocaine and electrical DC cardio-version should be performed if haemodynamic compromise occurs. DC cardio-version is safe in pregnancy and is a quick and useful tool for rapidly terminating potentially troublesome tachyarrhythmias [40].

## Implantable cardioverter defibrillators

Women with implantable cardioverter defibrillators (ICDs) implanted should not be discouraged from becoming pregnant. The data is favourable for both maternal and fetal outcomes in the presence of cardiac conditions necessitating ICDs. A study of 44 pregnant women with structural heart disease and ICDs, found that none received inappropriate shocks during pregnancy. Indeed, 75% received no shocks at all. Fetal outcomes were: 89% born healthy, 4% small for dates, and 2% stillborn [42].

## Long QT syndrome

Inherited LQTS is seen more commonly in women. However, women who are pregnant experience most cardiac events in the immediate post-partum period (9%), as opposed to during pregnancy (1.8–4.5%) [43]. Especially relevant to those with type 2 LQTS. The recommendation for this group is therefore to continue beta-blocker therapy throughout the pregnancy and post-partum period. There is a small risk of beta-blocker entering breast milk and causing neonatal bradyarrhythmia. However, the maternal risk is greater and takes precedence.

Cardiac Risk in the Young (CRY) a charity for cardiomyopathy and sudden cardiac death in the young has published a list of medications to avoid in LQTS [SADS: drugs to avoid. https://www.sads.org.uk/drugs-to-avoid/] [44].

Gene defects coding for cardiac ion channels have been identified as associated with inherited LQTS. There is an association with LQTS and sudden infant death syndrome, so referral for genetic review should be a priority in the post-partum period.

The options available in antiarrhythmic therapy and safety in pregnancy and breast-feeding are shown in **Table 4.2**.

| Table 4.2 Antiarrhythmic medications in pregnancy and breastfeeding | | |
|---|---|---|
| Drug | Safe in pregnancy | Safe during breastfeeding |
| Adenosine | ✔ Fetal toxicity with high doses | ✔ |
| Amiodarone | ✔ Suitable for emergency use only | ✘ Avoid as risk of neonatal hypothyroidism |
| Beta-blockers | ✔ Possible association with IUGR | ✔ |
| Digoxin | ✔ Fetal toxicity with high doses | ✔ |
| Flecainide | ✔ Insufficient data likely to be safe | ✔ Not known to be harmful |
| Lidocaine | ✔ Fetal toxicity with high doses | ✔ |
| Verapamil | ✔ Avoid rapid injection | ✔ |
| IUGR, intrauterine growth restriction. | | |

## Bradyarrhythmias

Patients with symptomatic bradycardia or congenital complete heart block should have a permanent pacemaker implanted prior to conception [45,46]. Most arrhythmias in women with a structurally normal heart are not associated with concerns around pregnancy or delivery [37]. The placing of temporary wires should be discouraged peri-delivery [45,46].

## ISCHAEMIC HEART DISEASE

Acute coronary syndrome (ACS) is a rare presentation in women of reproductive age, but pregnancy itself increases the risk of an acute myocardial infarct (MI) by three to four times. The incidence is 6 per 100,000 deliveries in the Western World, but is increasing, probably in the current climate of increased maternal age, smoking, and obesity. Mortality from MI in pregnancy is in the range of 37–50% [47].

Factors such as maternal age over 40 years, diabetes, hypertension, thrombophilia, transfusion, smoking, and peri-partum infection are significant risk factors for acute MI in pregnancy [48]. Indeed, the odds of MI in one study were 30-fold increased for a maternal age of 40 years and above [49], and cardiac death four times increased when compared to those for maternal age of <20 years [50,51].

The presentation of ACS is three times more likely to be as an ST-elevation MI (STEMI) as opposed to a non-ST-elevation MI (NSTEMI) [52]. Most occur in the third trimester or post-partum, making management difficult as thrombolysis is contraindicated pre-delivery and for 10 days post-delivery. Hence, the treatment of choice is immediate (primary) angioplasty, although there is little evidence to support this choice. Atherosclerotic disease accounts for a significant proportion of ACS in pregnancy, although other causations include coronary artery thrombotic occlusion and coronary artery spasm and spontaneous coronary artery dissection (SCAD) [53].

Spontaneous coronary artery dissection is a process of coronary artery dissection, due to intramural haematoma resulting in vessel occlusion. It is more common in young women, without conventional coronary artery risk factors. The classic presentation in pregnancy is with an anterior STEMI. It is hypothesised that the hormonal effects of pregnancy result in changes in vessel structure, and that, combined with the increased haemodynamic burden in late pregnancy, puts stress on the vessel architecture.

## Management of ACS in pregnancy

This is a medical emergency, so all care should be coordinated with an interventional cardiologist, obstetrician, and obstetric anaesthetist. The management of ACS in the pregnant woman should be the same as for the non-pregnant woman.

Patients should be given aspirin 75 mg stat and also clopidogrel (no data to suggest fetal toxicity) as dual anti-platelet therapy (DAPT). The fetus in the pelvis should be shielded using lead aprons and a radial arterial approach followed to allow optimal positioning of the mother to prevent vena caval compression, reducing venous return and further haemodynamic compromise (left lateral position). Consideration should be given to the type of stent used as drug-eluting stents require longer DAPT (>3 months) than bare metal stents (1 month).

## Pregnancy in women with existing coronary artery disease

Generally, maternal outcomes are favourable in this group [54], but registries have shown that there are higher than expected pre-term deliveries and lower birth weights. However, if there is evidence of significant impairment of LV function, pregnancy should be discouraged [37]. The suitability and safety of ACS medications in pregnancy and breastfeeding are shown in **Table 4.3**.

| Table 4.3 ACS cardiac medications in pregnancy and breastfeeding [55] | | | | |
|---|---|---|---|---|
| Drug | Pregnancy | Dose adjustments | Delivery | Breastfeeding |
| Aspirin | • Yes<br>• Crosses placenta and can cause pregnancy loss and congenital defects | Nil – 300 mg stat and then 75 mg od maintenance | Yes | Yes |
| Clopidogrel | • Yes<br>• Crosses placenta | Nil – 300 mg stat and then 75 mg od maintenance | Discontinue 7 days pre-delivery | Not recommended |
| Ticagrelor | Not recommended | | | Not recommended |
| Heparin (unfractionated UFH) | • Yes<br>• Increased maternal bleeding | Nil | Discontinue during delivery or spinal anaesthesia | Yes |
| Heparin (low molecular weight LMW) | • Yes<br>• Increased maternal bleeding | Dose according to booking weight | Discontinue during delivery or spinal anaesthesia<br>Consider switching to UFH in last weeks of pregnancy | Yes |
| NOAC | Not recommended | | | Not recommended |
| Beta-blockers | • Yes<br>• Risk of IUGR and fetal bradycardia<br>• Atenolol not recommended | Nil | Yes | Yes |
| Statins | Not recommended | | | Not recommended |
| ACE inhibitor/ARB | Contraindicated in pregnancy | | | Yes |
| ACS, acute coronary syndrome; ARB, angiotensin II receptor blocker; NOAC, non-vitamin K oral anticoagulant. | | | | |

# CARDIOMYOPATHY

Cardiomyopathy is a congenital or acquired disease of the heart muscle. It describes a group of disorders in which the heart muscle is structurally and functionally abnormal in the absence of coronary artery disease, hypertension, valvular disease, and congenital heart disease, sufficient to cause the observed abnormality. Cardiomyopathy exists in different forms: dilated, hypertrophic, ARVC, peripartum, restrictive, and LV non-compaction cardiomyopathies [55].

## Dilated cardiomyopathy

Dilated cardiomyopathy (DCM) can be idiopathic or secondary to a number of different conditions including myocarditis, alcohol or other toxins, endocrine and autoimmune disorders, and nutritional factors. Pregnancy in women with DCM is associated with poor outcomes, especially those with more than moderate LV impairment [LV ejection fraction (LVEF) < 45%]. The haemodynamic changes of pregnancy, specifically the increase in cardiac work, may provoke ventricular failure, pulmonary oedema, and fetal loss in women with DCM. Those with symptoms New York Heart Association (NYHA) class III and above should be counselled against pregnancy as there is an associated maternal mortality of 7% [56,57].

Adverse events occurring in pregnancy with DCM include heart failure, VT, aborted sudden death, AF, transient ischaemic attack, and stroke and death. Women with no history of previous cardiac events, and a good NYHA class with only mild LV impairment has a reasonable chance of an event-free pregnancy [56].

Some medications for ventricular failure are teratogenic: patients should be counselled pre-pregnancy regarding the risk of both poor maternal and fetal outcomes and any ACE inhibitor or ARBs should be withdrawn if the decision is made to continue with pregnancy. The cardiac function should be reassessed prior to conception, and advice against pregnancy given if the LVEF further deteriorates.

Beta-blockers should be maintained throughout pregnancy, with the appropriate fetal monitoring for intrauterine growth restriction (IUGR). Other drugs that can be used are diuretics (to manage fluid balance), nitrates, and hydralazine (to reduce preload).

Further management is discussed below with PPCM.

## Peri-partum cardiomyopathy

Peri-partum cardiomyopathy is heart failure secondary to LV systolic dysfunction, with an EF <45%, presenting between the last month of pregnancy and 5 months post-partum in a woman without previously known structural heart disease. The aetiology is unknown. The LV systolic dysfunction that occurs can be reversible [58].

Cardiomyopathy presenting earlier in pregnancy is defined as pregnancy-associated cardiomyopathy. Worldwide there is a huge variation in the incidence of PPCM with high rates in Haiti (1 in 299 livebirths) [59] and only 1 per 4,000 livebirths in the USA [60]. The lowest rates are found in Scandinavia and Japan [61,62]. The mortality rates are reported between <2 and 50%. Risk factors for developing PPCM can be seen in **Box 4.5**.

There are many hypotheses as to the aetiology of PPCM and include causes such as selenium deficiency, immune-mediated mechanism, myocarditis, and viral triggers (such as enteroviruses – *Coxsackie, Parvovirus B19*, adenovirus, and herpes). The role of fetal microchimerism (fetal cells enter the maternal circulation apparently to enhance maternal

> **Box 4.5 Risk factors for the development of peri-partum cardiomyopathy**
> - Increasing gravidity and age
> - Primiparous
> - Hypertension/Pre-eclampsia
> - African race
> - Twin pregnancy
> - Malnutrition
> - Diabetes
> - Smoking

tolerance of the fetus) is still under discussion. It is probable that no one factor is directly contributory and that PPCM is multifactorial [58]. Further research is awaited.

## Management of DCM and PPCM

In DCM, specific treatment may be targeted against the causation, if identified.

The first step in management is assessing the sustainability of the pregnancy. If pregnancy continues, therapy must be adjusted so that the fetus is not exposed to additional therapy-related risk. The management is similar to the management of DCM and includes ACE inhibitors or hydralazine if PPCM occurs during pregnancy, mineralocorticoid receptor antagonists, beta-blockers, digoxin, and diuretics. Anticoagulation should be considered in those with significantly impaired LVEF (<35%) [58] (**Table 4.4**).

Angiotensin-converting enzyme inhibitors/ARB should be started as soon as possible after delivery as these drugs are safe in breastfeeding. Bromocriptine, a dopamine-receptor antagonist, blocks the production of prolactin and has been shown to facilitate the recovery of the EF in a small study of 63 patients with PPCM [63,64]. There is a small chance of coronary thrombosis as a cardiac complication, so it should be prescribed with a prophylactic dose of low molecular weight heparin (LMWH) [65].

Cardiac defibrillators (both wearable and implantable) should be considered post-partum as the risk of dangerous ventricular tachyarrhythmia persists in PPCM.

Treatment of PPCM should continue for at least 12 months after recovery of LVEF. The removal of therapies should be monitored with LVEF on echocardiography. The suggested approach is to taper the magnetic resonance angiography (MRA), then ACE inhibitor or ARB and beta-blockers [66].

## Hypertrophic cardiomyopathy

In HCM, abnormal thickening of the heart muscle renders the muscle stiff and non-compliant. The hypertrophy often affects the LV outflow tract and may cause outflow tract obstruction. It predominantly affects diastolic function and patients present with palpitations and breathlessness, or arrhythmias (atrial and ventricular). AF, a consequence of the left atrial dilatation is common and predisposes to thromboembolism. Pregnancy in patients with HCM is considered to be lower risk than in those with severe DCM [67,68]. However, 48% report symptoms such as dyspnoea, heart failure, arrhythmia, angina, pre-syncope, and syncope [54,57,69,70]. However, those patients with end-stage hypertrophy that has progressed to dilatation and thinning of the LV wall, are classed as high risk for

| Table 4.4 Cardiac medications in DCM and PPCM during and after pregnancy | | | | |
|---|---|---|---|---|
| Drug | Pregnancy concerns? | During pregnancy? | Breastfeeding? | Post-partum? |
| ACE/ARB | Teratogenic | ✗ | Captopril, benazepril and enalapril considered safe | ✔ |
| Beta-blockers | Some concerns re: IUGR and fetal bradycardia | • Metoprolol, carvedilol, and bisoprolol considered safe<br>• Atenolol contraindicated | Metoprolol considered safe | ✔ |
| Mineralocorticoid receptor antagonist | Can cause post-implantation loss in animal studies | ✗ | ✗ | ✔ |
| Diuretics | Electrolyte disturbance and oligohydramnios | Furosemide and bumetanide considered safe | Furosemide considered safe | ✔ |
| Inotropes | Recommended | Levosimendan may be preferred | Unknown | ✔ |
| Vasodilators | Hydralazine and long-acting nitrates recommended | Conflicting data | Hydralazine considered safe | Convert to ACE/ARB |
| Ivabradine | Teratogenic in animals | | Unknown | ✔ |
| Anticoagulation - LMWH | Recommended – varying by trimester | ✔ | ✔ | ✔<br>Review 4–6 weeks post-partum |
| Digoxin | Recommended | ✔ | ✔ | ✔ |
| Bromocriptine | In post-partum period | | | ✔ |

sudden death [68,70]. Maternal mortality is increased by factors including family history of sudden death, extreme hypertrophy, unexplained syncope, non-sustained VT, and an abnormal BP response to exercise.

## Management of pregnancy in HCM

Beta-blockers, or verapamil if beta-blockers are not tolerated, and diuretics are advised for those who develop dyspnoea and exertional limitations. Anticoagulation and then DC cardioversion should be considered if AF occurs.

Normal delivery is advised as the risk of haemorrhage and hence excessive fluid loss is reduced. Hypovolaemia secondary to blood loss is poorly tolerated. General anaesthesia is discouraged due to a higher risk of complications.

## Restrictive cardiomyopathy

The key features of this cardiomyopathy are increased myocardial stiffness, and impaired relaxation that culminate in reduced ventricular filling. The process can affect both right and left ventricles. The increase in plasma volume in pregnancy may lead to volume overload and either right or LV failure.

Beta-blockers and diuretics should be considered therapies. Attempts should be made for normal delivery if possible [71].

## LV non-compaction cardiomyopathy

This is thought to be an inherited condition with hypertrabeculation of the myocardium, with deep clefts in the myocardium. There is an increased risk of thromboembolism. In 25% of pregnancies, there is a transient increase of LV trabeculation, so a confirmed diagnosis should not be made during pregnancy [72].

Pregnancy may be complicated by heart failure and arrhythmias, but mortality has not been reported. Anticoagulation is recommended in patients with a history of thromboembolism, AF, intra-cardiac thrombi, or LV impairment [66].

## Arrhythmogenic right ventricular cardiomyopathy

Arrhythmogenic right ventricular cardiomyopathy is an inherited cardiomyopathy where cardiac myocytes are replaced by fibrofatty infiltration. This process results in arrhythmia and right heart failure. Occasionally, the left ventricle may be affected too.

Generally, pregnancy is well-tolerated, but dizziness, dyspnoea, and palpitations are frequent, with the main concern being VT. Beta-blockers and flecainide are effective and ICDs should be considered during pre-pregnancy counselling. Symptomatic patients are advised to avoid pregnancy [73].

# VALVULAR HEART DISEASE

Valvular heart disease is the main acquired cardiac defect likely to cause problems for women during childbirth, across the world. The most common cause of maternal mortality is rheumatic valve disease: the main lesion being mitral stenosis (up to 90% of cases). Other conditions include congenital abnormalities or previous endocarditis. Rheumatic heart disease is rare in the UK, and if seen, is primarily in non-UK born mothers. The main valvular conditions in UK-born mothers are a consequence of bicuspid aortic valve and mitral valve prolapse [38,74].

Risk of pregnancy in valvular heart disease can be classified by using the World Health Organization (WHO) scale (**Table 4.5**) [37].

Risks are additive, and in particular if the patient has other high risk features such as hypertension, high body mass index (BMI), diabetes, or renal disease, the risks compound further.

## Preconception counselling

All patients with existing valve disease should be assessed before conception. It is important that cardiac assessment and counselling are considered pre-pregnancy. Consideration of pregnancy allows optimisation of any medications or interventions to enhance the success of pregnancy. Ideally, the antenatal care and review should be planned locally with specialist input as necessary, but some valve conditions will require specialist care from the outset. Delivery of high WHO risk score patients (see **Box 4.1**) should be discussed and planned with an obstetric anaesthetist, so that the delivery carries the lowest cardiovascular stress.

Risk of pregnancy in valvular heart disease can be classified by using the WHO scale (**Table 4.5**).

| Table 4.5 WHO risk score in valvular heart disease | | | | | |
|---|---|---|---|---|---|
| WHO risk score | | Mitral valve | Aortic valve | Tricuspid valve | Pulmonary valve |
| 1 | Pregnancy carries the same risk as the general population | Trivial MR | Trivial AR | Mild TR | • Mild PS<br>• Mild PR |
| 2 | Pregnancy carries a small increased risk of mortality and morbidity | • Mild MS<br>• Mild MR | • Mild AS<br>• Mild AR | • Mild TS<br>• Moderate TR | • Moderate PS<br>• Moderate PR |
| 2–3 | Pregnancy carries a moderately increased risk of mortality and morbidity | Moderate MR | • Moderate AR<br>• Bicuspid aortic valve with aorta <45 mm | | Severe PR |
| 3 | Pregnancy carries a significantly increased risk – expert obstetric and cardiology care required | • Severe MR<br>• Moderate MS | • Severe AR<br>• Moderate-severe AS<br>• Bicuspid aortic valve with aorta <45–50 mm | • Severe TR and TS | |
| 4 | Pregnancy carries a very high risk of maternal morbidity and mortality and is contraindicated. Termination of pregnancy should be discussed. If pregnancy continues, then care should be as for Level 3 | Severe MS | • Severe-critical AS<br>• Bicuspid aortic valve with aorta >50 mm | | |

The preconception assessment should include a full history (including exercise capacity, history of heart failure, or arrhythmia), an exercise test and echocardiogram (looking at pulmonary pressures, valve dysfunction, and LV dimensions and function).

Once pregnant, the patient should be assessed during each trimester and at any time a change of symptoms occurs.

## Mitral stenosis

The natural history of mitral stenosis typically starts with a 20–25 year asymptomatic period. As a result, many patients may first present in pregnancy when the haemodynamic demands on the heart, make the valve stenosis more apparent. Classically, pregnant women with mitral stenosis present in the second or third trimester with pulmonary congestion, pulmonary oedema, and atrial arrhythmias. The pregnancy-related rise in cardiac output makes the pressure gradient across the valve more critical and leads to an increase in left atrial volume and pressure, elevated pulmonary filling pressures, and results in increasing symptoms of dyspnoea and diminishing exercise capacity. Pregnancy-induced tachycardia further increases left atrial pressure by decreasing diastolic filling time. The development of secondary pulmonary hypertension (PH) may result in right ventricular failure presenting with peripheral oedema, ascites, and hepatic engorgement [75,76].

Predictors of maternal mortality include a valve area <1.5 cm$^2$ and NYHA functional class II, III, or IV. Fetal mortality increases with increasing NYHA class.

## Medical management

This should be directed at reducing volume overload. Diuretic therapy, reduced salt intake and reduced physical activity are the mainstay of this approach.

Beta-blockers reduce tachycardia, improving diastolic filling time and hence help to reduce left atrial pressure. If AF occurs, this requires anticoagulation and prompt correction with cardioversion, as the loss of atrial 'kick' can result in pulmonary oedema and cardiovascular collapse. Prevention of recurrence of AF is best performed using procainamide and quinidine. Digoxin in combination with beta-blockers is used for rate control in permanent AF. Anticoagulation is essential in the pro-thrombotic pregnant state with AF and mitral stenosis.

## Percutaneous ballon mitral valvuloplasty/commissurotomy

Ideally performed prior to conception on patients with valve areas <1 cm$^2$, this procedure can improve complication rates of pregnancy in women with mitral stenosis, compared to medically treated women.

If necessary, the procedure can be performed during pregnancy, ideally in the second trimester in patients with NYHA III-IV symptoms. Mitral valvuloplasty has a proven track record of normal subsequent deliveries and excellent fetal outcomes. However, it is contraindicated in women with moderate-severe mitral regurgitation (MR), calcification of the mitral valve or clot in the left atrium. Risks of radiation exposure can be avoided by performing the procedure purely under TOE (transoesophageal echocardiogram) control. Open surgical commissurotomy is an option, but is associated with higher rates of fetal loss.

If a woman with mitral valve disease who is pregnant becomes significantly symptomatic, valve replacement is an option and is best performed in the second trimester. However, this is not without increased risk. Maternal outcomes are virtually the same as the non-pregnant patient but fetal loss can be anything between 10 and 30% [74].

## Delivery

Delivery and the immediate post-partum period are very high risk. Difficult fluid balance and tachycardia can result in pulmonary congestion and a low-output state. Vaginal delivery is recommended but with epidural anaesthesia and a short second stage of labour, with assisted delivery devices. Oxygen will reduce pulmonary pressures, and fluid restriction. The use of diuretics will help to reduce peripartum rises in left atrial and pulmonary pressure due to fluid shifts [74].

## Mitral regurgitation

In the UK, this is most commonly due to mitral valve prolapse. This is usually well tolerated in pregnancy, particularly if the left ventricle is within normal dimensions and the function is normal. With MR, the left ventricle is offloaded as a result of the reduced SVR. This results in a diminution of MR.

Symptoms may include exertional dyspnoea, orthopnoea, and paroxysmal nocturnal dyspnoea. Some patients will present with AF-associated heart failure [75].

## Medical management

In the presence of impaired systolic function treatment, with hydralazine, and diuretics can help to further off load the left ventricle. In addition, digoxin is well tolerated in pregnancy and can be a helpful and well-tolerated positive inotrope.

## Surgical management

If symptoms are very limiting and the MR severe, surgical repair of the mitral valve is a good option and obviates the need for on-going anticoagulant therapy. Mitral valve replacement is possible, with good maternal and fetal outcomes, although any LV dysfunction present prior to surgery is unlikely to recover following surgery. Ideally, with women of child-bearing age consideration should be given to a tissue valve replacement as opposed to a mechanical valve in the mitral position, as this removes the need for anticoagulation challenges during pregnancy [77].

## Aortic stenosis

Symptomatic aortic stenosis is less common than mitral valve disease in the pregnant population. The most common cause for aortic valve disease is congenital valvular abnormalities, usually a bicuspid aortic valve. Surgical correction prior to conception is advised for all symptomatic patients and those with a peak gradient over 80 mmHg. Patients already symptomatic in the first trimester, will fall into the WHO IV risk score, and are classed as extremely high risk [77].

It is important to remember that in women with congenital aortic stenosis, there is a 15% risk of a similar anomaly in the fetus.

During pregnancy, patients with bicuspid aortic valves are at increased risk of aortic dissection due to pregnancy-related hormonal effects on the connective tissue of the aorta.

In aortic stenosis, the need to maintain the pressure gradient across the obstructed LV outflow tract puts an increased stress on the LV wall. As a result, LV hypertrophy and diastolic dysfunction develop which can progress on to fibrosis, resulting in diminished coronary flow reserve, and finally systolic heart failure. For this reason, women with severe aortic stenosis may first present in pregnancy.

Women with aortic valve areas >1 cm$^2$ (moderate-severe AS) should tolerate pregnancy well, but will need regular specialist review (WHO III). The main symptoms with more severe aortic stenosis are predominantly exertional chest pain, light-headedness, or syncope. Echocardiography should be performed every 6 weeks, to assess the LV function, pulmonary arterial hypertension, and no new ischaemia. The gradient across the aortic valve should increase during pregnancy, but failure to do so may suggest that the LV is failing, and imminent decompensation awaits [78,79].

## Medical management

Those with mild-moderate stenosis and asymptomatic are best managed medically. It is important to protect LV output by avoiding strenuous exercise/bed rest with oxygen, beta-blockers, and diuretics.

## Percutaneous balloon valvuloplasty

This procedure can be used as a bridge to aortic valve replacement in patients too unwell to undergo the procedure. It is advisable to use only in those valves that have no obvious calcification, and no regurgitation. The current quoted mortality rate in non-pregnant patients is 5%. There is obviously considerable risk to the fetus during the procedure as the fetal circulation is transiently occluded. If significant aortic regurgitation (AR) results from the procedure, emergency surgical aortic valve replacement is necessary.

## Surgical management

Patients with calcific aortic valves or with significant AR are best treated with an aortic valve replacement. In women of childbearing age, a bioprosthetic valve would be advisable as the need for anticoagulation is obviated. However, cardiopulmonary bypass during pregnancy carries a mortality of up to 15%, and a risk of fetal loss of 30% [80].

## Delivery

Vaginal delivery is suggested. However, in women with moderate-severe AS, caesarean section may need to be considered. Careful fluid balance and protection against vasodilatation are advised in order to avoid perilous BP drops that may compromise cardiac output. High-dependency care is essential for 48 hours post-delivery [75].

# Aortic regurgitation

Acute AR may be seen in aortic dissection, infective endocarditis, or prosthetic valve malfunction. Marfan's syndrome, bicuspid aortic valve, and hypertension are conditions that predispose to aortic dissection. Acute AR is a surgical emergency. Meticulous fluid balance and an urgent cardiothoracic opinion are essential. Patients may present with pulmonary oedema and cardiogenic shock as the ventricle has no time to adapt to the sudden increase in LV volume overload.

Chronic AR like MR, and well tolerated in pregnancy. It is usually seen in the presence of a bicuspid aortic valve or rheumatic heart disease. The peripheral vasodilatation of pregnancy helps to offload the overloaded left ventricle by reducing the volume of regurgitant blood.

Patients with AR and LV dilatation, present with dyspnoea, exertional fatigue and chest pain (WHO III/IV). If there is a significant degree of systolic dysfunction (NYHA II or III), the pregnancy may not be well tolerated.

## Management

Angiotensin-converting enzyme inhibitors are contraindicated throughout pregnancy so alternative vasodilating agents including nifedipine, nitrates, diuretics, and hydralazine should be used. Careful echocardiographic monitoring during pregnancy is recommended [75].

# Pulmonary valve disease

The most common problem is pulmonary stenosis and is often associated with Noonan's syndrome or tetralogy of Fallot. Patients become symptomatic with moderate or severe stenosis. Pregnancy is generally well tolerated in those with mild pulmonary stenosis, but even severe pulmonary stenosis with good right ventricular function may be well tolerated.

Echocardiographic surveillance is important. If the right ventricular function begins to suffer during pregnancy, then percutaneous balloon valvotomy can be performed from the second trimester [74].

Non-cardiac complications including hypertensive disorders, prematurity, and thromboembolic complications have been reported.

It should be remembered, that like in congenital aortic stenosis, there is a considerable risk of the fetus being affected (20%).

## Tricuspid valve disease

Tricuspid regurgitation (TR) is usually a result of endocarditis-related damage or related to Ebstein's anomaly [low-seated tricuspid valve, atrial septal defect (ASD), and TR]. Patients with Ebstein's anomaly should be assessed prior to conception and treated for the presence of abnormal conduction pathways causing tachyarrhythmias. TR is usually well-tolerated and unless associated with RV dilatation and dysfunction is associated with low-risk pregnancy.

Tricuspid stenosis (TS) is very rare and usually congenital. TS is often part of more complex underlying disease and should be managed in a specialist centre [74].

## Prosthetic valves

Prosthetic valves are used to treat patients with either congenital or acquired valve lesions and may be mechanical [require anticoagulation with vitamin K antagonists (VKAs) such as warfarin] or tissue/bioprostheses (porcine/bovine pericardium). The management of anticoagulation during pregnancy is problematic and without a clear evidence-base. Bioprostheses are most likely the best solution in women of childbearing age. Nevertheless, pregnancy with bioprosthetic valves is not completely risk-free and still renders the pregnancy in WHO II category [69]. Whilst bioprostheses do not have the longevity of mechanical prostheses, the elimination of the need for anticoagulation reduces both maternal and fetal risk. The deterioration of bioprostheses is mildly exacerbated by pregnancy (15 years vs. 13.5 years) [81]. Pregnancy with mechanical heart valve falls into WHO III, where pregnancy carries a significant risk of maternal mortality or severe morbidity.

Pre-pregnancy counselling is essential for women with mechanical and tissue prosthetic valves to discuss the risks to mother and fetus and the plans for anticoagulation during the pregnancy. Pregnancy is a pro-thrombotic state not only due to venous stasis because of the pressure of the pregnant uterus on the venous circulation but also because of the increased levels of thrombogenic factors. The risk of venous thromboembolism is five times higher in pregnancy than in the non-pregnant population [82]. Warfarin, a VKA, crosses the placenta and is associated with embryopathy, especially when used in the first 6–12 weeks. Metallic valves require warfarin anticoagulation. The risk factors for thromboembolism of prosthetic valves in pregnancy are shown in **Box 4.6**. Discussions should be had at the time of valve replacement when the consideration of bioprosthetic valves should be stressed in women of child-bearing age.

For patients with mechanical valves, the safest option for the mother seems to be to maintain warfarin therapy throughout pregnancy, with an elective caesarean section to reduce time off warfarin.

---

**Box 4.6 Risk factors for thromboembolism of prosthetic valves in pregnancy**

- Valve type – Bjork–Shiley
- Valve position – mitral valve
- Left atrial dilatation
- Additional arrhythmias – AF
- Previous thromboembolism
- Inadequate anticoagulation

---

**Table 4.6 Rates of thromboembolism and death with differing anticoagulant strategies in prosthetic heart valve pregnancy [88]**

| Anticoagulant strategy during pregnancy | Rate of thromboembolism (%) | Rate of maternal death (%) |
|---|---|---|
| Warfarin throughout | 3.9 | 1.8 |
| Heparin for first trimester, subsequent warfarin | 9.2 | 4.2 |
| Dose-adjusted heparin throughout | 25 | 7 |

There is still some discussion as to when to restart warfarin post-partum. Some suggest that it should be restarted immediately post-partum, and others at day 10, when the risk of post-partum haemorrhage is significantly lowered. Warfarin and both forms of heparin are safe in breastfeeding.

The risk of fetal anomalies with this strategy would be in the range of about 6%. These include nasal and musculoskeletal hypoplasia, mental impairment, chondrodysplasia punctata, epithelial, and central nervous system abnormalities. There is also an increased risk of fetal haemorrhage as warfarin crosses the placenta. The critical time for warfarin embryopathy is between 6 and 12 weeks of gestation [83,84].

With this strategy, the maternal thromboembolism risk is estimated to be 3.9%, with a risk of death of 1.8%. Interestingly, warfarin embryopathy seems to be dose-related: the critical level being 5 mg. The European Society of Cardiology (ESC) [37] and American Heart Association (AHA)/American College of Cardiology (ACC) guidance [77] suggest continuing warfarin throughout pregnancy if the dose required is <5 mg/day. If the dose required for adequate anticoagulation is higher than 5 mg, then the suggestion is to replace warfarin with LMWH between 6 and12 weeks, the time of embryogenesis. However, at least half of valve thromboses occur in this vulnerable time [85] and even low dose warfarin is associated with fetal mortality in some studies [86]. **Table 4.6** shows the spread of thromboembolism rates with differing anticoagulation strategies.

Further discussion is necessary to plan anticoagulation from 36 weeks of gestation, as some women may prefer to use LMWH versus warfarin 2 weeks before anticipated delivery.

Other alternatives include heparin (LMWH – twice daily) plus aspirin between 6–12 weeks of gestation, converting to warfarin from the second trimester. With this strategy, the maternal thromboembolism risk increased to 9.2%, with a risk of death of 4.2% [87].

The use of dose-adjusted heparin alone for the duration of the pregnancy was linked to a maternal thromboembolism risk of 25%, with a risk of death of 7%.

There is insufficient data on the use of LMWH in this situation although it is known that there is a lower risk of maternal heparin-induced thrombocytopoenia and osteopoenia. In addition, LMWH is associated with low neonatal mortality, and low rates of spontaneous abortion and intrauterine death.

The AHA/ACC recommends aspirin 75–100 mg daily in association with warfarin during the second and third trimester [77]. Compliance with whichever anticoagulant strategy is chosen is essential.

## Complications during pregnancy

Prosthetic valve thrombosis can be life-threatening. The risk of prosthetic valve thrombosis is higher in women with older mechanical valves (i.e. ball and cage valves), with mechanical valves in the mitral position, with >1 mechanical valve and when the valve is not working normally. An accurate and speedy diagnosis is key. The symptoms on presentation can include acute shortness of breath, pulmonary oedema, arrhythmia, or it can present as an acute thromboembolic event. The mechanical heart sounds may sound muffled. The investigation of choice should include urgent echocardiography or fluoroscopy (with lead shielding of the fetus). Management should involve a cardiologist and obstetrician and be akin to that of a non-pregnant patient [88]. Management ranges from medical therapy with intravenous heparin for a small thrombus burden, to fibrinolysis and surgical intervention, in acute life-threatening prosthetic valve thrombosis. Fibrinolytics (low-dose tPA) do not cross the placenta but do increase the risk of peri-partum and placental bleeding [88].

## Endocarditis

Infective endocarditis is rare in pregnancy affecting 1 per 100,000 pregnancies. Care should be managed by a multidisciplinary team of cardiologists, microbiologists and obstetricians, with special care taken to ensure that the antibiotics are safe in pregnancy and not associated with teratogenicity [89].

## CONGENITAL HEART DISEASE

About 1% of all livebirths will have some form of congenital heart disease. With improving and focussed healthcare, 85% of infants with congenital heart disease will survive into adulthood. Congenital heart disease ranges from relatively simple lesions (i.e. ASDs) to moderate (i.e. tetralogy of Fallot) to complex congenital heart disease (i.e. transposition of the great arteries).

For women with congenital heart disease, there is a risk varying between 3 and 12% of the fetus having a similar structural cardiac defect [90]. Therefore, specialist fetal ultrasound scanning should be mandatory at 14–16 weeks and may need to be repeated at 18–22 weeks. If the nuchal fold thickness is normal on a scan, it suggests a significantly lower incidence of CHD (1 in 1,000) [90].

As with patients with valvular heart disease, all patients with congenital heart disease should be counselled pre-pregnancy. Predictors of poor outcome are shown in **Box 4.7**. Effective discussions regarding contraception should take place in those in whom pregnancy is classed as high risk [91]. The modified WHO risk scores for congenital heart disease are shown in **Table 4.7**.

## Box 4.7 Predictors of poor outcome in simple congenital heart disease and pregnancy

- Pulmonary hypertension
- Severe systemic ventricular impairment (EF < 30%)
- Moderate systemic right ventricular dysfunction
- Severe left-sided outflow tract obstruction
- Severe symptomatic aortic stenosis
- Severe mitral stenosis
- Severe aortic root dilatation (>50 mm)
- Severe coarctation
- Severe tricuspid regurgitation
- Severe right ventricular dysfunction
- Marfan's syndrome with a dilated root (>45 mm)

### Table 4.7 Modified WHO risk score for congenital heart disease

| WHO risk score | Interpretation | Congenital heart disease |
|---|---|---|
| 1 | Pregnancy carries the same risk as the general population | • Mild pulmonary stenosis<br>• Small patent ductus arteriosus (PDA)<br>• Repaired ASD, VSD, and PDA |
| 2 | Pregnancy carries a small increased risk of mortality and morbidity | • Unrepaired ASD and VSD<br>• Repaired tetralogy of Fallot<br>• Turner syndrome without aortic root dilatation<br>• Mild LV impairment |
| 2–3 | Pregnancy carries a moderately increased risk of mortality and morbidity | • Marfan syndrome without aortic root dilatation<br>• Repaired coarctation without aneurysm<br>• Atrioventricular septal defect |
| 3 | Pregnancy carries a significantly increased risk: Expert obstetric and cardiology care required | • Mechanical valve<br>• Systemic right ventricle (transposition of great arteries – TGA, tetralogy of Fallot – ToF)<br>• Fontan/Single ventricle physiology<br>• Unrepaired cyanotic disease<br>• Moderate aortic dilatation |
| 4 | Pregnancy carries a very high risk of maternal morbidity and mortality and is contraindicated. Termination of pregnancy should be discussed. If pregnancy continues, then care should be as for Level 3 | • Pulmonary arterial hypertension (any cause)<br>• Severe LV dysfunction (EF < 30%)<br>• Ehlers–Danlos type IV<br>• Severe/Unrepaired coarctation<br>• Fontan with any complication |

ASD, atrial septal defect; EF, ejection fraction; LV, left ventricular; VSD, ventricular septal defect.

## Aortopathy

This term encompasses several conditions that predispose to aortic dissection, aneurysm formation, and rupture, including Marfan syndrome, Loeys–Dietz syndrome, Ehlers–Danlos type IV, and Turner syndrome, bicuspid aortic valve, and previous coarctation repair. Dissection can occur in pregnancy due to the hormonal effects of pregnancy on the

| Table 4.8 Relationship between aortic dimension and maternal risk of dissection | |
|---|---|
| Aorta size in mm | Maternal risk of dissection |
| <40 mm | 1% |
| >40 mm | 10% |

connective tissue of the aorta wall [92]. **Table 4.8** shows the relationship between aortic dimensions and risk of maternal dissection.

## Pre-pregnancy assessment

The aorta and dimensions should have been evaluated with echocardiography or CT/MRI within a year prior to conception. In those with high-risk dimensions, there should be consideration of elective aortic surgery, pre-pregnancy.

## Pregnancy management

Serial imaging of the aorta should be performed in each trimester and then until 6 months post-partum. BP management is imperative and should include beta-blocker therapy.

Rapid expansion of the aortic root may be grounds for termination of pregnancy (>5 mm), or early delivery if the fetus is viable.

## Delivery

A clear plan should be made, taking into consideration the risk of aortic dissection/rupture. Caesarean delivery should be considered, although in some cases a normal delivery can be planned with a shortened second stage. High-risk cases should be delivered in a centre with cardiothoracic surgery [92].

## Marfan's syndrome

There are over 2,000 women in the UK with Marfan's syndrome. The main risk during pregnancy is type A dissection, which is associated with a maternal mortality of 22%. It classically occurs in the third trimester or immediately post-partum, when wall stress of the aorta is maximal [93].

The Marfan patient with none of high-risk features shown in **Box 4.8** still has a 1% risk of pregnancy-related complications. A healthy UK woman has a 1 in 10,000 risk.

## Management

Patients with Marfan's syndrome should be treated with beta-blockers with regular fetal scanning to assess for intra-uterine growth retardation. An elective transthoracic echo should be performed between 6 and 10 weeks of gestation, followed by 4–6 weekly scans if the aorta is equal to or over 40 mm. MRI scanning can be used if further imaging is required.

## Delivery

Elective caesarean sections are suggested for high risk Marfan patients, especially those with an aorta over 45-mm diameter (ESC). However, some suggest a natural delivery advocating a short second stage of labour.

> **Box 4.8 High risk features for Marfan pregnancies**
> - Family history of sudden death
> - Aorta >40-mm diameter
> - Rapid rate of aortic dilatation

## Aortic dissection

Dissection can occur in pregnancy without pre-existing disease due to the hormonal effects of pregnancy on the connective tissue of the aorta wall.

Patients with bicuspid aortic valves have an increased risk of aortic dissection in pregnancy. Marfan's syndrome, bicuspid aortic valve, and hypertension are conditions that predispose to aortic dissection. Acute dissection is a surgical emergency. Patients present with pulmonary oedema and cardiogenic shock as the ventricle has no time to adapt to the sudden increase in LV volume overload.

## Management and delivery

As this is usually an emergency presentation, management will depend on the viability of the fetus. Emergency caesarean section and surgical aortic root correction are usually necessary [94].

## Coarctation

Most women with coarctation will have had a repair fashioned. MRI can be used to accurately assess the site of repair and to check for re-coarctation or aneurysm formation safely during pregnancy. Pregnancy is classed as low risk as long as there is no aneurysm at the repair site [95].

## Management

Beta-blockers can control BP well. The target BP should be equal to or lower than 130/80. Stenting of the coarctation is not recommended during pregnancy as there is a high risk of dissection at this time.

## Delivery

Normal delivery is fine, as long as the second stage is assisted and not prolonged. In the presence of an aneurysm, an elective caesarean section should be performed.

If a patient presents with a newly diagnosed coarctation, BP should be aggressively lowered with beta-blockers and delivery organised at 35 weeks, by elective caesarean section.

## Septal defects

### Atrial septal defect/patent foramen ovale

In the presence of a small shunt with normal pulmonary pressures, pregnancy is usually well tolerated.

Problems can occur due to paradoxical emboli, as pregnancy itself is a procoagulant state (five-fold increased risk of thromboembolism) and the presence of an arterial-venous connection facilitates the passage of thrombus.

With a more significant shunt, the concern is similarly for paradoxical emboli but also right ventricular dilatation and right heart failure. Serial echocardiography, each trimester should be used for monitoring the right heart dimensions and function [90].

## Management

As a result, compression stockings and prophylactic heparin should be used in late pregnancy. Device closure of the ASD should be considered prior to conception. Antibiotic prophylaxis is not necessary for delivery. Normal delivery should be the preference unless there is significant elevation of pulmonary pressures.

## Ventricular septal defect/patent ductus arteriosus

A small defect is generally better tolerated than ASDs as the pressure gradient across the ventricular septal defect (VSD) does not allow the passage of paradoxical emboli. However, there is a risk of infective endocarditis, so prophylactic antibiotics should be considered for instrumented or complicated deliveries [90].

# COMPLEX CONGENITAL HEART DISEASE

Counselling, contraception, and risk prediction should be discussed pre-pregnancy, and really as soon as the woman acquires reproductive ability. Several risk scores for pregnancy are available [Cardiac Disease in Pregnancy Risk Score (CARPREG), Zwangerschap bij Aangeboren Hartafwijking (ZAHARA), and WHO Classification]. The WHO classification has been shown to be the most helpful in women with congenital heart disease [96,97]. The essential investigations are shown in **Box 4.9**.

There are certain features in the patient history (shown in **Box 4.10**) that should be assessed in the pre-pregnant state and that gives an indication for increased risk and the need for further assessment.

## Repaired tetralogy of fallot

In the presence of good LV function and no significant RV outflow tract obstruction, pregnancy is well tolerated. Even with significant pulmonary regurgitation, pregnancy is

---

**Box 4.9 Pre-pregnancy investigations**

- History
- Physical examination
- Electrocardiogram (ECG)
- Echocardiogram
- Exercise ECG

---

**Box 4.10 Pre-pregnancy high-risk features in history**

- Reduced exercise capacity
- Symptoms of heart failure
- Palpitations
- Family history of sudden death or aortic dissection

generally trouble free apart from an increase in complaints of fatigue and breathlessness. However, significant impairment of LV function, implies high risk, and delivery should be by elective caesarean section, with avoidance of labour.

## Congenitally corrected transposition of the great arteries

Transposition of the great arteries occurs when the pulmonary artery and aorta are switched. The pulmonary artery is then connected to the left ventricle and the aorta to the right ventricle. This results in oxygenated blood returning to the lungs and not to the rest of the body. In congenitally corrected transposition of the great arteries (CCTGA), the AV node is absent and hence complete heart block can occur at any time. Patients with complete heart block should have a pacemaker implanted prior to conception [98].

Generally, pregnancy is well tolerated if the patient is symptom free prior to pregnancy. The systemic tricuspid valve may become more regurgitant during pregnancy due to the dilatation of the systemic ventricle (morphologically right ventricle). Furthermore, the systemic ventricle can easily fail with the significant haemodynamic demands of pregnancy. Delivery should then be by elective caesarean section.

## Transposition of the great arteries

The Mustard or Senning repair comprises an atrial rerouting, so that the tricuspid valve and right ventricle support the systemic circulation. Pregnancy is tolerated similarly to those with CCTGA, although the risk of CHB is less as the AV node is intact. However, the extensive scar tissue can lead to sinus node disease with its resultant atrial arrhythmias. The patients who undergo arterial switch procedures are at risk of myocardial ischaemia as the coronary arteries are reimplanted as part of the switch procedure [99].

Pulmonary venous pathways should be imaged pre-pregnancy by transoesophageal echocardiography or MRI scanning. It is important to demonstrate no obstruction as any obstruction produces a clinical presentation similar to severe mitral stenosis in the pregnant patient.

In the presence of good systemic ventricular function (EF > 40%), symptoms of NYHA class II or less, and unobstructed pulmonary venous pathways, pregnancy is classed as low risk [98,100].

## Fontan

In congenital heart disease with a single ventricle, both the systemic and pulmonary circulations are maintained by the single ventricle. This results in significant arterial desaturation and volume overload of the single ventricle.

In a Fontan circulation, the systemic venous return is connected to the pulmonary arteries, without connection to a ventricle. For patients with a functional single ventricle, the Fontan procedure creates two separate circulations in series. The patients are therefore, oxygenated and no longer cyanotic. The ventricle supports only the systemic circulation, so there is a propensity to low output states. The pulmonary circulation is not facilitated by a ventricular pump resulting in free drainage of venous blood into the pulmonary artery without pulsatile flow. However, certain problems ensue due to this novel circulation [99,101] (**Box 4.11**).

As a result, patients are anti-coagulated with warfarin long term. If ventricular function is good and patients are in NYHA I-II, pregnancy is not contraindicated. However, there is still a 30% risk of fetal loss in the first trimester.

> **Box 4.11 The Fontan circulatory problems in pregnancy**
>
> - Limited ability to increase cardiac output
> - Atrial arrhythmias
> - Prothrombotic circulation

> **Box 4.12 Conditions particularly relevant to the cyanotic patient during pregnancy**
>
> - Haemorrhage – due to impaired clotting factors and reduced platelet function
> - Paradoxical embolism – because of right to left shunt
> - Heart failure – as a result of pregnancy volume loading on an already overloaded ventricle
> - Increased cyanosis – because of the vasodilatation of pregnancy
> - Fetal loss – particularly if oxygen saturation below 85%

Fontan patients with impaired ventricular function, severe atrioventricular regurgitation or protein-losing enteropathy should be counselled against pregnancy [37,102].

## Delivery

Normal delivery is possible but meticulous planning and close supervision of labour is mandatory. Emergency caesarean section is often required [103].

## Cyanotic heart disease without pulmonary hypertension

Cyanotic heart disease may exist in the presence of uncorrected or persisting shunts. The fetal circulation is dependent on maternal oxygen saturation. Maternal saturations below 85% are associated with a 12% chance of fetal survival. Maternal saturations over 90% are associated with a 92% chance of fetal survival [104]. The underlying maternal cardiac lesion will predict the maternal and fetal risk.

The cyanotic patient is at increased risk of a number of problems during pregnancy (**Box 4.12**).

## Management

This should include prolonged bed rest, which will result in increased maternal oxygenation, and subsequent increased fetal survival. Pregnancy in women with oxygen saturations below 85% should be discouraged.

## Delivery

Normal delivery should be attempted, if possible, but there are often fetal problems that necessitate a caesarean section.

## Eisenmenger's syndrome

Over the last 40 years, the maternal mortality from Eisenmenger's syndrome has remained at 40%. No single medical or obstetric intervention has changed the excessively high level of mortality associated with this condition. Currently, the only treatment possible is heart transplantation. Patients with Eisenmenger's syndrome need to be fully informed of the increased risk of death both ante and post-partum and also the risk of severe morbidity. Sterilisation (using an irreversible method such as tubal ligation) or termination should be advised with this level of risk. If pregnancy is chosen, strict bed rest for the third trimester is essential. In addition, patients should be monitored in hospital for at least 2 weeks post-partum due to the on-going risk of sudden death [105].

### Fetal outcomes

The fetal and perinatal mortality rates associated with mothers with significant PH are approximately 30%. One third of infants born suffer from IUGR and only 25% of pregnancies reach term.

## Pulmonary hypertension

Pulmonary hypertension is defined as a mean pulmonary artery systolic pressure of over 25 mmHg. PH in pregnancy is associated with an extremely poor prognosis, classified as WHO-IV with a maternal mortality of 20–30%. The best prognosis is seen in idiopathic PH, receiving therapy: the mortality is 9%. Patients with PH should be advised not to consider pregnancy [106].

### Management

In patients stable on calcium channel blocker therapy, there is a relatively good prognosis. Pulmonary vasodilator therapy used pre-pregnancy should be continued during pregnancy, except for endothelin-receptor antagonists (ERAs – bosentan, macitentan, and ambrisentan) that are teratogenic. ERAs should be replaced by sildenafil and/or prostacyclin derivatives. Due to the high-risk nature of these patients, they should be managed in a specialist centre throughout pregnancy.

### Delivery

Delivery should be by caesarean section, with epidural/spinal anaesthesia as general anaesthetic agents reduce RV contractility, and laryngoscopy and positive pressure ventilation increase PVR leading to increased likelihood of RV failure [106].

## MEDICATIONS IN PREGNANCY

There is understandably, a limited evidence base of which medications are safe in pregnancy and breastfeeding. Therefore, evidence is garnered from animal studies and limited experience in humans. **Table 4.9** shows the current best evidence-based guidance for a variety of medications including, anti-hypertensives, anticoagulant, and anti-arrhythmics in addition to medications for patients presenting with ACSs [48,77,88,93,99,107]. The FDA Drug Classification is shown in **Table 4.10**.

### Final thoughts

Pregnancy is a very natural process and as we continue to make huge strides in human development, we are pushing the boundaries of human ability. But it is also the highest risk period in any woman's life. We should not shy away from the fact that some risk is too great to take, and these difficult conversations must be had. Most cardiac conditions can support pregnancy and as cardiologists, obstetricians, and obstetric anaesthetists, it is important that we work collaboratively to make every pregnancy as safe and supported as possible.

**Table 4.9 Safety of cardiac medications in pregnancy and breastfeeding.** *Continues on pages 91–92*

| Drug category | Examples | FDA pregnancy category | Adverse effects/ concerns during pregnancy | Suggested precautions | Breast-feeding |
|---|---|---|---|---|---|
| **Anti-hypertensives** | | | | | |
| Alpha-adrenergic inhibitors | Methyldopa | B | Induction of positive Coombs test | Stop immediately post-partum as high risk of postnatal depression | Yes |
| | Clonidine | C | Rare neonatal hypertension | | Probably |
| Angiotensin II receptor blockers (ARBs) | Losartan | D | Teratogenicity and fetal death | Stop immediately in pregnancy | No |
| | Valsartan | D | Teratogenicity and fetal death | Stop immediately in pregnancy | |
| Angiotensin-converting enzyme (ACE) inhibitors | Enalapril | D | Teratogenicity and fetal death | Stop immediately in pregnancy | Yes |
| | Captopril | D | Teratogenicity and fetal death | Stop immediately in pregnancy | |
| | Lisinopril | D | Teratogenicity and fetal death | Stop immediately in pregnancy | |
| Beta-blockers | Metoprolol | C | Fetal IUGR | Regular fetal growth scans | Preferred |
| | Propranolol | C | Fetal IUGR | Regular fetal growth scans | Preferred |
| | Carvedilol | C | Fetal IUGR | Regular fetal growth scans | Yes |
| | Bisoprolol | C | Fetal IUGR | Regular fetal growth scans | Yes |
| | Atenolol | D | Teratogenicity | Avoid | No |
| Combined alpha and beta blockers | Labetalol | C | Requires up to QDS dosing | Nil | Yes |
| Calcium-channel blockers | Nifedipine | C | | Caution if used with magnesium sulphate | Yes |
| | Verapamil | C | | | Yes |
| | Diltiazem | C | Teratogenicity | | Yes |
| Vasodilators | Hydralazine | C | | | Yes |
| | Nitroprusside | B | Possible transient fetal bradycardia | | Unknown |
| | Sildenafil | B | | | Unknown |

| | | Table 4.9 *Continued* | | | |
|---|---|---|---|---|---|
| Drug category | Examples | FDA pregnancy category | Adverse effects/ concerns during pregnancy | Suggested precautions | Breast-feeding |
| **Diuretics** | | | | | |
| | Furosemide | C | Possible association with neonatal PDA and sensorineural hearing loss | Maternal electrolyte monitoring | No |
| | Hydrochlorothiazide | C | Possible increased risk of neonatal hypoglycaemia and thrombocytopaenia reported | Neonatal bloods include FBC and electrolytes | |
| | Spironolactone | C | None reported | | Probably but not recom-mended |
| Anticoagulants | Warfarin | X | • Embryopathy with fetal warfarin syndrome at doses over 5 mg. <br>• Maternal risk of haemorrhage at delivery or anaesthesia | Fetal scan at 18–20 weeks | Yes |
| | Heparin UFH and LMWH | C | Potential risk of maternal osteoporosis, heparin-induced thrombocytopaenia and bleeding | Consider peri-delivery with mode of delivery | Yes |
| | Aspirin | B | Premature closure of PDA | Low dose probably acceptable | |
| | Clopidogrel | B | Premature closure of PDA | Discontinue 7 days pre-delivery | Unknown |
| Direct thrombin inhibitors | Dabigatran | B | Teratogenic in animal studies and theoretical risk of maternal haemorrhage | | Unknown |
| Direct factor Xa inhibitors | Rivaroxaban | C | Teratogenic in animal studies and theoretical risk of maternal haemorrhage | | Unknown |
| **Fibrinolytics** | Streptokinase | C | Increased maternal risk and risk of placental bleeding | | Unknown |

## Table 4.9 *Continued*

| Drug category | Examples | FDA pregnancy category | Adverse effects/ concerns during pregnancy | Suggested precautions | Breast-feeding |
|---|---|---|---|---|---|
| | Tissue plasminogen activator | C | Increased maternal risk and risk of placental bleeding | | Unknown |
| Inotropic agents | Digoxin | C | None reported | | Yes |
| | Epinephrine | C | | | Unknown |
| | Norepinephrine | C | | | Unknown |
| | Dopamine | C | | | Probably |
| Anti-arrhythmics | | | | | |
| Beta-blockers | Metoprolol | C | Fetal IUGR | Serial fetal growth scans | Yes |
| | Propranolol | C | Fetal IUGR | Serial fetal growth scans | Yes |
| | Carvedilol | C | Fetal IUGR | Serial fetal growth scans | Yes |
| | Bisoprolol | C | Fetal IUGR | Serial fetal growth scans | Yes |
| | Atenolol | D | Fetal IUGR and bradycardia | | NO |
| Class 1A | Quinidine | C | None reported | | Yes |
| | Procainamide | C | None reported | | Yes |
| Class 1C | Flecainide | C | None reported | | Yes |
| Class III | Sotalol | B | | | No |
| | Amiodarone | D | Thyroid dysfunction | | No |
| Purine nucleosides | Adenosine | C | | | |

IUGR, intrauterine growth restriction; PDA, patent ductus arteriosus.

## Table 4.10 FDA drug classification

| A | No evidence of risk to fetus in controlled studies of women |
|---|---|
| B | Animal studies may not have shown risk, but no studies in women |
| C | Animal studies may have demonstrated risk so drugs should be given only if benefit outweighs risk to the fetus |
| D | Confirmed evidence of fetal risk but benefits in pregnant women may be acceptable, in certain scenarios (life-threatening conditions/no other drug available) |
| X | Confirmed evidence of fetal risk in human and animal studies. The drug is contraindicated in women who are or may become pregnant |

FDA, Food and Drug Administration.

# REFERENCES

1.	Knight M, Bunch K, Tuffnell D, et al. (2020). Saving Lives, Improving Mothers' Care Maternal, Newborn and Infant Clinical Outcome Review Programme. [online] Available from: www.hqip.org.uk/national-programmes [Last accessed May, 2022].

2.	Laopaiboon M, Lumbiganon P, Intarut N, et al. Advanced maternal age and pregnancy outcomes: a multicountry assessment. BJOG 2014; 121:49–56.

3.	Jamal A, King BA, Neff LJ, et al. Current cigarette smoking among adults—United States, 2005–2015. MMWR Morb Morta Wkly Rep 2016; 65:1205–1212.

4.	Creamer MR, Wang TW, Babb S, et al. Tobacco product use and cessation indicators among adults — United States, 2018. MMWR Morb Mortal Wkly Rep 2019; 68:1013–1019.

5.	Albrecht SS, Kuklina EV, Bansil P, et al. Diabetes trends among delivery hospitalizations in the U.S., 1994-2004. Diabetes Care 2010; 33:768–773.

6.	Kuklina EV, Ayala C, Callaghan WM. Hypertensive disorders and severe obstetric morbidity in the United States. Obstet Gynecol 2009; 113:1299–1306.

7.	Fisher SC, Kim SY, Sharma AJ, et al. Is obesity still increasing among pregnant women? Prepregnancy obesity trends in 20 states, 2003–2009. Prevent Med 2013; 56:72–78.

8.	Hinkle SN, Sharma AJ, Kim SY, et al. Prepregnancy obesity trends among low-income women, United States, 1999–2008. Matern Child Health J 2012; 16:1339–1348.

9.	Johnson M, von Klemperer K. Cardiovascular changes in normal pregnancy. In: Steer SJ, Gatzoulis MA (Eds). Heart Disease and Pregnancy. Cambridge: Cambridge University Press; 2016. pp. 19–28.

10.	Capeless EL, Clapp JF. Cardiovascular changes in early phase of pregnancy. Am J Obstet Gynecol 1989; 161:1449–1453.

11.	Duvekot JJ, Cheriex EC, Pieters FAA, et al. Early pregnancy changes in hemodynamics and volume homeostasis are consecutive adjustments triggered by a primary fall in systemic vascular tone. Am J Obstet Gynecol 1993; 169:1382–1392.

12.	Meah VL, Cockcroft JR, Backx K, et al. Cardiac output and related haemodynamics during pregnancy: a series of meta-analyses. Heart 2016; 102:518–526.

13.	Sanghavi M, Rutherford JD. Cardiovascular physiology of pregnancy. Circulation 2014; 130:1003–1008.

14.	Robson SC, Hunter S, Boys RJ, et al. Serial study of factors influencing changes in cardiac output during human pregnancy. American J Physiol Heart Circ Physiol 1989; 256:H1060–H1065.

15.	Hunter S, Robson SC. Adaptation of the maternal heart in pregnancy. Heart 1992; 68:540–543.

16.	Mahendru AA, Everett TR, Wilkinson IB, et al. A longitudinal study of maternal cardiovascular function from preconception to the postpartum period. J Hypertens 2014; 32:849–856.

17.	Sunitha M. Electrocradiographic QRS Axis, Q Wave and T-wave Changes in 2nd and 3rd Trimester of Normal Pregnancy. J Clin Diagn Res 2014; 8:BC17–BC21.

18.	NICE. Hypertension in pregnancy: diagnosis and management NICE guideline [NG133]. 2019.

19.	Magee LA, Ornstein MP, von Dadelszen P. Management of hypertension in pregnancy. BMJ 1999; 318:1332–1336.

20.	Behrens I, Basit S, Melbye M, et al. Risk of post-pregnancy hypertension in women with a history of hypertensive disorders of pregnancy: Nationwide Cohort Study. BMJ 2017; 358:j3078.

21.	Bramham K, Nelson-Piercy C, Brown MJ, et al. Postpartum management of hypertension. BMJ 2013; 346:f894.

22.	Ayoubi. Pre-eclampsia: pathophysiology, diagnosis, and management. Vascular Health and Risk Management. 2011; 7:467–474.

23.	Duley L. The Global Impact of Pre-eclampsia and Eclampsia. Semin Perinatol 2009; 33130–33137.

24.	Duley L, Gülmezoglu AM, Henderson-Smart DJ. Magnesium sulphate and other anticonvulsants for women with pre-eclampsia. In: Duley L (Ed). Cochrane Database of Systematic Reviews. Chichester, UK: John Wiley & Sons, Ltd; 2003.

25.	Hernandez-Diaz S, Toh S, Cnattingius S. Risk of pre-eclampsia in first and subsequent pregnancies: prospective cohort study. BMJ 2009; 338:b2255.

26.	Bellamy L, Casas JP, Hingorani AD, et al. Pre-eclampsia and risk of cardiovascular disease and cancer in later life: systematic review and meta-analysis. BMJ 2007; 335:974.

27.	Skjaerven R, Wilcox AJ, Klungsoyr K, et al. Cardiovascular mortality after pre-eclampsia in one child mothers: prospective, population based cohort study. BMJ 2012; 345:e7677.

28.	Trivedi N. A meta-analysis of low-dose aspirin for prevention of preeclampsia. J Postgrad Med 2011; 57:91–95.

29. Rolnik DL, Wright D, Poon LC, et al. Aspirin versus Placebo in Pregnancies at High Risk for Preterm Preeclampsia. N Eng J Med 2017; 377:613–622.

30. Hoffman MK, Goudar SS, Kodkany BS, et al. Low-dose aspirin for the prevention of preterm delivery in nulliparous women with a singleton pregnancy (ASPIRIN): a randomised, ouble-blind, placebo-controlled trial. Lancet 2020; 395:285–293.

31. Adamson DL, Nelson-Piercy C. Managing palpitations and arrhythmias during pregnancy. Postgrad Med J 2008; 84:17584280.

32. Shotan A, Ostrzega E, Mehra A, et al. Incidence of Arrhythmias in Normal Pregnancy and Relation to Palpitations, Dizziness, and Syncope. Am J Cardiol. 1997; 79:1061–1064.

33. Tawam M, Levine J, Mendelson M, et al. Effect of pregnancy on paroxysmal supraventricular tachycardia. Am J Cardiol 1993; 72:838–840.

34. Shih-Huang L, Shih-Ann C, Tsu-Juey W, et al. Effects of pregnancy on first onset and symptoms of paroxysmal supraventricular tachycardia. Am J Cardiol 1995; 76:675–678.

35. Elkayam U, Goodwin TM. Adenosine therapy for supraventricular tachycardia during pregnancy. Am J Cardiol 1995; 75:521–523.

36. Silversides CK, Harris L, Haberer K, et al. Recurrence Rates of Arrhythmias During Pregnancy in Women With Previous Tachyarrhythmia and Impact on Fetal and Neonatal Outcomes. The American J Cardiol 2006; 97:1206–1212.

37. Regitz-Zagrosek V, Roos-Hesselink JW, Bauersachs J, et al. 2018 ESC Guidelines for the management of cardiovascular diseases during pregnancy. Euro Heart J 2018; 39:3165–3241.

38. Emmanuel Y, Thorne SA. Heart disease in pregnancy. Best Prac Res Clin Obstet Gynaecol 2015; 29:579–597.

39. Roberts A, Mechery J, Mechery A, et al. Management of palpitations and cardiac arrhythmias in pregnancy. Obstet Gynaecol 2019; 21:263–270.

40. Knotts RJ, Garan H. Cardiac arrhythmias in pregnancy. Semin Perinatol 2014; 38:285–288.

41. Nakagawa M, Katou S, Ichinose M, et al. Characteristics of new-onset ventricular arrhythmias in pregnancy. J Electrocardiol 2004; 37:47–53.

42. Natale A, Davidson T, Geiger MJ, et al. Implantable Cardioverter-Defibrillators and Pregnancy. Circulation. 1997; 96:2808–2812.

43. Rashba EJ, Zareba W, Moss AJ, et al. Influence of Pregnancy on the Risk for Cardiac Events in Patients With Hereditary Long QT Syndrome. Circulation 1998; 97:451–456.

44. Cardiac Risk in the Young. (2022). Drugs to Avoid in Long Qt syndrome. [online] Available from: https://www.sads.org.uk/drugs-to-avoid/ [Last accessed May, 2022].

45. Dalvi BV, Chaudhuri A, Kulkarni HL, et al. Therapeutic guidelines for congenital complete heart block presenting in pregnancy. Obstet Gynaecol 1992; 79:802–804.

46. Abramovici H, Faktor JH, Gonen Y, et al. Maternal permanent bradycardia: Pregnancy and delivery. Obstet Gynaecol 1984; 63:381–383.

47. Webber MD, Halligan RE, Schumacher JA. Acute infarction, intracoronary thrombolysis, and primary PTCA in pregnancy. Cathet Cardiovascr Diagn 1997; 42:38–43.

48. Ramlakhan KP, Johnson MR, Roos-Hesselink JW. Pregnancy and cardiovascular disease. Nat Rev Cardiol 2020; 17:718–31.

49. Paulson RJ, Boostanfar R, Saadat P, et al. Pregnancy in the Sixth Decade of Life. JAMA 2002; 288:2320–2323.

50. Ladner HE, Danielsen B, Gilbert WM. Acute myocardial infarction in pregnancy and the puerperium: A population-based study. Obstetr Gynecol 2005; 105:480–488.

51. James AH, Jamison MG, Biswas MS, et al. Acute myocardial infarction in pregnancy. Circulation 2006; 113:1564–1571.

52. Elkayam U, Jalnapurkar S, Barakkat MN, et al. Pregnancy-associated acute myocardial infarction. Circulation 2014; 129:1695–1702.

53. Roth A, Elkayam U. Acute myocardial infarction associated with pregnancy. J Am Coll Cardiol 2008; 52:171–180.

54. Roos-Hesselink JW, Ruys TPE, Stein JI, et al. Outcome of pregnancy in patients with structural or ischaemic heart disease: results of a registry of the European Society of Cardiology. Euro Heart J 2013; 34:657–665.

55. McKenna WJ, Maron BJ, Thiene G. Classification, epidemiology, and global burden of cardiomyopathies. Circ Res 2017; 121:722–730.

56. Grewal J, Siu SC, Ross HJ, et al. Pregnancy Outcomes in Women With Dilated Cardiomyopathy. J Am Coll Cardiol 2009; 55:45–52.

57. Billebeau G, Etienne M, Cheikh-Khelifa R, et al. Pregnancy in women with a cardiomyopathy: Outcomes and predictors from a retrospective cohort. Arch Cardiovasc Dis 2018; 111:199–209.

58. Sliwa K, Hilfiker-Kleiner D, Petrie MC, et al. Current state of knowledge on aetiology, diagnosis, management, and therapy of peripartum cardiomyopathy: a position statement from the Heart Failure Association of the European Society of Cardiology Working Group on peripartum cardiomyopathy. Euro J Heart Fail 2010; 12:767–778.

59. Fett JD, Christie LG, Carraway RD, et al. Five-Year Prospective Study of the Incidence and Prognosis of Peripartum Cardiomyopathy at a Single Institution. Mayo Clin Proc 2005; 80:1602–1606.

60. Pearson GD, Veille JC, Rahimtoola S, et al. Peripartum Cardiomyopathy. JAMA 2000; 283:1183–1188.

61. Kamiya CA, Kitakaze M, Ishibashi-Ueda H, et al. Different Characteristics of Peripartum Cardiomyopathy Between Patients Complicated With and Without Hypertensive Disorders—Results From the Japanese Nationwide Survey of Peripartum Cardiomyopathy. Circ J 2011; 75:1975–1981.

62. Sliwa K, Mebazaa A, Hilfiker-Kleiner D, et al. Clinical characteristics of patients from the worldwide registry on peripartum cardiomyopathy (PPCM). Euro J Heart Fail 2017; 19:1131–1141.

63. Hilfiker-Kleiner D, Haghikia A, Berliner D, et al. Bromocriptine for the treatment of peripartum cardiomyopathy: a multicentre randomized study. Euro Heart J 2017; 38:2671–2679.

64. Haghikia A, Schwab J, Vogel-Claussen J, et al. Bromocriptine treatment in patients with peripartum cardiomyopathy and right ventricular dysfunction. Clin Res Cardiol 2019; 108:290–927.

65. Duncker D, Westenfeld R, Konrad T, et al. Risk for life-threatening arrhythmia in newly diagnosed peripartum cardiomyopathy with low ejection fraction: a German multi-centre analysis. Clin Res Cardiol 2017; 106:582–589.

66. Schaufelberger M. Cardiomyopathy and pregnancy. Heart 2019; 105:1543–1551.

67. Oakley GD, McGarry K, Limb DG, et al. Management of pregnancy in patients with hypertrophic cardiomyopathy. BMJ 1979; 1:1749–1750.

68. Thaman R, Varnava A, Hamid MS, et al. Pregnancy related complications in women with hypertrophic cardiomyopathy. Heart 2003; 89:752–756.

69. Goland S, van Hagen IM, Elbaz-Greener G, et al. Pregnancy in women with hypertrophic cardiomyopathy: data from the European Society of Cardiology initiated Registry of Pregnancy and Cardiac disease (ROPAC). Eur Heart J 2017; 38:2683–2690.

70. Autore C, Conte MR, Piccininno M, et al. Risk associated with pregnancy in hypertrophic cardiomyopathy. J Am Coll Cardiol 2002; 40:1864–1869.

71. Faksh A, Codsi E, Barsoum M, et al. Pregnancy in Desmin-Related Cardiomyopathy. Ame J Perinatol Rep 2015; 5:e165–167.

72. Gati S, Papadakis M, Papamichael ND, et al. Reversible De Novo Left Ventricular Trabeculations in Pregnant Women. Circulation 2014; 130:475–483.

73. Bauce B, Daliento L, Frigo G, et al. Pregnancy in women with arrhythmogenic right ventricular cardiomyopathy/dysplasia. Eur J Obstet Gynecol Reprod Biol 2006; 127:186–189.

74. Thorne S. Pregnancy and native heart valve disease. Heart 2016; 102:1410–1417.

75. Elkayam U, Goland S, Pieper PG, et al. High-risk cardiac disease in pregnancy. Jo Am Coll Cardiol 2016; 68:396–410.

76. Silversides CK, Colman JM, Sermer M, et al. Cardiac risk in pregnant women with rheumatic mitral stenosis. Am J Cardiol 2003; 91:1382–1385.

77. Nishimura RA, Otto CM, Bonow RO, et al. 2014 AHA/ACC Guideline for the Management of Patients With Valvular Heart Disease: Executive Summary. Circulation 2014; 129:2440–2492.

78. Tzemos N, Silversides CK, Colman JM, et al. Late cardiac outcomes after pregnancy in women with congenital aortic stenosis. Am Heart J 2009; 157:474–480.

79. Silversides CK, Colman JM, Sermer M, et al. Early and intermediate-term outcomes of pregnancy with congenital aortic stenosis. Am J Cardiol 2003; 91:540–545.

80. Yates MT, Soppa G, Smelt J, et al. Perioperative management and outcomes of aortic surgery during pregnancy. J Thorac Cardiovasc Surg 2015; 149:607–610.

81. Elkayam U, Goland S, Pieper PG, et al. High-risk cardiac disease in pregnancy. J Am Coll Cardiol 2016; 68:396–410.

82. Rodger M, Sheppard D, Gándara E, et al. Haematological problems in obstetrics. Best Prac Res Clin Obstet Gynaecol 2015; 29:671–684.

83. Goland S, Elkayam U. Anticoagulation in Pregnancy. Cardiol Clin 2012; 30:395–405.

84. Elkayam U, Singh H, Irani A, et al. Anticoagulation in Pregnant Women With Prosthetic Heart Valves. J Cardiovasc Pharmacol Ther 2004; 9:107–115.

85. van Hagen IM, Roos-Hesselink JW, Ruys TPE, et al. Pregnancy in women with a mechanical heart valve. Circulation 2015; 132:132–142.

86. Basu S, Aggarwal P, Kakani N, et al. Low-dose maternal warfarin intake resulting in fetal warfarin syndrome: In search for a safe anticoagulant regimen during pregnancy. Birth Defects Res A Clin Mol Teratol 2016; 106:142–147.

87. Chan WS, Anand S, Ginsberg JS. Anticoagulation of Pregnant Women With Mechanical Heart Valves. Arc Int Med 2000; 160:191–196.

88. Vahanian A, Alfieri O, Andreotti F, et al. Guidelines on the management of valvular heart disease (version 2012). Eur Heart J 2012; 33:2451–2496.

89. Bhagra CJ, D'Souza R, Silversides CK. Valvular heart disease and pregnancy part II: management of prosthetic valves. Heart 2017; 103:244–252.

90. Head CEG, Thorne SA. Congenital heart disease in pregnancy. Postgrad Med J 2005; 81:292–298.

91. Stout K. Pregnancy in women with congenital heart disease: the importance of evaluation and counselling. Heart 2005; 91:713–714.

92. Kamel H, Roman MJ, Pitcher A, et al. Pregnancy and the Risk of Aortic Dissection or Rupture. Circulation 2016; 134:527–533.

93. Lindley KJ, Bairey Merz CN, Asgar AW, et al. Management of women with congenital or inherited cardiovascular disease from pre-conception through pregnancy and postpartum. J Am Coll Cardiol 2021; 77:1778–1798.

94. Braverman AC, Mittauer E, Harris KM, et al. Clinical features and outcomes of pregnancy-related acute aortic dissection. JAMA Cardiol 2020; 6:58–66.

95. Ramlakhan KP, Tobler D, Greutmann M, et al. Pregnancy outcomes in women with aortic coarctation. Heart 2021; 107:290–298.

96. van Hagen IM, Boersma E, Johnson MR, et al. Global cardiac risk assessment in the Registry Of Pregnancy And Cardiac disease: results of a registry from the European Society of Cardiology. Eur J Heart Fail 2016; 18:523–533.

97. Balci A, Sollie-Szarynska KM, van der Bijl AGL, et al. Prospective validation and assessment of cardiovascular and offspring risk models for pregnant women with congenital heart disease. Heart 2014; 100:1373–1381.

98. Warnes CA. Transposition of the Great Arteries. Circulation 2006; 114:2699–2709.

99. Canobbio MM, Warnes CA, Aboulhosn J, et al. Management of Pregnancy in Patients with Complex Congenital Heart Disease: A Scientific Statement for Healthcare Professionals from the American Heart Association. Circulation 2017; 135:e50–87.

100. Clarkson PM, Wilson NJ, Neutze JM, et al. Outcome of pregnancy after the mustard operation for transposition of the great arteries with intact ventricular septum. J Am Coll Cardiol 1994; 24:190–193.

101. Drenthen W. Pregnancy and delivery in women after Fontan palliation. Heart 2006; 92:1290–1294.

102. Garcia Ropero A, Baskar S, Roos Hesselink JW, et al. Pregnancy in Women With a Fontan Circulation. Circulation 2018; 11:6–11.

103. Cauldwell M, Steer PJ, Bonner S, et al. Retrospective UK multicentre study of the pregnancy outcomes of women with a Fontan repair. Heart 2018; 104:401–406.

104. Presbitero P, Somerville J, Stone S, et al. Pregnancy in cyanotic congenital heart disease. Outcome of mother and fetus. Circulation 1994; 89:2673–2676.

105. Bishop L, Lansbury A, English K. Adult congenital heart disease and pregnancy. BJA Educ 2018; 18:23–29.

106. Hemnes AR, Kiely DG, Cockrill BA, et al. Statement on pregnancy in pulmonary hypertension from the pulmonary vascular research institute. Pulm Circ 2015; 5:435–465.

107. Cauldwell M, Baris L, Roos-Hesselink JW, et al. Ischaemic heart disease and pregnancy. Heart 2019; 105:189–195.

# Chapter 5

# Preterm birth and the vaginal microbiomes

*Belen Gimeno-Molina, Phillip R Bennett, David A MacIntyre, Lynne Sykes*

## PRETERM BIRTH

### Definition

Preterm birth (PTB) refers to delivery before completing 37 weeks of gestation and is classified as extremely preterm (<28 + 0 weeks); very preterm (between 28 + 0 and 31 + 6 weeks); and moderate or late PTB (between 32 + 0 and 36 + 6 weeks). PTB rates vary between 5% and 18% depending on the country and it affects 14.9 million newborns across the world annually [1]. It is the leading cause of mortality and morbidity among children under-five [2]. The frequency and severity of neonatal complications are higher the earlier the preterm delivery, and a consistent inverse association also exists between gestational age at birth and economic costs [3]. During the first 2 years of age, moderate and late PTBs are estimated at £12,037 and £5,823 per birth, respectively; in contrast to an average of £2,056 of a term infant [4]. The burden increases further with earlier deliveries and can reach up to £317,166 in cases of extreme prematurity [5].

### Preterm birth causes and associative risk factors

Preterm birth can be classified as 'indicated' or 'spontaneous'. Around one-third of PTB is initiated by the obstetric care provider, also referred to as iatrogenic PTB. Common indications include obstetric cholestasis, pre-eclampsia, and intrauterine growth. Most cases are spontaneous, presenting either in labour, or with preterm pre-labour rupture of

**Belen Gimeno-Molina** BSc MSc, March of Dimes Prematurity Research Center, Institute of Reproductive and Developmental Biology, Department of Metabolism, Digestion and Reproduction, Imperial College London, UK
Email: b.gimeno-molina@imperial.ac.uk

**Phillip R Bennett** BSc PhD MD FRCOG FMedSci, March of Dimes Prematurity Research Center, Institute of Reproductive and Developmental Biology, Department of Metabolism, Digestion and Reproduction, Imperial College London, UK
Email: p.bennett@imperial.ac.uk

**David A MacIntyre** PhD, March of Dimes Prematurity Research Center, Institute of Reproductive and Developmental Biology, Department of Metabolism, Digestion and Reproduction, Imperial College London, UK
Email: d.macintyre@imperial.ac.uk

**Lynne Sykes** BSc MBBS PhD MRCOG, March of Dimes Prematurity Research Center, Institute of Reproductive and Developmental Biology, Department of Metabolism, Digestion and Reproduction, Imperial College; The Parasol Foundation Centre for Women's Health and Cancer Research, St Mary's Hospital, Imperial College Healthcare NHS Trust, London, UK
Email: l.sykes@imperial.ac.uk

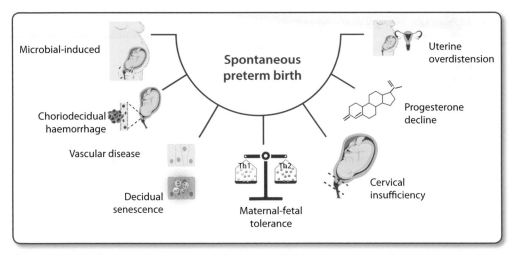

**Figure 5.1** Causes of spontaneous preterm birth. Spontaneous PTB is a syndrome caused by multiple aetiologies including microbial-induced inflammation, choriodecidual haemorrhage, vascular disease, decidual senescence, imbalanced maternal fetal tolerance, cervical insufficiency, a proposed decline in progesterone activity, and uterine overdistension.
*Source:* Image created with BioRender.com.

the membranes (PPROM). Spontaneous PTB (sPTB) should be considered as a syndrome with multiple aetiological factors, including microbial-induced (traditionally referred to as infection), choriodecidual haemorrhage and vascular disease, decidual senescence, disruption of maternal-fetal tolerance, cervical insufficiency, presumed decline in progesterone action, and uterine overdistension (**Figure 5.1**). Several associative risk factors have also been identified (**Table 5.1**), including maternal characteristics (such as ethnicity, smoking status, and socio-economic class), obstetric history (such as previous PTB or mid trimester loss), and specific pregnancy-related factors (such as multiple pregnancies, vaginal bleeding, and asymptomatic bacteriuria). Despite multiple associative risk factors, understanding of the mechanisms underpinning the varied aetiologies of PTB is still lacking. This has hampered the ability to correctly target interventions to prevent PTB and has hampered the development of new therapeutic strategies.

Although neonatal survival rates have been improved over the last few decades, this is predominantly due to the advances in neonatal care and the use of antenatal corticosteroids for fetal lung maturity [6]. Importantly, there has been no decline in the incidence of PTB either nationally or globally [1,7]. There is a global and national drive to reduce the rates of PTB and its related morbidity and mortality. The sustainable development goal 3 has set a target to reduce neonatal and under-five mortality to 12 and 25 per 1,000 births respectively in all countries by 2030. Recently, the department of health issued a target of reducing PTB in England and Wales from 8 to 6% by 2025 [8], and as a result the Saving Babies' Lives Care Bundle Version 2 (SBLCBv2) introduced Element 5, with recommendations on three areas of intervention to improve outcomes; prediction and prevention of PTB, and better preparation when PTB is unavoidable [9].

| Table 5.1 Risk factors associated with preterm birth (PTB) | | | |
|---|---|---|---|
| | **Risk factor** | | **Comment** |
| **Maternal characteristics** | Ethnicity | | Africans and Afro-Caribbeans are at higher risk than Caucasians |
| | Socio-demographic factors | | Socio-economic status (poverty), maternal age (adolescents and advanced age), educational attainment (low level), marital status (singleton), and access to healthcare services |
| | Nutritional status | | Low BMI and overweight and obese women |
| | Lifestyle | Behavioural | Depression, stress, and anxiety. Although psychosocial traits are interrelated to other parameters |
| | | Smoking | Correlated to the number of cigarettes smoked per day. Associated with a systemic inflammatory response |
| | | Drugs, alcohol | Heavy alcohol consumption during pregnancy increases the risk of low birthweight and PTB |
| | | Air pollution | Exposure to particulate air pollution |
| | Medical history | | Periodontal disease: Haematogenous transmission of oral microbial pathogens<br>Gestational diabetes, anaemia, and low levels of vitamin D |
| **Cervical history** | Cervical surgery | | Cone biopsy<br>Large excision transformation zone (LLETZ) |
| | Cervical insufficiency | | Cervical length: higher risk when mid-pregnancy short cervix (<25 mm) |
| **Pregnancy history** | Short interpregnancy interval | | Less than 6 months |
| | Previous preterm birth or mid-trimester loss | | ~20% risk of recurrence |
| **Current gestation** | Multiple gestation | | PTB accounts for half of the complications observed in this obstetrical population (for both spontaneous and induced deliveries) |
| | In vitro fertilisation | | Assisted reproductive technologies involved implantation of multiple embryos and advanced maternal age |
| | Vaginal bleeding | | Placental abruption, placenta praevia, but also first and mid-trimester haemorrhages without placental complications |
| | Bacterial vaginosis<br>Asymptomatic bacteriuria | | Overgrowth of atypical micro-organisms in the vagina, with or without symptomatology |

# Current strategies and recent advances in PTB prediction, prevention, and preparation

## Prediction

The SBLCBv2 Element 5 recommends all pregnant women to be assessed for risk of PTB by the beginning of the second trimester, and stratified to low, intermediate, or high-risk care pathways based on the following history: previous fully dilated caesarean section or history of cervical excisional treatment (intermediate risk) or previous PTB/PPROM/cervical cerclage, uterine anomaly, and trachelectomy for cervical cancer (high risk). Intermediate and high-risk care pathways advocate the use of transvaginal cervical length monitoring and the biomarker fetal fibronectin (fFN) to improve prediction of PTB and to guide intervention.

In a study of 2,915 women, the relative risk of PTB was 6.19 and 9.57-fold in women with a cervical length <26 mm (10th percentile) when measured at 24 and 28 weeks of gestation, respectively [10]. Although the risk of PTB is inversely proportional to the length of the cervix, 25 mm is usually considered as the threshold to recommend intervention. More recently, it is being acknowledged that cervical length surveillance rather than single time point assessments appears to be more predictive of PTB [11], and efforts should be made to assess if the rate of cervical change provides added predictive value. fFN is an extracellular matrix glycoprotein present at the maternal fetal interface. Usually, its levels are low during mid-pregnancy; in contrast, a high value (≥50 ng/mL) from 22 weeks of gestation is associated with an increased risk of PTB [12]. More recently quantitative fFN has been introduced to guide management in asymptomatic women at risk of PTB. A study of 1,448 women showed that sPTB < 34 weeks increased from 2.7% to 11.0%, 14.9%, 33,9%, and 47.6% with increasing concentration of cervico-vaginal fFN <10, 10–49, 50–199, 200–499, and ≥500 ng/mL, respectively [13]. The rationale for using cervical length monitoring and/or fFn is that regardless of aetiology, cervical ripening and fetal membrane disruption are processes that occur prior to symptoms and onset of labour. Nevertheless, the limitations of these strategies are the lack of evidence to support their use in a low-risk population, and the lack of contribution to understanding the mechanism underpinning PTB, and thus further hampering the development of new and more targeted preventative strategies. Furthermore, given that most women who deliver preterm have no prior identifiable risk factor, development of predictive tools is required that can be applied to all pregnant women.

## Prevention

The SBLCBv2 Element 5 recommends all pregnant women are assessed for treatment of modifiable PTB risk factors such as offering smoking cessation support, antibiotics for asymptomatic bacteriuria, and commencing aspirin for those at risk due to placental disease. In addition, it recommends that all women should have access to preterm prevention services lead by clinicians able to provide intervention such as high vaginal and trans-abdominal cerclage and progesterone. However, the guideline acknowledges that at present, the evidence base cannot determine precisely in which women, and under what circumstances each intervention would be the most effective. This highlights the urgent need for understanding the precise mechanisms underpinning each aetiological factor that drives PTB.

Cervical cerclage was first described by Shirodkar [14] and later by McDonald [15]. Cervical cerclage is offered as a prophylactic measure based on previous obstetric history suggestive of cervical insufficiency (elective cerclage) or if a short cervix is detected by ultrasound or vaginal examination (emergency cerclage). The technique is thought to work by maintaining and/or restoring structural support, and by providing an immunological barrier between the vagina and uterine cavity. Cervical cerclage can reduce the risk of PTB by 30% in women with singleton pregnancy, short cervix, and previous history of sPTB [16]. However, cervical cerclage is not always a successful operation. Sakai et al showed that in patients with short cervix but with cervical inflammation (higher levels of IL-8 in cervical mucus), cervical cerclage was less effective than in those without signs of inflammation [17]. This suggests that cerclage may be least effective in women with inflammation/ infection driven cervical shortening and PTB. Recent advances in understanding the role of cerclage in PTB prevention reveal that cerclage material appears to influence its efficacy, with monofilament leading to lower rates of PTB compared to braided cerclage material [18,19]. Results of the C-STICH study (ISRCTN 15373349), a multicentre randomised controlled trial of monofilament versus braided, powered to compare pregnancy loss and PTB rates between cerclage material, are due to be reported shortly.

Progesterone is also widely used as a prophylactic measure and is thought to act predominantly by promoting uterine quiescence. Although many studies have shown that progesterone can reduce the risk of preterm labour [20,21], there are also many studies which have shown it to be ineffective [22–24]. It is likely that this is due to the multifactorial aetiology of PTB, the heterogeneity of women recruited into these studies and method/ timing of administration, and that progesterone may only provide benefit in a certain population, for which we are yet to clearly define [25]. There have been no recent advances in determining which women would benefit the most from progesterone use, neither has there been any new significant evidence to suggest causing harm.

## Preparation

The SBLCBv2 Element 5 focuses on optimising place of birth, time-critical administration of antenatal corticosteroids for fetal lung maturation, magnesium sulphate for neuroprotection, and a multidisciplinary team approach for improving preparation and care for women and babies at high risk of imminent PTB. Recent advances in preparation include the introduction of international recommendations for administration of magnesium sulphate for neuroprotection [26], and the development of an antenatal optimisation toolkit for PTB < 34 weeks by the British Association of Perinatal Medicine [27].

To achieve our national and global targets of reducing PTB, neonatal and childhood morbidity and mortality, we need to adapt our approach away from managing PTB as one syndrome, but to invest in understanding the mechanisms underpinning each aetiological factor. This will enable us to develop improved techniques to more accurately risk stratify, and to develop more targeted, and thus more effective preventative strategies. In this chapter, we summarise the recent advances in understanding the role of the vaginal microbiome in PTB, and how this can be used to develop future novel predictive and preventative strategies.

## The role of infection and inflammation in PTB

Although the aetiology of preterm labour is unknown in approximately half of cases, infection has been acknowledged as the most common causal aetiology for more than half a century [28,29]. Evidence of causality comes from demonstrating the presence of intra-amniotic infection and/or inflammation in women who subsequently deliver preterm [30] and animal models demonstrating that intrauterine or systemic administration of bacterial and viral products lead to preterm delivery [31]. The biochemical processes required to initiate infection-induced parturition have been widely studied in both human and animal models. Pattern recognition receptors (PRRs) such as toll-like receptors (TLRs) initiate the innate immune response by recognising pathogen-associated molecular patterns (PAMPs) such as foreign, viral, and microbial products, but also endogenous signals [damage-associated molecular patterns (DAMPs)]. TLR activation is coupled to the activation of the transcriptional factor NF-κβ, initiating a pro-inflammatory cascade of cytokines, chemokines, cyclo-oxygenase-2 (COX-2), prostaglandins, and matrix metalloproteinases that participate in several processes of labour including cervical remodelling, uterine contractility, and rupture of fetal membranes [30,32] (**Figure 5.2**).

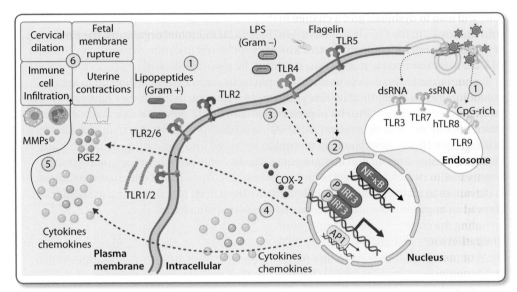

**Figure 5.2** Infectious mechanism leading to labour. (1) Bacterial and viral pathogens are recognised by different TLR receptors. (2) Activation of TLRs leads to the activation of transcription factor NF-κB, IRF-3, and AP-1, (3) which increases TLR expression and (4) promotes the production COX-2 (5) as well as cytokines, chemokines, and PGE2. These events lead to the recruitment and infiltration of immune cells, release of MMPs and an augmented pro-inflammatory response. In turn this leads to rupture of fetal membranes, cervical ripening, uterine contractility, and ultimately preterm labour.
TLR, toll-like receptor; dsRNA, double strand RNA (from virus); ssRNA, single strand RNA (from virus); PGE2, prostaglandin E2; MMPs, matrix metalloproteinases.
*Source:* Image created with BioRender.com.

Inflammation in the absence of infection, known as 'sterile inflammation', has also been widely reported in association with PTB [33,34]. However, it is plausible that this inflammation is not sterile, but instead driven by fastidious bacteria or viral infections that are not culturable with traditional culture-based techniques. With the advent of next generation sequencing (NGS), advances in our understanding of infection driven PTB are no longer dependent on culture-based techniques. We now have a more detailed understanding of microbial communities that reside in the vagina, including commensals (microbes causing benefit or no harm) and pathobionts (microbes with potential to cause harm), and their influence on PTB risk.

# THE VAGINAL MICROBIOMES AND PRETERM BIRTH

## Microbiome: Definition

The term microbiome is used to describe micro-organisms, their genomes and their milieu conditions [35]. Microbiota represents the whole diversity of micro-organisms that inhabit the human body, including bacteria, archaea, eukaryote-fungi, yeast, and protozoa's, and viruses [36]. Each of the different body sites harbours a multiple and sophisticated ecological community [37]. A healthy microbiota usually involves a diversity of species providing a benefit to the host development and health. A disruption of the homeostatic state will lead to dysbiosis and a change in the composition of the resident commensal communities. This can be due to the loss of beneficial microbial organisms, the expansion of pathogenic microorganism, and/or loss of overall microbial diversity [38]. Over the past decade, there has been a growing interest to better understand the complexity and function of the human microbiota in health and disease by many research groups and the Human Microbiome Project (HMP). The first phase of the HMP started in 2007 and consisted of the characterisation of microbial community sites to establish 'healthy' composition of different body sites (mainly vagina, skin, and gut). A second phase of the HMP, known as integrative HMP (iHMP) focuses on exploring the host-microbiome interplay, and the biological properties and the relationship between immunity, metabolism, and molecular activity within the microbiome [39].

Advances in culture-independent characterisation of microbial communities have allowed us to gain a greater knowledge of the diversity of the human microbiome, including the cervico-vaginal composition collected with swabs (**Figure 5.3**). Next-generation molecular techniques rely on the amplification and sequencing of the *16S rRNA* or metagenomics approaches, in which sequences the bacterial communities' genes and genomes are obtained [40,41]. The use of high-throughput sequencing and NGS techniques has made it possible to identify bacteria by their genetic signature [40,42]. The bacterial *16S rRNA* gene contains nine hyper-variable regions (V1–V9) that demonstrate considerable sequence diversity among different bacteria (**Figure 5.3**). Universal primers target the conserved regions flanking the hyper-variable regions; allowing amplification and further sequencing to finally assign a taxonomy [43]. Selection of primers will affect the further classification. For example, V1–V3 region robustly classifies the most common *Lactobacillus* species, but it might fail to represent *G. vaginalis* communities. The V6 region is biased against *Sneathia, Ureaplasma*, and *Mycoplasma* species [44].

## The vaginal microbiome

The vaginal microbiome plays a key role in health and disease. Vaginal microbial composition is in part hormonally regulated. Prior to menarche, low levels of circulating oestrogen are associated with high diversity microbial composition, consisting of aerobic, anaerobic, and enteric bacteria [45]. Following menarche, which is associated with higher circulating oestrogen, there is proliferation of vaginal epithelial cells and glycogen deposition. The cell-free glycogen serves a carbohydrate substrate for the growth of *Lactobacillus* species in the genital tract leading to lactic acid release, provoking a pH decrease ideal for the proliferation of acidophilic bacteria such as *Lactobacillus* [46].

The *Lactobacillus* genus has long been associated with promoting vaginal health, due to the production of lactic acid and the maintenance of a low pH, establishing a protective barrier that avoids and inhibits the growth of endogenous pathogenic bacteria [47,48]. Moreover, *Lactobacillus* species is able to produce hydrogen peroxide and bacteriocins (such as acidolin, lactacin B, and lactocin 160) that also inhibits the growth of micro-organisms like *Gardnerella* species [49,50]. The vaginal microbiome of reproductive-age women using NGS-based technology was first described by Ravel et al [47]. They described five different cervicovaginal community state types (CSTs), identified according to the community composition. Four were predominated by *Lactobacillus* genus: CST-I: *L. crispatus*; CST-II: *L. gasseri*; CST-III: *L. iners*; and CST-V: *L. jensenii*. However, CST-IV was characterised by the presence of heterogeneous anaerobic bacteria (*Prevotella, Dialister, Atopobium, Gardnerella, Megasphaera, Peptoniphilus, Sneathia, Aerococcus*, and *Mobiluncus*).

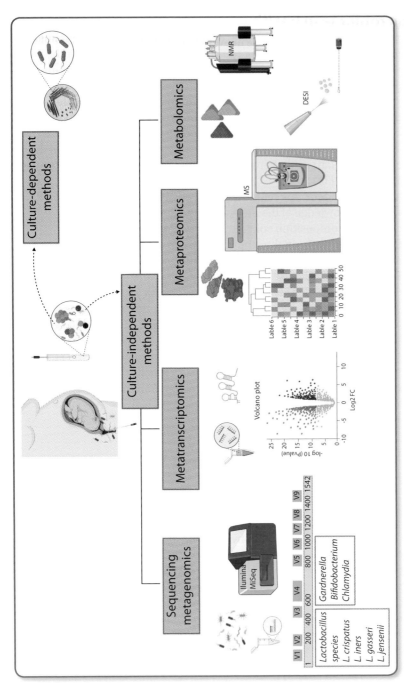

**Figure 5.3** Methodologies for detection of the vaginal microbiome. Traditionally, the study of vaginal microbiome relies on culture-dependent methods. Recent advances have been made developing culture-independent methodologies for a more comprehensive understanding of the complexities of the human microbiome. Sequencing of the *16S rRNA* gene is the most common molecular technique to assess the vaginal microbiome, assigning a taxonomy to the sequences observed. Other methods include metatranscriptomics, based on RNA approaches to understand activated pathways. Metaproteomics and metabolomics rely on technologies such as MS, nuclear magnetic resonance (NMR) or Desorption electrospray ionisation (DESI) to understand which proteins and metabolites reflect microbial activity.
*Source:* Image created with BioRender.com.

## The vaginal microbiome in healthy pregnancy

During pregnancy, there is a significant decrease in overall diversity and increased stability in the vaginal microbiota; mainly with enrichment of *Lactobacillus* species [51–54]. In contrast, women who begin pregnancy with high diversity tend to shift towards a homogeneous lactobacilli-dominated microbiome by the second trimester [54,55]. At the end of pregnancy (as oestrogen levels decline fast after parturition), there is a shift of the vaginal microbiota at delivery, characterised by a reduction in *Lactobacillus* species and an increase in alpha-diversity [53]. We have demonstrated that these changes persist post-partum [56]. Collectively, these data support the potential importance and the protective role of *Lactobacillus* species for successful pregnancy.

## The vaginal microbiome and preterm birth

Since 2014, many research groups across the world have reported on the association between vaginal microbial composition and PTB outcome. In broad terms, studies have consistently reported on the dominance of *Lactobacillus* species, especially of *L. crispatus* (CST-I) being associated with term delivery, whereas a heterogeneous and anaerobic community deplete in *Lactobacillus* being associated with PTB [57]. There is also evidence in some populations that dominance of *L. iners* (CST-III) is also associated with PTB [58].

It is clear that the association between microbial composition and risk of PTB is influenced by ethnicity; however, the mechanism for this is not yet established. The earliest study by Romero et al did not find differences in vaginal microbial composition between preterm and term deliveries in a largely predominant African American population, although the numbers of participants were small ($n = 72$, of which 18 delivered preterm) [52]. These findings were consistent with a later study in 2016 of 40 African American women by Nelson et al [59]. However, in contrast, a study with similar numbers demonstrated that bacterial diversity was higher in Caucasian women who subsequently delivered preterm PTB [60]. Several studies have confirmed the association between increased diversity, dysbiosis, and CST-IV with PTB in populations of predominantly white or mixed ethnicities [53,61–65]. The most commonly reported taxa associated with PTB risk are *Gardnerella*, *Ureaplasma*, *Prevotella*, and *Mycoplasma* [53,61,63]. Furthermore, recent studies have demonstrated these taxa and others such as *Mobiluncus curtisii/mulieris*, *Sanguinegens*, *Atopobium*, and *Megasphaera* are also associated with PTB in African American women, adding to the complexity of the effect of population specific PTB risk [55,66,67].

A clearer influence of ethnicity on the associations between vaginal microbial composition and PTB risk is seen in the case of colonisation with *L. iners*. Although several studies have consistently shown this species to be associated with increased risks of PTB, this relationship appears to be predominantly in Anglo Saxons/White Caucasians [50,66,68,69]. In contrast, this association is not seen in Chinese or in African American women [66,70].

## The vaginal microbiome in preterm rupture of membranes

Preterm premature rupture of membranes (PPROM) is described as rupture of membranes before 37 weeks and precedes approximately 30% of sPTBs. If there are no clinical signs of chorioamnionitis, expectant management aims to prolong the pregnancy to gain fetal maturity. Around 50–60% of pregnant women with PPROM will deliver within a week;

however, the longer the latency, the higher the risk of developing signs of intrauterine infection [29,71]. Hence, clinical management is a challenging balance between prolonging the pregnancy to gain fetal maturity against the increased risk of adverse neonatal outcome.

Advances have been made in understanding the role of the vaginal microbial composition in influencing the risk of PPROM. Several studies have reported on the vaginal microbiome at the time of PPROM. A cohort study of 36 women presenting with PPROM between 24 and 34 weeks found that the vaginal microbiome was highly diverse. *Megasphaera* and *Prevotella* were detected in all samples; and only half of the samples were *Lactobacillus* dominant (considering a cut-off of >50% relative abundance), from which *L. iners* was the most common [72]. The rest were characterised by heterogeneous typical non-lactobacilli (usually classified as CST-IV). Longitudinal profiling during the latency period confirmed that this diversity was maintained until delivery.

Baldwin et al also evaluated the vaginal microbial profile in PPROM during latency period, from presentation until delivery in 15 women who experienced PPROM, and compared them to gestational age-matched controls with uncomplicated pregnancies [73]. At the time of rupture, lactobacilli species were underrepresented and there was high diversity, compared to controls. In this cohort, *Prevotella* and *Peptoniphilus* were the most prevalent species detected is association with PPROM. A larger cohort of women experiencing PPROM ($n = 61$) was studied by Kacerobski et al [74]. Analysis of the cervical microbiota by 16SrRNA sequencing (V4–V6 region) showed four bacterial CSTs, two dominated by *Lactobacillus* (*L. crispatus* and *L. iners*) and two diverse. They found a higher incidence of microbial invasion of the amniotic cavity (MIAC) and histological chorioamnionitis in women with CST-IVB (dominated by *G. vaginalis* and *S. sanguinegens*), and a lower incidence in women with CSTs dominated by *Lactobacillus*.

There are limited studies describing the vaginal microbiome leading up to PPROM. We reported on a prospective study of 250 at predefined increased risk of PTB (previous PTB, previous PPROM, and/or previous cervical treatment) [75]. We sampled women at four time points between 8 and 36 weeks, and 15 of these women experience PPROM. Women that delivered at term were characterised by low richness and diversity, and dominance of *Lactobacillus* at mid-gestation; however, at the same matched gestational age, women who ultimately experienced PPROM had a microbial profile characterised by a high diversity and an intermediate or low *Lactobacillus* species dominance. Those samples were enriched in bacteria from *Bacteroides*, *Fusobacteria,* and *Clostridiales* classes. Interestingly, 50% of women who were *Lactobacillus* dominant before PPROM event, became dysbiotic after rupture of membranes, suggesting the rupture event can significantly affect the microbial signature. To further explore the vaginal microbiota in early pregnancy prior to PPROM, we examined a study population of 1,500 women, of which 60 experienced PPROM [76]. Compared to 36 gestational aged-matched controls, the women with PPROM were characterised by a reduction of *Lactobacillus* species, and increased richness. The longitudinal evaluation revealed instability of bacterial community and a shift towards a higher diversity whereas uncomplicated term deliveries were characterised by a stable alpha diversity, reduced richness, and *Lactobacillus crispatus* dominance.

In keeping with the concept of ascending inflammation and infection driving adverse neonatal outcome, we also demonstrated an enrichment for *Prevotella*, *Sneathia*, *Peptostreptococcus,* and *Catonella* species; as well as a reduced levels of *Lactobacillus* species in women who had chorioamnionitis and funisitis [75]. In addition, colonisation with *Lactobacillus crispatus* was protective of early onset neonatal sepsis.

## The vaginal microbiome and cervical shortening

Cervical remodelling is a physiological process that consists of softening, ripening, dilation, and post-partum repair phases [77,78]. However, premature cervical remodelling leading to cervical shortening is a risk factor for PTB. We have shown that *L. iners* dominance at as early as 16 weeks of gestation is associated with developing a short cervix (<25 mm) [68]. As well as seeing an increase in the proportion of women with *L. iners* dominance and *L. iners* abundance in women with a short cervix, there are also increased concentrations of cervicovaginal fluid (CVF) immunoglobulin M (IgM) and interleukin-6 (IL-6) compared to those with a long cervix, implying activation of both the adaptive and innate immune response [19].

## The vaginal microbiome and first-trimester miscarriage

Miscarriage affects 25% of pregnancies, with up to half of cases being due to aneuploidy or chromosomal aberrations. Many miscarriages occur with unknown aetiology, and infection has long been considered as a potential cause [79]. Advances in NGS have enabled us to understand more about the association between vaginal microbiota and early miscarriage. In 78 women who went on to have a miscarriage, bacterial composition prior to the event (<8 weeks of gestation) was associated with *Lactobacillus* depletion and a higher proportion of samples were dominated by CST-IV [80]. Furthermore, Grewal et al studied 93 women who had miscarriages, showing a significantly higher prevalence of *Lactobacillus* species deplete vaginal microbial composition in euploid compared to aneuploid miscarriage [81].

# IMMUNE ACTIVATION AS A MECHANISM OF MICROBIAL DRIVEN PTB

Historically, the immunological status of pregnancy has been compared to a 'host-graft' concept, conceived by Medawar, in which some degree of immunosuppression was required in order to tolerate the semi-allogenic fetus [82]. However, it is now clear that a constant immunosuppression would not be desirable during pregnancy, but that successful pregnancy requires a dynamic and responsive immune system. The most simplistic description refers to a dynamic Th1/Th2 balance [83], with a pro-inflammatory Th1-driven phase occurring during implantation and placentation, transitioning to an anti-inflammatory Th2-biased phase in the second trimester, and finally to a Th1 pro-inflammatory phase in preparation for labour and delivery [84]. The hypothesis of Th2 pre-dominance and down regulation of the Th1 response originated from Wegmann and colleagues [85] and is supported by a general improvement in autoimmune conditions involving the Th1 spectrum in pregnancy but relapsing following delivery, whereas Th2-driven conditions generally worsen in pregnancy [83].

Significant evidence exists to support the role of both systemic and local immune activation in PTB. Systemic conditions such as inflammatory bowel disease, systemic lupus erythematosus (SLE), appendicitis, and viral illnesses predispose to higher PTB rates [83]. Local inflammation, characterised by immune cell infiltration and pro-inflammatory cytokine release at the maternal-fetal and cervico-vaginal interface, is also seen in women who deliver preterm [83,86]. Furthermore, murine studies confirm the importance of inflammation in driving PTB, as preterm delivery can be induced with the administration of cytokines such as IL-1 and tumour necrosis factor-alpha (TNF-$\alpha$) [31,86].

Many studies have demonstrated higher concentrations of cytokines such as IL-6, IL-8, monocyte chemotactic protein-1 (MCP-1), and granulocyte-macrophage colony-stimulating factor (GM-CSF) in cervico-vaginal fluid of women who go on to develop a short cervix and/or deliver preterm [17,87–89]. However, recent advances in our understanding of microbial composition have allowed us to determine more specifically the relationship between local inflammation, the vaginal microbiome, and preterm delivery. Early studies utilising *16S rRNA* gene sequencing revealed that a dysbiotic microbial composition was associated with higher concentrations of cytokines such as IL-1$\beta$, TNF-$\alpha$, and interferon-gamma (IFN-$\gamma$) in pregnant women at high risk of delivering preterm [18]. Kacerovski and colleagues demonstrated how the concentration of IL-6 in CVF varied significantly between the different CST in women with pregnancies complicated by PPROM [90]. Higher concentrations were detected in women with CST-IVA (mixed non-lactobacilli group with presence of *Ureaplasma*, *Propionibacterium*, *Fusobacterium*, and *Streptococcus* species) and CST-IVB (also non-lactobacilli but dominated by *G. vaginalis* and *S. sanguinegens*) compared to women with CST-I (*L. crispatus*) and CST-III (*L. iners*). Fettweis et al also found that IL-1$\beta$, IL-6, eotaxin, and MIP-1$\beta$ were increased in women who delivered preterm compared to term [55]. Furthermore, the pro-inflammatory cytokines were positively correlated with dysbiotic taxa, such as *A. vaginae*, *G. vaginalis,* and *Megasphaera* type 1, in women who delivered preterm.

We and others have acknowledged that the immune response involves more than merely cytokine production. Elovitz et al have demonstrated that cervico-vaginal concentrations of $\beta$-defensin-2 (a host-derived anti-microbial peptide, produced by epithelial cells) are lower in women who deliver preterm compared to term, with the relationship more pronounced in women with CST-III, CST-IVA, and CST-V [66]. We have more recently demonstrated that women with CST-III and CST-IV who subsequently deliver preterm have an augmented local adaptive and innate immune response compared to women who deliver at term. We believe that *L. iners* and CST-IV-associated taxa such as *G. vaginalis* are recognised by mediators such as IgM, IgG, and mannose-binding lectin (MBL), which leads to activation of the complement system via the classical and lectin pathways [19]. Downstream effects of this are seen, resulting in increased IL-8, IL-6, and IL-$\beta$. C3a, C5a, and IL-8 are chemoattractants of neutrophils. It is likely that neutrophils contribute to the local release of COX-2, prostaglandins, and matrix metalloproteinases, contributing to cervical and fetal membrane remodelling, and ultimately cervical dilation and fetal membrane rupture (**Figure 5.4**).

We have shown that cervical vaginal fluid concentrations of MBL, IgM, IgG$_{1-4}$, C3b, and C5 are lowest in women colonised with *L. crispatus* (CST-I). This immune suppressive effect is consistent in vitro findings that vaginal epithelial cells stimulated with the TLR3 agonist poly IC and TLR2/6 agonist FSL show inhibition of IL-6, IL-8, and TNF-$\alpha$ production if cultured with *L. crispatus* [91].

# ADVANCES IN TARGETING MICROBIAL DRIVEN PTB AS A PREVENTATIVE STRATEGY

## Prediction: Detection of the vaginal microbiome and its associated immunome

In clinical settings, the most established techniques for evaluating the microbial composition are the Amsel [92] and the Nugent score [93], which rely on measuring pH and the presence of clue cells and bacterial morphotypes on gram stain smears. Clinical settings also rely on culture-based methods, but these methods are limited, as not all microorganisms can be cultured. Although culture-independent characterisation with NGS techniques provides more detail of the vaginal microbiome composition, it is time

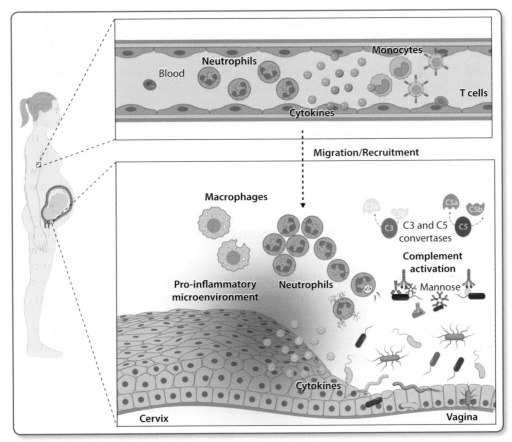

**Figure 5.4** Immunological mechanism of microbial-driven preterm birth. Preterm birth is associated with both systemic and local immune activation. Women with a high-risk vaginal microbial signature are dominated by *L. iners* (CST-III) or dysbiotic/anaerobic bacteria (CST-IV). These taxa can be recognised by immune mediators such as IgM, IgG and/or MBL, leading to the activation of the complement cascade and the recruitment of immune cells such as neutrophils. This further amplifies the local pro-inflammatory environment by the release of cytokines and matrix metalloproteinases.
*Source:* Image created with BioRender.com.

consuming, expensive, and currently only available in the context of research. Studies are underway that aim to develop more accessible methodologies for point of care testing that can be used in the clinical setting.

Recently, Oliver and colleagues evaluated the cervicovaginal microbiome (both bacterial and fungal composition) and metabolic profile of healthy pregnancies using GC-TOF MS (gas chromatography-time of flight mass spectrometry) and LC-MS/MS (liquid chromatography-tandem MS) [94]. The metabolome of cervico-vaginal fluid was found to be stable across gestation, and some metabolites were associated with the microbial composition (e.g. higher abundance of indole-3-lactate and mannitol in *L. crispatus* dominant communities).

An alternative to assess the mucosal metabolome is desorption electrospray ionisation MS (DESI-MS). Pruski et al have developed a rotating device where swabs can be applied with minimum sample preparation to evaluate the metabolites from cervico-vaginal fluid [95]. This technique allows discrimination of amino acids, peptides, carbohydrates and fatty acids, among others; and takes only 3 minutes to obtain a result. Mass spectra reveal changes in the lipid mass range of m/z 700–900, and these alterations are associated with phospholipid metabolism and fatty acid oxidation, particularly sphingolipids, which are implicated in innate immunity during pregnancy. They further assessed the use of DESI-MS as a point of care diagnostic tool, evaluating swab samples from women diagnosed with bacterial vaginosis (BV). The technique, combined with multivariate analyses, showed that samples from women with BV, had higher levels of cadaverine, putrescine, and tyramine compared to healthy controls. The most recent advances in the development of this technology now allow for robust prediction of the composition of the vaginal microbiome as well as the local immune milieu. The direct on swab-metabolic profiling is able to discriminate those who are *Lactobacillus* species deplete with immune activation in women who subsequently delivered preterm [96]. This technique offers great potential for a rapid point of care test for improved PTB risk stratification to determine which women are at risk of microbial driven PTB.

## Prevention – modulation of the vaginal microbiome and the immune milieu

### Cerclage, progesterone and the vaginal microbiome

Cerclage for the prevention of PTB is not always effective. It is possible that the success of cerclage is predominantly via its mechanism of providing mechanical and structural support. Recently, there have been reports of higher rates of preterm delivery in women who receive a braided (polyester ethylene terephthalate fibres braided together) rather than monofilament (single strand of non-absorbable polyamide polymer) suture. We have demonstrated that braided material appears to be associated with a shift towards a high-risk microbial profile and immune activation, whereas monofilament appears to be immunologically inert. We studied prospectively collected samples from 49 women pre-cerclage insertion and for 16 weeks of post-cerclage to determine if any alterations to the vaginal microbiome composition was seen following monofilament ($n = 24$) or braided ($n = 25$) cerclage insertion. Prior to cerclage, intermediate and dysbiosis microbial profiles were similar in both groups; however, insertion of the braided cerclage led to a five-fold increase in microbial dysbiosis within 4 weeks of insertion, which persisted until at least 16 weeks. In contrast, insertion of monofilament cerclage did not disrupt microbial composition, and women maintained high *Lactobacillus* abundance and stability [18]. In addition, insertion of braided cerclage was associated with an increase in cervico-vaginal cytokine concentration (IL-1$\beta$, IL-6, IL-8, TNF-$\alpha$, and MMP-1). We have subsequently validated the adverse effect on the innate immune response in a separate study cohort, and additionally identified an increase in complement proteins and immunoglobulins following braided cerclage. This was also associated with higher PTB rates of 57% in women who received braided compared to monofilament cerclage (20%) [19].

Since the composition of vaginal CSTs can be influenced by hormone levels, menses, and oral contraceptives, we have also assessed if vaginal progesterone influences the vaginal microbial composition and the local immune milieu. Use of vaginal progesterone does not have an effect on the microbial composition, richness or diversity [68], or on the local innate and adaptive immune response [19].

## Antibiotics

Given that vaginal microbial composition and microbial invasion of the intra-amniotic cavity play a clear role in the aetiology of PTB, a substantial amount of effort has been made to examine the efficacy of antibiotics for the prevention of PTB. Much of the research has focussed on treating women with BV, or in the context of PPROM. However, there remains no clear evidence that antibiotic prophylaxis reduces the risk of PTB [97], and in some studies, there is evidence that empirical treatment with antibiotics can cause harm. The largest study to date is a randomised controlled trial where 84,530 women were screened for BV in early pregnancy, and 3,105 women with BV were randomised to oral clindamycin or placebo. No reduction in labour miscarriage or spontaneous PTB < 32 weeks were seen [98]. The PREMET study of women at high risk of PTB was stopped early by the trial steering committee, due to an increased risk of PTB noted in the metronidazole treatment group (21%) compared to the placebo group 11% [99]. In the context of PPROM, although the Oracle I study reported on a reduction in a composite of short-term respiratory function, chronic lung disease, and major neonatal cerebral abnormality with erythromycin, it also showed a significant increase in the occurrence of neonatal necrotising enterocolitis in women receiving co-amoxiclav [100]. We recently reported that the use of erythromycin in women with PPROM tended to convert a healthy *Lactobacillus* dominant vaginal composition to one of *Lactobacillus* depletion, a composition that was related to early onset neonatal sepsis [75]. Therefore, advancing the potential for antibiotics as a preventative strategy requires more detailed analyses of the vaginal microbial composition pre and post-treatment to correctly phenotype and decide in whom antibiotics may benefit.

## Live bio-therapeutics and probiotics

Rather than using empirical antibiotics to modulate the vaginal microbiome, interest is growing for the potential use of live bio-therapeutics (live microorganisms used for prevention or treatment of disease) and probiotics (non-pathogenic microorganisms of human origin given to provide health benefit). A recent Cochrane review and meta-analysis concluded that there is no benefit or detrimental effect of probiotic use in the context of PTB prevention [101,102]. This is unsurprising, as recent studies using oral probiotics administered in early pregnancy have failed to modify the vaginal microbiota [103,104].

It is likely that local administration, in the form of a vaginal pessary, would offer more promise for modulation of the microbiome and PTB prevention. Recently, a systematic review revealed the potential of vaginally applied probiotics for the treatment of BV [105], a risk factor for PTB. In 2020, a phase 2b randomised placebo-controlled trial of vaginal *L. crispatus* CTV-05 (LACTIN- V) reported successful colonisation and a reduction in rates of recurrent BV in non-pregnant women [106]. Promisingly, a study of 106 women with PPROM were randomised to receive a vaginal probiotic (containing *L. rhamnosus* and *L. gasseri*) in addition to standard antibiotics or antibiotics alone, and showed that the gestational age, the latency period from PPROM to delivery and birth weight was higher in the women who received the combination of *Lactobacillus* and antibiotics, compared to women who only received antibiotic treatment [107]. We have recently completed recruitment to a phase 1 trial seeking to determine the feasibility, safety, and tolerance of LACTIN-V in a cohort of pregnant women at risk of PTB, with analyses of results underway (ClinicalTrials.gov Identifier: NCT03992534).

## Immunomodulation as a therapeutics potential

The immune response to microbes relies on host recognition, immune cell infiltration and activation, and release of pro-inflammatory mediators such as cytokines and chemokines. We have recently demonstrated that the complement system is also activated in the context of microbial driven cervical shortening and PTB [19]. Women with CST-III (*L. iners* dominated) and CST-IV (diverse composition) have higher concentrations of cervico-vaginal MBL, IgM, $IgG_{1-4}$, C3b, C5, IL-8, and IL-1β compared to women with CST-I (*L crispatus* dominated). Therefore, by administration vaginal *L. crispatus* to modulate composition to CST-I, it is highly likely that a secondary beneficial effect would lead to immune quiescence.

An alternative strategy is to repurpose biologics and complement therapeutics to inhibit local cervico-vaginal inflammation. Compelling evidence of the role of the complement system in PTB exists in both animal and human studies. Murine studies using intravaginal LPS demonstrate a role for C3 and C5a in cervical ripening and PTB [108,109], and C5a knock-out mice are resistant to LPS induced PTB [110]. Evidence of systemic activation of the complement system in human pregnancy has also been linked to miscarriage [111] and sPTB [112–115] in humans. We have shown that cervicovaginal C3b and C5 are increased in women who are CST-III and undergo cervical shortening and sPTB, and in women who are CST-IV who subsequently deliver preterm [19]. It is plausible that defragmentation of C3 and C5 leads to C3a and C5a driven chemoattraction of cervico-vaginal neutrophils to aid phagocytosis and microbial clearance. Neutrophils are a major source of pro-labour and pro-inflammatory mediators for example prostaglandins, matrix metalloproteinases, and IL-8, which are required for cervical remodelling and fetal membrane rupture. Significant advances in complement therapeutics have been made over the last decade targeting the classical, lectin, and alternative pathways [116]. Eculizumab, a C5a inhibitor, has United States Food and Drug Administration (USFDA) approval for use in pregnancy for the treatment of paroxysmal nocturnal haemoglobinuria and is used off label for other conditions such as anti-phospholipid syndrome, sickle cell anaemia, and haemolysis elevated liver enzymes and low platelets (HELLP) syndrome [117]. Future studies examining the potential for repurposing complement therapeutics for PTB prevention should be considered.

We and many others have also demonstrated the significant increase in cervico-vaginal IL-6 and IL-1β in women who subsequently deliver preterm. This raises the potential for considering the use of biologics targeting cytokines and their receptors. Although caution has traditionally been applied to the use of biologics in pregnancy, especially from the third trimester onward, there has been extensive use of tocilizumab (IL-6) in pregnant women with severe COVID-19 during the pandemic, many of whom were in their third trimester, with no safety alerts been issued.

## Pregnancy interval and the vaginal microbiome

One of the most simplistic and feasible strategies for modulating the risk of PTB is to ensure the interval until the next pregnant exceeds a year. Several studies have reported that an interpregnancy interval < 12 months is associated with an increased risk of PTB, regardless of the first pregnancy being a preterm or term [118,119]. Term labour is characterised by a reduction in *Lactobacillus* species and an increased alpha diversity that persists post-partum, even up to a year later [53,87]. It is plausible that a short interpregnancy interval does not allow enough time for the vaginal microbiome to be restored to a more favourable composition for a subsequent successful pregnancy.

# OTHER VAGINAL MICROBIOMES

The mycobiota makes reference to the fungal organisms present at body sites. It is outnumbered by its bacterial counterparts, and its study has faced the intrinsic problem of culture-based approaches, so its contribution to health and disease has been underrepresented [120] and characterised the mycobiome in women of reproductive age women. Using sequencing Drell et al techniques on *n* = 494 vaginal samples from healthy asymptomatic women [121]. *Candida albicans* was the most predominant fungi, where much higher (65% of *Candida* species), compared to what has been traditionally consider basic colonisation in asymptomatic women. There is evidence that bacteria and fungi have a commensalism relationship on the vagina. Tortelli et al showed similar rates of *Candida* colonisation between lactobacillus-dominant or non-dominant signatures, yet *L. iners* was more likely to cohabit with *Candida* species [122]. However, there are no studies exploring the mycobiome in the context of PTB.

Advances in studying the vaginal virome in the context of pregnancy and PTB have recently been made since the introduction of high-throughput sequencing and metagenomic approaches. As part of the HMP data recovery, Wylie and colleagues studied viruses from several body sites (nose, skin, mouth, vagina, and stool) from healthy individuals; and found at least one virus in 92% of samples. Papillomaviruses were the most dominant in the vaginal milieu (38%) [123]. Even in the absence of disease, they described how viruses and bacteria have a dynamic relationship: the alpha papillomavirus detected was more common in samples with vaginal bacterial dysbiosis/diversity compared to *Lactobacillus* dominated environments. More recently, the same group evaluated the vaginal virome component in the context of pregnancy and PTB and found that almost all women (80% of *n* = 60) harbour at least one virus in the vagina [124]. A higher viral richness, seen as early as the first trimester, was associated with preterm labour, and the risk of PTB was even higher when combining both bacterial and viral diversity. Significant evidence exists in both animal and human studies to support a double hit hypothesis, whereby priming of the immune system by exposure to viruses can lead to a more severe response to subsequent bacterial infection [125,126]. It is therefore plausible that future work exploring the virome in women who subsequently deliver preterm may lead to increased understanding of the role viruses, and the potential for antivirals as a novel target for PTB prevention.

# CONCLUSION

In summary, PTB should be considered as a syndrome, with multiple aetiological factors. To succeed in our global drive to reduce PTB rates and neonatal morbidity and mortality, significant advances in understanding the mechanism of each aetiological factors are needed. We have summarised the main advances in our understanding of the role of the vaginal microbiome in spontaneous PTB. A vaginal composition which is diverse or dominated by *Lactobacillus iners* is associated with an increase in cervical shortening, PPROM, and preterm labour. This is likely to be due to a dysregulated immune response involving both the adaptive and innate immune response, and the complement system. In contrast, women with a vaginal microbial composition rich in *Lactobacillus crispatus* are more likely to be protected from local immune activation and PTB. These advances provide promise for the development of new tools to improve risk stratification, and new therapeutic strategies such as live bio-therapeutics and complement therapeutics to better individualise preventative therapies.

# REFERENCES

1. Blencowe H, Cousens S, Oestergaard MZ, et al. National, regional, and worldwide estimates of preterm birth rates in the year 2010 with time trends since 1990 for selected countries: a systematic analysis and implications. Lancet 2012; 379:2162–2172.
2. Liu L, Oza S, Hogan D, et al. Global, regional, and national causes of child mortality in 2000-13, with projections to inform post-2015 priorities: an updated systematic analysis. Lancet.2015; 385:430–440.
3. Petrou S, Yiu HH, Kwon J. Economic consequences of preterm birth: a systematic review of the recent literature (2009-2017). Arch Dis Child 2019; 104:456–465.
4. Khan KA, Petrou S, Dritsaki M, et al. Economic costs associated with moderate and late preterm birth: a prospective population-based study. BJOG 2015; 122:1495–1505.
5. Petrou S, Eddama O, Mangham L. A structured review of the recent literature on the economic consequences of preterm birth. Arch Dis Child Fetal Neonatal Ed 2011; 96:F225–232.
6. Shapiro-Mendoza CK, Lackritz EM. Epidemiology of late and moderate preterm birth. Semin Fetal Neonatal Med 2012; 17: 120–125.
7. Sykes L, MacIntyre D, Teoh T, et al. Targeting Immune Activation in the Prevention of Preterm Labour. Eur Obstet Gynaecol 2011; 6:100–106.
8. Department of Health. Safer Maternity Care—The National Maternity Safety Strategy—Progress and Next Steps, 2017. [online] Available from: https://assets.publishing.service.gov.uk/government/uploads/system/uploads/attachment_data/file/662969/Safer_maternity_care_-_progress_and_next_steps.pdf [Last accessed May, 2022].
9. England NHS. Saving Babies' Lives Care Bundle Version 2, 2019. [online] Available from: https://www.england.nhs.uk/wp-content/uploads/2019/03/Saving-Babies-Lives-Care-Bundle-Version-Two-Updated-Final-Version.pdf [Last accessed May, 2022].
10. Iams JD, Goldenberg RL, Meis PJ, et al. The length of the cervix and the risk of spontaneous premature delivery. National Institute of Child Health and Human Development Maternal Fetal Medicine Unit Network. N Engl J Med 1996; 334:567–572.
11. Hughes K, Kane SC, Araujo Junior E, et al. Cervical length as a predictor for spontaneous preterm birth in high-risk singleton pregnancy: current knowledge. Ultrasound Obstet Gynecol 2016; 48:7–15.
12. Glover AV, Manuck TA. Screening for spontaneous preterm birth and resultant therapies to reduce neonatal morbidity and mortality: A review. Semin Fetal Neonatal Med 2018; 23:126–132.
13. Abbott DS, Hezelgrave NL, Seed PT, et al. Quantitative fetal fibronectin to predict preterm birth in asymptomatic women at high risk. Obstet Gynecol 2015; 125:1168–1176.
14. Shirodkar VN. A new method of operative treatment for habitual abortions in the second trimester of pregnancy. Antiseptic 1955; 52:299–300.
15. McDonald IA. Suture of the cervix for inevitable miscarriage. J Obstet Gynaecol Br Emp 1957; 64:346–350.
16. Berghella V, Rafael TJ, Szychowski JM, et al. Cerclage for short cervix on ultrasonography in women with singleton gestations and previous preterm birth: a meta-analysis. Obstet Gynecol 2011; 117:663–671.

17. Sakai M, Shiozaki A, Tabata M, et al. Evaluation of effectiveness of prophylactic cerclage of a short cervix according to interleukin-8 in cervical mucus. Am J Obstet Gynecol 2006; 194:14–19.
18. Kindinger LM, MacIntyre DA, Lee YS, et al. Relationship between vaginal microbial dysbiosis, inflammation, and pregnancy outcomes in cervical cerclage. Sci Transl Med 2016; 8:350ra102.
19. Chan D, Bennett PR, Lee YS, et al. Microbial-driven preterm labour involves crosstalk between the innate and adaptive immune response. Nat Commun 2022; 13:975.
20. da Fonseca EB, Bittar RE, Carvalho MH, et al. Prophylactic administration of progesterone by vaginal suppository to reduce the incidence of spontaneous preterm birth in women at increased risk: a randomized placebo-controlled double-blind study. Am J Obstet Gynecol 2003; 188:419–424.
21. Hassan SS, Romero R, Vidyadhari D, et al. Vaginal progesterone reduces the rate of preterm birth in women with a sonographic short cervix: a multicenter, randomized, double-blind, placebo-controlled trial. Ultrasound Obstet Gynecol 2011; 38:18–31.
22. O'Brien JM, Adair CD, Lewis DF, et al. Progesterone vaginal gel for the reduction of recurrent preterm birth: primary results from a randomized, double-blind, placebo-controlled trial. Ultrasound Obstet Gynecol 2007; 30:687–696.
23. Norman JE, Marlow N, Messow CM, et al. Vaginal progesterone prophylaxis for preterm birth (the OPPTIMUM study): a multicentre, randomised, double-blind trial. Lancet 2016; 387:2106–2116.
24. Crowther CA, Ashwood P, McPhee AJ, et al. Vaginal progesterone pessaries for pregnant women with a previous preterm birth to prevent neonatal respiratory distress syndrome (the PROGRESS Study): A multicentre, randomised, placebo-controlled trial. PLoS Med 2017; 14:e1002390.
25. Sykes L, Bennett PR. Efficacy of progesterone for prevention of preterm birth. Best Pract Res Clin Obstet Gynaecol 2018; 52:126–136.
26. Chollat C, Marret S. Magnesium sulfate and fetal neuroprotection: overview of clinical evidence. Neural Regen Res 2018; 13:2044–2049.
27. British Association of Perinatal Medicine. Antenatal optimisation for preterm infants less than 34 weeks. A quality improvement tool kit. 2020.
28. Romero R, Quintero R, Oyarzun E, et al. Intraamniotic infection and the onset of labor in preterm premature rupture of the membranes. Am J Obstet Gynecol 1988; 159:661–666.
29. Goldenberg RL, Culhane JF, Iams JD, et al. Epidemiology and causes of preterm birth. Lancet 2008; 371:75–84.
30. Romero R, Espinoza J, Goncalves LF, et al. The role of inflammation and infection in preterm birth. Semin Reprod Med 2007; 25:21–39.
31. Elovitz MA, Mrinalini C. Animal models of preterm birth. Trends Endocrinol Metab 2004; 15:479–487.
32. Lindstrom TM, Bennett PR. The role of nuclear factor kappa B in human labour. Reproduction 2005; 130:569–581.
33. Romero R, Dey SK, Fisher SJ. Preterm labor: one syndrome, many causes. Science 2014; 345:760–765.
34. Gilman-Sachs A, Dambaeva S, Salazar Garcia MD, et al. Inflammation induced preterm labor and birth. J Reprod Immunol 2018; 129:53–58.
35. Marchesi JR, Ravel J. The vocabulary of microbiome research: a proposal. Microbiome 2015; 3:31.
36. Human Microbiome Project C. A framework for human microbiome research. Nature 2012; 486:215–221.
37. Human Microbiome Project C. Structure, function and diversity of the healthy human microbiome. Nature 2012; 486:207–214.
38. Petersen C, Round JL. Defining dysbiosis and its influence on host immunity and disease. Cell Microbiol 2014; 16:1024–1033.
39. Integrative HMPRNC. The Integrative Human Microbiome Project. Nature 2019; 569:641–648.
40. Barb JJ, Oler AJ, Kim HS, et al. Development of an Analysis Pipeline Characterizing Multiple Hypervariable Regions of 16S rRNA Using Mock Samples. PLoS One 2016; 11:e0148047.
41. Belizario JE, Napolitano M. Human microbiomes and their roles in dysbiosis, common diseases, and novel therapeutic approaches. Front Microbiol 2015; 6:1050.
42. Van Der Pol WJ, Kumar R, Morrow CD, et al. In Silico and Experimental Evaluation of Primer Sets for Species-Level Resolution of the Vaginal Microbiota Using 16S Ribosomal RNA Gene Sequencing. J Infect Dis 2019; 219:305–314.
43. Chakravorty S, Helb D, Burday M, et al. A detailed analysis of 16S ribosomal RNA gene segments for the diagnosis of pathogenic bacteria. J Microbiol Methods 2007; 69:330–339.
44. Pruski P, Lewis HV, Lee YS, et al. Assessment of microbiota:host interactions at the vaginal mucosa interface. Methods 2018; 149:74–84.
45. Hill GB, St Claire KK, Gutman LT. Anaerobes predominate among the vaginal microflora of prepubertal girls. Clin Infect Dis 1995; 20:S269–270.

46. Linhares IM, Summers PR, Larsen B, et al. Contemporary perspectives on vaginal pH and lactobacilli. Am J Obstet Gynecol 2011; 204:120.e1–e5.
47. Ravel J, Gajer P, Abdo Z, et al. Vaginal microbiome of reproductive-age women. Proc Natl Acad Sci U S A 2011; 108:4680–4687.
48. Witkin SS, Ledger WJ. Complexities of the uniquely human vagina. Sci Transl Med 2012; 4:132fs11.
49. Aroutcheva A, Gariti D, Simon M, et al. Defense factors of vaginal lactobacilli. Am J Obstet Gynecol 2001; 185:375–379.
50. Petricevic L, Domig KJ, Nierscher FJ, et al. Characterisation of the vaginal *Lactobacillus* microbiota associated with preterm delivery. Sci Rep 2014; 4:5136.
51. Aagaard K, Riehle K, Ma J, et al. A metagenomic approach to characterization of the vaginal microbiome signature in pregnancy. PLoS One 2012; 7:e36466.
52. Romero R, Hassan SS, Gajer P, et al. The vaginal microbiota of pregnant women who subsequently have spontaneous preterm labor and delivery and those with a normal delivery at term. Microbiome 2014; 2:18.
53. DiGiulio DB, Callahan BJ, McMurdie PJ, et al. Temporal and spatial variation of the human microbiota during pregnancy. Proc Natl Acad Sci U S A 2015; 112:11060–11065.
54. Serrano MG, Parikh HI, Brooks JP, et al. Racioethnic diversity in the dynamics of the vaginal microbiome during pregnancy. Nat Med 2019; 25:1001–1011.
55. Fettweis JM, Serrano MG, Brooks JP, et al. The vaginal microbiome and preterm birth. Nat Med 2019; 25:1012–1021.
56. MacIntyre DA, Chandiramani M, Lee YS, et al. The vaginal microbiome during pregnancy and the postpartum period in a European population. Sci Rep 2015; 5:8988.
57. Grewal K, MacIntyre DA, Bennett PR. The reproductive tract microbiota in pregnancy. Biosci Rep 2021; 41:BSR20203908.
58. Bayar E, Bennett PR, Chan D, et al. The pregnancy microbiome and preterm birth. Semin Immunopathol 2020; 42:487–499.
59. Nelson DB, Shin H, Wu J, et al. The Gestational Vaginal Microbiome and Spontaneous Preterm Birth among Nulliparous African American Women. Am J Perinatol 2016; 33:887–893.
60. Hyman RW, Fukushima M, Jiang H, et al. Diversity of the vaginal microbiome correlates with preterm birth. Reprod Sci 2014; 21:32–40.
61. Freitas AC, Bocking A, Hill JE, et al. Increased richness and diversity of the vaginal microbiota and spontaneous preterm birth. Microbiome 2018; 6:117.
62. Tabatabaei N, Eren AM, Barreiro LB, et al. Vaginal microbiome in early pregnancy and subsequent risk of spontaneous preterm birth: a case-control study. BJOG 2019; 126:349–358.
63. Brown RG, Chan D, Terzidou V, et al. Prospective observational study of vaginal microbiota pre- and post-rescue cervical cerclage. BJOG 2019; 126:916–925.
64. Flaviani F, Hezelgrave NL, Kanno T, et al. Cervicovaginal microbiota and metabolome predict preterm birth risk in an ethnically diverse cohort. JCI Insight 2021; 6:e149257.
65. Sarmento SGP, Moron AF, Forney LJ, et al. An exploratory study of associations with spontaneous preterm birth in primigravid pregnant women with a normal cervical length. J Matern Fetal Neonatal Med 2021; 1–6.
66. Elovitz MA, Gajer P, Riis V, et al. Cervicovaginal microbiota and local immune response modulate the risk of spontaneous preterm delivery. Nat Commun 2019; 10:1305.
67. Dunlop AL, Satten GA, Hu YJ, et al. Vaginal Microbiome Composition in Early Pregnancy and Risk of Spontaneous Preterm and Early Term Birth Among African American Women. Front Cell Infect Microbiol 2021; 11:641005.
68. Kindinger LM, Bennett PR, Lee YS, et al. The interaction between vaginal microbiota, cervical length, and vaginal progesterone treatment for preterm birth risk. Microbiome 2017; 5:6.
69. Payne MS, Newnham JP, Doherty DA, et al. A specific bacterial DNA signature in the vagina of Australian women in midpregnancy predicts high risk of spontaneous preterm birth (the Predict1000 study). Am J Obstet Gynecol 2021; 224:635–636.
70. Ng S, Chen M, Kundu S, et al. Large-scale characterisation of the pregnancy vaginal microbiome and sialidase activity in a low-risk Chinese population. NPJ Biofilms Microbiomes 2021; 7:89.
71. Mercer BM. Preterm premature rupture of the membranes. Obstet Gynecol 2003; 101:178–193.
72. Paramel Jayaprakash T, Wagner EC, van Schalkwyk J, et al. High Diversity and Variability in the Vaginal Microbiome in Women following Preterm Premature Rupture of Membranes (PPROM): A Prospective Cohort Study. PLoS One 2016; 11:e0166794.
73. Baldwin EA, Walther-Antonio M, MacLean AM, et al. Persistent microbial dysbiosis in preterm premature rupture of membranes from onset until delivery. Peer J 2015; 3:e1398.

74. Kacerovsky M, Musilova I, Andrys C, et al. Prelabor rupture of membranes between 34 and 37 weeks: the intraamniotic inflammatory response and neonatal outcomes. Am J Obstet Gynecol 2014; 210:325.e1–e10.

75. Brown RG, Marchesi JR, Lee YS, et al. Vaginal dysbiosis increases risk of preterm fetal membrane rupture, neonatal sepsis and is exacerbated by erythromycin. BMC Med 2018; 16:9.

76. Brown RG, Al-Memar M, Marchesi JR, et al. Establishment of vaginal microbiota composition in early pregnancy and its association with subsequent preterm prelabor rupture of the fetal membranes. Transl Res 2019; 207:30–43.

77. Word RA, Li XH, Hnat M, et al. Dynamics of cervical remodeling during pregnancy and parturition: mechanisms and current concepts. Semin Reprod Med 2007; 25:69–79.

78. Yellon SM. Immunobiology of Cervix Ripening. Front Immunol 2019; 10:3156.

79. Hay PE, Lamont RF, Taylor-Robinson D, et al. Abnormal bacterial colonisation of the genital tract and subsequent preterm delivery and late miscarriage. BMJ 1994; 308:295–298.

80. Al-Memar M, Bobdiwala S, Fourie H, et al. The association between vaginal bacterial composition and miscarriage: a nested case-control study. BJOG 2020; 127:264–274.

81. Grewal K, Lee YS, Smith A, et al. Chromosomally normal miscarriage is associated with vaginal dysbiosis and local inflammation. BMC Med 2022; 20:38.

82. Rendell V, Bath NM, Brennan TV. Medawar's Paradox and Immune Mechanisms of Fetomaternal Tolerance. OBM Transplant 2020; 4:26.

83. Sykes L, MacIntyre DA, Yap XJ, et al. The Th1:th2 dichotomy of pregnancy and preterm labour. Mediators Inflamm 2012; 2012:967629.

84. Mor G, Aldo P, Alvero AB. The unique immunological and microbial aspects of pregnancy. Nat Rev Immunol 2017; 17:469–482.

85. Wegmann TG, Lin H, Guilbert L, et al. Bidirectional cytokine interactions in the maternal-fetal relationship: is successful pregnancy a TH2 phenomenon? Immunol Today 1993; 14:353–356.

86. Agrawal V, Hirsch E. Intrauterine infection and preterm labor. Semin Fetal Neonatal Med 2012; 17:12–19.

87. Chandiramani M, Seed PT, Orsi NM, et al. Limited relationship between cervico-vaginal fluid cytokine profiles and cervical shortening in women at high risk of spontaneous preterm birth. PLoS One 2012; 7:e52412.

88. Taylor BD, Holzman CB, Fichorova RN, et al. Inflammation biomarkers in vaginal fluid and preterm delivery. Hum Reprod 2013; 28:942–952.

89. Tornblom SA, Klimaviciute A, Bystrom B, et al. Non-infected preterm parturition is related to increased concentrations of IL-6, IL-8 and MCP-1 in human cervix. Reprod Biol Endocrinol 2005; 3:39.

90. Kacerovsky M, Vrbacky F, Kutova R, et al. Cervical microbiota in women with preterm prelabor rupture of membranes. PLoS One 2015; 10:e0126884.

91. Rose WA 2nd, McGowin CL, Spagnuolo RA, et al. Commensal bacteria modulate innate immune responses of vaginal epithelial cell multilayer cultures. PLoS One 2012; 7:e32728.

92. Amsel R, Totten PA, Spiegel CA, et al. Nonspecific vaginitis. Diagnostic criteria and microbial and epidemiologic associations. Am J Med 1983; 74:14–22.

93. Nugent RP, Krohn MA, Hillier SL. Reliability of diagnosing bacterial vaginosis is improved by a standardized method of gram stain interpretation. J Clin Microbiol 1991; 29:297–301.

94. Oliver A, LaMere B, Weihe C, et al. Cervicovaginal Microbiome Composition Is Associated with Metabolic Profiles in Healthy Pregnancy. mBio 2020; 11:e01851–20.

95. Pruski P, MacIntyre DA, Lewis HV, et al. Medical Swab Analysis Using Desorption Electrospray Ionization Mass Spectrometry: A Noninvasive Approach for Mucosal Diagnostics. Anal Chem 2017; 89:1540–1550.

96. Pruski P, Correia GDS, Lewis HV, et al. Direct on-swab metabolic profiling of vaginal microbiome host interactions during pregnancy and preterm birth. Nat Commun 2021; 12:5967.

97. Simcox R, Sin WT, Seed PT, et al. Prophylactic antibiotics for the prevention of preterm birth in women at risk: a meta-analysis. Aust N Z J Obstet Gynaecol 2007; 47:368–377.

98. Subtil D, Brabant G, Tilloy E, et al. Early clindamycin for bacterial vaginosis in pregnancy (PREMEVA): a multicentre, double-blind, randomised controlled trial. Lancet 2018; 392:2171–2179.

99. Shennan A, Crawshaw S, Briley A, et al. A randomised controlled trial of metronidazole for the prevention of preterm birth in women positive for cervicovaginal fetal fibronectin: the PREMET Study. BJOG 2006; 113:65–74.

100. Kenyon SL, Taylor DJ, Tarnow-Mordi W, et al. Broad-spectrum antibiotics for preterm, prelabour rupture of fetal membranes: the ORACLE I randomised trial. ORACLE Collaborative Group. Lancet 2001; 357:979–988.

101. Grev J, Berg M, Soll R. Maternal probiotic supplementation for prevention of morbidity and mortality in preterm infants. Cochrane Database Syst Rev 2018; 12:CD012519.

102. Jarde A, Lewis-Mikhael AM, Moayyedi P, et al. Pregnancy outcomes in women taking probiotics or prebiotics: a systematic review and meta-analysis. BMC Pregnancy Childbirth 2018; 18:14.

103. Husain S, Allotey J, Drymoussi Z, et al. Effects of oral probiotic supplements on vaginal microbiota during pregnancy: a randomised, double-blind, placebo-controlled trial with microbiome analysis. BJOG 2020; 127:275–284.

104. Yang S, Reid G, Challis JRG, et al. Effect of Oral Probiotic Lactobacillus rhamnosus GR-1 and Lactobacillus reuteri RC-14 on the Vaginal Microbiota, Cytokines and Chemokines in Pregnant Women. Nutrients 2020; 12:368.

105. van de Wijgert J, Verwijs MC, Agaba SK, et al. Intermittent Lactobacilli-containing Vaginal Probiotic or Metronidazole Use to Prevent Bacterial Vaginosis Recurrence: A Pilot Study Incorporating Microscopy and Sequencing. Sci Rep 2020; 10:3884.

106. Cohen CR, Wierzbicki MR, French AL, et al. Randomized Trial of Lactin-V to Prevent Recurrence of Bacterial Vaginosis. N Engl J Med 2020; 382:1906–1915.

107. Daskalakis GJ, Karambelas AK. Vaginal Probiotic Administration in the Management of Preterm Premature Rupture of Membranes. Fetal Diagn Ther 2017; 42:92–98.

108. Gonzalez JM, Franzke CW, Yang F, et al. Complement activation triggers metalloproteinases release inducing cervical remodeling and preterm birth in mice. Am J Pathol 2011; 179:838–849.

109. Gonzalez JM, Pedroni SM, Girardi G. Statins prevent cervical remodeling, myometrial contractions and preterm labor through a mechanism that involves hemoxygenase-1 and complement inhibition. Mol Hum Reprod 2014; 20:579–589.

110. Denny KJ, Coulthard LG, Mantovani S, et al. The Role of C5a Receptor Signaling in Endotoxin-Induced Miscarriage and Preterm Birth. Am J Reprod Immunol 2015; 74:148–155.

111. Ohmura K, Oku K, Kitaori T, et al. Pathogenic roles of anti-C1q antibodies in recurrent pregnancy loss. Clin Immunol 2019; 203:37–44.

112. Lynch AM, Gibbs RS, Murphy JR, et al. Complement activation fragment Bb in early pregnancy and spontaneous preterm birth. Am J Obstet Gynecol 2008; 199:354.e1–e8.

113. Soto E, Romero R, Vaisbuch E, et al. Fragment Bb: evidence for activation of the alternative pathway of the complement system in pregnant women with acute pyelonephritis. J Matern Fetal Neonatal Med 2010; 23:1085–1090.

114. Vaisbuch E, Romero R, Erez O, et al. Activation of the alternative pathway of complement is a feature of pre-term parturition but not of spontaneous labor at term. Am J Reprod Immunol 2010; 63:318–330.

115. Kim YJ, Kim KH, Ko EJ, et al. Complement C3 Plays a Key Role in Inducing Humoral and Cellular Immune Responses to Influenza Virus Strain-Specific Hemagglutinin-Based or Cross-Protective M2 Extracellular Domain-Based Vaccination. J Virol 2018; 92:e00969–18 .

116. Zelek WM, Xie L, Morgan BP, et al. Compendium of current complement therapeutics. Mol Immunol 2019; 114:341–352.

117. Stefanovic V. The Extended Use of Eculizumab in Pregnancy and Complement Activation(-)Associated Diseases Affecting Maternal, Fetal and Neonatal Kidneys-The Future Is Now? J Clin Med 2019; 8:407.

118. Hsieh TT, Chen SF, Shau WY, et al. The impact of interpregnancy interval and previous preterm birth on the subsequent risk of preterm birth. J Soc Gynecol Investig 2005; 12:202–207.

119. Marinovich ML, Regan AK, Gissler M, et al. Associations between interpregnancy interval and preterm birth by previous preterm birth status in four high-income countries: a cohort study. BJOG 2021; 128:1134–1143.

120. Bradford LL, Ravel J. The vaginal mycobiome: A contemporary perspective on fungi in women's health and diseases. Virulence 2017; 8:342–351.

121. Drell T, Lillsaar T, Tummeleht L, et al. Characterization of the vaginal micro- and mycobiome in asymptomatic reproductive-age Estonian women. PLoS One 2013; 8:e54379.

122. Tortelli BA, Lewis WG, Allsworth JE, et al. Associations between the vaginal microbiome and Candida colonization in women of reproductive age. Am J Obstet Gynecol 2020; 222:471.e1–e9.

123. Wylie KM, Mihindukulasuriya KA, Zhou Y, et al. Metagenomic analysis of double-stranded DNA viruses in healthy adults. BMC Biol 2014; 12:71.

124. Wylie KM, Wylie TN, Cahill AG, et al. The vaginal eukaryotic DNA virome and preterm birth. Am J Obstet Gynecol 2018; 219:189.e1–e12.

125. Ilievski V, Hirsch E. Synergy between viral and bacterial toll-like receptors leads to amplification of inflammatory responses and preterm labor in the mouse. Biol Reprod 2010; 83:767–773.

126. Rasheed ZBM, Lee YS, Kim SH, et al. Differential Response of Gestational Tissues to TLR3 Viral Priming Prior to Exposure to Bacterial TLR2 and TLR2/6 Agonists. Front Immunol 2020; 11:1899.

# Chapter 6

# Current management of endometriosis: Diagnosis to surgical treatment

*Miguel Luna Russo, Rosanne M Kho*

## INTRODUCTION

Endometriosis is defined as the presence of endometrial-type tissue outside of the endometrial cavity [1,2]. This chronic inflammatory and oestrogen-dependent disease can be present in 1 out of 10 women of reproductive age. The average age of diagnosis is 28 years of age. Despite being more common in the reproductive age, endometriosis can be present in the pre-menarchal and post-menopausal females. Approximately 87% of patient with endometriosis will suffer from chronic pelvic pain. Endometriosis is also a known contributor to infertility and can be present in approximately 47% of women presenting with difficulty in conceiving. Unfortunately, this disease carries a delay in diagnosis that has been reported to up to 9 years. This delay has contributed to the decline in quality of life and productivity in patients with this disease. Quality of life of women with endometriosis has been reported to be similar to women with terminal cancer. The combination of poor quality of life and delay of diagnosis has led to an increase in healthcare expenditure  and estimated societal economic burden estimated as high as 49 billion USD per year in the United States alone [1,2].

The pathophysiology and management of this chronic and debilitating disease is complex, and its diagnosis can be confounded due to its significant overlap with other pain syndromes. The lack of standardised medical and surgical treatment patterns can also lead to suboptimal management. The management of endometriosis requires specialised and multidisciplinary care that should be centred around the patients' goals for fertility and improvement of pain. Endometriosis literature is robust in observational research, unfortunately, and there is a paucity of randomised controlled trials in the management of this disease.

## PATHOGENESIS

The pathogenesis of endometriosis continues to be controversial as no one single theory can explain all the phenotypic variations of this disease. Currently, the origin of

**Miguel Luna Russo** MD FACOG, Director of Endometriosis, Department of Ob Gyn, Women's Health Institute, Cleveland Clinic, Cleveland, OH
Email: Lunarum@ccf.org

**Rosanne M Kho** MD, Department of Ob Gyn and Women's Health Institute, Cleveland Clinic, Cleveland, OH
Email: Khor@ccf.org

endometriosis can be explained by the following three concepts: (1) Sampson's theory of retrograde menstruation, (2) coelomic metaplasia, and (3) the Müllerianosis theory.

Retrograde menstruation remains the most popular theory of pathogenesis of endometriosis [3]. It was initially proposed by Dr John A Sampson in the 1920. This theory began with the study of "chocolate cyst" and was proposed after noticing menstrual blood in the pelvis during laparotomies in women before, during, and after their menstrual cycle. This phenomenon exposes the pelvis to endometrial stem cells that may then implant over the surface of the pelvic peritoneum, ovaries, bladder and rectum and continue to proliferate and shed with every menstrual cycle [3]. Haematogenous and lymphatic spread of these endometrial stem cells that later implant and proliferate in areas outside of the pelvis has been described as one of the possible causes of extra-pelvic endometriosis [4]. This theory has been contested in the past as it is unable to explain endometriosis occurring in the pre-menarchal period and endometriosis reported in males [5].

Metaplasia of coelomic epithelium has also been proposed as a theory and is described as differentiation and transformation of peritoneal and superficial ovarian epithelium into endometrioid cells types likely resulting from menstrual debris and oestrogen exposure [6]. Stems cells arising from extra-uterine sites such as the bone marrow has also been suggested to undergo transformation into endometrioid type cell lines. The peritoneal lining, pleura, and Müllerian ducts share the same embryologic cell origin, the coelomic epithelium [7], potentially explaining the rare cases of endometriosis in males, extra-pelvic site, and in pre-pubertal females.

The Müllerianosis theory describes the presence of Müllerian tissue remnants after migration of the Müllerian ducts [3]. This has been proposed as the one of the mechanisms in the origin of deep infiltrating endometriosis of the posterior and anterior cul-de-sac.

A single theory of pathogenesis alone is unable to explain the totality of phenotypic presentations of endometriosis. To this date the literature is lacking in the basic science research that could explain all presentations of this disease.

Endometriosis lesions are responsive to oestrogen and progesterone. Generally, lesions are responsive to female sex hormones in the same ways as endometrial tissue. Endometriotic lesions have a tropic response to serum circulating oestrogens but are also capable of oestrogen production driven by expression of aromatase at a cellular level. Implants differ in oestrogen receptor expression compared to eutopic endometrium. Endometriosis implants are characterised by a higher expression of oestrogen receptor beta, this phenomenon is considered pathological and leads to a suppression of progesterone receptors in the lesion itself. This has been postulated as a mechanism of progesterone resistance causing lesions to proliferate despite endogenous and exogenous progesterone exposure [3]. Continued genome methylation within the implants contributes to increased endogenous oestrogen and prostaglandin production, creating a highly inflammatory environment. This inflammatory milieu creates an influx of cytokines (i.e. IL-6, TNF-$\alpha$) in addition for nerve and vascular growth factors (i.e. VEGF, NGF) that later contribute to chronic pain, adhesion formation and infertility [1] (**Figure 6.1**).

## MECHANISM OF SUBFERTILITY

Decreased fertility in endometriosis is a multifactorial phenomenon where chronic inflammation, adhesion formation, and ovarian tissue damage can play a role both independently and in unison. It is often difficult to differentiate the exact culprit as there has not been a clear correlation between disease burden and subfertility [3].

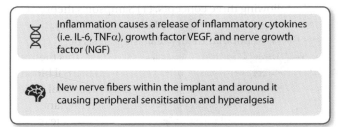

**Figure 6.1** Mechanisms of pain.

Inflammation causes a release of inflammatory cytokines (i.e. IL-6, TNFα), growth factor VEGF, and nerve growth factor (NGF)

New nerve fibers within the implant and around it causing peripheral sensitisation and hyperalgesia

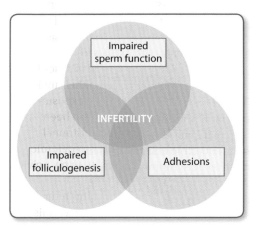

**Figure 6.2** Mechanisms of subfertility.

The chronic inflammatory environment created by endometriosis may play a large contributing role in the mechanism of subfertility. Pelvic adhesions can result from the inflammatory insult to the peritoneal lining, later leading to anatomic distortion and impairment of tubal function by obstruction preventing oocyte and sperm transit for conception to occur. Oocyte capture by the distal end of the fallopian tube may also be hindered by adhesions and fibrosis potentially caused by ovarian endometriomas [8]. This environment also causes gamete oxidative stress. Inflammatory cell enlistment by endometriosis lesions physiology leads to an immune response that signals macrophage recruitment that then leads to an increase in cytokine release, this cascade then causes damage to gamete cell structure. In in-vitro studies, human sperm and mice oocytes have been incubated in peritoneal fluid with endometriosis [9]. When compared to cells incubated in peritoneal fluid from non-endometriosis patients, 60% of cells incubated in peritoneal fluid of patients with endometriosis were noted to have structural DNA damage while only 20% of cells were noted to be affected in the non-disease group [10] (**Figure 6.2**).

Ovarian endometriomas (**Figure 6.3**) are a known cause of ovarian cortical damage and lead by mass effect and continued inflammation that leads to fibrosis. Constant injury to the ovarian cortex can lead to decrease in ovarian reserve. In a study of women undergoing endometriosis surgery anti-Müllerian hormone (AMH) levels were measured all patients. In patients with endometriomas present at the time of surgery, AMH levels were lower than those without endometriomas. There was a significantly lower level in those patients with bilateral endometriomas present [11].

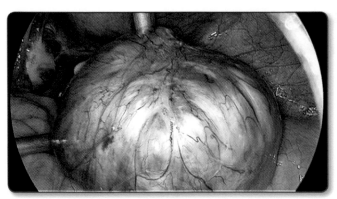

**Figure 6.3** Large ovarian endometrioma.

## MECHANISM OF PAIN

Cyclic and non-cyclic pelvic pain are the most common presenting symptoms in patients with endometriosis. A patient reporting cyclic pain that evolves into constant non-cyclic pelvic pain should prompt immediate evaluation for possible endometriosis. Severe dysmenorrhoea is often the dominant initial present pain symptom in patients with endometriosis [12]. In a study of adolescents with pelvic pain, up to 75% of those who underwent laparoscopy were noted to have endometriosis [13].

Chronic pelvic pain (CPP) is a common finding in patients with endometriosis. In women with CPP who underwent diagnostic laparoscopy, endometriosis was found to be present in up to 87% of cases [14]. Chronic pelvic pain is often multi-factorial and symptoms vary arising from the urinary tract, sexual organs, bowel, and pelvic floor. Chronic pelvic pain is debilitating and often exacerbated by depressive and anxious episodes. Anxiety and depression have been reported in 87% of patients with endometriosis regardless of the stage of disease [15].

## TYPES OF ENDOMETRIOSIS

Endometriosis lesions are categorised by lesion appearance, lesion type and location. Implants can appear pigmented and non-pigmented. Pigmented lesions are often red or black in colour with or without associated hyperaemia and haemorrhagic tissue. Non-pigmented lesions are often areas of fibrosis over the peritoneal surface. Both pigmented and non-pigmented lesions can be vesicular or papillary. All endometriotic implants can been superficial or deep infiltrating, superficial lesions are implants that do not infiltrate surrounding tissue (**Figure 6.4**). Deep infiltrating implants are defined as lesions that are >5 mm in size and depth of infiltration of tissue. Ovarian endometriosis lesions can be both superficial and deep lesions, ovarian endometriomas are cystic lesions of the ovary that are considered deep lesions of the ovary. Ovarian endometriomas are a consequence of superficial endometriosis lesions that become encapsulated secondary to surrounding fibrosis later developing into cystic lesions of the ovary [16].

Endometriosis is most found in the confines of the pelvis but can be found outside of the pelvic cavity. Extra-pelvic lesions are most commonly found in the upper abdomen but have been reported affecting distant sites such as the spinal cord and central nervous system [17]. The spread and implantation of endometriosis within the abdominal cavity

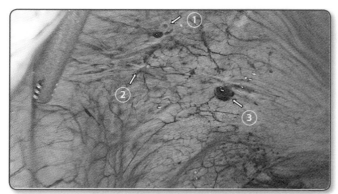

**Figure 6.4** (1) Pigmented dark lesions that are both deep infiltrating and superficial papillary; (2) Non-pigmented 'powder burn' lesion with a papillary component; (3) Pigmented red papillary lesion.

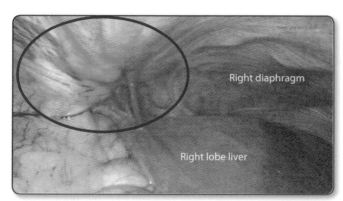

**Figure 6.5** Deep endometriosis of the abdominal portion of the right diaphragm.

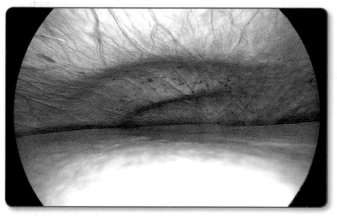

**Figure 6.6** Superficial endometriosis of the abdominal portion of the right diaphragm.

has been attributed to the direction of flow of peritoneal fluid in a clockwise fashion with stasis in dependent areas [18], this supports the findings of a systematic review of extra-pelvic endometriosis by Andres MP et al. noting that 80% of diaphragmatic endometriosis cases were located on the right side of the diaphragm where peritoneal fluid flow is partially obstructed by the falciform ligament [17] (**Figures 6.5** and **6.6**).

# DIAGNOSIS

Laparoscopy with histologic diagnosis of gland and stroma continues to be the gold standard for the diagnosis of endometriosis. Despite advances in preoperative imaging for endometriosis this gold standard continues to be supported by gynaecologic specialty governing bodies [19]. This requirement of histologic confirmation of endometriosis has likely contributed to the delay in diagnosis in patients with endometriosis. Experts in the field of endometriosis have proposed a path for clinical diagnosis of endometriosis by combining clinical history, physical examination findings and imaging with the goal of reducing time to diagnosis [20]. Early diagnosis of endometriosis without the need of a diagnostic invasive procedure followed by referral to a gynaecologic surgeon experienced in the management of endometriosis should be the norm.

## Symptomatology

The presentation of endometriosis is highly variable depending on the burden of disease and location of deep implants. Dysmenorrhoea is often the dominant symptom but patients commonly present with chronic pelvic pain, dyspareunia, and pain during defecation. Cyclic menstrual pelvic pain that transitions into constant pain is highly suspicious of endometriosis. Deep infiltrating endometriosis of the pelvic compartments involving the bladder, sigmoid or rectum can present with dysuria, haematuria, loose stools, constipation, and pseudo-obstructive symptoms [21,22]. Endometriosis of the diaphragm and thoracic cavity can be associated with cyclic shoulder pain, catamenial pneumothorax, and pleural effusions [23].

## Role of imaging in the diagnosis of endometriosis

Diagnostic imaging is an integral step in the management of patients with endometriosis and should be included as the second step of the diagnostic algorithm of this disease process (**Figure 6.7**). MRI and pelvic ultrasound can be helpful in the pre-operative diagnosis of deep, ovarian, and extra-pelvic endometriosis while also serving as an invaluable tool for preoperative planning and counselling. Diagnostic imaging should be a complement to a clinical history and physical examination, imaging alone should not be used as a sole method of diagnosis. Findings during diagnostic imaging should be reported in a standardised specific structured report. Structured reporting compartmentalises the pelvis in anterior, middle, and posterior compartments while also reporting lesions size, location, and distance from key anatomic structures [24].

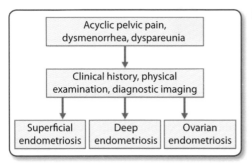

**Figure 6.7** Endometriosis diagnostic algorithm.

This reporting system allows for accurate preoperative planning and standardises imagining results for future research endeavours.

Transvaginal ultrasound in combination with physical examination has been shown to be precise in the preoperative diagnosis of endometriosis [25]. Transvaginal ultrasound has been shown to have a sensitivity and specificity of approximately 95% in the diagnosis of deep infiltrating endometriosis of the pelvis [12]. Recent advances in this modality have led to the diagnosis of superficial endometriosis but further studies are needed to validate this method as an adequate diagnostic tool [26]. Pelvic ultrasound is inexpensive and can be performed by gynaecologists experienced in ultrasound during the evaluation of patients with endometriosis. Unfortunately its accuracy in diagnosis is associated with a steep learning curve [27].

Magnetic resonance imaging (MRI) shares a similar accuracy in sensitivity and specificity in the diagnosis of deep infiltrating and extra-pelvic endometriosis with TVUS (>95%) [28]. MRI carries a less steep learning curve for reading physicians. Unfortunately, it is not as available in all institutions and is more an expensive imaging modality than pelvic ultrasound. The use of vaginal contrast and rectal contrast to perform MRI has been noted to increase the sensitivity and sensitivity of the diagnosis of deep infiltrating endometriosis of the posterior pelvic compartment involving the lower rectum and upper vagina [29].

## MEDICAL MANAGEMENT OF ENDOMETRIOSIS

Pharmacologic management of endometriosis has been based on suppression of endometrial tissue proliferation and shedding, as well as prostaglandin regulation [30]. Because of this, oestrogen suppression and pain control have been the leading target in the medical management of endometriosis. Medical therapy continues to be recommended as a first-line treatment by societies like the American College of Obstetricians and Gynecologist and Society for Reproductive Medicine [19,30].

Current available medical therapies for the management of endometriosis include, combined oestrogen and progesterone formulations, progesterone alone, gonadotropin-releasing hormone (GnRH) antagonists and agonist, androgenic steroids, antiandrogens, aromatase inhibitors, and selective progesterone receptor modulators. These medical therapeutic options overall are suppressive therapies as medical therapy alone is unable to resolve deep and ovarian endometriosis. Generally, medical therapy in endometriosis requires long-term use therefore, when choosing a pharmacologic option, this option should be low cost and have a tolerable side effect profile. Ideally, surgical and medical suppression should be combined as surgery alone without subsequent medical suppression has been associated with a 50% pain symptom recurrence in a 5-year period post surgery [31].

Non-steroidal anti-inflammatory drugs are often used as a first-line treatment of endometriosis-related pain, specifically for the alleviation of dysmenorrhoea. These drugs may be helpful in combination with hormonal therapies, but data is lacking to show a significant improvement of pain when used alone [30].

Combined oestrogen and progesterone formulations are commonly used as first-line therapies for patients with endometriosis and pain. They are usually prescribed with the goal of suppressing menses and therefore can aid in cyclic pelvic pain relief. In patients undergoing suppressive therapy after surgical excision of endometriosis, continuous administration with the goal of amenorrhea was shown to be more effective then cyclic administration in reduction of menstrual associated pelvic pain [32]. Harada et al. compared combined oral contraceptives versus placebo in a double-blind randomised control trial that noted a significant decreased in dysmenorrhoea in the contraceptive group compared to placebo. In patients who presented with ovarian endometriomas, this study also noted a reduction in size of endometriomas in the contraceptive pill group [33]. Other studies comparing oral contraceptive versus placebo have shown a significant reduction in pain, as well as deep infiltrating implants of the posterior pelvic compartment [31]. It is important to note that the benefits of these therapeutic regimens disappear when therapy is discontinued, and endometriosis excision is not performed.

Progestin-only formulations are effective in the reduction of pain in patients with endometriosis. The most used progestin options include, norethindrone acetate (NETA), depot medroxyprogesterone acetate, etonogestrel-releasing implant, and levonorgestrel-releasing intrauterine device (LNG-IUD). Both NETA and depot medroxyprogesterone have received FDA approval for use in the management of endometriosis related pain. The most common side effect of these progestin formulations is breakthrough bleeding that can resolve spontaneously or with oestrogen add-back therapy for up to 14 days. All these formulations have been studied and noted to be effective in reducing pelvic pain and in some cases endometrioma and size of deep infiltrating nodules of the posterior compartment. Depot medroxyprogesterone acetate has been shown to have similar efficacy as GnRH agonist in the reduction of pelvic pain associated with endometriosis, unfortunately this method is known to cause a reduction in bone mineral density as well as causing undesired side effects such as bleeding and weight gain limiting its long-term use. NETA has been shown to improve endometriosis-related pain and decrease in deep infiltrating disease burden without causing significant bleeding side effects or bone loss [34]. Etonogestrel-releasing implant has been shown to sustain relief of pain during defecation and intercourse consistently for a 2-year period of use [35]. LNG-IUDs are as effective as GnRH agonist in preventing the recurrence of pain after endometriosis resection. When compared head to head in a randomised control trial, LNG-IUD was similar to depot GnRH analogue in preventing pain recurrence postoperatively with the added benefit of less vasomotor symptoms, no need for add-back therapy, and ability for long-term use (5 years) without need of bone mineral density assessment [36].

Gonadotropin-releasing hormone agonist should be reserved for patients who have failed other medical therapies who have been diagnosed with endometriosis histologically or those who have severe extra-pelvic disease that are not amendable to surgery. GnRH agonists are not optimal for long-term use because of their side effect profile. These drugs are associated with menopausal symptoms such as hot flashes, depressed mood, fatigue, hair loss, bone loss and vaginal dryness. When prolonged therapy is indicated, add-back therapy with NETA or combined oestrogen and progesterone contraceptive pills should be administered to ameliorate menopausal symptoms. These drugs have been studied extensively and improve endometriosis-associated pain, especially when used for suppression in the post-operative period. Because of the high side effect profile, GnRH agonist should not be used as a first line drug. Studies have not shown GnRH agonist to be superior to progestins or combination oral contraceptives [37,38].

Most recently GnRH antagonists have and are being studied as a first-line therapy for patients with endometriosis. GnRH antagonist can be administered orally and do not produce FSH and LH surges as the drug binds to receptors in the anterior pituitary [39]. The first randomised trial versus placebo was published in 2017 with the goal of assessing the response of the drug on menstrual and non-menstrual pelvic pain. Patients noted a decrease in dysmenorrhoea in as high as 76% and decrease in non-menstrual pelvic pain in as high as 50% during the study period [40]. Unfortunately only 48% of patients completed treatment after 12 months of use in a follow-up study from the same group [41]. When compared to progestin formulations, GnRH agonist has not been found to be superior for the improvement of endometriosis-related pain [39].

## Surgical management of endometriosis

The inflammatory environment and adhesiogenic nature of endometriosis can cause significant anatomical distortion. Surgery for endometriosis is complex and requires expert knowledge of anatomy and minimally invasive techniques. Laparoscopic surgery is the preferred approach for the surgical management of endometriosis [2]. Laparoscopy provides improved visualisation as well as improved postoperative outcomes [42]. Robotic surgery has not been shown to have improved outcomes when compared to traditional laparoscopy [43].

Indications for surgical management vary and should be tailored to specific patient goals for fertility and pain control. Most common indications for surgery are persistent pain that is not improved with medical therapy, need for tissue diagnosis or to facilitate infertility treatments.

## Surgery for ovarian endometriomas

Ovarian endometriomas are a known cause of pelvic pain and decreased ovarian reserve [16]. Persistent pain, rapid size increase, and suspicion of atypical presentation on imaging are indications for surgical removal. They are rarely isolated lesions and are present concomitantly with other deep endometriosis lesions in 85% of cases. If an endometrioma is identified on basic ultrasound, targeted imaging for endometriosis (MRI or ultrasound) should be considered to evaluate for other sites of deep endometriosis prior to surgical management [44]. Asymptomatic endometriomas <4 cm should be managed expectantly, especially in patients who have immediate fertility desires to avoid further ovarian tissue damage caused by surgery [45] (**Figure 6.8**). Endometrioma cystectomy is the preferred approach to removal. Endometrioma cystectomy is associated with increased spontaneous conception and decreased cyst recurrence [46]. Proper surgical technique is vital during endometrioma cystectomy, normal anatomy should be restored prior to ovarian cystectomy to clearly identify ovarian blood supply and avoid inadvertent injury. Endometriomas often rupture during

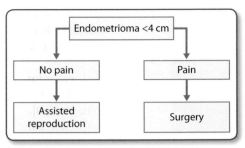

**Figure 6.8** Management algorithm of patient diagnosed with endometriomas that desire immediate fertility.

restoration of anatomy. Once chocolate fluid is drained, the cyst wall can be separated from the ovarian stroma using traction alternating with blunt and sharp dissection. If the endometrioma remains intact during the initial dissection, injectable saline or dilute vasopressin injected under the ovarian stroma has been described. Hydro-dissection can aid in facilitating dissection and create more haemostatic cystectomy. During ovarian cystectomy judicious use of electrosurgical energy is encouraged to decrease the amount of tissue damage. Surgical haemostatic materials can be used over the cystectomy bed to control bleeding. In a study comparing haemostatic materials versus bipolar electrosurgical energy in controlling bleeding after cystectomy, bipolar energy was associated with a significant drop in anti-Müllerian hormone compared to the haemostatic material group (41% vs. 18%) [47]. If haemostatic agents are not available, suture of the cystectomy bed is preferred to avoid the use of energy. If immediate fertility is not desired, post-operative suppression should be considered with the goal of decreasing potential recurrence (**Figure 6.9**).

## Surgery for deep infiltrating endometriosis

Deep infiltrating endometriosis (DIE) lesions are defined as lesions that are >5 mm in size and depth of infiltration. Medical therapy can improve pain in patients with DIE but is unable to be curative [42] (**Figure 6.10**). DIE lesions are often surrounded by fibrotic tissue and tend to cause significant anatomic distortion. These infiltrating lesions affect

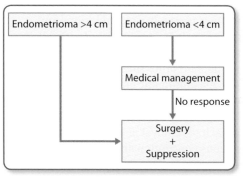

**Figure 6.9** Management algorithm of patient diagnosed with endometriomas without immediate fertility desire.

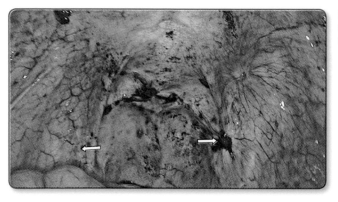

**Figure 6.10** Deep infiltrating endometriosis of bilateral utero-sacral ligaments.

retroperitoneal structures by causing significant fibrosis. DIE should be excised completely; ablation is not recommended in these cases due to the proximity of lesions to important anatomical structures of the pelvis. Safe surgical excision of DIE require advanced surgical experience as extensive pelvis dissections are often needed [48].

## Surgical management of bowel endometriosis

Endometriosis involving the bowel is present in approximately 10–12% of all patients with endometriosis. Lesions can involve all layers of the bowel wall and can cause angulation of the lumen, retractions, and strictures (**Figure 6.11**). Symptoms can include cyclic and non-cyclic nausea, vomiting, bloating, haematochezia, constipation, dyschezia, and intestinal obstruction [49].

Bowel lesions are often nodular with surrounding fibrosis. The rectum and sigmoid are the portions of the large bowel most involved (85% of patients with advanced disease) and usually present with symptoms of constipation, dyschezia, dyspareunia and bloating. Painful nodularity of the retro-cervical area on examination should raise suspicion of lower left colon involvement. Recto-sigmoid lesions seldom cause intestinal obstruction. Right sided bowel lesions are less frequent and usually involve the ileo-cecal junction and are frequently associated with cyclic pseudo-obstructive symptoms. Intestinal obstruction is more common with right-sided lesions [50].

Excision of symptomatic endometriosis lesions of the rectum and sigmoid has been shown to provide significant relief of dyspareunia in patients with retro-cervical disease [51]. Removal of bowel endometriosis has also been associated with increased spontaneous pregnancy rates in patients with advanced endometriosis and infertility [52]. Adequate resection of bowel lesions can be achieved via conservative or definite approaches. Rectal shaving and discoid excisions are considered conservative surgical methods, while segmental resection are deemed definitive excisions [53].

### Bowel shaving

Shaving is defined by the removal of active endometriosis tissue and fibrosis from the visceral surface of the bowel. This method is not a full-thickness excision of the bowel wall. In order for shaving to be considered and be successful, the lesion should not infiltrate beyond the muscularis externa and should involve < 50% of the lumen circumference.

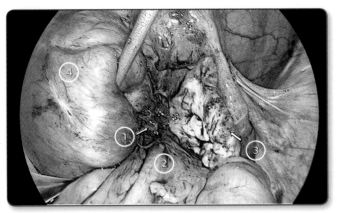

**Figure 6.11** Retro-cervical nodule leading to 'kissing ovaries'. The following can be appreciated: (1) Endometriosis nodule involving bilateral ovaries and the recto-sigmoid junction; (2) Recto-sigmoid Junction; (3) Right ovary; (4) Left ovary and tube. Large endometrioma and hydro-salpinx noted.

If the muscularis of the rectum or sigmoid is visible after resection, the serosa should be re-approximated over the defect to provide structural support and potentially prevent stool leakage in the post-operative period. A bowel wall integrity test (bubble test) should be performed after shaving in order to assure the bowel lumen was not breached during shaving [54].

## Discoid excision

Discoid excision is a partial full thickness excision of the bowel wall. Disk excision can be performed when lesions up to 3 cm in size that infiltrate beyond the muscularis layer towards the bowel mucosa. The full thickness defect should be repaired in two layers of absorbable suture in a direction perpendicular to the bowel lumen [54]. An airtight closure is required, if the bowel integrity test fails a loop ileostomy or colostomy is indicated. Ostomy should be considered if suture repair line is at a distance of 5 cm or less from the anal verge [55].

## Segmental resection

Complete segmental resection is the most common type of bowel endometriosis excision performed in patient with advanced disease. Lesions that cause significant bowel lumen stenosis, infiltrating lesions that involve the rectal mucosa and have an intra-luminal component or lesions >3 cm with a >50% luminal involvement are indications for segmental resection. Ostomy is indicated for low laying anastomotic staple line. This method of excision is associated with the lowest rates of lesion recurrence but can carry higher rates of diversion, bowel and bladder dysfunction, and post-operative complications [56–58].

## CONCLUSION

Endometriosis is a chronic disease that commonly affects women of reproductive age but is not exclusive of pre-menarchal and post-menopausal period. Major negative impacts on patients' quality of life, mental health, sexual function, bowel function, and fertility are commonly associated with a diagnosis of endometriosis. Treatment strategies for women with endometriosis should be multidisciplinary and tailored to the patients' needs, including future reproductive goals.

## REFERENCES

1.    Luna Russo MA, Chalif JN, Falcone T. Clinical management of endometriosis. Minerva Ginecol 2020; 72.
2.    Falcone T, Flyckt-Rebecca R. Clinical management of endometriosis. Obstet Gynecol 2018 ;131:557–571.
3.    Vercellini P, Viganò P, Somigliana E, et al. Endometriosis: pathogenesis and treatment. Nat Rev Endocrinol 2014; 10:261–275.
4.    Hill CJ, Fakhreldin M, Maclean A, et al. Clinical Medicine Endometriosis and the Fallopian Tubes: Theories of Origin and Clinical Implications. J Clin Med 2020; 9:1905.
5.    Sourial S, Tempest N, Hapangama DK. Theories on the Pathogenesis of Endometriosis. Int J Reprod Med 2014:179515.
6.    Rolla E. Open Peer Review Endometriosis: advances and controversies in classification, pathogenesis, diagnosis, and treatment [version 1; peer review: 4 approved] 2019; 8:529.
7.    Sasson IE, Taylor HS. Stem Cells and the Pathogenesis of Endometriosis. Ann N Y Acad Sci 2008; 1127:106–115.
8.    Anatomy DP, Function AP. Endometriosis and infertility. Fertil Steril 2006; 86:S156–S160.

9. Mansour G, Sharma RK, Agarwal A, et al. Endometriosis-induced alterations in mouse metaphase II oocyte microtubules and chromosomal alignment: a possible cause of infertility. Fertil Steril 2010; 94:1894–1899.

10. Mansour G, Aziz N, Sharma R, et al. The impact of peritoneal fluid from healthy women and from women with endometriosis on sperm DNA and its relationship to the sperm deformity index. Fertil Steril 2009; 92:61–67.

11. Goodman LR, Goldberg JM, Flyckt RL, et al. Effect of surgery on ovarian reserve in women with endometriomas, endometriosis and controls. Am J Obstet Gynecol 2016; 215:589.e1–589.e6.

12. Abrao MS, Gonçalves MODC, Dias JA, et al. Comparison between clinical examination, transvaginal sonography and magnetic resonance imaging for the diagnosis of deep endometriosis. Hum Reprod 2007; 22:3092–3097.

13. Chapron C, Borghese B, Streuli I, et al. Markers of adult endometriosis detectable in adolescence. J Pediatr Adolesc Gynecol 2011; 24:S7–S12.

14. Aredo JV, Heyrana KJ, Karp BI, et al. Relating Chronic Pelvic Pain and Endometriosis to Signs of Sensitization and Myofascial Pain and Dysfunction. Semin Reprod Med 2017; 35:88–97.

15. Laganà AS, La Rosa VL, Rapisarda AMC, et al. Anxiety and depression in patients with endometriosis: Impact and management challenges. Int J Womens Health 2017; 9:323–330.

16. Muzii L, Di Tucci C, Di Mascio D, et al. Current management of ovarian endometriomas. Minerva Ginecol 2018; 70:286–294.

17. Andres MP, Arcoverde FVL, Souza CCC, et al. Extrapelvic Endometriosis: A Systematic Review. J Minim Invasive Gynecol 2020; 27:373–389.

18. Vercellini P, Abbiati A, Viganò P, et al. Asymmetry in distribution of diaphragmatic endometriotic lesions: Evidence in favour of the menstrual reflux theory. Hum Reprod Hum Reprod 2007; 22:2359–2367.

19. ACOG Committee on Practice Bulletins--Gynecology. ACOG Practice Bulletin No. 11: Medical management of endometriosis. Obstet Gynecol 1999; 94:1–14.

20. Agarwal SK, Chapron C, Giudice LC, et al. Clinical diagnosis of endometriosis: a call to action. Am J Obstet Gynecol 2019; 220:354.e1–354.e12.

21. Ballard KD, Seaman HE, De Vries CS, et al. Can symptomatology help in the diagnosis of endometriosis? Findings from a national case-control study – Part 1. BJOG 2008; 115:1382–1391.

22. Seracchioli R, Mabrouk M, Guerrini M, et al. Dyschezia and Posterior Deep Infiltrating Endometriosis: Analysis of 360 Cases. J Minim Invasive Gynecol 2008; 15:695–699.

23. Nezhat C, Lindheim SR, Backhus L, et al. Thoracic endometriosis syndrome: A review of diagnosis and management. J Soc Laparoendosc Surg 2019; 23:e2019.00029.

24. Feldman MK, VanBuren WM, Barnard H, et al. Systematic interpretation and structured reporting for pelvic magnetic resonance imaging studies in patients with endometriosis: value added for improved patient care. Abdom Radiol 2020; 45:1608–1622.

25. Hudelist G, Oberwinkler KH, Singer CF, et al. Combination of transvaginal sonography and clinical examination for preoperative diagnosis of pelvic endometriosis. Hum Reprod 2009; 24:1018–1024.

26. Leonardi M, Espada M, Lu C, et al. A Novel Ultrasound Technique Called Saline Infusion SonoPODography to Visualize and Understand the Pouch of Douglas and Posterior Compartment Contents: A Feasibility Study. J Ultrasound Med 2019; 38:3301–3309.

27. Young SW, Dahiya N, Patel MD, et al. Initial Accuracy of and Learning Curve for Transvaginal Ultrasound with Bowel Preparation for Deep Endometriosis in a US Tertiary Care Center. J Minim Invasive Gynecol 2017; 24:1170–1176.

28. Bazot M, Bornier C, Dubernard G, et al. Accuracy of magnetic resonance imaging and rectal endoscopic sonography for the prediction of location of deep pelvic endometriosis. Hum Reprod 2007;22:1457–1463.

29. Chassang M, Novellas S, Bloch-Marcotte C, et al. Utility of vaginal and rectal contrast medium in MRI for the detection of deep pelvic endometriosis. Eur Radiol 2010; 20:1003–1010.

30. Treatment of pelvic pain associated with endometriosis: A committee opinion. Fertil Steril 2014;101:927–935.

31. Harada T, Kosaka S, Elliesen J, et al. Ethinylestradiol 20 µg/drospirenone 3 mg in a flexible extended regimen for the management of endometriosis-associated pelvic pain: a randomized controlled trial. Fertil Steri 2017; 108:798–805.

32. Muzii L, Di Tucci C, Achilli C, et al. Continuous versus cyclic oral contraceptives after laparoscopic excision of ovarian endometriomas: A systematic review and metaanalysis. Am J Obstet Gynecol 2016; 214:203–211.

33. Harada T, Momoeda M, Taketani Y, et al. Low-dose oral contraceptive pill for dysmenorrhea associated with endometriosis: a placebo-controlled, double-blind, randomized trial. Fertil Steril 2008; 90:1583–1588.

34. Casper RF. Progestin-only pills may be a better first-line treatment for endometriosis than combined estrogen-progestin contraceptive pills. Fertil Steril 2017; 107:533–536.

35. Ferrero S, Scala C, Ciccarelli S, et al. Treatment of rectovaginal endometriosis with the etonogestrel-releasing contraceptive implant. Gynecol Endocrinol 2020; 36:540–544.
36. Petta CA, Ferriani RA, Abrao MS, et al. Randomized clinical trial of a levonorgestrel-releasing intrauterine system and a depot GnRH analogue for the treatment of chronic pelvic pain in women with endometriosis. Hum Reprod 2005; 20:1993–1998.
37. Somigliana E, Vercellini P, Vigano P, et al. Postoperative Medical Therapy After Surgical Treatment of Endometriosis: From Adjuvant Therapy to Tertiary Prevention. J Minim Invasive Gynecol 2014; 21:328–334.
38. Vlahos N, Vlachos A, Triantafyllidou O, et al. Continuous versus cyclic use of oral contraceptives after surgery for symptomatic endometriosis: A prospective cohort study. Fertil Steril 2013; 100:1337–1342.
39. Vercellini P, Viganò P, Barbara G, et al. Elagolix for endometriosis: all that glitters is not gold. Hum Reprod 2019; 34:193–199.
40. Taylor HS, Giudice LC, Lessey BA, et al. Treatment of endometriosis-associated pain with elagolix, an oral GnRH antagonist. N Engl J Med 2017; 377:28–40.
41. Surrey E, Taylor HS, Giudice L, et al. Long-Term Outcomes of Elagolix in Women With Endometriosis. Obstet Gynecol 2018; 132:147–160.
42. Flyckt R, Kim S, Falcone T. Surgical Management of Endometriosis in Patients with Chronic Pelvic Pain. Semin Reprod Med 2017; 35:54–64.
43. Soto E, Luu TH, Liu X, et al. Laparoscopy vs. Robotic Surgery for Endometriosis (LAROSE): a multicenter, randomized, controlled trial. Fertil Steril 2017; 107:996–1002.e3.
44. Exacoustos C, De Felice G, Pizzo A, et al. Isolated Ovarian Endometrioma: A History Between Myth and Reality. J Minim Invasive Gynecol. 2018; 25:884–891.
45. Llarena NC, Falcone T, Flyckt RL. Fertility Preservation in Women With Endometriosis. Clin Med Insights Reprod Heal 2019; 13:117955811987338.
46. Hart R, Hickey M, Maouris P, et al. Excisional surgery versus ablative surgery for ovarian endometriomata: A Cochrane Review. Hum Reprod 2008: CD004992.
47. Choi C, Kim WY, Lee DH, et al. Usefulness of hemostatic sealants for minimizing ovarian damage during laparoscopic cystectomy for endometriosis. J Obstet Gynaecol Res 2018; 44:532–539.
48. Gingold JA, Falcone T. The Retroperitoneal Approach to Endometriosis. J Minim Invasive Gynecol 2017; 24:896.
49. De Cicco C, Corona R, Schonman R, et al. Bowel resection for deep endometriosis: A systematic review. BJOG 2011; 118:285–291.
50. Vercellini P, Sergenti G, Buggio L, et al. Advances in the medical management of bowel endometriosis. Best Pract Res Clin Obstet Gynaecol 2021; 71:78–99.
51. Fedele L, Bianchi S, Zanconato G, et al. Long-term follow-up after conservative surgery for rectovaginal endometriosis. Am J Obstet Gynecol 2004; 190:1020–1024.
52. Roman H, Chanavaz-Lacheray I, Ballester M, et al. High postoperative fertility rate following surgical management of colorectal endometriosis. Hum Reprod 2018; 33:1669–1676.
53. Roman H, Bubenheim M, Huet E, et al. Conservative surgery versus colorectal resection in deep endometriosis infiltrating the rectum: A randomized trial. Hum Reprod 2018; 33:47–57.
54. Abrão MS, Petraglia F, Falcone T, et al. Deep endometriosis infiltrating the recto-sigmoid: Critical factors to consider before management. Hum Reprod Update 2015; 21:329–339.
55. Shiomi A, Ito M, Saito N, et al. The indications for a diverting stoma in low anterior resection for rectal cancer: A prospective multicentre study of 222 patients from Japanese cancer centers. Color Dis 2011; 13:1384–1389.
56. Abrão MS, Andres MP, Barbosa RN, et al. Optimizing Perioperative Outcomes with Selective Bowel Resection Following an Algorithm Based on Preoperative Imaging for Bowel Endometriosis. J Minim Invasive Gynecol 2020; 27:883–891.
57. Roman H, Bridoux V, Tuech JJ, et al. Bowel dysfunction before and after surgery for endometriosis. Am J Obstet Gynecol 2013; 209:524–530.
58. Vesale E, Roman H, Moawad G, et al. Voiding Dysfunction after Colorectal Surgery for Endometriosis: A Systematic Review and Meta-analysis. J Minim Invasive Gynecol 2020; 27:1490–1502.e3.

# Chapter 7

# Polycystic ovary syndrome: Prevention and management of cardiometabolic risk

*Ophelia Millar, Nikoleta Papanikolaou, Channa N Jayasena*

## INTRODUCTION

Polycystic ovary syndrome (PCOS) is a complex, heterogeneous endocrine disorder with long-term effects on menstruation, fertility, metabolism and quality of life (QoL). PCOS is one of the most common metabolic disorders in women and the leading cause of infertility. Its worldwide prevalence ranges from 6 to 10% in reproductive-aged women depending on which diagnostic criteria are used [1].

Polycystic ovary syndrome is characterised by disordered ovulation, hyperandrogenism (HA), hyperinsulinaemia and/or polyfollicular ovarian morphology. Clinical manifestations vary greatly but include oligomenorrhoea or amenorrhoea, hirsutism, acne, and obesity. The International evidence-based guideline for the assessment and management of polycystic ovarian syndrome 2018 recommends investigations for PCOS in the form of biochemical tests to calculate free androgen index, testosterone, sex hormone-binding globulin (SHBG), luteinising hormone (LH), follicle-stimulating hormone (FSH), prolactin and thyroid function tests. Ultrasound scan is required in adult women when diagnosis is not clear based on clinical and biochemical features. Ultrasound is not recommended in adolescence because of the high prevalence of ovarian polyfollicular morphology. Typical management aims to alleviate symptoms, improve fertility, reduce risk of cardiovascular outcomes and improve QoL through lifestyle intervention, medical management and psychological therapy.

Although PCOS is diagnosed in reproductive-aged women, the effects extend far beyond menopause due to the broad spectrum of associated morbidities including

**Ophelia Millar** MBBS, Section of Investigative Medicine, Imperial College, Commonwealth Building, Hammersmith Hospital, London, UK
Email: o.millar@nhs.net

**Nikoleta Papanikolaou** MBBS MRCP, Section of Investigative Medicine, Imperial College, Commonwealth Building, Hammersmith Hospital, London, UK
Email: n.papanikolaou@imperial.ac.uk

**Channa N Jayasena** PhD FRCP FRCPath, Reader in Reproductive Endocrinology/Andrology, Imperial College London, Consultant, Hammersmith and St Mary's Hospital, London, UK
Email: c.jayasena@imperial.ac.uk

type 2 diabetes mellitus (T2DM), cardiovascular disease (CVD), endometrial cancer and psychological disorders. Recent interest focusses on the cardiometabolic risks associated with PCOS such as stroke and myocardial infarction, some of the leading causes of mortality [2]. This chapter provides a summary of PCOS and discusses the associated cardiometabolic risk factors and their management.

## HERITABILITY, PATHOPHYSIOLOGY AND DIAGNOSIS OF POLYCYSTIC OVARY SYNDROME

The exact aetiology of this multifactorial syndrome is largely unknown. It is likely a complex interplay of proteins and genes influenced by epigenetic and environmental factors, including diet and lifestyle. This results in the neuroendocrine, metabolic and ovarian dysfunction characteristic of PCOS.

Abnormalities of the hypothalamic–pituitary axis have been observed in women with PCOS (**Figure 7.1**). Gonadotropin-releasing hormone (GnRH) pulsatile secretion is impaired, promoting LH production and causing a relative decrease in FSH. Progesterone is implicated from this impairment, whereby its normal negative feedback on the hypothalamus is reduced, which is considered to be mediated by androgen [3,4]. LH stimulates androgen secretion from ovarian theca cells and thus raised LH results in HA [5]. In vitro studies have shown that multiple enzymes of the steroidogenesis pathway within the ovary are upregulated, contributing to this androgen excess [6].

In parallel, decreased FSH production interferes with normal folliculogenesis. Furthermore, an imbalance between FSH and other intraovarian factors such as anti-müllerian hormone

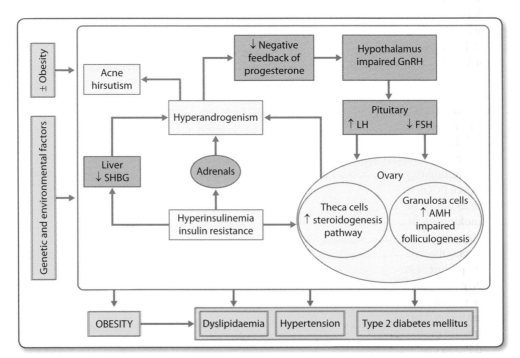

**Figure 7.1** The pathophysiological mechanism and metabolic risks of polycystic ovary syndrome.

(AMH) leads to the abnormal ovarian follicular development seen in PCOS. AMH, produced by granulosa cells, inhibits the transition from primordial to primary follicles while FSH stimulates the maturation of follicles.

Since the 1980s, insulin has attracted interest as the key player in the pathophysiology of PCOS. It is now known that insulin resistance and compensatory hyperinsulinaemia are common in women with PCOS, irrespective of obesity. Although around 65% of women with PCOS are classified as overweight or obese, both overweight and lean women with PCOS may demonstrate insulin resistance (95% vs. 75%) [7]. However, insulin resistance is selective, affecting metabolic but not mitogenic pathways and thus is known as the 'insulin signalling paradox': where adipose tissue, skeletal muscle and the liver express insulin resistance, but steroid-producing tissues maintain insulin sensitivity [5]. Hyperinsulinaemia further contributes to HA via two main mechanisms: (1) augmentation of androgen production in the theca cells and adrenal glands, and (2) reduction of SHBG production in the liver, thus further enhancing androgen action [8,9].

Population studies increasingly show familial aggregation of PCOS. Approximately 20–40% of first-degree female relatives of women with PCOS also have PCOS compared to 4–6% prevalence in those without a family history [10]. However, a genetic marker is yet to be established. Likely genes involved include those encoding for the synthesis, transport and regulation of androgens or those related to insulin metabolism such as insulin receptors [11]. Studies first hypothesised an autosomal dominant inheritance pattern for PCOS, linked to a single gene defect [12]. However, most researchers now describe PCOS as polygenic, and recent small-cohort twin studies of monozygotic and dizygotic pairs have suggested an X-linked polygenic pattern. Twin studies suggest the heritability of PCOS to be 72% which would support a largely genetic epidemiology [12].

A proposed evolutionary origin known as the "thrifty gene hypothesis" offers an explanation as to the increased prevalence of PCOS in certain populations. The "thrifty gene hypothesis" is controversial, and its accuracy has been criticised due to lack of evidence. However, it may explain the propensity of obesity and T2DM in certain populations where historically, carriers of the "thrifty gene" had increased survival by accumulating adipose stores between famines. Similarly, characteristics of PCOS may have historically provided evolutionary survival advantages. Oligo-ovulation often results in greater intervals between pregnancies and higher maternal age at pregnancy, favouring maternal and infant survival [11]. Furthermore, insulin resistance increases glucose availability for cerebral metabolism and increases sympathetic tone, favouring survival during environmental stressors [11].

In addition to gene mutations, environmental factors such as diet and lifestyle may influence PCOS and further account for familial aggregation. These may begin as early in life as before birth, with insults during pregnancy such as maternal hypertension or smoking leading to intrauterine growth restriction [13]. This is associated with a predisposition to insulin resistance and metabolic dysfunction. When combined with a sedentary lifestyle and poor diet, this may induce obesity later in life and subsequently development of PCOS [13].

Diagnosis of PCOS can be difficult and lengthy owing to the variability of clinical presentation and the multistep process required. More than one-third of women report a time interval of over 2 years before establishing diagnosis and often three or more healthcare professionals were involved [14]. The Rotterdam criteria are the most widely used PCOS classification. It states that for diagnosis of PCOS, women must have any two of the following three features: Chronic oligo/anovulation (oligo), HA and polycystic ovarian morphology (PCOM) [15]. HA may be clinical (hirsutism, acne) or biochemical (elevated free testosterone, free androgen index). PCOM is viewed on transvaginal ultrasound by the presence of >20 follicles in each ovary and/or ovarian volume >10 mL$^3$ [15].

Four phenotypes of PCOS exist based on the Rotterdam criteria, each with their own metabolic implications: Type A (oligo + HA + PCOM), Type B (oligo + HA), Type C (HA + PCOM) and Type D (oligo + PCOM). Phenotypes A and B are referred to as "Classic" PCOS. Population studies show these women have marked menstrual dysfunction, insulin resistance, obesity, dyslipidaemia and are at greater risk of developing metabolic syndrome. Phenotype C is described as "Ovulatory" PCOS, with less pronounced hyperinsulinaemia, HA, hirsutism and metabolic syndrome compared with "Classic" PCOS. Interestingly, one study observed women with this phenotype to have a higher socioeconomic status, although explanations for this are unknown. Finally, phenotype D is known as "non-hyperandrogenic" PCOS. It has the mildest metabolic and endocrine dysfunction and is the least common phenotype, although this may reflect a difficulty in diagnosis due to its milder clinical presentation [16].

An older criterion from 1990 by the National Institute of Health exists, but this typically identifies more severe forms of PCOS, requiring both HA and oligo/anovulation for diagnosis [15]. Thus, this criterion has become less popular in recent years. It is also important to note that use of these diagnostic criteria in adolescents is controversial due to differences in clinical presentation and biochemistry between teenage and adult women [17]. New international guidelines aim to balance the importance of timely diagnosis for early lifestyle intervention with managing the risk of overdiagnosis in this cohort [17].

## CARDIOMETABOLIC RISK FACTORS

There is an established association between PCOS and future adverse cardiometabolic health. Women with PCOS have increased prevalence of traditional cardiometabolic risk factors compared to healthy controls [18]. These risk factors include obesity, T2DM, impaired glucose tolerance, dyslipidaemia and hypertension. Meta-analyses have found women with PCOS to have a greater risk of cardiovascular outcomes such as coronary heart disease and stroke, yet evidence is limited [19,20]. Given the well-established association between PCOS and CVD risk factors, early detection and management of CVD risk factors is vital to improve the long-term health of women with PCOS.

The most prevalent of these cardiometabolic risk factors is being overweight or obese. A meta-analysis of 35 studies found that women with PCOS were more likely to be overweight or have central obesity than women without PCOS [21]. Interestingly, this prevalence was even higher in Caucasian women compared with Asian women [21]. Studies in the United States have found an 80% prevalence of obesity in women with PCOS, although outside of the United States this figure is around 50% [22]. Obesity is likely attributable to chronic HA from insulin resistance. This constant exposure to androgens over a long period of time can lead to the accumulation of visceral fat, causing central obesity [18]. Furthermore, central obesity exacerbates insulin resistance and so a cumulative cycle ensues of worsening HA and increased visceral adiposity [21].

Polycystic ovary syndrome is a leading risk factor for the development of T2DM in women [22]. The severity of insulin resistance varies between PCOS phenotypes, with the "Classic" phenotype demonstrating the most insulin resistance independent of body mass index (BMI) [23]. Insulin resistance leads to dysglycaemia, which typically presents with impaired glucose tolerance. Approximately 40% of women with the "Classic" PCOS phenotype have impaired glucose tolerance and T2DM by age 40 [24]. Obesity and family history of T2DM are independently additive risk factors for this development [22]. A prospective study assessing the prevalence of T2DM in women with PCOS found the prevalence for all phenotypes to be 2.2%, rising to 39.3% at 19 year follow up [23]. With the well-established association between T2DM and increased risk of heart disease and cardiovascular events, this is an important risk factor to identify and manage in PCOS patients. Women with PCOS are also at increased risk of pregnancy complications [25]. This includes a 3-fold increased risk of developing gestational diabetes mellitus (GDM) which in turn is associated with additional complications such as preeclampsia and premature delivery [25].

Dyslipidaemia is another cardiometabolic risk factor that is found in 70% of women with PCOS [23]. This typically manifests as raised levels of low-density lipoprotein (LDL) and very low-density lipoprotein (VLDL) cholesterol with high serum triglycerides and free fatty acids [23]. Additionally, there are decreased levels of the protective high-density lipoprotein (HDL) cholesterol. Women with PCOS have increased oxidised LDL cholesterol which further increases risk of CVD [23]. As with T2DM, obesity further exacerbates this dyslipidaemia. Research suggests that this is caused by HA rather than insulin resistance [22].

Emerging data suggest that women with PCOS are at greater risk of hypertension (blood pressure $\geq 140/90$ mmHg) [26]. This is thought to be through hyperandrogenic activation of the renin–angiotensin–aldosterone system [23] and visceral adipose cells contributing to endothelial dysfunction [27]. Prevalence of hypertension in women with PCOS of reproductive age is 19.2% compared with 11.9% in age-matched controls [26]. This is further increased in post-menopausal women with some studies reporting prevalence as high as 25.7% [23]. Hypertensive women with PCOS exhibit greater additional cardiovascular risk factors such as obesity and dyslipidaemia and thus it is important to control blood pressure to reduce risk of future cardiovascular events [26].

Due to the high prevalence of these cardiometabolic risk factors in women with PCOS and their associated morbidity and mortality, the International evidence-based guideline published in 2018 recommend regular screening [28]. In particular, monitoring for weight should be offered at a minimum 6–12 monthly, including height, BMI and waist circumference. Glycaemic status assessment should be offered at diagnosis in all women with PCOS and thereafter every 1–3 years based on risk assessment. Oral glucose tolerance test (OGTT), HbA1c and fasting plasma glucose can all be used. In the high-risk subgroup, such as women with a BMI >25, history of GDM or family history of T2DM the OGTT is the preferred method of testing. Additionally, OGTT should be offered to all women at preconception stage when planning pregnancy. All overweight and obese women should have a fasting lipid profile including cholesterol, LDL, HDL and serum triglycerides at diagnosis and based on their overall cardiovascular risk thereafter. Blood pressure should be measured at least annually.

Non-conventional risk factors for cardiometabolic health in PCOS are emerging but need further research in order to be established. These include chronic inflammation, oxidative stress, activation of the sympathetic nervous system and vitamin D deficiency [27].

## CARDIOMETABOLIC HEALTH

Evidence suggests that PCOS is increasingly associated with markers of subclinical CVD such as carotid intima media thickness (CIMT), coronary artery calcium, endothelial dysfunction and pulse wave velocity (PWV). CIMT is a marker of vascular structural change and is viewed by ultrasound. A meta-analysis found women with the "Classic" PCOS phenotype to have a significantly thicker CIMT (0.072 mm) compared with healthy controls [27]. This corresponds with a CIMT progression of 5 years, as the expected average increase in the general population is 0.015 mm per year [27]. Further research has found a significant increase in coronary artery calcifications between women with "Classic" PCOS and controls (23.6% vs. 10.3%) [29]. However, this risk was not present when comparing women with either anovulation or HA alone, despite a high prevalence of CVD risk factors in these cohorts [29]. These findings suggest that women with both anovulation and HA have an increased risk of premature atherosclerosis, an important marker of CVD.

Additional markers of subclinical disease include functional changes of the vascular system such as endothelial dysfunction and PWV. Normal endothelial function is important for maintenance of vascular tone and oxidative stress regulation. However, this mechanism is pathological in women with PCOS. This is likely attributable to the presence of insulin resistance and its associated increase in oxidative stress and pro-inflammatory cytokines (which are known to damage the endothelium) [30]. Endothelial dysfunction can be non-invasively measured by ultrasound flow-mediated dilatation (FMD) of the brachial artery. Research has found that coronary dilation in women with PCOS is approximately 4.1% lower than healthy controls and that for every 3.5% decrease in FMD, the risk of a cardiovascular event increases by 21% [30]. Thus, FMD may be a useful marker in screening women with PCOS for subclinical CVD. PWV is a marker of arterial stiffness and is predictive of cardiovascular mortality in conditions such as essential hypertension and chronic renal failure [31]. Increased PWV and therefore greater arterial stiffness has been found in PCOS compared to women without PCOS although further research is needed to clarify the absolute risk of CVD events in this cohort [31].

Despite the increased CVD risk factors and markers of sub-clinical disease in women with PCOS, there is limited evidence for CVD related morbidity and mortality. The diagnostic criteria of PCOS have changed throughout the past few decades. Much of the research on CVD end points have included young women with retrospective diagnoses of PCOS that no longer meet the current definition [32]. Few studies have used long-term follow up that may reveal increased life-time CVD risk in these women [32]. The recent International evidence-based guideline has reported no significant difference between women with and without PCOS for CVD outcomes such as myocardial infarction, angina, stroke or CVD related deaths [28]. However, the guideline also reports methodological and reporting bias as possible reasons for this and therefore limit the interpretation of the data [28]. Uncertainty currently remains around the risk of clinical cardiovascular events in women with PCOS and large prospective longitudinal studies are required. However, the well-documented CVD risk factors suggest that women with PCOS are a high-risk cohort and CVD screening and risk prevention should form a critical part of management.

## LIFESTYLE MODIFICATIONS

Lifestyle modifications including behavioural, dietary and exercise interventions are often incorporated in high-risk cardiometabolic populations for CVD risk reduction and weight loss. Due to the high prevalence of CVD risk factors in PCOS, lifestyle modification is also first-line management in this cohort. Aside from reducing CVD, lifestyle modification is thought to improve weight loss, metabolic, reproductive, fertility and QoL outcomes in these women [33].

Excess weight in women with PCOS exacerbates insulin resistance and increases the prevalence and severity of the cardiometabolic, reproductive and psychological features of PCOS [33]. The International evidence-based guideline recommends reducing BMI by 5% in order to reduce serum insulin and testosterone levels and improve menstrual function [28]. Specific dietary approaches include a low carbohydrate diet, low glycaemic index diet, increased dietary fibre and vitamin D supplementation. Increased dietary fibre intake has been associated with reduced CVD and T2DM in the general population by regulating blood glucose and increasing insulin sensitivity [34]. It may also reduce caloric consumption by increasing satiety, thereby promoting weight loss [34]. Increasing dietary fibre in women with PCOS has produced varying results, however this is still a reasonable recommendation due to the health benefits seen in the general population [33].

'A variety of balanced dietary approaches can be recommended to reduce dietary energy intake and induce weight loss in women with PCOS' according to the International evidence-based guideline [28]. Additionally, there is no evidence that any specific energy equivalent diet type is better than another and so general healthy eating principles should be followed in order to achieve an energy deficit of 500–750 kcal/day [28]. Similar to in the general population, health care providers should tailor dietary changes to the patient's food preferences and avoid nutritionally unbalanced diets.

Exercise is well known to induce health benefits in the general population. This becomes even more important in high CVD risk populations for weight loss, lowering blood pressure and improving glycaemic control and blood lipid profile [35]. Physical activity may include aerobic/endurance activities, resistance/weight bearing activities or a combination, further sub-grouped into intensities ranging from light to high. Aerobic exercise is particularly important for BMI reduction in women with PCOS. A recent systematic review found a 4.5–10% weight loss from moderate intensity exercise intervention in premenopausal women, independent of the type, frequency or duration of exercise sessions [36]. Weight loss from exercise was also associated with improved cardiometabolic features including fasting insulin [36]. Moderate aerobic exercise has been shown to improve short-term glucose disposal and insulin sensitivity by reducing inflammatory responses and improving insulin signalling transduction [33]. Consistent moderate physical activity at least three times per week reduces the risk of T2DM in high-risk populations and improves CVD risk factors, hence this may be beneficial in PCOS [36].

The International evidence-based guideline recommends varying intensity and duration of physical activity in women with PCOS depending on age and weight loss goals [28]. However, they also acknowledge the motivation required for this and so highlight the importance of behavioural therapy in addition to dietary and exercise interventions. There were no studies assessing behavioural therapy for weight loss in PCOS and so recommendations were informed form general populations. Behavioural change techniques included goal setting, self-monitoring, stimulus control, slowing the rate of eating and family/social support. A systematic review found that dietary and exercise interventions, when combined with these behavioural change techniques, significantly improved weight loss in populations at risk of CVD and T2DM compared with diet and/ or exercise alone [37]. As such, management of cardiometabolic risk in women with PCOS should emphasise self-management components for efficient weight loss alongside dietary and exercise interventions.

Despite the potential for benefit, 45% of women with PCOS report having received no lifestyle modification advice [33]. The above recommendations may increase consultation times with associated healthcare costs, however the long-term benefits from weight loss and reduced cardiometabolic risk are expected to reduce the burden on healthcare systems [28].

## PHARMACOLOGICAL AND SURGICAL MANAGEMENT OF CARDIOMETABOLIC RISK

When dietary and exercise interventions alone do not prove effective, medical therapies are indicated for second line management of PCOS. Commonly used medical therapies such as the combined oral contraceptive pill (COCP) and metformin are "off label" for the management of PCOS. These recommendations are predominantly evidence-based and are still allowed in many countries. As with any prescription, it is important to inform patients and discuss the evidence of possible benefits and adverse effects before commencing pharmacological treatment. It is recommended that a holistic approach is taken and that medical therapies should be used in conjunction with lifestyle modifications and patient education.

Clinical and biochemical findings of PCOS such as menstrual irregularities, signs of HA, elevated testosterone, hyperlipidaemia and dysglycaemia are commonly managed with both COCP and lifestyle changes in both adult and adolescent women [38]. The efficacy of COCPs for the management of PCOS varies greatly depending on the type, duration of use, severity and phenotype of PCOS and adherence to treatment [38]. Thus, systematic reviews have been used to assess the evidence of COCPs versus lifestyle, placebo and metformin treatments alone and in combination therapies.

A recent systematic review and meta-analyses which directly informed the International evidence-based guideline included 56 studies to evaluate the effect of the COCP and metformin on the clinical, hormonal and metabolic features of PCOS [38]. Overall, the COCP was found to be effective at alleviating menstrual cycle irregularity and HA in both adult women and adolescents, regardless of the subtype of COCP [38]. It is recommended that the lowest effective oestrogen dose is prescribed in order to balance efficacy and side effects [28]. There is no evidence that the COCP alone is effective at reducing the prevalence of metabolic parameters of PCOS such as excess weight, dysglycaemia and lipid profile, although it is not associated with worsening insulin resistance [39]. The increased risk of venous thromboembolism with COCP use in the general population should also be considered in PCOS. However, there is no evidence for increased risk in PCOS and long-term use of COCPs in PCOS are not associated with increased cardiovascular events [39]. Several metabolic parameters represent relative or absolute contraindications to initiate COCP and therefore individualised treatment is required [38].

Metformin, a biguanide, acts in the liver to inhibit gluconeogenesis and lipogenesis and increase glucose uptake, and in the gut lumen to increase insulin sensitivity [40]. It is largely regarded as a safe drug due to its ability to improve glycaemic control without inducing hypoglycaemia and there are no apparent severe adverse effects associated with long-term use [40]. The side effects of oral metformin are common and include gastrointestinal disturbances such as nausea, vomiting, diarrhoea and abdominal pain which are self-limiting and mostly reported to be mild to moderate in severity [28]. Gastrointestinal disturbances may be minimised with a lower metformin starting dose, extended release preparations and administration with food [28].

Metformin plays an important role in reducing the cardiometabolic risk of women with PCOS. Meta-analyses demonstrate a significant reduction in BMI, cholesterol and triglyceride levels across all BMI ranges with metformin therapy [38]. Further studies have found improvements in blood pressure, insulin resistance and waist-hip ratio with metformin compared to placebo or COCP [39]. A recent systematic review reports that lifestyle intervention combined with 1.5–2 g daily oral metformin reduced BMI by 0.73 kg/m$^2$ after 6 months compared with lifestyle intervention plus placebo in PCOS [41]. It is important to manage weight gain and obesity in women with PCOS to reduce the risk of T2DM development and metformin combined with lifestyle intervention appears to be the most effective for this [41]. Subsequently, the International evidence-based guideline recommends metformin in addition to lifestyle intervention in adult women with PCOS for weight loss, hormonal and metabolic outcomes.

Additional pharmacological agents including anti-obesity drugs, anti-androgen drugs and inositol have been suggested for weight management in PCOS with varying results. Anti-obesity agents such as sibutramine and orlistat are increasingly being used for weight loss and maintenance in obesity in the general population, but accessibility is low and costs are high [42]. There is an absence of evidence for these drugs in women with PCOS and so guidelines have been informed by evidence in non-PCOS obese adults. Weight loss is challenging for most patients and so the addition of anti-obesity agents may be helpful by decreasing appetite and increasing satiety [42]. However, patients should be made aware that gradual weight gain typically occurs upon stopping the anti-obesity drugs and so caloric restriction and behaviour modification remain crucial [42].

Anti-androgen agents have no efficacy in weight loss in PCOS but may be considered in the treatment of hirsutism where COCPs are contraindicated [28]. There is no evidence that inositol, an insulin sensitising agent, is effective for weight loss or the management of hormonal features of PCOS and thus should be regarded as experimental therapy [28]. Meta-analysis has found no significant difference in BMI with inositol compared with placebo and further research is needed to assess the efficacy of this drug in PCOS [28].

There is a paucity of studies assessing the impact of surgery on the cardiometabolic risks associated with PCOS. As such, the International evidence-based guideline did not include bariatric surgery as a treatment option for the management of cardiometabolic risk. Since then, a review looking into the impact of bariatric surgery in women with PCOS has reported a significant reduction in BMI in all 10 studies reviewed [43]. Following this weight loss, resolution of metabolic syndrome and either total resolution of T2DM or normalisation of insulin levels was observed in nearly all studies measuring insulin resistance [43]. However, mean follow-up was at one year and thus it is unknown if weight loss was maintained long-term. It is clear that bariatric surgery results in short-term effective weight loss with beneficial effects on reduction of metabolic syndrome and insulin resistance. However, longitudinal studies with longer follow-up time are needed to assess if these initial results translate to cardiometabolic risk reduction in the long-term. A recent Cochrane systematic review has reported that laparoscopic ovarian drilling (LOD) does not improve symptoms of PCOS compared to medical management [44]. There may be some benefits of LOD on fertility management of women with PCOS but there is no role for LOD in management of cardiometabolic risk [44].

## Key points for clinical practice

- PCOS represents one of the most common metabolic disorders in women
- There is a well-established association between PCOS and cardiometabolic risk factors
- Regular screening and reduction of cardiovascular risk is recommended
- Lifestyle modification remains the mainstay of cardiometabolic risk management; metformin has been shown to offer metabolic benefits, particularly in women with an increased BMI
- COCP and anti-androgen agents have no role in improving cardiometabolic health
- Large prospective longitudinal studies are required to prove CVD related events in the PCOS cohort

# CONCLUSION

Polycystic ovary syndrome is an important endocrine disorder affecting up to 10% of reproductive-aged women with widespread adverse effects. There is a well-established association between PCOS and cardiometabolic risk factors, particularly being overweight or obese. Additionally, impaired glucose tolerance, T2DM and gestational diabetes are more prevalent in PCOS. Therefore, all women with PCOS should be screened for cardiovascular risk factors. Lifestyle modifications are recommended to improve cardiometabolic health and reduce adverse outcomes such as coronary heart disease and stroke. Metformin as an adjunctive therapy may also improve cardiometabolic health in women with PCOS, however, other pharmacological agents have not yielded significant results.

# REFERENCES

1. Bozdag G, Mumusoglu S, Zengin D, et al. The prevalence and phenotypic features of polycystic ovary syndrome: A systematic review and meta-Analysis. Hum Reprod 2016; 31:2841–2855.
2. Wekker V, van Dammen L, Koning A, et al. Long-term cardiometabolic disease risk in women with PCOS: a systematic review and meta-analysis. Hum Reprod Update 2020; 26:942–960.
3. Azziz R, Carmina E, Chen Z, et al. Polycystic ovary syndrome. Nat Rev Dis Prim 2016; 2.
4. Eagleson CA, Gingrich MB, Pastor CL, et al. Polycystic Ovarian Syndrome: Evidence that Flutamide Restores Sensitivity of the Gonadotropin-Releasing Hormone Pulse Generator to Inhibition by Estradiol and Progesterone 1. J Clin Endocrinol Metab 2000; 85:4047–4052.
5. Azziz R. Reproductive endocrinology and infertility: Clinical expert series polycystic ovary syndrome. Obstet Gynecol 2018; 132:321–336.
6. Nelson VL, Legro RS, Strauss JF, McAllister JM. Augmented androgen production is a stable steroidogenic phenotype of propagated theca cells from polycystic ovaries. Mol Endocrinol 1999; 13:946–957.
7. Witchel SF, Oberfield SE, Peña AS. Polycystic Ovary Syndrome: Pathophysiology, Presentation, and Treatment with Emphasis on Adolescent Girls. J Endoc Soc 2019; 3:1545–1573.
8. Nestler JE, Jakubowicz DJ, Falcon de Vargas A, et al. Insulin Stimulates Testosterone Biosynthesis by Human Thecal Cells from Women with Polycystic Ovary Syndrome by Activating Its Own Receptor and Using Inositolglycan Mediators as the Signal Transduction System 1. J Clin Endocrinol Metab 1998; 83:2001–2005.
9. Nestler JE, Powers LP, Matt DW, et al. A direct effect of hyperinsulinemia on serum sex hormone-binding globulin levels in obese women with the polycystic ovary syndrome. J Clin Endocrinol Metab 1991; 72:83–89.
10. Goodarzi MO, Dumesic DA, Chazenbalk G, et al. Polycystic ovary syndrome: Etiology, pathogenesis and diagnosis. Nat Rev Endocrinol 2011; 7:219–231.

11. De Leo V, Musacchio MC, Cappelli V, et al. Genetic, hormonal and metabolic aspects of PCOS: An update. Reprod Biol Endocrinol2016; 14.

12. Khan MJ, Ullah A, Basit S. Genetic basis of polycystic ovary syndrome (PCOS): Current perspectives. Appl Clin Genet 2019; 12:249–260.

13. Escobar-Morreale HF. Polycystic ovary syndrome: Definition, aetiology, diagnosis and treatment. Nat Rev Endocrinol 2018; 14:270–284.

14. Gibson-Helm M, Teede H, Dunaif A, Dokras A. Delayed diagnosis and a lack of information associated with dissatisfaction in women with polycystic ovary syndrome. J Clin Endocrinol Metab 2017; 102:604–612.

15. Dewailly D. Diagnostic criteria for PCOS: Is there a need for a rethink? Best Practice and Research. Clin Obstet Gynaecol 2016; 37:5–11.

16. Lizneva D, Suturina L, Walker W, et al. Criteria, prevalence, and phenotypes of polycystic ovary syndrome. Fertil Steril 2016; 106:6–15.

17. Vassalou H, Sotiraki M, Michala L. PCOS diagnosis in adolescents: The timeline of a controversy in a systematic review. J Pediatr Endocrinol Metab 2019; 32:549–559.

18. Osibogun O, Ogunmoroti O, Michos ED. Polycystic ovary syndrome and cardiometabolic risk: Opportunities for cardiovascular disease prevention. Trends Cardiovasc Med 2020; 30:399–404.

19. de Groot PCM, Dekkers OM, Romijn JA, et al. PCOS, coronary heart disease, stroke and the influence of obesity: A systematic review and meta-analysis. Hum Reprod Update 2011; 17:495–500.

20. Zhou Y, Wang X, Jiang Y, et al. Association between polycystic ovary syndrome and the risk of stroke and all-cause mortality: insights from a meta-analysis. Gynecol Endocrinol 2017; 33:904–910.

21. Lim SS, Davies MJ, Norman RJ, et al. Overweight, obesity and central obesity in women with polycystic ovary syndrome: A systematic review and meta-analysis. Hum Reprod Update 2012; 18:618–637.

22. Torchen LC. Cardiometabolic Risk in PCOS: More than a Reproductive Disorder. Curr Diab Rep 2017; 17.

23. Anagnostis P, Tarlatzis BC, Kauffman RP. Polycystic ovarian syndrome (PCOS): Long-term metabolic consequences. Metabolism 2018; 86:33–43.

24. Studen KB, Pfeifer M. Cardiometabolic risk in polycystic ovary syndrome. Endoc Connect 2018; 7:R238–R251.

25. Palomba S, De Wilde MA, Falbo A, et al. Pregnancy complications in women with polycystic ovary syndrome. Hum Reprod Update 2015; 21:575–592.

26. Shi Y, Cui Y, Sun X, et al. Hypertension in women with polycystic ovary syndrome: Prevalence and associated cardiovascular risk factors. Eur J Obstet Gynecol Reprod Biol 2014; 173:66–70.

27. Kakoly NS, Moran LJ, Teede HJ, et al. Cardiometabolic risks in PCOS: a review of the current state of knowledge. Expert Rev Endocrinol Metab 2019; 14:23–33.

28. Teede H, Misso M, Costello M, et al. International evidence based guideline for the assessment and management of polycystic ovary syndrome. Clin Endocrinol (Oxf) 2018; 89:251–268.

29. Calderon-Margalit R, Siscovick D, Merkin SS, et al. Prospective association of polycystic ovary syndrome with coronary artery calcification and carotid-intima-media thickness the coronary artery risk development in young adults women's study. Arterioscler Thromb Vasc Biol 2014; 34:2688–2694.

30. Dambala K, Paschou SA, Michopoulos A, et al. Biomarkers of Endothelial Dysfunction in Women with Polycystic Ovary Syndrome. Angiology 2019; 70:797–801.

31. Meyer C, McGrath BP, Cameron J, et al. Vascular dysfunction and metabolic parameters in polycystic ovary syndrome. J Clin Endocrinol Metab 2005; 90:4630–4635.

32. Dokras A. Cardiovascular disease risk in women with PCOS. Steroids 2013; 78:773–776.

33. Aly JM, Decherney AH. Lifestyle Modifications in PCOS. Clin Obstet Gynecol 2021; 64:83–9.

34. Weickert MO, Pfeiffer AFH. Metabolic effects of dietary fiber consumption and prevention of diabetes. J Nutr 2008; 138:439–442.

35. Hansen D, Niebauer J, Cornelissen V, et al. Exercise Prescription in Patients with Different Combinations of Cardiovascular Disease Risk Factors: A Consensus Statement from the EXPERT Working Group. Sports Med 2018; 48:1781–1797.

36. Harrison CL, Lombard CB, Moran LJ, et al. Exercise therapy in polycystic ovary syndrome: A systematic review. Hum Reprod Update 2011; 17:171–183.

37. Greaves CJ, Sheppard KE, Abraham C, et al. Systematic review of reviews of intervention components associated with increased effectiveness in dietary and physical activity interventions. BMC Public Health 2011; 11.

38. Teede H, Tassone EC, Piltonen T, et al. Effect of the combined oral contraceptive pill and/or metformin in the management of polycystic ovary syndrome: A systematic review with meta-analyses. Clin Endocrinol 2019; 91:479–489.

39. Tay CT, Joham AE, Hiam DS, et al. Pharmacological and surgical treatment of nonreproductive outcomes in polycystic ovary syndrome: An overview of systematic reviews. Clin Endocrinol 2018; 89:535–553.
40. Flory J, Lipska K. Metformin in 2019. JAMA 2019; 321:1926–1927.
41. Naderpoor N, Shorakae S, De Courten B, et al. Metformin and lifestyle modification in polycysticovary syndrome: Systematic review and meta-analysis. Hum Reprod Update 2015; 21:560–574.
42. Apovian CM, Aronne LJ, Bessesen DH, et al. Pharmacological management of obesity: An endocrine society clinical practice guideline. J Clin Endocrinol Metab 2015; 100:342–362.
43. Lee R, Joy Mathew C, Jose MT, et al. A Review of the Impact of Bariatric Surgery in Women With Polycystic Ovary Syndrome. Cureus 2020; 12.
44. Bordewijk EM, Ng KYB, Rakic L, et al. Laparoscopic ovarian drilling for ovulation induction in women with anovulatory polycystic ovary syndrome. Cochrane Database Syst Rev 2020; 2020.

# Chapter 8

# Update on recurrent miscarriage

*Danai Balfoussia, Raj Rai*

## INTRODUCTION

Miscarriage, the loss of a pregnancy under 24 weeks' gestation, complicates one in five clinically recognised pregnancies. It is increasingly recognised as being a cause of significant psychological morbidity spanning the spectrum of depression, anxiety and post-traumatic stress disorder (PTSD). Studies have identified an almost 40% incidence of PTSD three months following pregnancy loss [1].

Sporadic miscarriage occurs in 15–25% of pregnancies [2]. In contrast, recurrent pregnancy loss, the loss of three or more consecutive pregnancies, complicates 1% of pregnancies. Recurrent and sporadic miscarriages are thought to represent distinct clinical entities as the probability of three consecutive sporadic miscarriages by chance alone should mathematically occur in approximately 0.34% pregnancies whereas the rate of recurrent miscarriage is almost three times that suggesting a separate pathophysiological process altogether.

There is no consensus agreement among international societies on the definition of recurrent miscarriage. The American Society for Reproductive Medicine (ASRM) uses the term 'recurrent pregnancy loss' following the loss of two or more clinical pregnancies [3]. The European Society of Human Reproduction and Embryology (ESHRE) distinguishes between recurrent pregnancy loss and recurrent miscarriage, defining the former as the loss of two more, consecutive or non-consecutive, pregnancies excluding molar or ectopic gestations [4]. It uses the term 'recurrent miscarriage' in the context of two or more losses of confirmed intra-uterine pregnancies. By contrast, the Royal College of Obstetricians and Gynaecologists (RCOG) uses only the term 'recurrent miscarriage' and defines this as the loss of three or more consecutive pregnancies [5]. The recently published updated draft guideline retains the same definition but allows for clinician discretion for earlier investigation when there is a suspicion that the miscarriages are unlikely to be sporadic.

**Danai Balfoussia** BSc MBBS MRCOG, Department of Reproductive Medicine, Wolfson Fertility Centre, Hammersmith Hospital, Imperial College Healthcare NHS Trust, London, UK
Email: danai.balfoussia04@ic.ac.uk

**Raj Rai** MBBS MD MRCOG, Department of Reproductive Medicine, St Mary's Hospital, Imperial College Healthcare NHS Trust, London, UK
Email: r.rai@ic.ac.uk

# PARENTAL AGE

Advancing maternal age has consistently been shown to be a risk factor for miscarriage, likely secondary to declining oocyte quality. A population-based study of 421,201 pregnancies demonstrated a 10% risk of miscarriage for those aged 25–29%, rising rapidly after age 30 years and reaching 53% from age 45 years onwards [6,7].

Paternal age is increasingly recognised as a risk factor for miscarriage. Its effect is more pronounced from age 40 years onwards with a meta-analysis of over 71,500 pregnancies demonstrating a relative risk of miscarriage of 1.06 (95% CI 1.06–1.43) and 1.43 (95% CI 1.13–1.81) for those aged 40–44 years and ≥45 years, respectively. This effect is thought to be mediated through a combination of age-related changes which include accumulation of reactive oxygen species, reduced antioxidant capacity and impaired DNA repair pathways [8].

Combined parental age is also likely to be a significant contributor due to the impaired oocyte repair mechanisms with advancing maternal age and therefore a more pronounced effect of the impact of sperm oxidative damage on embryo quality and subsequent pregnancy outcome.

# BEHAVIOURAL FACTORS

There is conflicting evidence regarding the impact of smoking with studies supporting a detrimental effect of active and passive smoking [6] while others were unable to confirm a significant association [9]. Obesity has also been linked to recurrent miscarriage [10]. A systematic review showed that body mass index (BMI) >30 kg/m$^2$ and BMI >25 kg/m$^2$ were associated with an increased risk of future miscarriage (OR 1.77; 95% CI 1.25–2.50 and OR 1.35; 95% CI 1.07–1.72, respectively) [9]. Being underweight also increased the odds of recurrent miscarriage, but not of future miscarriage [9]. Evidence regarding a link between caffeine intake and recurrent miscarriage is conflicting. A study of 52 women with a history of recurrent miscarriage showed an increased risk of miscarriage for each caffeine intake of 100 mg/day [11]. These findings were not replicated in a meta-analyses with the authors acknowledging the poor quality of available evidence [9].

# THROMBOPHILIA

The role of the haemostatic pathways in recurrent miscarriage has been extensively explored. Thrombophilias, a group of disorders that result in a prothrombotic state, can be divided into acquired and inherited.

## Acquired thrombophilias

Anti-phospholipid syndrome (APS) is an acquired thrombophilic defect. Fifteen per cent of couples with recurrent miscarriage have obstetric APS. This results in the loss of chromosomally normal pregnancies, typically between 7 and 12 weeks' gestation [12]. In untreated pregnancies, the miscarriage rate is as high as 90% [12].

The mechanism of APS-related pregnancy loss is not simply one of placental thrombosis. Placental histopathology of pregnancies affected by APS has demonstrated a prevalence of intervillous thrombosis comparable to that of non-APS pregnancies suggesting that thrombosis is not the main mechanism at play [13]. The adverse pregnancy outcomes linked to APS are thought to be mediated through three main pathways [13].

Firstly, anti-phospholipid antibodies negatively affect trophoblast proliferation and increase cell death. Secondly, these antibodies impact on trophoblast syncytialisation. Finally, anti-phospholipid antibodies affect signalling pathways involved in trophoblast invasion resulting in impaired maternal decidual invasion by the trophoblast and impaired transformation of the spiral arteries.

Diagnosis of APS is based on the modified Sapporo criteria and is reached if at least one of the clinical and laboratory criteria are met [14]. Clinical criteria include vascular thrombosis or any of the following adverse pregnancy outcomes: Three or more consecutive miscarriages under 10 weeks' gestation, one or more miscarriage over 10 weeks of a morphologically normal fetus or a preterm birth before 34 weeks due to pre-eclampsia, eclampsia or recognised features of placental insufficiency. Laboratory criteria are the presence of one or more of the following antibodies detected on two or more occasions 12 weeks apart: Lupus anticoagulant, anti-cardiolipin antibodies (IgM or IgG in serum or plasma in medium or high titre) or anti-$\beta$2 glycoprotein-I antibody (IgG and/or IgM in serum or plasma in titre greater than the 99% percentile).

## Inherited thrombophilias

Discovery of APS ignited interest in the role of inherited thrombophilias. It was theorised that micro-thrombotic events secondary to thrombophilia would affect placental invasion and subsequent placental function [15].

Factor V Leiden exerts its thrombogenic effect by producing a factor V variant that is resistant to breakdown by activated protein C. This mutation is inherited in an autosomal dominant pattern and is observed with a frequency of 3–8% in a Caucasian population [15]. It has been proposed that Factor V Leiden increases the risk of placental micro-thrombosis resulting in miscarriage. The data on its role in recurrent miscarriage is contentious but meta-analyses appear to support an association between FVL [16–18] and recurrent miscarriage and late pregnancy loss [16].

Prothrombin gene mutation G20210A results in elevated levels of plasma prothrombin, a precursor of thrombin. Meta-analyses have demonstrated a consistent but weak association between prothrombin gene mutation and recurrent miscarriage [16,18]. By contrast, anti-thrombin deficiency, a strong risk factor for venous thrombosis, does not appear to be associated with recurrent miscarriage as shown by two meta-analyses [16,18].

Protein S acts as a cofactor to activated Protein C and together the two inhibit coagulation by degrading FVIIIa and FVa, thereby inhibiting thrombin generation. While Protein S deficiency has been shown to be associated with recurrent miscarriage [16,18], this does not appear to be the case for Protein C deficiency [16,18].

5,10-methylenetetrahydrofolate reductase (MTHFR) mutations result in reduced MTHFR enzyme activity and subsequent blockage of conversion of 10-methylenetetrahydrofolate to 5-methylenetetrahydrofolate affecting the conversion of cysteine to methionine and ultimately resulting in increased serum homocysteine levels [19]. Data for the association between this mutation and risk of recurrent miscarriage are conflicting [18–20].

## Investigations

Women, who fulfil the clinical criteria for APS, should undergo laboratory testing. More recently, it has been argued that testing should be extended to women who have had two or more miscarriages, irrespective of whether they are consecutive. A study of 1,719 patients showed that there is no increased diagnostic yield for APS after three miscarriages rather than two, and no increased diagnostic yield after consecutive versus non-consecutive miscarriages [21].

Lupus anticoagulant, as suggested by its name, was first studied in patients with systemic lupus erythematosus (SLE). While in-vitro it has an anticoagulant effect and is associated with prolonged clotting time, in vivo it is associated with thrombosis. Testing for lupus anticoagulant lacks standardisation and is based on reaction with reagents containing phospholipids or phospholipid-binding proteins. The two tests typically used are dilute Russell's viper venom time and a lupus anticoagulant sensitive activated partial thrombin time (APTT) assay [22]. Whilst either of these two tests can be used to reach a diagnosis, they are often used in combination as no single test is 100% sensitive [14].

Anti-cardiolipin antibodies (IgG or IgM) in serum or plasma in a medium or high titre (>40 GPL or MPL, or >99th percentile) present on two or more occasions 12 weeks apart can also be used for diagnosis. Inter-laboratory variations in results are observed and the IgM variant is also subject to false positive results, especially in the low-positive range [14].

Anti-$\beta$2 glycoprotein-I antibody (IgG or IgM) in serum or plasma with a titre greater than the 99th percentile and present on two or more occasions at least 12 weeks apart is sufficient to diagnose APS. Compared to anti-cardiolipin antibodies, these antibodies have a higher specificity for APS and lower inter-laboratory variation in result interpretation [14].

International organisations including ESHRE and ASRM caution against routine testing for inherited thrombophilias as although there is evidence to suggest an association with recurrent miscarriage, no treatment to date has been shown to be effective in reducing this risk [4,22].

## Treatment

Aspirin, heparin (unfractionated and low molecular) and steroids have all been trialled in the treatment of APS. Aspirin alone has been shown to increase the live birth rate by 42%, while aspirin in combination with unfractionated heparin resulted in 71% increase in live birth rate [23]. In a recent meta-analysis, the relative risk of live birth was significantly increased in the aspirin with heparin group versus aspirin alone (RR 1.27; 95% CI 1.09–1.49). Importantly, there was no statistically significant difference in live birth when comparing low molecular with aspirin versus unfractionated heparin with aspirin (RR 1.44; 95% CI 0.80–2.62) [24]. Considering the significant advantages of low molecular weight heparin over unfractionated heparin, the former combined with aspirin should be recommended in pregnancy. This is in line with guidance from ESHRE [4], ASRM [22] and the RCOG [5].

There is significant variation in the published literature regarding timing of commencement of aspirin and heparin. In most trials aspirin was commenced pre-conceptually. Heparin was started in the luteal phase in some trials and after detection of fetal cardiac pulsations in others. Interestingly, a recent study comparing heparin initiation at 5 weeks versus following detection of fetal cardiac activity at 7 weeks, showed significantly different on-going pregnancy rates of 81% and 61%, respectively at 12 weeks [25]. This study highlighted the importance of early initiation of both aspirin and heparin.

Evidence on treatment with anticoagulants for inherited thrombophilias is less compelling. A Cochrane meta-analysis, published in 2014, examined the impact of aspirin, low molecular weight heparin, or combined aspirin and low molecular weight heparin in women with two or more unexplained miscarriages with or without an inherited thrombophilia. None of these interventions improved the live birth rate. A more recent meta-analysis comparing low-molecular weight heparin to no treatment in women with two or more losses under 10 weeks' gestation, showed no difference in live birth rates [26]. The evidence to date does not support the routine use of anticoagulants in pregnancy to prevent miscarriage in women with inherited thrombophilias and a history of recurrent miscarriage. The ALIFE2 trial, which randomised pregnant women with a history of inherited thrombophilia and recurrent miscarriage to low molecular weight heparin starting at before 7 weeks or no treatment at all is ongoing. Finally, when considering thromboprophylaxis the risk of thrombosis, and not just that of miscarriage, should be reviewed as the former may be an indication for anticoagulant treatment.

## UTERINE ABNORMALITIES

Congenital uterine abnormalities are associated with adverse obstetric outcomes such as second trimester loss, preterm labour, growth restriction, malpresentation and increased risk of caesarean section. These abnormalities arise from defects in one of the three phases of Müllerian duct development: Organogenesis, fusion of Müllerian ducts, and septal resorption or canalisation. Developmental abnormalities at the organogenesis stage can lead to a unicornuate uterus. Defects in the fusion of the two Müllerian ducts can be divided into vertical – resulting in uterus didelphys or bicornuate uterus, and horizontal – resulting in an imperforate hymen or transverse horizontal septum. Incomplete or absent septal resorption or canalisation leads to a complete or partial septate uterus or an arcuate uterus. A number of theories have been proposed to explain how the presence of a septum may contribute to miscarriage. These focus predominantly on the septal endometrium, septal subendometrial blood flow and on the reduced uterine capacity [27].

One of the main challenges in determining the role of congenital uterine abnormalities in recurrent miscarriage is the use of multiple classification systems. This is illustrated by the fact that 30% of women meet either the ESHRE [27], ASRM [28] or Congenital Uterine Malformations by Expert [29] criteria for a septate uterus but <3% will meet the criteria for all three [30].

Notwithstanding the above, epidemiological studies suggest an association between congenital uterine abnormalities and recurrent miscarriage. The prevalence of these abnormalities in the general population is 4.6–6.7% while that in the recurrent miscarriage population is 12.6–18.2% [31–33]. This correlation was confirmed in the largest-to-date meta-analysis which showed an association between congenital uterine abnormalities and first trimester pregnancy loss (RR 1.56; 95% CI 1.17–2.08) [34]. In the subgroup analysis, only septate and bicornuate morphology were associated with increased risk of first trimester loss (RR 2.65; 95% CI 1.39–5.06 and RR 2.32; 95% CI 1.05–5.13, respectively). This effect was more pronounced with second trimester loss.

The same study looked at the recurrent miscarriage population and demonstrated an association between congenital uterine abnormalities and future first or second trimester miscarriage. There were not enough studies to perform a subgroup analysis to examine the impact of individual abnormalities.

Less data is available on the effect of fibroids on miscarriage but it is generally accepted that non-cavity distorting fibroids are unlikely to impact on fertility [35]. A systematic literature review published in 2017 showed a trend towards an increased risk of miscarriage from 22% to 47% in women with submucosal fibroids [36]. Removal of cavity-distorting fibroids reduced the risk of second trimester miscarriage in a retrospective study of 264 women [37]. In the same study, women with non-cavity distorting fibroids had similar subsequent pregnancy rates to women with unexplained recurrent miscarriage.

Intra-cavity adhesions, usually secondary to curettage of the gravid uterus, have been studied in the context of miscarriage. It is postulated they may be associated with a subsequent increased risk of miscarriage. The proposed pathway is multifactorial and includes absence of sufficient healthy endometrium for implantation and on-going pregnancy development, impaired subendothelial vascularisation resulting in endometrial fibrosis, and constriction of the uterus [38]. Although, there are no randomised studies to support a correlation, clinical experience suggests an association.

## Investigations

Women with recurrent pregnancy loss should undergo imaging to assess the uterus for structural abnormalities. Congenital uterine abnormalities can be diagnosed with a number of imaging modalities: two-dimensional (2D) or three-dimensional (3D) ultrasound, saline infusion sonohysterography (SIS), hysterosalpingography (HSG), magnetic resonance imaging (MRI) or combined hysteroscopy and laparoscopy. Combined hysteroscopy and laparoscopy was initially proposed as the gold-standard diagnostic tool [33]. This has been largely superseded by less invasive alternatives. Two-dimensional ultrasound in the secretory phase of the cycle has a high specificity but low sensitivity [39,40]. Three-dimensional ultrasound has the benefit of allowing for assessment of the internal and external contour of the uterus and has a similar diagnostic accuracy to MRI [39,40].

There is no international consensus on what should be the primary imaging modality. ASRM recommend either HSG or SIS with use of MRI or 3D ultrasound for further assessment when required, whilst ESHRE recommends 3D ultrasound as first-line, with MRI reserved for more complex cases [27,28]. The benefit of 3D ultrasound compared to SIS or HSG is that it is relatively inexpensive, less invasive and is not associated with a risk of infection. It also allows accurate measurements and classification of abnormalities based on the ESGE-ESHRE classification system [27,41]. MRI is useful in the diagnosis of complex uterine abnormalities and for the assessment of the presence of functional endometrium in a rudimentary non-communicating horn. Importantly, it is a non-invasive investigation and is therefore suitable for women who are not sexually active. Overall, either SIS or 3D ultrasound is appropriate diagnostic tool with MRI reserved for more complex cases.

Magnetic resonance imaging and ultrasound can be used for the assessment of uterine myomas. SIS, 3D ultrasound and MRI can assess for uterine cavity distortion. SIS is particularly useful for the diagnosis of intra-uterine synechiae.

## Treatment

Septate and bicornuate uterine morphology are associated with an increased risk of miscarriage. Open or laparoscopic metroplasty has been used for bicornuate uterus but has not been shown to reduce the risk of future miscarriage and is therefore not recommended [42].

Hysteroscopic metroplasty has been described in the context of septate and subseptate uterine morphology. This can be performed using cold scissors or an electrosurgical loop or needle. No one technique has been demonstrated to be superior [40,43]. Laparoscopic and ultrasound guidance to ensure complete septal division and reduce the risk of perforation have also been suggested with variable uptake [40,44]. Furthermore, there is a 1% risk of subsequent adhesion formation [44] and to mitigate for this, insertion of copper coils, intra-uterine balloons and adhesions barriers have been described in the literature, as well as use of HRT. There is no evidence to clearly support this practice, although common sense would dictate that trying to separate the uterine walls post-operatively should reduce the risk of adhesion formation. This principle is often applied in fibroid resection where concurrent resection of fibroids on opposite sides of the uterine cavity is avoided to reduce the risk of scar tissue formation. The evidence suggests that even following surgery, women remain at increased risk of adverse obstetric outcomes with one study showing an increased risk of fetal malpresentation, growth restriction and caesarean section compared to women with normal uterine anatomy [45].

Data on the effectiveness of hysteroscopic metroplasty on miscarriage was up to recently limited to non-randomised studies. A meta-analysis of observational, predominantly retrospective, studies demonstrated a reduced probability of miscarriage post-operatively (RR 0.37; 95% CI 0.25–0.55) [34]. The study was criticised because the population was heterogeneous and included women with no history of subfertility or recurrent miscarriage. A prospective non-randomised study in women with recurrent miscarriage showed that surgery was associated with a higher subsequent live birth rate [42].

There is only one randomised controlled study (TRUST) which examined the role of hysteroscopic metroplasty [46]. This study recruited 80 women with a history of subfertility, miscarriage or preterm labour over an 8-year period. There was no difference in subsequent risk of miscarriage, preterm birth or live birth rate between the two groups. There was one case of uterine perforation at hysteroscopy acting as a reminder that this intervention is not without risk. The study was criticised for not using a consistent threshold for uterine septum size as an inclusion criterion, for the use of multiple different resection techniques and for lack of standardisation of how complete resection was identified (bleeding from the myometrium versus by comparing the level of resection to the level of the ostia) [43]. The patient population limits the generalisability of any results from this study to the recurrent miscarriage patient population. The pilot randomised controlled trial (RCT) of hysteroscopic septal resection is currently recruiting [47].

The American Society for Reproductive Medicine guidance remains that septal resection 'may be beneficial' and 'should be considered' in women with recurrent pregnancy loss [22]. The committee commented on the lack of evidence from RCTs. The TRUST trial, that was subsequently published, is unlikely to result in a change in international guidance. In the UK, the National Institute for Health and Care Excellence (NICE) concluded that the evidence supported hysteroscopic septal resection in women with recurrent pregnancy loss but recommended that specialists in reproductive medicine, uterine imaging and hysteroscopic surgery should be used to identify suitable patients and to perform the procedure [48].

# GENETICS

## Fetal aneuploidy

Fetal aneuploidy is the most common cause of sporadic miscarriage. The risk of aneuploidy increases primarily with advancing female age. Up to 70% of sporadic miscarriages are due to aneuploidy, the most common of which is trisomy followed by polyploidy, monoploidy and chromosomal structural abnormalities [49,50].

The traditional view that aneuploidy contributes to only a minority of cases of recurrent miscarriage is largely driven by studies [51,52] using older cytogenetic analysis technologies, namely G-banding. This technique is limited by a high incidence of culture failure in up to 10–30% of cases [53] and maternal contamination in 20–30% [54]. Newer technologies, array comparative genomic hybridisation (aCGH) and single nucleotide polymorphism (SNP), have significantly lower failure rates and have been recently used in recurrent miscarriage. A 2018 study using 24 chromosome microarray analysis (CMA) on products of conception showed a 67% fetal aneuploidy rate in the recurrent miscarriage population [55]. This rate is comparable to that encountered in sporadic miscarriage, suggesting that earlier work using G-banding technology underestimated the contribution of fetal aneuploidy to recurrent pregnancy loss.

A follow-up study confirmed similar rates of aneuploidy and found that approximately 25% of couples with aneuploidy on products of conception detected with CMA had at least one concomitant abnormal finding on the ASRM workup highlighting the importance of a complete work-up [56].

Looking at the in-vitro fertilisation (IVF) population, aneuploidy rates of 60% were confirmed in a study of 2,282 PGT-A tested embryos of couples with a history of recurrent miscarriage [57]. A further study performing PGT using FISH to analyse chromosomes 13, 16, 18, 21, 22, X and Y in patients with recurrent miscarriage versus those undergoing assisted conception treatment for monogenic disorders showed a higher rate of aneuploidy in the first group (56.5% vs. 33.9%; $p$ <0.0001) [58], confirming that fetal aneuploidy is a significant contributor to recurrent miscarriage.

## Parental translocations

Parental translocations account for a minority of patients with recurrent miscarriage. Balanced reciprocal and Robertsonian translocations are found in 2–5% of couples with recurrent miscarriage [59,60]. Studies following up carrier couples over a 10-year period showed that in the long-term 83% had at least one healthy child. This was comparable to non-carrier couples [61]. Of those with a reciprocal translocation, 54% had at least one miscarriage but 83% later had a healthy child. This compares to a 49% and 34% risk of miscarriage in couples with inversions and Robertsonian translocations, respectively. In the above two groups, 78% and 82% respectively had at least one healthy live birth during the ten year follow-up period.

## Investigations

Fetal chromosomal analysis is recommended following three miscarriages [5]. Diagnostic techniques have significantly evolved over time as outlined earlier. Conventional cytogenetic analysis was initially performed using the G-banding for metaphase spread after culture of villous cells [53]. Other techniques such as fluorescence in-situ hybridisation (FISH) and multiplex ligation-dependent probe amplification (MLPA) are limited by the probes used. Newer molecular techniques, aCGH and SNP have failure rates of 2% and 4% respectively [62].

Some have argued that cytogenetic analysis should not routinely be performed as it may not change management. However, it has multiple benefits. Firstly, considering the significant parental psychological morbidity associated with miscarriage, identifying a cause can be helpful for the couple. Secondly, fetal karyotype is important for prognosis and to help predict risk of future miscarriage. Finally, identification of a fetal unbalanced structural translocation should prompt parental karyotyping. Couples with abnormal karyotypes should be referred onwards for counselling and to discuss the implications for future pregnancies.

## Treatment

In-vitro fertilisation with pre-implantation chromosome testing for aneuploidy has been explored in women with recurrent miscarriage. A distinction needs to be made between couples with a parental balanced translocation and those with unexplained recurrent miscarriage.

When a parental balanced translocation is detected, the couple should be referred to a geneticist to discuss the significance of the identified translocation. The two options thereafter are to persevere with natural conception or to proceed with IVF using pre-implantation genetic testing for chromosomal structural re-arrangements (PGT-SR) or for single gene defects/monogenic (PGT-M). Some studies argue that couples should be encouraged to continue with natural conception as there is evidence to suggest that carrier couples have the same chance of having a healthy child over a 10-year period compared to parents with normal karyotypes [61], although they do remain at increased risk of miscarriage. Others recommend PGT. This is based on the evidence that while this technique may not increase the live birth rate [61,63,64], it does appear to reduce the risk of miscarriage [63–66]. Studies also suggest a shorter time to achieve an on-going pregnancy [63,65–67]. On this basis, couples with a balanced translocation should be counselled about the option of PGT, bearing in mind that given the financial cost of this intervention, this may not be a suitable option for everyone.

For women with unexplained recurrent miscarriage the treatment options are natural conception or PGT IVF. A case series of women undergoing PGT showed a miscarriage rate of 6.9% compared with the expected rate of 33.5% in a recurrent pregnancy loss control population [57]. The authors concluded that these results suggested that 'idiopathic' recurrent miscarriage is due predominantly to chromosomal abnormalities in embryos.

A recent study reviewed cases from the Society of Assisted Reproductive Technologies Clinical Outcomes Reporting System and analysed data from 12,631 autologous frozen embryo treatment (FET) performed between 2010 and 2016 [68]. They analysed cycles of women with three or more miscarriages undergoing FET with or without PGT-A and cycles of women with tubal infertility undergoing IVF with or without PGT-A. The live birth and clinical pregnancy rates with FET-PGT-A in women with recurrent miscarriage versus those with tubal infertility were comparable.

In the recurrent miscarriage group, the PGT-A group had higher clinical pregnancy and live birth rates [(59% vs. 47%; $p < 0.001$) and (48% vs. 34%; $p < 0.001$) respectively] and lower miscarriage rates (11% vs. 13%; $p = 0.02$). The difference in live birth rate was more pronounced with advancing maternal age [(RR 1.31; 95% CI 1.12–1.52) for age <35 years vs. (RR 3.80; 95% CI 2.52–5.72) for ages >42 years].

A retrospective intention-to-treat analysis comparing women with expectant management versus PGT IVF showed no difference in live birth or miscarriage [69]. Subgroup analysis comparing the expectant management group with those having a transfer of a euploid embryo demonstrated a higher live birth rate in the latter [69]. A retrospective study comparing frozen embryo-replacement cycle with or without PGT-A in women with unexplained recurrent miscarriage also showed a rise in on-going pregnancy and live birth rates but with no difference in miscarriage rates [68]. Higher live birth rates were more pronounced with advancing maternal age (live birth outcome was 1.31; 95% CI 1.12, 1.52 for age <35 years vs. 3.80; 95% CI 2.52–5.72 for ages >42 years). This suggests that aneuploidy is likely to be the main contributory factor in recurrent miscarriage with advancing maternal age. This age-related benefit of PGT-A was also found in the STAR trial [70].

The evidence suggests that women undergoing IVF PGT-A and having a transfer of a euploid embryo, have a higher chance of achieving a live birth compared to age-matched controls attempting natural conception. It is important that women are informed of the risk of cycle cancelation and of evidence from intention-to-treat studies. Considering the emotional burden of recurrent miscarriage, it is likely that despite the uncertainties of PGT-A, a significant proportion of women may still choose to proceed with this treatment. Couples should be supported in their decision.

## IMMUNOLOGICAL

The contemporary view of reproductive immunology is that a pregnancy far from being a conflict between mother and fetus for survival is in fact a cooperative venture between the two. The concept of immune rejection is a false one. Currently the tensions are focussed on the role of NK cells, both peripheral and uterine, in the pathogenesis of pregnancy loss and other adverse pregnancy outcomes.

Uterine NK cells perform a role of targeting and clearing inflammatory stress cells. Their numbers fluctuate, increasing in the secretory phase of the menstrual cycle and in early pregnancy, suggesting a protective role in endometrial decidualisation and pregnancy implantation [71]. The uterine NK cell population expresses the CD56 and CD 16 surface markers and are referred to as $CD56^{Bright}CD16^{+}$ [72].

Some studies have demonstrated higher levels of endometrial NK cells in women with recurrent miscarriage compared to healthy parous controls [73]. Looking at CD56 NK cell subgroup, there was a higher proportion of $CD56^{Dim}$, which unlike $CD56^{Bright}$, is associated with cytotoxic activity.

Peripheral blood NK cells predominantly express CD56 and CD16 at low density ($CD56^{dim}CD16^{-}$ cells) and have cytotoxic activity [72]. Peripheral blood NK cell testing has been suggested as a surrogate marker for uterine NK cell levels [74]. Major limitations of this approach are the lack of correlation between peripheral and uterine NK cell populations and more importantly the lack of standardisation of testing methodologies for these two cell populations.

Notwithstanding these limitations, a recent meta-analysis showed a higher peripheral NK cell percentage and absolute numbers in women with recurrent miscarriage compared to healthy controls. There was no difference in uterine NK cells numbers in the two groups [75]. More importantly, a further meta-analysis showed that neither uterine nor peripheral NK cell count were predictive of future miscarriage [76]. The evidence to date does not consistently support a correlation between uterine or peripheral NK cell number and recurrent miscarriage or risk of future miscarriage [72].

The HLA system is thought to play a key role in maternal immunomodulation and has been studied in the context of 'failed' immune tolerance and subsequent miscarriage. Research has focussed predominantly on HLA-B, HLA-C, HLA-G, HLA-DR and HLA-B. A meta-analysis showed an association between recurrent miscarriage and maternal HLA-DRB1*4 and HLA-DRB1*15(77). By contrast, HLA-DRB1*13 and HLA-DRB1*14 were associated with a lower risk of recurrent miscarriage. HLA sharing between couples is thought to be a risk factor for miscarriage due to a dampened immunomodulatory response [77]. Indeed, couple sharing of HLA-B or HLA-DR was associated with an increased risk of recurrent miscarriage [77]. Significant limitations of the study were high levels of information and selection bias, and relatively low observed odds ratios.

Cytokine responses have also been studied in recurrent miscarriage. T helper 1 (Th1) responses have a deleterious effect on the placenta and pregnancy, while T helper 2 (Th2) responses are considered protective of pregnancy [78]. A study of 47 women showed a higher concentration of cytokines associated with a Th1 response in women with recurrent pregnancy loss diagnosed with a miscarriage compared to parous women with on-going pregnancies [78]. A further study of 81 women attempted to answer whether the observed cytokine shift was a cause or a consequence of miscarriage. The group demonstrated a shift towards a Th1 response in women diagnosed with miscarriage but not in those with on-going pregnancy, suggesting that the cytokine shift is a result, rather than a cause, of miscarriage [79].

## Investigations

Immunological testing remains perhaps one of the most contentious areas of recurrent miscarriage. Natural killer (NK) cells by virtue of their emotive name are often perceived by patients as a de facto significant contributor to miscarriage and a necessary investigation. This, however, poses multiple ethical and practical challenges. Firstly, although an association with recurrent miscarriage has been demonstrated, no intervention has conclusively been shown to alter pregnancy outcome. Secondly, there is no standardisation of measurement (flow cytometry versus immunohistochemistry) of uterine or peripheral NK cells and no agreed normal range or reporting system with some reporting absolute values and others reporting NK cells as a percentage of the whole white cell population. Furthermore, testing for uterine NK cells is an invasive test, and with natural fluctuations in NK cell numbers, it is unclear what the optimal sampling time is. While peripheral NK cell testing has been proposed as a less invasive alternative, it is not entirely clear whether this represents an accurate surrogate marker given the differing antigen (CD56, CD16) expression on these two NK cell populations [72]. Evidence for the effectiveness of monitoring NK cell levels is lacking and considering the significant cost of testing and of unproven medical interventions, routine testing cannot currently be recommended. Similarly, the evidence does not support cytokine or HLA parental testing.

## Treatment

Uterine NK cells express glucocorticoid receptors. Steroids, and in particular prednisolone, have been explored as potential treatment options. While chronic exposure to prednisolone can have maternal side effects, it has the significant benefit that it is almost entirely metabolised by the placenta with minimal placental transfer to the fetus [80]. A recent meta-analysis showed that prednisolone did not increase the live birth rate or reduce the risk of miscarriage in women with recurrent miscarriage [81].

Intravenous immunoglobulin (IVIG) has an immunomodulatory role which in the context of recurrent miscarriage and high NK cells is thought to be mediated by inhibition of NK cell cytotoxicity, control of cytokine secretion, and reduction and neutralisation of autoantibodies [82]. An observational study of 217 women with recurrent miscarriage showed that use of IVIG resulted in a live birth rate of 96% in subsequent pregnancy compared to 31% in those who did not receive IVIG. These results were replicated in a meta-analysis of 557 women, which found higher live birth rates (RR 2.57; 95% CI 1.79–3.69) and lower miscarriage rates in women treated with IVIG. There was significant heterogeneity in the data (I2 = 62% and 83%, respectively) [81]. Importantly, a Cochrane meta-analysis showed that use of IVIG did not increase the live birth rates in the recurrent miscarriage population [81]. These findings are reflected in the guidance published by the RCOG, ASRM and ESHRE who do not recommend treatment with IVIG. Considering the treatment cost and risks of anaphylaxis and transmission of infection, its use in the recurrent miscarriage population cannot be supported.

Intralipid is a synthetic product composed of 10% soybean oil, 1.2% egg yolk phospholipids, 2.25% glycerine, and water [81]. Use of intralipid was not associated with a higher clinical pregnancy in a retrospective cohort study [83] and in a subsequent meta-analysis [81]. Evidence does not support its use in recurrent miscarriage.

## ENDOCRINE

Progesterone is essential for pregnancy until 8 weeks' gestation. Serum progesterone is lower in pregnancies that miscarry compared to those that are on-going. Luteal phase deficiency is defined by the ASRM as a luteal phase of <10 days in length [84]. This is thought to be due to lower progesterone production by the corpus luteum. One of the main challenges of making an association between a luteal phase defect and recurrent pregnancy loss is the lack of consensus on diagnostic criteria. Use of histological and biochemical endpoints as diagnostic criteria for endometrial dating is unreliable [84]. Notwithstanding this, studies have used a combination of endometrial sampling and serum progesterone levels and have shown an association between luteal phase deficiency and recurrent miscarriage [85-87]. A follow-up study, however, did not demonstrate a predictive value of this diagnosis in terms of risk of further miscarriage [88]. Therefore, while luteal phase deficiency may be implicated in some cases of recurrent miscarriage, its clinical applicability is limited.

Levothyroxine is important for in-utero fetal neurodevelopment with overt thyroid disease being linked to poor obstetric outcomes. Hypo- and hyper-thyroidism should be treated. The data for subclinical hypothyroidism is less clear. This has been studied in the context of subfertility with some observational studies suggesting a beneficial effect of levothyroxine supplementation but there is a lack of validation from RCTs [89]. In the context of recurrent miscarriage, the prevalence of subclinical hypothyroidism was found to be between 12.6% and 16% [90,91] compared to 4.3% in the general population and 3.5% in pregnancy [92,93]. The authors commented on the high heterogeneity and wide confidence intervals when reporting on the recurrent miscarriage population. A subsequent meta-analysis did not support an association between subclinical hypothyroidism and recurrent miscarriage [91].

Thyroid autoimmunity, defined by the presence of thyroid peroxidase or thyroglobulin antibodies, has also been studied in recurrent miscarriage. A meta-analysis comparing women with recurrent pregnancy loss to a control population demonstrated an association with thyroid autoimmunity (OR 1.94; 95% CI 1.43–2.64) [91]. Six studies examined the predictive value of thyroid autoantibodies on future risk of miscarriage with three of these showing that presence of antibodies conferred an increased risk of miscarriage [94,95]. This was supported by a subsequent meta-analysis [96]. A significant limitation of multiple studies is that they do not screen for anti-phospholipid antibodies, which are known to be more prevalent in women with thyroid autoimmunity [97] and in the recurrent miscarriage population can be associated with a diagnosis of APS.

Polycystic ovarian syndrome (PCOS) has been studied in the context of recurrent miscarriage. A meta-analysis confirmed an association with recurrent miscarriage demonstrating a higher incidence of future miscarriage in the PCOS subgroup but with no difference in the overall live birth rate [98]. It was hypothesised that the adverse early pregnancy outcomes were due to raised luteinising hormone and testosterone levels but this has not been confirmed in subsequent studies [99]. Insulin resistance is observed in women with PCOS and has also been suggested as a possible mechanism for miscarriage in this population. This is supported by the association between insulin resistance and recurrent pregnancy loss in healthy non-diabetic women [100]. The evidence is clear that an association between PCOS and recurrent miscarriage exists but the pathophysiology remains poorly understood.

## Investigations

Thyroid function tests are recommended in those with a history of recurrent miscarriage. In those with subclinical hypothyroidism, thyroid peroxidase antibodies should be checked.

## Management

Progesterone has historically been used empirically in women with recurrent miscarriage as a low risk intervention, although data on its effectiveness is conflicting. The PROMISE trial is the largest to-date multi-centre, double-blind, placebo-controlled randomised trial looking at the effect of progesterone supplementation on live birth in the recurrent miscarriage population [101]. A total of 836 women were randomised to 400 mg twice daily vaginal micronised progesterone versus placebo from positive urinary pregnancy test through 12 weeks' gestation. There was no difference in live birth rate or miscarriage. A subsequent Cochrane meta-analysis looking at 1,684 women showed that progestogen supplementation may lead to a reduction in the number of miscarriages (average RR 0.73; 95% CI 0.54–1.00) [102].

Following on from this, the PRISM trial, another multi-centre, double-blind, placebo-controlled randomised trial looked at vaginal micronised progesterone supplementation versus placebo in 4,153 women presenting with bleeding in early pregnancy [103]. There was no difference in overall live birth rate but subgroup analysis demonstrated a higher live birth rate in the progesterone group in those with at least one previous miscarriage. This has since been incorporated in the miscarriage guidance published by the NICE [104].

A further challenge in interpreting the data from published studies is the use of different progestogen preparations. A Cochrane meta-analysis showed that of all progestogens, only vaginal micronised progesterone may increase the live birth rate for women with a history of one or more previous miscarriages and presenting with bleeding in early pregnancy [105].

Studies have looked at whether there is a role for levothyroxine supplementation in women with thyroid antibodies. A recent meta-analysis attempted to address this exact question and demonstrated a lower miscarriage rate (OR 0.49; 95% CI 0.39–0.96) in those with thyroid autoantibodies receiving levothyroxine [106]. Importantly, this meta-analysis included only four studies one of which started levothyroxine supplementation at 10 weeks by which point the majority of losses in the control group had already occurred.

The TABLET trial, a prospective RCT of levothyroxine 50 μg versus placebo started before conception and continued throughout pregnancy in euthyroid women with thyroid peroxidase antibodies and infertility or history of miscarriage, did not demonstrate a difference in miscarriage or live birth rates [107]. The study was underpowered to examine the recurrent miscarriage population separately. A criticism of this study is that it did not screen for the presence of anti-phospholipid antibodies, which can be found in association with thyroid autoantibodies and left untreated are likely to lead to further miscarriage.

The T4-life trial, a multi-centre, placebo controlled randomised trial in euthyroid women with recurrent miscarriage and thyroid peroxidase antibodies has completed recruitment and results are awaited [108]. Based on the current evidence, the American Thyroid Association has concluded that there is insufficient evidence to recommend levothyroxine supplementation in pregnant women with thyroid peroxidase antibodies but that as this is a low risk intervention, it may be considered in women with a history of recurrent pregnancy loss. By contrast, the RCOG does not recommend routine levothyroxine supplementation in this patient group.

Regarding subclinical hypothyroidism, the data also remains unclear with no RCTs in the recurrent miscarriage population. A meta-analysis showed that levothyroxine supplementation in the general population reduced the risk of miscarriage by 57%. Subgroup analysis validated this result in women undergoing IVF but not in those who conceived spontaneously [106]. The American Thyroid Association strongly recommends levothyroxine treatment in those with thyroid peroxidase antibodies and a TSH >4 mU/L. It also suggests 'consideration' of levothyroxine if the TSH is >2.5 mU/L. In those with no thyroid autoimmunity, levothyroxine supplementation is recommended for a TSH >4 mU/L [89].

## MALE FACTOR

Advancing paternal age is associated with an increased risk of recurrent miscarriage. This is thought to be due to an increased rate of sperm DNA fragmentation with advancing age.

Sperm DNA is highly compact with a volume typically 10% or less to that of a somatic cell nucleus [70]. To achieve this most of the DNA is tightly bound to protamine, a much smaller protein than histones. Supercompaction is thought to be protective from oxidative stress. The residual DNA is loosely bound to histones and thereby susceptible to genotoxic factors [109,110] associated with advancing age, obesity and varicocoeles. Oxidative stress results in DNA fragmentation. Low grades of sperm DNA fragmentation can be corrected by oocyte repair mechanisms following fertilisation. By contrast, more extensive DNA fragmentation is resistant to repair mechanisms and may affect early embryonic development following the activation of the paternal genome. Another important consideration is that with advancing maternal age, the oocyte's ability to correct for sperm DNA fragmentation is impaired [111]. This translates into poorer quality embryos in older women, compared to younger ones, using sperm with comparable levels of DNA fragmentation.

High sperm DNA fragmentation has been linked to infertility, lower assisted conception success rates and miscarriage [112]. Studies have shown higher sperm DNA fragmentation in males whose partners had a history of recurrent pregnancy loss [113,114]. One study comparing males with partners with a history of recurrent pregnancy loss, to fertile men and infertile men, showed higher DNA fragmentation in the first group [113]. Interestingly, their semen analysis parameters were superior to those observed in sub-fertile men but comparable to fertile healthy men in terms of sperm concentration and motility. The morphology was poorer in the recurrent pregnancy loss group compared to the fertile controls. This study suggests that the semen in the recurrent pregnancy loss group is suitable for oocyte fertilisation, contrary to the infertile group, but that the high levels of DNA fragmentation are beyond the oocyte's capacity for repair resulting in miscarriage.

A meta-analysis of 901 couples showed that male partners of women with recurrent pregnancy loss had significantly higher sperm DNA fragmentation levels compared to fertile controls [110]. A recognised limitation of this study was the high heterogeneity secondary to the inconsistent definition of recurrent pregnancy loss, the use of frozen sperm in some studies and the variation in periods of abstinence.

Studies are further limited by the use of different techniques to assess DNA fragmentation. The main assays used are the sperm chromatin dispersion (SCD) test, the sperm chromatin structure assay (SCSA) and the terminal deoxynucleotidyl transferase–mediated dUTP nick-end labelling (TUNEL) assay. SCD uses fluorescent microscopy and has the benefit of visualising sperm directly. Its significant disadvantage is that it can be harder to interpret [114]. THE SCSA and TUNEL assays rely on flow cytometry. The former measures the susceptibility of sperm DNA to denaturation [110] while the latter measures the quantity of DNA strand breaks [110,113]. Specific cut-off values for each assay have not been agreed.

While there appears to be an association between high levels of sperm DNA fragmentation and recurrent miscarriage, routine testing cannot be recommended in view of the paucity of prospective data on effective interventions. Considering the established association between obesity, smoking, sedentary lifestyle, diabetes and oxidative stress, lifestyle modifications should be recommended. There may also be a role for antioxidants, although prospective data is lacking.

## CONCLUSION

Research into recurrent miscarriage has moved into the mainstream. Recurrent miscarriage is associated with long-term psychological and physical morbidity. It is becoming increasingly apparent that this patient group experiences not only worse short-term outcomes – risk of growth restriction, placental abruption and stillbirth, but also long-term non-gynaecological sequelae. There is a clear and consistent link with psychological morbidity including depression, anxiety and symptoms of PTSD [115]. Recurrent miscarriage has also been linked to premature death [116], cardiovascular disease [116–118] and thrombosis [118,119]. There is an almost 40% increased risk of premature death (hazard ratio 1.39; 95% CI 1.03–1.86) and almost double the risk of cardiovascular disease (hazard ratio 1.84; 95% CI 0.76–4.49). Postulated mechanisms for these associations include insulin resistance, immune disorders and endothelial dysfunction [116]. Women should be counselled about the above risks and medical intervention should be considered where relevant to prevent long-term morbidity and mortality.

# REFERENCES

1. Farren J, Jalmbrant M, Ameye L, et al. Post-traumatic stress, anxiety and depression following miscarriage or ectopic pregnancy: a prospective cohort study. BMJ Open 2016; 6:e011864.
2. Blohm F, Fridén B, Milsom I. A prospective longitudinal population-based study of clinical miscarriage in an urban Swedish population. BJOG 2007; 115:176–183.
3. Definitions of infertility and recurrent pregnancy loss: a committee opinion. Fertil Steril 2020; 113:533–535.
4. The ESHRE Guideline Group on RPL, Bender Atik R, Christiansen OB, Elson J, et al. ESHRE guideline: recurrent pregnancy loss. Hum Reprod Open 2018; 2018:hoy004.
5. Royal College of Obstetricians and Gynaecologists. (2011) Recurrent Miscarriage, Investigation and Treatment of Couples. [online] Available from: https://www.rcog.org.uk/en/guidelines-research-services/guidelines/gtg17/. [Last Accessed May, 2022]
6. Magnus MC, Wilcox AJ, Morken NH, et al. Role of maternal age and pregnancy history in risk of miscarriage: prospective register based study. BMJ 2019; 364:l869.
7. Franssen MTM, Korevaar JC, van der Veen F, et al. Management of recurrent miscarriage: evaluating the impact of a guideline. Hum Reprod 2007; 22:1298–1303.
8. du Fossé NA, van der Hoorn M-LP, van Lith JMM, et al. Advanced paternal age is associated with an increased risk of spontaneous miscarriage: a systematic review and meta-analysis. Hum Reprod Update 2020; 26:650–669.
9. Ng KYB, Cherian G, Kermack AJ, et al. Systematic review and meta-analysis of female lifestyle factors and risk of recurrent pregnancy loss. Sci Rep 2021; 11:7081.
10. Cavalcante MB, Sarno M, Peixoto AB, et al. Obesity and recurrent miscarriage: A systematic review and meta-analysis: Obesity and recurrent miscarriage. J Obstet Gynaecol Res 2019; 45:30–38.
11. Stefanidou EM, Caramellino L, Patriarca A, et al. Maternal caffeine consumption and sine causa recurrent miscarriage. Eur J Obstet Gynecol Reprod Biol 2011; 158:220–224.
12. Rai RS. Antiphospholipid syndrome and recurrent miscarriage. J Postgrad Med 2002; 48:3–4.
13. Tong M, Viall CA, Chamley LW. Antiphospholipid antibodies and the placenta: a systematic review of their in vitro effects and modulation by treatment. Hum Reprod Update 2015; 21:97–118.
14. Miyakis S, Lockshin MD, Atsumi T, et al. International consensus statement on an update of the classification criteria for definite antiphospholipid syndrome (APS). J Thromb Haemost 2006; 4:295–306.
15. Ormesher L, Simcox L, Tower C, et al. Management of inherited thrombophilia in pregnancy. Womens Health (Lond Engl) 2016; 12:433–441.
16. Liu X, Chen Y, Ye C, et al. Hereditary thrombophilia and recurrent pregnancy loss: a systematic review and meta-analysis. Hum Reprod 2021;36:1213–1229.
17. Eslami MM, Khalili M, Soufizomorrod M, et al. Factor V Leiden 1691G > A mutation and the risk of recurrent pregnancy loss (RPL): systematic review and meta-analysis. Thrombosis J 2020; 18:11.
18. Rey E, Kahn SR, David M, et al. Thrombophilic disorders and fetal loss: a meta-analysis. Lancet 2003; 361:901–908.
19. Xu Y, Ban Y, Ran L, et al. Relationship between unexplained recurrent pregnancy loss and 5,10-methylenetetrahydrofolate reductase) polymorphisms. Fertil Steril 2019; 111:597–603.
20. Chen H, Yang X, Lu M. Methylenetetrahydrofolate reductase gene polymorphisms and recurrent pregnancy loss in China: a systematic review and meta-analysis. Arch Gynecol Obstet 2016; 293:283–290.
21. van den Boogaard E, Cohn DM, Korevaar JC, et al. Number and sequence of preceding miscarriages and maternal age for the prediction of antiphospholipid syndrome in women with recurrent miscarriage. Fertil Steril 2013; 99:188–192.
22. Evaluation and treatment of recurrent pregnancy loss: a committee opinion. Fertil Steril 2012; 98:1103–111.
23. Rai R, Cohen H, Dave M, et al. Randomised controlled trial of aspirin and aspirin plus heparin in pregnant women with recurrent miscarriage associated with phospholipid antibodies (or antiphospholipid antibodies). BMJ 1997; 314:253–257.
24. Hamulyák EN, Scheres LJJ, Goddijn M, et al. Antithrombotic therapy to prevent recurrent pregnancy loss in antiphospholipid syndrome—What is the evidence? J Thromb Haemost 2021; 19:1174–1185.
25. Eid MI, Abdelhafez MS, El-refaie W, et al. Timing of initiation of low-molecular-weight heparin administration in pregnant women with antiphospholipid syndrome: a randomized clinical trial of efficacy and safety. Int J Womens Health 2019; 11:41–47.
26. Skeith L, Carrier M, Kaaja R, et al. A meta-analysis of low-molecular-weight heparin to prevent pregnancy loss in women with inherited thrombophilia. Blood 2016; 127:1650–1655.

27. Grimbizis GF, Gordts S, Di Spiezio Sardo A, et al. The ESHRE/ESGE consensus on the classification of female genital tract congenital anomalies. Hum Reprod 2013; 28:2032–2044.

28. Pfeifer S, Butts S, Dumesic D, et al. Uterine septum: a guideline. Fertil Steril 2016; 106:530–540.

29. Ludwin A, Martins WP, Nastri CO, et al. Congenital Uterine Malformation by Experts (CUME): better criteria for distinguishing between normal/arcuate and septate uterus?: Septate and normal/arcuate uterus. Ultrasound Obstet Gynecol 2018; 51:101–109.

30. Ludwin A. Septum resection does not improve reproductive outcomes: truly? Hum Reprod 2020; 35:1495–1498.

31. Grimbizis GF. Clinical implications of uterine malformations and hysteroscopic treatment results. Hum Reprod Update 2001; 7:161–174.

32. Chan YY, Jayaprakasan K, Zamora J, et al. The prevalence of congenital uterine anomalies in unselected and high-risk populations: a systematic review. Hum Reprod Update 2011; 17:761–771.

33. Saravelos SH, Cocksedge KA, Li TC. Prevalence and diagnosis of congenital uterine anomalies in women with reproductive failure: a critical appraisal. Hum Reprod Update 2008; 14:415–429.

34. Venetis CA, Papadopoulos SP, Campo R, et al. Clinical implications of congenital uterine anomalies: a meta-analysis of comparative studies. Reprod BioMed Online 2014; 29:665–683.

35. Guo XC, Segars JH. The Impact and Management of Fibroids for Fertility. Obstet Gynecol Clin North Am 2012; 39:521–533.

36. Klatsky PC, Tran ND, Caughey AB, et al. Fibroids and reproductive outcomes: a systematic literature review from conception to delivery. Am J Obstet Gynecol 2008; 98:357–366.

37. Saravelos SH, Yan J, Rehmani H, et al. The prevalence and impact of fibroids and their treatment on the outcome of pregnancy in women with recurrent miscarriage. Hum Reprod 2011; 26:3274–3279.

38. Yu D, Wong YM, Cheong Y, et al. Asherman syndrome—one century later. Fertil Steril 2008; 89:759–779.

39. Graupera B, Pascual MA, Hereter L, et al. Accuracy of three-dimensional ultrasound compared with magnetic resonance imaging in diagnosis of Müllerian duct anomalies using ESHRE-ESGE consensus on the classification of congenital anomalies of the female genital tract: 3D-US to diagnose MDA. Ultrasound Obstet Gynecol 2015; 46:616–622.

40. Budden A, Abbott JA. The Diagnosis and Surgical Approach of Uterine Septa. J Minim Invas Gynecol.2018; 25:209–217.

41. Akhtar M, Saravelos S, Li T, et al. the Royal College of Obstetricians and Gynaecologists. Reproductive Implications and Management of Congenital Uterine Anomalies: Scientific Impact Paper No. 62 November 2019. BJOG 2022; 127.

42. Sugiura-Ogasawara M, Lin BL, Aoki K, et al. Does surgery improve live birth rates in patients with recurrent miscarriage caused by uterine anomalies? J Obstet Gynaecol 2015; 35:155–158.

43. Alvero R, Burney RO, Khorshid A, et al. Surgical treatment of uterine septum to improve reproductive outcomes—resect or not? Fertil Steril 2021; 116:298–305.

44. Valle RF, Ekpo GE. Hysteroscopic Metroplasty for the Septate Uterus: Review and Meta-Analysis. J Minim Invas Gynecol 2013; 20:22–42.

45. Agostini A, De Guibert F, Salari K, et al. Adverse Obstetric Outcomes at Term after Hysteroscopic Metroplasty. J Minim Invas Gynecol 2009; 16: 454–457.

46. Rikken JFW, Kowalik CR, Emanuel MH, et al. Septum resection versus expectant management in women with a septate uterus: an international multicentre open-label randomized controlled trial. Hum Reprod 2021; 36:1260–1267.

47. Cochrane Central Register of Controlled Trials. Pilot randomised controlled trial of hysteroscopic septal resection. [online] Available from: https://www.cochranelibrary.com/central/doi/10.1002/central/CN-01869130/full. [Last Accessed May, 2022]

48. National Institute for Health and Care Excellence. Hysteroscopic metroplasty of a uterine septum for recurrent miscarriage. Interventional procedures guidance [IPG510]. London: National Institute for Health and Care Excellence; 2015.

49. Stephenson MD. Cytogenetic analysis of miscarriages from couples with recurrent miscarriage: a case-control study. Hum Reprod 2002; 17:446–451.

50. Stephenson M, Kutteh W. Evaluation and Management of Recurrent Early Pregnancy Loss. Clin Obstet Gynecol 2007; 50:132–145.

51. Ogasawara M, Aoki K, Okada S, et al. Embryonic karyotype of abortuses in relation to the number of previous miscarriages. Fertil Steril 2000; 73:300–304.

52. Sugiura-Ogasawara M, Ozaki Y, Katano K, et al. Abnormal embryonic karyotype is the most frequent cause of recurrent miscarriage. Hum Reprod 2012; 27:2297–2303.

53. Ozawa N. Cytogenetic Analysis of Spontaneous Miscarriage. In: The Human Embryo [Internet]. London: InTechOpen; 2019.
54. Jobanputra V, Esteves C, Sobrino A, et al. Using FISH to increase the yield and accuracy of karyotypes from spontaneous abortion specimens: accuracy of karyotypes from spontaneous abortions. Prenat Diagn 2011; 31:755–759.
55. Popescu F, Jaslow CR, Kutteh WH. Recurrent pregnancy loss evaluation combined with 24-chromosome microarray of miscarriage tissue provides a probable or definite cause of pregnancy loss in over 90% of patients. Hum Reprod 2018; 33:579–587.
56. Papas RS, Kutteh WH. A new algorithm for the evaluation of recurrent pregnancy loss redefining unexplained miscarriage: review of current guidelines. Curr Opin Obstet Gynecol 2020; 32:371–379.
57. Hodes-Wertz B, Grifo J, Ghadir S, et al. Idiopathic recurrent miscarriage is caused mostly by aneuploid embryos. Fertil Steril 2012; 98:675–680.
58. Rubio C, Simon C, Vidal F, et al. Chromosomal abnormalities and embryo development in recurrent miscarriage couples. Hum Reprod 2003; 18:182–188.
59. Braekeleer MD, Dao TN. Cytogenetic studies in couples experiencing repeated pregnancy losses. Hum Reprod 1990; 5:519–528.
60. Clifford K, Rai R, Watson H, et al. Pregnancy: an informative protocol for the investigation of recurrent miscarriage: preliminary experience of 500 consecutive cases. Hum Reprod 1994; 9:1328–1332.
61. Franssen MTM, Korevaar JC, van der Veen F, et al. Reproductive outcome after chromosome analysis in couples with two or more miscarriages: case-control study. BMJ 2006; 332:759–763.
62. Smits MAJ, van Maarle M, Hamer G, et al. Cytogenetic testing of pregnancy loss tissue: a meta-analysis. Reprod BioMed Online 2020; 40:867–879.
63. Fischer J, Colls P, Escudero T, et al. Preimplantation genetic diagnosis (PGD) improves pregnancy outcome for translocation carriers with a history of recurrent losses. Fertil Steril 2010; 94:283–289.
64. Ikuma S, Sato T, Sugiura-Ogasawara M, et al. Preimplantation Genetic Diagnosis and Natural Conception: A Comparison of Live Birth Rates in Patients with Recurrent Pregnancy Loss Associated with Translocation. PLoS ONE 2015; 10:e0129958.
65. Chang EM, Han JE, Kwak IP, et al. Preimplantation genetic diagnosis for couples with a Robertsonian translocation: practical information for genetic counseling. J Assist Reprod Genet 2012; 29:67–75.
66. El Hachem H, Crepaux V, May-Panloup P, et al. Recurrent pregnancy loss: current perspectives. Int J Womens Health 2017; 9:331–345.
67. Keymolen K, Staessen C, Verpoest W, et al. Preimplantation genetic diagnosis in female and male carriers of reciprocal translocations: clinical outcome until delivery of 312 cycles. Eur J Hum Genet 2012; 20:376–380.
68. Bhatt SJ, Marchetto NM, Roy J, et alG. Pregnancy outcomes following in vitro fertilization frozen embryo transfer (IVF-FET) with or without preimplantation genetic testing for aneuploidy (PGT-A) in women with recurrent pregnancy loss (RPL): a SART-CORS study. Hum Reprod 2021; 36:2339–2344.
69. Murugappan G, Shahine LK, Perfetto CO, et al. Intent to treat analysis of in vitro fertilization and preimplantation genetic screening versus expectant management in patients with recurrent pregnancy loss. Hum Reprod 2016; 31:1668–1674.
70. Munné S, Kaplan B, Frattarelli JL, et al. Preimplantation genetic testing for aneuploidy versus morphology as selection criteria for single frozen-thawed embryo transfer in good-prognosis patients: a multicenter randomized clinical trial. Fertil Steril 2019; 112:1071–1079.e7.
71. Chong HP, Quenby SM. Natural killer cells and reproductive health. Obstet Gynecol 2016; 18:91–97.
72. Royal College of Obstetricians and Gynaecologists. (2016). The Role of Natural Killer Cells in Human Fertility. Scientific Impact Paper No. 53. [online] Available from: https://www.rcog.org.uk/globalassets/documents/guidelines/scientific-impact-papers/sip_53.pdf. [Last Accessed May, 2022]
73. Quenby S, Bates M, Doig T, et al. Pre-implantation endometrial leukocytes in women with recurrent miscarriage. Hum Reprod 1999; 14:2386–2391.
74. Kitaya K, Yamaguchi T, Yasuo T, et al. Post-ovulatory rise of endometrial CD16(−) natural killer cells: in situ proliferation of residual cells or selective recruitment from circulating peripheral blood? J Reprod Immunol 2007; 76:45–53.
75. Seshadri S, Sunkara SK. Natural killer cells in female infertility and recurrent miscarriage: a systematic review and meta-analysis. Hum Reprod Update 2014; 20:429–438.
76. Tang AW, Alfirevic Z, Quenby S. Natural killer cells and pregnancy outcomes in women with recurrent miscarriage and infertility: a systematic review. Hum Reprod 2011; 26:1971–1980.

77. Meuleman T, Lashley LELO, Dekkers OM, et al. HLA associations and HLA sharing in recurrent miscarriage: A systematic review and meta-analysis. Hum Immunol 2015; 76:362–373.

78. Raghupathy R, Makhseed M, Azizieh F, et al. Cytokine production by maternal lymphocytes during normal human pregnancy and in unexplained recurrent spontaneous abortion. Hum Reprod 2000; 15:713–718.

79. Bates MD. Aberrant cytokine production by peripheral blood mononuclear cells in recurrent pregnancy loss? Hum Reprod 2002; 17:2439–2444.

80. Tang AW, Alfirevic Z, Turner MA, et al. Prednisolone Trial: Study protocol for a randomised controlled trial of prednisolone for women with idiopathic recurrent miscarriage and raised levels of uterine natural killer (uNK) cells in the endometrium. Trials 2009; 10:102.

81. Woon EV, Day A, Bracewell-Milnes T, et al. Immunotherapy to improve pregnancy outcome in women with abnormal natural killer cell levels/activity and recurrent miscarriage or implantation failure: a systematic review and meta-analysis. J Reprod Immunol 2020; 142:103189.

82. Yang X, Meng T. Is there a Role of Intravenous Immunoglobulin in Immunologic Recurrent Pregnancy Loss? J Immunol Res 2020; 2020:1–14.

83. Martini AE, Jasulaitis S, Fogg LF, et al. Evaluating the Utility of Intralipid Infusion to Improve Live Birth Rates in Patients with Recurrent Pregnancy Loss or Recurrent Implantation Failure. J Hum Reprod Sci 2018; 11:261–268.

84. Diagnosis and treatment of luteal phase deficiency: a committee opinion. Fertil Steril 2021; 115:1416–1423.

85. Balasch J, Creus M, Márquez M, et al. The significance of luteal phase deficiency on fertility: a diagnostic and therapeutic approach. Hum Reprod 1986; 1:145–147.

86. Jordan J, Craig K, Clifton DK, et al. Luteal phase defect: the sensitivity and specificity of diagnostic methods in common clinical use **Supported by grants RO1 HD 18967 (M.R.S.) and MO1 RR00037 (Clinical Research Center, University of Washington, Seattle, Washington). Fertil Steril 1994; 62:54–62.

87. Li TC, Spuijbroek MDEH, Tuckerman E, et al. Endocrinological and endometrial factors in recurrent miscarriage. BJOG 2000; 107: 1471–1479.

88. Ogasawara M, Kajiura S, Katano K, et al. Are serum progesterone levels predictive of recurrent miscarriage in future pregnancies? Fertili Steril 1997; 68:806–809.

89. Alexander EK, Pearce EN, Brent GA, et al. 2017 Guidelines of the American Thyroid Association for the Diagnosis and Management of Thyroid Disease During Pregnancy and the Postpartum. Thyroid 2017; 27: 315–389.

90. Liu Y, Liu Y, Zhang S, et al. Etiology of spontaneous abortion before and after the demonstration of embryonic cardiac activity in women with recurrent spontaneous abortion. Int J Gynecol Obstet 2015; 129:128–132.

91. Dong AC, Morgan J, Kane M, al. Subclinical hypothyroidism and thyroid autoimmunity in recurrent pregnancy loss: a systematic review and meta-analysis. Fertil Steril 2020; 113: 587–600.e1.

92. Hollowell JG, Staehling NW, Flanders WD, et al. Serum TSH, T4, and Thyroid Antibodies in the United States Population (1988 to 1994): National Health and Nutrition Examination Survey (NHANES III). J Clin Endocrinol Metab 2002; 87:489–499.

93. Dong AC, Stagnaro-Green A. Differences in Diagnostic Criteria Mask the True Prevalence of Thyroid Disease in Pregnancy: A Systematic Review and Meta-Analysis. Thyroid 2019; 29:278–289.

94. Pratt DE, Kaberlein G, Dudkiewicz A, et al. The association of antithyroid antibodies in euthyroid nonpregnant women with recurrent first trimester abortions in the next pregnancy. Fertil Steril 1993; 60:1001–1005.

95. Vissenberg R, Fliers E, van der Post JAM, et al. Live-birth rate in euthyroid women with recurrent miscarriage and thyroid peroxidase antibodies. Gynecol Endocrino 2016; 32:132–135.

96. Thangaratinam S, Tan A, Knox E, et al. Association between thyroid autoantibodies and miscarriage and preterm birth: meta-analysis of evidence. BMJ 2011; 342:d2616.

97. Alecsandru D, Garcia Velasco JA. Levothyroxine and thyroid peroxidase antibodies in women with recurrent pregnancy loss. Fertil Steril 2020; 113:546.

98. Mayrhofer D, Hager M, Walch K, et al. The Prevalence and Impact of Polycystic Ovary Syndrome in Recurrent Miscarriage: A Retrospective Cohort Study and Meta-Analysis. J Clin Med 20201; 9:2700.

99. Rai R, Backos M, Rushworth F, et al. Polycystic ovaries and recurrent miscarriage—a reappraisal. Hum Reprod 2000; 15:612–615.

100. Craig LB, Ke RW, Kutteh WH. Increased prevalence of insulin resistance in women with a history of recurrent pregnancy loss. Fertil Steril 2002; 78:487–490.

101. Coomarasamy A, Williams H, Truchanowicz E, et al. A Randomized Trial of Progesterone in Women with Recurrent Miscarriages. N Engl J Med 2015; 373:2141–2148.

102. Haas DM, Hathaway TJ, Ramsey PS. Progestogen for preventing miscarriage in women with recurrent miscarriage of unclear etiology. Cochrane Pregnancy and Childbirth Group. Cochrane Database Syst Rev 2018; 10:CD003511.

103. Coomarasamy A, Devall AJ, Cheed V, et al. A Randomized Trial of Progesterone in Women with Bleeding in Early Pregnancy. N Engl J Med 2019; 380:1815–1824.

104. National Institute for Health and Care Excellence. Ectopic pregnancy and miscarriage: diagnosis and initial management. NICE guideline [NG126] [Internet]. London: NICE; 2019.

105. Devall AJ, Papadopoulou A, Podesek M, et al. Progestogens for preventing miscarriage: a network meta-analysis. Cochrane Pregnancy and Childbirth Group. Cochrane Database Syst Rev 2021; 4:CD013792.

106. Rao M, Zeng Z, Zhou F, et al. Effect of levothyroxine supplementation on pregnancy loss and preterm birth in women with subclinical hypothyroidism and thyroid autoimmunity: a systematic review and meta-analysis. Hum Reprod Update 2019; 25:344–361.

107. Dhillon-Smith RK, Middleton LJ, Sunner KK, et al. Levothyroxine in Women with Thyroid Peroxidase Antibodies before Conception. N Engl J Med 2019; 380:1316–1325.

108. Vissenberg R, van Dijk MM, Fliers E, et al. Effect of levothyroxine on live birth rate in euthyroid women with recurrent miscarriage and TPO antibodies (T4-LIFE study). Contemp Clin Trial 2015; 44:134–138.

109. Miller D, Brinkworth M, Iles D. Paternal DNA packaging in spermatozoa: more than the sum of its parts? DNA, histones, protamines and epigenetics. Reproduction 2010; 139:287–301.

110. McQueen DB, Zhang J, Robins JC. Sperm DNA fragmentation and recurrent pregnancy loss: a systematic review and meta-analysis. Fertil Steril 2019; 112:54–60.e3.

111. Setti AS, Braga DP de AF, Provenza RR, et al. Oocyte ability to repair sperm DNA fragmentation: the impact of maternal age on intracytoplasmic sperm injection outcomes. Fertil Steril 2021; 116:123–129.

112. Robinson L, Gallos ID, Conner SJ, et al. The effect of sperm DNA fragmentation on miscarriage rates: a systematic review and meta-analysis. Hum Reprod 2012; 27:2908–2917.

113. Carlini T, Paoli D, Pelloni M, et al. Sperm DNA fragmentation in Italian couples with recurrent pregnancy loss. Reprod BioMed Online 2017; 34:58–65.

114. Brahem S, Mehdi M, Landolsi H, et al. Semen Parameters and Sperm DNA Fragmentation as Causes of Recurrent Pregnancy Loss. Urology 2011; 78:792–796.

115. Farren J, Mitchell-Jones N, Verbakel JY, Tet al. The psychological impact of early pregnancy loss. Hum Reprod Update 2018; 24:731–749.

116. Wang YX, Mínguez-Alarcón L, Gaskins AJ, et al. Association of spontaneous abortion with all cause and cause specific premature mortality: prospective cohort study. BMJ 2021; n530.

117. Wagner MM, Beshay MM, Rooijakkers S, et al. Increased cardiovascular disease risk in women with a history of recurrent miscarriage. Acta Obstet Gynecol Scand 2018; 97:1192–1199.

118. Quenby S, Gallos ID, Dhillon-Smith RK, et al. Miscarriage matters: the epidemiological, physical, psychological, and economic costs of early pregnancy loss. Lancet 2021; 397:1658–1667.

119. Quenby S, Farquharson RG, Dawood F, et al. Recurrent miscarriage and long-term thrombosis risk: a case–control study. Hum Reprod 2005; 20:1729–1732.

# Chapter 9

# Recent advances in the efficacy and safety of progesterone for the prevention of miscarriages

*Rumana Rahman, Mausumi Das*

Miscarriage is generally defined as the loss of a pregnancy before viability. Globally, about 44 pregnancy losses occur each minute – a statistic which represents approximately 23 million miscarriages every year [1]. Threatened miscarriage is defined as vaginal bleeding, with a closed cervix that occurs before the gestational age at which a fetus would be viable ex utero [2]. The estimated overall reported miscarriage rate is 10–20% with about 80% of all cases of early pregnancy losses occurring in the first trimester [1,2]. Miscarriage can lead to complications resulting from excessive bleeding or infection, as well as devastating psychological impact on the couple, including anxiety, depression, or post-traumatic stress disorder. It is further challenging in those with recurrent pregnancy loss with no plausible explanation [1]. Most first trimester miscarriages can be attributed to a genetic cause, however, anatomical, infectious, hormonal, immunological, or metabolic factors can also play a role [3].

## ROLE OF PROGESTERONE IN THE PREVENTION OF MISCARRIAGES

Progesterone is an essential hormone for conception and maintenance of a pregnancy. Secreted by the corpus luteum in the ovary, it is needed to prepare the endometrium for implantation of the embryo and thus plays a crucial role in achieving a successful pregnancy (**Figure 9.1**) [3,4]. After implantation, progesterone contributes to the maintenance of pregnancy by modulating the maternal immune response, reducing uterine contractility, and regulating the uteroplacental circulation. Therefore, progesterone deficiency can be associated with early pregnancy loss and its supplementation in such cases may help to maintain the pregnancy through its anti-inflammatory, immunomodulatory and uterine relaxant benefits, prevent pre-term birth and enable fetal viability and maturity [4,5].

**Rumana Rahman** MBBS, BSc, MRCOG, Specialist Registrar in Obstetrics and Gynaecology, The Hillingdon Hospital, Uxbridge, UK
Email: rumana.rahman@nhs.net

**Mausumi Das** MD MRCOG MPH, Queen Charlotte and Hammersmith Hospitals, Imperial College Healthcare NHS Trust, and Chelsea and Westminster Hospital NHS Foundation Trust, London, UK
Email: mausumidas@nhs.net

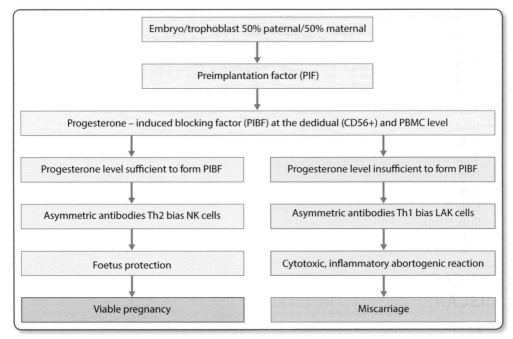

**Figure 9.1** The role of progesterone in successful pregnancy.
LAK cells, lymphokine-activated killer cell; NK, natural killer cells; PBMC, peripheral blood mononuclear cells
*Source:* Adapted from Di Renzo GC, Giardina I, Clerici G, et al. Progesterone in normal and pathological pregnancy. Horm Mol Biol Clin Investig 2016; 27:35–48.

After around 12 weeks of pregnancy, the placenta takes over the role of progesterone production. The essential role of progesterone in pregnancy has led researchers to hypothesise that low progesterone levels could lead to increased risk of miscarriage. Progesterone deficiency has been associated with an increased risk of euploid miscarriages, pre-term births, and infertility [4,6].

## PROGESTERONE FORMULATIONS

A variety of natural and synthetic progestogens are available for therapeutic use. Whereas, micronised progesterone has an identical molecular structure to natural progesterone, synthetic progestogens, which include dydrogesterone (6-dehydro-retroprogesterone) and 17α-hydroxyprogesterone caproate have a different chemical structure, pharmacologic effects, and safety profile [7–10].

Micronisation and sustained release formulations improve the bioavailability and limit hepatic first-pass metabolism [7,10,11]. Vaginally administered progesterone avoids hepatic first-pass metabolism, has high bioavailability, and has been reported to induce adequate endometrial secretory transformation [12]. In contrast to the intramuscular and vaginal routes of administration, oral formulations are rapidly metabolised in the gastrointestinal tract [7,12]. Oral natural micronised progesterone preparations require multiple daily dosing to achieve adequate therapeutic effect [10]. It has been suggested that sustained-release formulations of natural micronised progesterone may have advantages over conventional oral natural micronised progesterone preparations due to better bioavailability and improved compliance [10].

In clinical practice, it is imperative to discuss the information generated from well-designed studies with women at high risk of miscarriages to encourage informed and shared decision-making. Guidelines and recommendations should carefully assess the evidence available, the uncertainty around treatment effects, and available safety data. Clinical studies of progesterone use during pregnancy support its tolerability and relatively minimal adverse effects [13–15].

Evidence suggests that progesterone therapy should be considered in women with threatened miscarriage and a history of one or more previous early pregnancy loss. There has been a recent update in the NICE guidelines to standardise the use of progesterone in threatened miscarriage. The recommendation suggests that vaginal micronised progesterone at the dose of 400 mg twice daily should be prescribed to women with a confirmed intrauterine pregnancy and previous history of miscarriage who present with vaginal bleeding [16].

# EFFICACY OF PROGESTERONE THERAPY IN THREATENED MISCARRIAGE AND RECURRENT MISCARRIAGE

Progesterone supplementation has been considered by researchers, physicians, and patients during early pregnancy to prevent miscarriages based on its physiological importance. Women at risk of miscarriage can be divided into two groups, those with a history of recurrent miscarriage and others with bleeding in early pregnancy [17]. Several studies have suggested a beneficial effect of progesterone use to prevent early pregnancy loss. These include two well-designed, randomised, multi-centre, placebo-controlled trials: (1) PROMISE (PROgesterone in recurrent MIScarriagE) trial conducted in women with unexplained recurrent miscarriages [18] and (2) PRISM (PRogesterone In Spontaneous Miscarriage) trial involving women with bleeding in early pregnancy (threatened miscarriage) [17].

The PROMISE trial was a randomised controlled trial (RCT) in women with unexplained recurrent miscarriages. The researchers randomly assigned 836 women with a history of three or more pregnancy losses in the first trimester, to receive twice-daily vaginal suppositories containing either 400 mg of micronised progesterone or matched placebo soon after a positive urinary pregnancy test until 12 weeks of gestation. The primary outcome was live birth after 24 weeks of gestation. The primary analysis of the trial found the live birth rate to be 66% in the progesterone group compared to 63% in the placebo group [relative rate (RR) 1.04; 95% confidence interval (CI) 0.94–1.15]. The difference was not statistically significant. A pre-specified sub-group analysis by the number of previous miscarriages showed a non-significant trend toward greater effectiveness with increasing number of previous miscarriages [18].

The PRISM trial was a large, multicentre, randomised, double-blind, placebo-controlled trial involving 4,153 women with vaginal bleeding in early pregnancy. Women were randomly allocated to receive vaginal suppositories containing either 400 mg of progesterone or placebo twice daily, from the time at which they presented with vaginal bleeding in the presence of an intrauterine pregnancy of <12 weeks' gestation and continued through to 16 weeks of gestation. The primary outcome was live birth after at least 34 weeks of gestation. The authors reported a live birth rate of 75% in the progesterone group and 72% in the placebo group (RR 1.03; 95% CI 1.00–1.07; $p = 0.08$). Pre-specified sub-group analysis by the number of previous miscarriages, showed that the effectiveness of progesterone was more prominent in the sub-group of women with three or more previous miscarriages and bleeding in current pregnancy with a live birth rate of 72% with progesterone and 57% in the placebo group (RR 1.28; 95% CI 1.08–1.51; $p = 0.007$) [17].

These results suggest that treatment with vaginal micronised progesterone 400 mg twice daily was associated with increasing live birth rates according to the number of previous miscarriages [11,17,18]. Treatment with progesterone did not result in any significant improvement in live birth rates among women with vaginal bleeding in early pregnancy but no previous miscarriages. This led the authors to conclude that women with a history of miscarriage who present with bleeding in early pregnancy may benefit from the use of vaginal micronised progesterone 400 mg twice daily [17]. The authors noted that as the trials studied a vaginal preparation of progesterone, at a dose of 400 mg twice daily, it was possible that the results may not be generalisable to women receiving other doses and preparations by other routes [11,17,18].

A meta-analysis of 10 trials involving 1,684 women, suggested that progesterone supplementation therapy may reduce the rate of miscarriages in subsequent pregnancies [RR 0.73; 95% CI 0.54–1.00]. Although the authors reported a probable slight improvement in the live birth rate for women receiving progestogen, they were unclear about the effect on the rate of pre-term birth [14].

A Cochrane review of seven randomised trials, involving 696 women, investigated the safety and efficacy of progesterone therapy in patients with threatened miscarriage. It found that the risk of miscarriage was lower in women receiving progestogen therapy. Progesterone reduced the risk of miscarriage in comparison to those receiving placebo or no treatment (RR 0.64; 95% CI 0.47–0.87). Three of these trials investigated oral progesterone and four trials evaluated vaginal progesterone. The authors concluded that the level of evidence was of moderate quality for the primary outcome of miscarriage versus successful pregnancy mainly due to limitations in study design (**Table 9.1**). In the sub-group analysis, the authors found that treatment with oral progesterone probably reduces the miscarriage rate compared to no treatment, while treatment with vaginal progesterone demonstrated a minimal reduction in the miscarriage rate. In addition, progesterone use in early pregnancy was not found to be harmful for either mother or baby [19].

| Table 9.1 Outcomes of progesterone versus placebo or no treatment for threatened miscarriages | | | | | |
|---|---|---|---|---|---|
| Outcomes of pregnancy | Probable outcome with placebo or no treatment | Probable outcome with progesterone treatment (95% CI) | Relative effect (95% CI) | Participants (studies) | Quality of evidence |
| Miscarriage | 242 per 1,000 | 138 per 1,000 (102 to 189) | RR 0.64 (0.47 to 0.87) | 696 (7) | Moderate |
| Pre-term birth | 91 per 1,000 | 84 per 1,000 (49 to 142) | RR 0.86 (0.52 to 1.44) | 588 (5) | Low |
| Congenital abnormalities | 13 per 1,000 | 9 per 1,000 (1 to 62) | RR 0.70 (0.10 to 4.82) | 337 (2) | Very low |

RR, risk ratio
*Source*: Adapted from Wahabi HA, Fayed AA, Esmaeil SA, et al. Progestogen for treating threatened miscarriage. Cochrane Database Syst Rev 2018; 8:CD005943.

A meta-analysis of 10 RCTs comparing progestogen with a placebo or no treatment in women with threatened miscarriage, found that progestogens increased live birth rates and reduced the risk of miscarriage, with benefit only seen with oral progestogen and not with vaginal progesterone [20].

A randomised study involving 150 women with threatened miscarriage found that oral micronised sustained release progesterone was as effective as vaginal micronised progesterone in preventing miscarriages [21]. Larger RCTs are needed to assess the efficacy of different progesterone formulations in the management of threatened miscarriages.

The authors of the TRoMaD (randomised controlled trial of micronised progesterone and dydrogesterone) study, investigated 141 women presenting with threatened miscarriage who were randomised to either micronised progesterone or dydrogesterone therapy. The post-treatment bleeding pattern and self-reported side effects on day 4–10 of treatment and the occurrence of spontaneous miscarriage at week 16 of gestation were evaluated. The results demonstrated that the extent of bleeding at day 4–10 of treatment and subsequent miscarriage rates were comparable between micronised progesterone and dydrogesterone. The study also showed that the risk of miscarriage in women with low serum progesterone levels was significantly higher than in women with high progesterone levels, regardless of treatment type (**Table 9.2**) [22].

In another RCT, Turgal et al. (2017) compared the effect of oral micronised progesterone on the first-trimester fetal and placental volumes using three-dimensional ultrasonography in 60 women with threatened abortion and a singleton pregnancy. After treatment, the oral natural micronised progesterone group had significantly higher placental volume than in the control group [(336%, 67–1,077 vs. 141%, 29–900) ($p = 0.007$)]. The mean differences in gestational sac, amniotic sac, and embryonic volumes between the oral natural micronised progesterone group and control groups were similar [23].

A recent network meta-analysis of seven RCTs involving 5,682 women, concluded that vaginal micronised progesterone may increase the live birth rate for women with a history of one or more previous miscarriages and early pregnancy bleeding compared to placebo (RR 1.08; 95% CI 1.02–1.15). However, in women with no previous miscarriages and early pregnancy bleeding, there was little or no improvement in the live birth rate (RR 0.99; 95% CI 0.95–1.04) when treated with vaginal micronised progesterone compared to placebo. The quality of evidence for dydrogesterone compared with placebo for women with recurrent miscarriage was of low certainty, therefore, the effects remain inconclusive. There was no data to assess the efficacy of 17α-hydroxyprogesterone or oral micronised progesterone for the outcome of live birth in women with recurrent miscarriage [13].

| Table 9.2 Comparison of miscarriage proportions between low and high serum progesterone group | | | | |
|---|---|---|---|---|
| Treatment groups | Serum progesterone <35 nmol/L | | Serum progesterone ≥35 nmol/L | |
| | Miscarriage (n, %) | Ongoing pregnancy (n, %) | Miscarriage (n, %) | Ongoing pregnancy (n, %) |
| Micronised progesterone | 5 (62.5) | 3 (37.5) | 1 (2.0) | 50 (98.0) |
| Dydrogesterone | 5 (50.0) | 5 (50.0) | 4 (8.2) | 45 (91.8) |
| p-value | <0.001 | | 0.005 | |

*Source*: Adapted from Siew JYS, Allen JC, Hui CYY, et al. The randomised controlled trial of micronised progesterone and dydrogesterone (TRoMaD) for threatened miscarriage. Eur J Obstet Gynecol Reprod Biol. 2018; 228:319–324.

## SAFETY OF PROGESTERONE IN PREGNANCY

Several studies have evaluated the safety profile of progesterone use in early pregnancy. A meta-analysis of seven RCTs involving 5,682 women, concluded that there is probably no difference in congenital abnormalities and adverse drug events with vaginal micronised progesterone for threatened or recurrent miscarriage compared with placebo [13].

In both the PROMISE and PRISM trials, there was no evidence of short-term harm or an increased risk of congenital malformations in women taking micronised vaginal progesterone. Although underpowered for this purpose, the findings are nevertheless reassuring [15,17,18]. The PROMISE trial involving 836 women did not find any difference in congenital anomaly between the progesterone and placebo groups [18]. The PRISM study that included 4,153 women showed no difference in congenital, familial, or genetic disorders between participants treated with vaginal micronised progesterone and those who received placebo [17]. Other studies have similarly found no increased risk of congenital abnormalities in women taking progesterone in early pregnancy [15].

Some studies have also evaluated the long-term effect of pre-natal progesterone treatment on child development. A systematic review based on five RCTs looked at studies comparing progesterone to placebo in second and/or third trimester for the prevention of pre-term birth. The review studied a multitude of developmental measurements in children aged 6 months–8 years and found that there was no evidence of benefit or harm in children exposed to progesterone prenatally for the prevention of pre-term birth [24].

In one of the largest fetal safety studies of natural progesterone in pregnancy, Hilgers et al., from the Pope Paul VI Institute for the Study of Human Reproduction examined the data of 1,310 pregnancies from a high-risk reproductive medicine/infertility population over a period of 35 years. The objective of the study was to compare the fetal outcomes between pregnancies that received natural progesterone supplementation and those that did not receive progesterone supplementation. The study showed that there was no significant difference in the incidence of fetal anomalies (both chromosomal and non-chromosomal) in the progesterone supplemented group versus the non-progesterone group [29 (2.2%) vs. 10 (2.2%); $p = 0.99$)]. The authors concluded that progesterone use in early pregnancy is not teratogenic or associated with an increased incidence of genital malformations or birth defects such as cardiac anomalies, limb reduction, neural tube defect, hydrocephalus, or oesophageal atresia. The study looked at the safety and tolerability of progesterone and supported a well-established benefit of using progesterone in pregnancy. It suggested that progesterone use in early pregnancy can be considered both safe and well-tolerated [25].

Similarly, another study based on the long-term effects of prenatal progesterone exposure on neurophysiological development and hospital admissions among twins up to 8 years of age showed that the use of progesterone in second and third trimester of pregnancy did not have any long-term harmful effects in children [26].

In contrast, synthetic progestins have been associated with safety concerns in some studies. A possible link between prenatal exposure to 17α-hydroxyprogesterone caproate, a synthetic progestogen, and risk of cancer in children has been reported. This study investigated a total of 1,008 offspring who were diagnosed with cancer over 730,817 person-years of follow-up. Among these individuals approximately 1% had prenatal exposure to 17α-hydroxyprogesterone caproate. First trimester use was associated with an increased risk of all cancers and the risk increased with the number of injections given. Exposure in the second or third trimester showed that male offspring had an additional risk of cancer when compared with females. The risk of certain cancers such as prostate, colorectal, and brain was higher in the offspring exposed to 17α-hydroxyprogesterone caproate in the first trimester of pregnancy compared to those not exposed [27].

Other studies have also suggested an adverse effect of synthetic progestins in early pregnancy. A systematic review and meta-analysis involving six studies of which four were cohort studies, reported that the incidence of abnormal glucose test result and gestational diabetes mellitus was higher in women with singleton pregnancies exposed to weekly 17α-hydroxyprogesterone caproate for the prevention of recurrent miscarriage when compared to unexposed control groups. But once the results from the cohort studies were excluded, this effect of progesterone was not significant in women who had been randomly allocated to 17α-hydroxyprogesterone caproate [28].

Several clinical studies have demonstrated safety concerns with the use of dydrogesterone in early pregnancy. In a case control study comparing 202 children born with congenital heart disease and a control group consisting of 200 children, the use of dydrogesterone in early pregnancy was found to be associated with congenital heart disease in the offspring (adjusted odds ratio 2.71; 95% CI 1.54–4.24; $p = 0.001$). However, this study was subject to selection and recall bias [29]. In another study that reviewed birth defects reported between 1977 and 2005, 28 cases of a potential link between maternal dydrogesterone use during pregnancy and congenital birth defects were found, although the type of defects did not show any specific pattern [30]. A case report also described the first case of Takotsubo cardiomyopathy associated with the initiation of dydrogesterone in a pre-menopausal woman [31]. It has been suggested that dydrogesterone may cause significant, albeit delayed, liver dysfunction in pregnancy necessitating the need for liver transplantation [32].

The most common adverse effects reported by women taking oral natural micronised progesterone for obstetric indications are drowsiness, somnolence, and dizziness [10]. Sustained release formulations of oral natural micronised progesterone have been reported to be well tolerated and associated with lower rates of drowsiness and dizziness, which were mild and transient [10].

## CONCLUSION

Progesterone is essential for the establishment and maintenance of pregnancy. As such, progesterone supplementation is used therapeutically for several obstetric indications associated with low progesterone levels including management of threatened spontaneous miscarriage, treatment of women with recurrent pregnancy loss, and women undergoing in vitro fertilisation. The current evidence regarding the efficacy of progesterone in miscarriage remains inconclusive. Data so far suggests that there is no benefit of using progesterone in women with threatened miscarriage without a history of previous miscarriage. However, in those presenting with bleeding in early pregnancy and a history of previous miscarriage, progesterone therapy may be effective in improving live birth rates. The apparent tolerability and safety profile of progesterone use in early pregnancy also makes it an acceptable treatment of choice for threatened miscarriage in clinical practice. It is essential to discuss the information obtained from these studies with women at high risk of miscarriages to encourage informed and shared decision-making. Further studies are required to answer questions such as the most appropriate indication for use, preferred dosage, route of administration, duration of treatment, and cost-effectiveness of using progesterone for threatened miscarriage.

# REFERENCES

1. Quenby S, Gallos ID, Dhillon-Smith RK, et al. Miscarriage matters: The epidemiological, physical, psychological, and economic costs of early pregnancy loss. Lancet 2021; 397:1658–1667.
2. Greene MF. Progesterone for threatened abortion. N Engl J Med 2019; 380:1867–1868.
3. Tsikouras P, Deftereou T, Anthoulaki X, et al. "Abortions in First Trimester Pregnancy, Management, Treatment". In: Lakhno I (Ed). Induced Abortion and Spontaneous Early Pregnancy Loss—Focus on Management. London: IntechOpen; 2019.
4. Di Renzo GC, Giardina I, Clerici G, et al. The role of progesterone in maternal and fetal medicine. Gynecol Endocrinol 2012; 28:925–932.
5. Di Renzo GC, Giardina I, Clerici G, et al. Progesterone in normal and pathological pregnancy. Horm Mol Biol Clin Investig 2016; 27:35–48.
6. Gandhi A, Wani R. Role of Oral Natural Micronized Progesterone Sustained Release in Threatened Miscarriage and Preterm Labor. Am J Perinatol 2020; 37:1–42.
7. Palshetkar N. Evidence-based clinical recommendations in the management of threatened miscarriage. Am J Perinatol 2019; 36:1–12.
8. Griesinger G, Tournaye H, Macklon N, et al. Dydrogesterone: pharmacological profile and mechanism of action as luteal phase support in assisted reproduction. Reprod Biomed Online 2019; 38:249–259.
9. Romero R, Stanczyk FZ. Progesterone is not the same as 17α-hydroxyprogesterone caproate: implications for obstetrical practice. Am J Obstet Gynecol 2013; 208:421–426.
10. Wagh GN, Kundavi Shankar KM, et al. A review of conventional and sustained-release formulations of oral natural micronized progesterone in obstetric indications. Drugs Context 2021; 10:2021-7-1.
11. Coomarasamy A, Devall AJ, Brosens JJ, et al. Micronized vaginal progesterone to prevent miscarriage: a critical evaluation of randomized evidence. Am J Obstet Gynecol 2020; 223:167–176.
12. Tavaniotou A, Smitz J, Bourgain C, et al. Comparison between different routes of progesterone administration as luteal phase support in infertility treatments. Human Reprod Update 2000; 6:139–148.
13. Devall AJ, Papadopoulou A, Podesek M, et al. Progestogens for preventing miscarriage: a network meta-analysis. Cochrane Database Syst Rev 2021; 4:CD013792.
14. Haas DM, Hathaway TJ, Ramsey PS. Progestogen for preventing miscarriage in women with recurrent miscarriage of unclear etiology. Cochrane Database Syst Rev 2018; 10:CD003511.
15. Feferkorn I, Tulandi T. The role of progesterone in miscarriage: Low progesterone levels have been associated with an increased rate of miscarriage. Contemp Obstet Gynecol 2021; 66:20.
16. Webster K, Eadon H, Fishburn S, et al. Ectopic pregnancy and miscarriage: diagnosis and initial management: summary of updated NICE guidance. BMJ 2019; 367:l6283.
17. Coomarasamy A, Devall AJ, Cheed V, et al. A Randomized Trial of Progesterone in Women with Bleeding in Early Pregnancy. New England J Med 2019; 380:1815–1824.
18. Coomarasamy A, Williams H, Truchanowicz E. A randomized trial of progesterone in women with recurrent miscarriages. N Engl J Med 2015; 373:2141–2148.
19. Wahabi HA, Fayed AA, Esmaeil SA, et al. Progestogen for treating threatened miscarriage. Cochrane Database Syst Rev 2018; 8:CD005943.
20. Li L, Zhang Y, Tan H, et al. Effect of progestogen for women with threatened miscarriage: a systematic review and meta-analysis. BJOG 2020; 127:1055–1063.
21. Wani R, Relwani H, Mistry N, et al. A prospective comparative study of oral NMP SR tablets and vaginal NMP capsules in women with threatened abortion and patients at risk of preterm labor. Am J Perinatol 2021; 38:12–18.
22. Siew JYS, Allen JC, Hui CYY, et al. The randomised controlled trial of micronised progesterone and dydrogesterone (TRoMaD) for threatened miscarriage. Eur J Obstet Gynecol Reprod Biol 2018; 228:319–324.
23. Turgal M, Aydin E, Ozyuncu O. Effect of micronized progesterone on fetal-placental volume in first-trimester threatened abortion. J Clin Ultrasound 2017; 45:14–19.
24. Simons NE, Leeuw M, van't Hooft J, et al. The long-term effect of prenatal progesterone treatment on child development, behaviour and health: a systematic review. BJOG 2021; 128:964–974.
25. Hilgers TW, Keefe CE, Pakiz KA. The use of isomolecular progesterone in the support of pregnancy and fetal safety. Issues Law Med 2015; 30:159–168.
26. Vedel C, Larsen H, Holmskov A, et al. Long-term effects of prenatal progesterone exposure: neurophysiological development and hospital admissions in twins up to 8 years of age. Ultrasound Obstet Gynecol 2016; 48:382–389.

27.  Murphy CC, Cirillo PM, Krigbaum NY, et al. In utero exposure to 17α-hydroxyprogesterone caproate and risk of cancer in offspring. Am J Obstet Gynecol 2022; 226:132.e1–132.e14.

28.  Eke AC, Sheffield J, Graham EM. 17α-Hydroxyprogesterone Caproate and the Risk of Glucose Intolerance in Pregnancy: A Systematic Review and Meta-analysis. Obstet Gynecol 2019; 133:468–475.

29.  Zaqout M, Aslem E, Abuqamar M, et al. The Impact of Oral Intake of Dydrogesterone on Fetal Heart Development During Early Pregnancy. Pediatr Cardiol 2015; 36:1483–1488.

30.  Queisser-Luft A. Dydrogesterone use during pregnancy: overview of birth defects reported since 1977. Early Hum Dev 2009; 85:375–377.

31.  Ioannou A. Takotsubo cardiomyopathy associated with dydrogesterone use. BMJ Case Rep 2021; 14:e246553.

32.  Malherbe JAJ, Garas G, Khor TS, et al. Delayed fulminant hepatic failure from dydrogesterone-related in vitro fertilization therapy requiring liver transplantation during pregnancy. Am J Case Rep 2020; 21:e925690.

# Chapter 10

# Management of intramural myoma and infertility

*Suha Arab, Togas Tulandi*

## INTRODUCTION

The effects of uterine myoma especially intramural myoma on reproduction remain unclear and results of published studies have been mixed. A meta-analysis in 2002 showed that intramural myoma that does distort the uterine cavity did not influence fertility outcome [1]. However, the authors of a systematic review and meta-analysis published in 2010 including 19 studies and 6,087 in-vitro fertilisation (IVF) cycles concluded that women with non-cavity distorting intramural myoma (IM) have lower IVF clinical pregnancy rate (RR 0.85; 95% CI 0.77–0.94; $p = 0.002$) and live birth rate (RR 0.79; 95% CI 0.70–0.88; $p < 0.0001$) when compared to those without myoma [2].

In a prospective study in 2011, 119 women with sub-serosal and intramural myomas (80 of 119 had IM myomas) were compared to 119 others without myoma. Ovarian stimulation did not increase the myoma volume. The results suggest that non-cavity distorting myoma of <5 cm do not affect IVF outcome. However, 36 of the 119 patients had sub-serosal myomas. They also found that there was no clear association between location (80 intramural vs. 36 sub-serosal), number (1 vs. >2 myomas) and dimension (<2 vs. > 2 cm) and the clinical outcome [3].

However, the results of a meta-analysis evaluating women with non-cavity distorting myoma including 28 studies and 9,189 IVF cycles showed that the clinical pregnancy (RR 0.86; 95% CI 0.80–0.93; $p = 0.0001$), live birth (RR 0.82; 95% CI 0.73–0.02; $p = 0.005$), and implantation rates (RR 0.9; 95% CI 0.83–1.0; $p = 0.04$) were significantly reduced among women with myoma [4–7]. Miscarriage rate was also significantly higher in the study group (RR 1.27; 95% CI 1.08–1.5; $p = 0.004$). The results confirmed the negative impact of IM myoma on IVF clinical outcomes [8]. Another meta-analysis including 15 studies and 5,029 patients also confirmed the adverse effects of intramural myoma on IVF clinical pregnancy rate and live birth rate [9,10].

- In term of myoma location and its relationship with the endometrial cavity, the closer to the uterine cavity (type 3), the worst the clinical outcome (Yan et al 2014) when he compared to that of type 4 and 5 myoma

**Suha Arab** MD MS, Department of Obstetrics and Gynecology, King Abdulaziz University Hospital, Obstetric and Gynecology Department, Jeddah, Saudi Arabia
Email: suhaarab@gmailcom

**Togas Tulandi** MD MHCM, Department of Obstetrics and Gynecology, McGill University, Montreal QC, Canada
Email: togas.tulandi@mcgill.ca

- In IVF population, live birth rate decreased in those with intramural myoma of over 5 cm in diameter
- Christopoulos et al reported that live birth rate reduced in women with multiple myomas
- Several studies reported the negative impact of intramural myoma on implantation rate (lower odds by 10%), clinical IVF pregnancy (lower odds by 20–32%), and live birth rates (lower odds by 20–44%). However, the impact on miscarriage rate remains unclear. Few studies showed that non-cavity distorting intramural myoma has no significant impact on the miscarriage rate (Guven et al. 2013 and Yan et al. 2018). However, a meta-analysis in 2018 showed a significant increase in miscarriage rate among women with the IM myoma

# INTRAMURAL MYOMA MANAGEMENT AND INFERTILITY

Uterine artery embolisation for the treatment of uterine myoma in women desiring to conceive is not recommended. It might affect ovarian reserve and is associated with increased miscarriage rate, preterm delivery, intrauterine growth restriction, placenta accreta and increased miscarriage rate [Society of Obstetricians and Gynaecologists of Canada (SOGC) guidelines 2015]. Decision for surgical intervention should be taken after careful counselling of advantages and disadvantages of the procedure.

- Expected management along with monitoring the size of intramural myoma in asymptomatic woman during ovarian stimulation in IVF treatment is the preferred options. The guidelines of the SOGC (2015) recommend against myomectomy for intramural myoma regardless the size of myoma
- Surgical intervention could be considered in women with intramural myoma and otherwise unexplained infertility, after failed multiple IVF-ICSI treatment and/or with multiple type 3 intramural myomas with diameter >5 cm and/or distorting the uterine cavity

## Role of myomectomy for intramural myoma in infertile population

In a study of 128 women with sub-serosal or non-cavity distorting intramural myomas who underwent myomectomy for fertility enhancement, 41 of 128 women were trying to conceive. Besides the presence of myoma, they did not have any other infertility factors. Prior to myomectomy, 19 of 41 women conceived spontaneously, 57% subsequently experienced a miscarriage. After myomectomy, 25 women conceived spontaneously. Compared to before myomectomy, the miscarriage rate after myomectomy was 13% ($p = 0.001$). In a sub-analysis, women who conceived after myomectomy were younger [32 vs. 35 years ($p = 0.0073$)] and the removed myoma was significantly larger than those who did not get pregnant (5.8 vs. 4.2 cm, $p = 0.027$) [10].

Surrey et al performed a retrospective study in the IVF population, 31 women had submucous myoma and 26 others had cavity-distorting intramural myomas. Following myomectomy, the on-going pregnancy rates (86% and 84%) were comparable to those among 896 women without myoma (77%). It suggests that pre-IVF myomectomy improved the outcome of IVF treatment [11].

In a randomised trial, Casini et al evaluated 181 women with different type of myomas; sub-mucosal ($n$ = 52), intramural ($n$ = 45), sub-serosal ($n$ = 11), mix sub-mucosal and intramural ($n$ = 42) and mix sub-serosal with intra-mural ($n$ = 32) groups. They were randomised into the myomectomy group and the non-myomectomy group (control group). Compared to the control group, the pregnancy rate among women with intramural or sub-serosal myoma group who underwent myomectomy were similar (40% vs. 56%). Yet, myomectomy improved the pregnancy rate in those in the submucosal group and the combined intramural and submucosal myoma (27% vs. 43%, $p \le 0.05$). The miscarriage rates in the non-treated sub-mucosal group and the control group were 50% and 30%, respectively. The miscarriage rates in the study group with intramural myoma and in the control group were comparable [12].

A meta-analysis including four randomised trial and 422 patients showed that myomectomy for intramural myoma did not improve the clinical pregnancy rate (OR 1.8; 95% CI 0.57–6.14) nor the miscarriage rate (OR 1.3; 95% CI 0.26–6.7) [13]. The authors also found that the results of laparoscopic myomectomy were comparable to those of myomectomy by laparotomy [14].

The role of myomectomy in infertile women with non-cavity distorting intra-mural myoma remains unclear. We recommend myomectomy in infertile women with full thickness myoma (from endometrium to the serosa) especially those with idiopathic infertility or myoma ≥5 cm in diameter.

## Predictive reproductive outcomes after myomectomy

- *Age*: As expected, age is a predictor factor for reproductive outcome after myomectomy [Campo et al. (2003)]
- *Myoma size*: Campo et al also found that removal of larger myoma is associated with a higher pregnancy rate (5.8 vs. 4.2 cm, $p$ = 0.027) [10]
- *Uterine cavity distortion*: In a prospective study, Tian et al evaluated 83 women with ($n$ = 38) or without cavity distorting intramural myoma ($n$ = 45). Post-operative spontaneous pregnancy was significantly higher in the cavity distorting group than non-cavity distorting group (70.5% vs. 47.6%, $p$ = 0.044) with RR of 3.7. Age was also found to be an important factor. Accordingly, young women with cavity distorting intramural myoma will have the best chance of conceiving following myomectomy [15]
- *Race*: Lebovits et al found that in a prospective study woman who conceived were significantly younger than who did not (35.4 vs. 37.2 years, $p$ = 0.02); 63.5% were white and 24.3% were African American ($p$ = 0.008). They suggested that white young women had a higher probability of conceiving following myomectomy of intramural myoma. Relative risk for age was 0.96; 95% CI 0.93–0.99; $p$ = 0.014 and for race was 0.58; 95% CI 0.38–0.88; $p$ = 0.011. They also found that women who conceived had larger intra-mural myoma pre-operative than who did not (7.3 vs. 6.1 cm, $p$ = 0.003) [16]

## MECHANISM OF INFERTILITY IN WOMEN WITH INTRAMURAL MYOMA

Non-cavity distorting intramural myoma can affect fertility in various mechanisms.
- *Alteration in uterine peristaltic*: Intramural myoma can alter the uterine peristalsis during embryo implantation stage leading to decreased implantation and pregnancy

rates [17]. Fanchin et al found that in the presence of myoma, uterine peristalsis diminished during the implantation stage [17]. Yoshino et al studied uterine peristalsis among 51 women with non-cavity distorting intramural myoma using MRI in the luteal phase (day 5–9). They found that women with lower frequency of uterine peristalsis had higher pregnancy rate than those with higher frequency of uterine peristalsis (34% vs. 0%) ($p < 0.005$). Although, the study was not done in IVF population, the results suggest that abnormal uterine peristalsis might negatively affect gamete or embryo migration during the implantation process [18]

- *Endometrial vascularity*: Specific vascular balance in the endometrium is needed during luteal phase of the cycle for normal endometrial function. Using three-dimensional ultrasound, Kamel et al studied endometrial vascularity in 182 women with non-cavity distorting intramural myomas and matched them to 182 controls. The results showed that women with myomas, especially over 4 cm ($n = 68$) had significantly increased endometrial vascularity when compared to those with myoma <4 cm ($n = 114$) [19]. The rates of pregnancy or implantation were not evaluated in their study

- *Diminished expression of specific gene*: Women with intramural myoma are associated with diminished expression of specific gene in their myometrium and endometrium during implantation period which might affect endometrial receptivity and decidualisation. For example, bone morphological protein 2 (BMP-2) is a multifunctional growth factor that plays a critical role in endometrial receptivity. Transforming growth factor-beta (TGF-β) is a growth factor that is produced by myoma with increased amount [20]. Sinclair et al found that TGF-β produced by myomas decreased the endometrial receptivity to BMP-2 by reducing the BMP receptor expression [21]. Doherty et al found that myoma-derived TGF-β was necessary and sufficient to change endometrial BMP-2 responsiveness and subsequently affecting embryo implantation process [22]. Unlu et al reported that after myomectomy, there was a significant increase in the endometrial genes receptivity expression. It is possible that myomectomy increases the endometrial receptivity and embryo implantation process through this mechanism [23]

- Cavity distorting myoma might affect gamete migration and/or embryo implantation similar to that of submucosal myoma. Non-cavity distorting intramural myoma affects fertility by different mechanisms including alteration of uterine peristalsis, high endometrial vascularity or increased in endometrial receptivity gene expression

## CONCLUSION

Submucous myoma, cavity-distorting myoma and non-cavity distorting uterine myoma of over 4 cm have a negative effect on fertility and fertility outcome. Myomectomy in those women is associated with increased live birth rate.

## REFERENCES

1. Donnez J, Jadoul P. What are the implications of myomas on fertility? A need for a debate? Hum Reprod 2002; 17:1424–1430.
2. Sunkara SK, Khairy M, El-Toukhy T, et al. The effect of intramural myomas without uterine cavity involvement on the outcome of IVF treatment: a systematic review and meta-analysis. Hum Reprod 2010; 25:418–429.

3.  Somigliana E, De Benedictis S, Vercellini P, et al. Myomas not encroaching the endometrial cavity and IVF success rate: a prospective study. Hum Reprod 2011; 26:834–839.
4.  Guven S, Kart C, Unsal MA, et al. Intramural leoimyoma without endometrial cavity distortion may negatively affect the ICSI-ET outcome. Reprod Biol Endocrinol 2013; 11:102.
5.  Yan L, Ding L, Li C, et al. Effect of myomas not distorting the endometrial cavity on the outcome of in vitro fertilization treatment: a retrospective cohort study. Fertil Steril 2014; 101:716–721.
6.  Christopoulos G, Vlismas A, Salim R, et al. Myomas that do not distort the uterine cavity and IVF success rates: an observational study using extensive matching criteria. BJOG 2017; 124:615–621.
7.  Yan L, Yu Q, Zhang YN, et al. Effect of type 3 intramural myomas on in vitro fertilization-intracytoplasmic sperm injection outcomes: a retrospective cohort study. Fertil Steril 2018; 109:817–822.e2.
8.  Wang X, Chen L, Wang H, et al. The Impact of Noncavity-Distorting Intramural Myomas on the Efficacy of In Vitro Fertilization-Embryo Transfer: An Updated Meta-Analysis. Biomed Res Int 2018; 2018:8924703.
9.  Rikhraj K, Tan J, Taskin O, et al. The Impact of Noncavity-Distorting Intramural Myomas on Live Birth Rate in In Vitro Fertilization Cycles: A Systematic Review and Meta-Analysis. J Womens Health (Larchmt) 2020; 29:210–219.
10. Campo S, Campo V, Gambadauro P. Reproductive outcome before and after laparoscopic or abdominal myomectomy for subserous or intramural myomas. Eur J Obstet Gynecol Reprod Biol 2003; 110:215–219.
11. Surrey ES, Minjarez DA, Stevens JM, et al. Effect of myomectomy on the outcome of assisted reproductive technologies. Fertil Steril 2005; 83:1473–1479.
12. Casini ML, Rossi F, Agostini R, et al. Effects of the position of myomas on fertility. Gynecol Endocrinol 2006; 22:106–109.
13. Brady PC, Stanic AK, Styer AK. Uterine myomas and subfertility: an update on the role of myomectomy. Curr Opin Obstet Gynecol 2013; 25:255–259.
14. Metwally M, Raybould G, Cheong YC, et al. Surgical treatment of myomas for subfertility. Cochrane Database Syst Rev 2020; 1:CD003857.
15. Tian YC, Wu JH, Wang HM, et al. Improved Fertility Following Enucleation of Intramural Myomas in Infertile Women. Chin Med J (Engl) 2017; 130:1648–1653.
16. Lebovitz O, Orvieto R, James KE, et al. Predictors of reproductive outcomes following myomectomy for intramural myomas. Reprod Biomed Online 2019; 39:484–491.
17. Fanchin R, Ayoubi JM. Uterine dynamics: impact on the human reproduction process. Reprod Biomed Online 2009; 18:57–62.
18. Yoshino O, Hayashi T, Osuga Y, et al. Decreased pregnancy rate is linked to abnormal uterine peristalsis caused by intramural myomas. Hum Reprod 2010; 25:2475–2479.
19. Kamel A, El-Mazny A, Ramadan W, et al. Effect of intramural myoma on uterine and endometrial vascularity in infertile women scheduled for in-vitro fertilization. Arch Gynecol Obstet 2018; 297:539–545.
20. Lee KY, Jeong JW, Wang J, et al. BMP-2 is critical for the murine uterine decidual response. Mol Cell Biol 2007; 27:5468–5478.
21. Sinclair DC, Mastroyannis A, Taylor HS. Leiomyoma simultaneously impair endometrial BMP-2-mediated decidualization and anticoagulant expression through secretion of TGF-β 3. J Clin Endocrinol Metab 2011; 96:412–421.
22. Doherty LF, Taylor HS. Leiomyoma-derived transforming growth factor-beta impairs bone morphogenetic protein-2-mediated endometrial receptivity. Fertil Steril 2015; 103:845–852.
23. Unlu C, Celik O, Celik N, et al. Expression of Endometrial Receptivity Genes Increase After Myomectomy of Intramural Leiomyomas not Distorting the Endometrial Cavity. Reprod Sci 2016; 23:31–41.

# Chapter 11

## Management of hydrosalpinx in women treated with in-vitro fertilisation

*Einav Kadour-Peero, Togas Tulandi*

## INTRODUCTION

Hydrosalpinx is the distension of a serous fluid-filled fallopian tube, in the presence of complete distal occlusion [1]. It may occur as an isolated tubal disorder or as a component of a complex adnexal lesion that causes distal tubal occlusion [2]. Hydrosalpinx is usually discovered in infertile women with tubal disease [1]. The prevalence of hydrosalpinx is 10–13% on ultrasound [3] and up to 30% on hysterosalpingography (HSG) or at surgery [4,5]. Although rarely needed, multiplanar magnetic resonance imaging (MRI) can confirm the presence of distal tubal dilatation [2].

## CAUSES AND CONSEQUENCES

There are many different causes of hydrosalpinx including pelvic inflammatory disease (PID), tubal pregnancy, tubal cancer, ruptured appendicitis, peritonitis or previous pelvic or abdominal surgery [2,6]. The most common cause is PID, usually resulting from prior sexually transmitted diseases such as *Chlamydia trachomatis* or *Neisseria gonorrhoeae* [6]. Tubal tuberculosis is an uncommon cause of hydrosalpinx especially in the Western world [7].

Primary hydrosalpinx could be found in relation to a rare congenital disorder Hirschsprung's disease [8]. Hydrosalpinx is rarely encountered in paediatric population. Beside infertility, hydrosalpinx is usually asymptomatic. However, torsion of hydrosalpinx will cause abdominal pain [9,10].

## EFFECT ON FERTILITY

Tubal factor accounts for up to 30% of infertility [11,12]. Women with bilateral hydrosalpinx will not be able to conceive spontaneously. They could conceive with in-vitro fertilisation (IVF) treatment. In the IVF population, hydrosalpinx is found in 10–30% of women [12].

**Einav Kadour-Peero** MD, Department of Obstetrics and Gynecology, McGill University, Montreal QC, Canada
Email: einavkadour@gmail.com

**Togas Tulandi** MD MHCM, Department of Obstetrics and Gynecology, McGill University, Montreal QC, Canada
Email: togas.tulandi@mcgill.ca

Its presence is associated with reduced IVF outcome. It is associated with decreased implantation and pregnancy rates and increased miscarriage rate [4]. The implantation and pregnancy rates in women with hydrosalpinx are a half and the miscarriage rate is double compared to those with non-hydrosalpinx tubal-factor infertility [13–15].

The unfavourable outcome of IVF treatment in women with hydrosalpinx could be due to leakage of the tubal fluid into the uterine cavity producing a hostile endometrium to implantation, toxic effect of the fluid to gametes and embryos [13,16,17] or to an altered nutrient environment in the tubal fluid affecting early stages of embryogenesis [16,18–20]. Prostaglandins and other inflammatory molecules in the hydrosalpinx fluid may negatively affect endometrial apposition and attachment of blastocyst [21]. It is also possible that the fluid flush out the embryo from the uterine cavity.

## MANAGEMENT

Traditionally, infertile women with hydrosalpinx are treated surgically with salpingostomy. However, the live birth rate after this surgical procedure is generally low of <30% within 1 year after surgery. Further, the risk of ectopic pregnancy is fairly high of about 5%. In this IVF era, the role of reconstructive tubal surgery for hydrosalpinx is minimal. Today, the purpose of hydrosalpinx treatment is to enhance IVF outcome. The treatment consists of salpingectomy, salpingostomy, proximal tubal occlusion, hydrosalpinx sclerotherapy or antibiotic treatment.

### Salpingectomy

Salpingectomy is the main treatment of hydrosalpinx before IVF treatment. In fact, the United Kingdom's National Institute of Health and Clinical Excellence (NICE) guidelines recommend laparoscopic salpingectomy before assisted reproductive technologies when hydrosalpinx is diagnosed by HSG or ultrasound [22]. These guidelines are supported by several meta-analyses that recommend salpingectomy for hydrosalpinx [23–25]. Johnson et al. showed that the on-going clinical pregnancy rates in the salpingectomy group were 31% and 17.6% in the control group (OR 2.2; 95% CI 1.26–3.82) [23].

With salpingectomy, chronically infected tube is removed reducing the chances of abscess formation and improving access to the ovaries during oocyte retrieval [26]. Instead of laparotomy, salpingectomy should be done by laparoscopy. A few authors reported that salpingectomy could be associated with impaired ovarian blood flow reducing response to ovarian stimulation [27,28]. A meta-analysis of 25 studies showed that the gonadotropin dose required for stimulation in IVF was increased, and the number of oocytes retrieved was decreased after salpingectomy [29]. However, it appears that this was only true after bilateral salpingectomy [30]. In order to mitigate this effect, salpingectomy should be done using minimally thermogenic instruments and very close to the tube.

### Salpingostomy

An alternative surgical option is salpingostomy similar to that for reconstructive tubal surgery [31]. A systematic review showed that salpingostomy for hydrosalpinx is associated with a spontaneous pregnancy rate of 27%, cumulative clinical pregnancy rate of 25.5% at 24 months after salpingostomy and a live birth rate of 25% [32]. Due to decreased ovarian reserve in women with advancing age, it could be considered only in women in the twenties or early thirties and in those who refuse treatment with IVF. The recurrence rate of hydrosalpinx after salpingostomy is as high as 70% [33]. Those women might need to undergo another surgery to remove the fallopian tube before IVF treatment.

## Proximal tubal occlusion

Proximal tubal occlusion is usually performed in women with frozen pelvis where the hydrosalpinx is buried in massive and dense adhesions. It could be performed hysteroscopically or laparoscopically. In laparoscopic tubal occlusion, the proximal part of the tube can be cauterised or occluded with a clip. In hysteroscopy, the placement of Essure intratubal devices occludes the tube and prevents leakage of hydrosalpingeal fluid into the uterine cavity. Proximal tubal occlusion is associated with reduced interference of the integrity of the ovarian blood supply.

A meta-analysis shows that the complication rate, clinical pregnancy rate, multiple pregnancy rate, miscarriage rate, ectopic pregnancy rate, mean number of oocytes and mean number of embryos after proximal tubal occlusion either by laparoscopy or hysteroscopy and after laparoscopic salpingectomy are comparable [34]. Evidence suggests that hysteroscopic tubal occlusion is associated with decreased live birth rate compared to laparoscopic salpingectomy. There is no difference in live birth rate between laparoscopic proximal tubal occlusion and laparoscopic salpingectomy [34]. Proximal tubal occlusion may be associated with on-going pelvic pain secondary to the pressure and presence of the diseased tube, and risks of adnexal torsion [35]. In addition, the resulting bipolar tubal blockage (proximal and distal) can be associated with further distension the hydrosalpinx. Due the presence of abdominal pain related to Essure necessitating removal of the device, Essure is no longer available in the market.

## Tubal embolisation by interventional radiology

Fallopian tube embolisation with fluoroscopic guidance was reported for tubal sterilisation for the first time in 2005 [36]. Placement of embolisation microcoil is comparable to hysteroscopic placement and results in a similar rate of contraception [37]. In a recent study by Yang et al., treating patient with hydrosalpinx by radiologically-guided tubal occlusion with embolisation microcoils, the procedure did not affect the ovarian blood supply [38]. Compared to laparoscopic salpingectomy, no difference was found in the basal follicle-stimulating hormone (FSH) and oestradiol levels before and after the treatment, and there were no significant differences in ovarian responsiveness to gonadotropins [38].

## Doxycycline treatment

Antibiotics treatment has been advocated for women with hydrosalpinx treated with IVF. However, the implantation, clinical pregnancy, on-going pregnancy and live birth rates were inferior to that after salpingectomy [39]. This treatment is not recommended.

## Hydrosalpinx sclerotherapy

Aspiration of hydrosalpinx fluid is a less invasive, simple and inexpensive. It can be performed under ultrasound guidance. However, the recurrence rate after fluid aspiration is as high as one-third of the cases [40]. In addition to aspiration, sclerotherapy can be done in which a sclerosing agent is instilled into the tube. The purpose of sclerotherapy is to decrease recurrence of hydrosalpinx after aspiration. First, the hydrosalpinx fluid is aspirated and 98% ethanol equal to a half volume of the aspirated fluid is injected into the dilated tube and left inside the tube for 5–10 minutes before removal. Antibiotic prophylaxis is prescribed during and after the procedure. Sclerotherapy is considered successful when the fallopian tube contains <10% of the original volume of fluid in 2 weeks follow-up sonography. The recurrence rate after sclerotherapy is up to 20% in 2 weeks follow up [40]. Two meta-analyses showed that IVF outcomes were similar between hydrosalpinx sclerotherapy and salpingectomy, including: ovarian response parameters, live birth rate and clinical pregnancy rate [40,41].

# CONCLUSION

Hydrosalpinx clearly affects IVF outcome by decreasing implantation and pregnancy rates, and increasing the risk of miscarriage. Treatment of hydrosalpinx by salpingectomy or proximal tubal occlusion improves the IVF outcome. However, treatment should be individualised, considering the patient's risk profile and desires. The newly suggested minimally invasive treatment with hydrosalpinx sclerotherapy or radiologically-guided tubal occlusion with embolisation microcoils might be promising; especially for patients who are not suitable candidates for surgery. Yet, further studies are still needed. **Table 11.1** shows advantages, disadvantages and IVF pregnancy rate after different treatment of hydrosalpinx.

| Table 11.1 Advantages, disadvantages and in-vitro fertilisation (IVF) pregnancy rate after different treatment of hydrosalpinx | | | |
|---|---|---|---|
| Treatment method | Advantages | Disadvantages | On-going pregnancy rate after IVF |
| Salpingectomy | Lower the chance of ectopic pregnancy | • Invasive<br>• Reduced ovarian response to stimulation | 31% |
| Salpingostomy | • Maintain the option of spontaneous pregnancy | • Requires surgical experience<br>• High rate of recurrence 70% | 25% |
| Proximal tubal occlusion | • Less invasive<br>• No effect on ovarian function | • On-going pelvic pain<br>• Further distension the hydrosalpinx<br>• Increased miscarriage rate | 30% |
| Tubal embolisation by interventional radiology | • Less invasive<br>• No effect on ovarian function | Exposure to radiation using fluoroscopic guidance | 35% |
| Doxycycline treatment | • Non-invasive<br>• Inexpensive | Lower implantation rate and, clinical pregnancy, and live birth rates | 17% |
| Sclerotherapy | • Less invasive<br>• Inexpensive | High rate of recurrence (up to 21%) | 42% |

# REFERENCES

1. Aboulghar MA, Mansour RT, Serour GI. Controversies in the modern management of hydrosalpinx. Hum Reprod Update 1998; 4:882e90.
2. Outwater EK, Siegelman ES, Chiowanich P. Dilated fallopian tubes: MR imaging characteristics. Radiology 1998; 208:463–469.
3. Katz E, Akman MA, Damewood MD, et al. Deleterious effect of the presence of hydrosalpinx on implantation and pregnancy rates with in vitro fertilization. Fertil Steril 1996; 66:122–125.
4. Strandell A, Waldenstrom U, Nilsson L, et al. Hydrosalpinx reduces in-vitro fertilization/embryo transfer pregnancy rates. Hum Reprod 1994; 9:861–863.
5. Blazar AS, Hogan JW, Seifer DB, et al. The impact of hydrosalpinx on successful pregnancy in tubal factor infertility treated by in vitro fertilization. Fertil Steril 1997; 67:517–520.
6. Puttemans PJ, Brosens IA. Salpingectomy improves in-vitro fertilization outcome in patients with a hydrosalpinx: blind victimization of the fallopian tube? Hum Reprod 1996; 11:2079–2081.
7. D'Arpe S, Franceschetti S, Caccetta J, et al. Management of hydrosalpinx before IVF: A literature review, J Obstet Gynaecol 2015; 35:547–550.
8. Palazón P, Saura L, de Haro I, et al. Bilateral hydrosalpinx in patients with Hirschsprung's disease. J Pediatr Surg 2018; 53:1945–1950.
9. Kazmi Z, Gupta S. Practice in management of paediatric and adolescent hydrosalpinges: a systematic review. Eur J Obstet Gynecol Reprod Biol 2015; 195:40–51.
10. Cabral MD, Siqueira L. Hydrosalpinx in postmenarchal nonsexually active girls: a review of 6 cases in a children's hospital. J Pediatr Adolesc Gynecol 2015; 28:203–207.
11. Evers JLH. Female subfertility. Lancet 2002; 360:151–159.
12. González JL, Castillo JE, Toro EP, et al. Essure a novel option for the treatment of hydrosalpinx: a case series and literature review. Gynecol Endocrinol 2016; 32:166–170.
13. Zeyneloglu HB, Arici A, Olive DL. Adverse effects of hydrosalpinx on pregnancy rates after in vitro fertilization-embryo transfer. Fertil Steril 1998; 70:492–499.
14. Camus E, Poncelet C, Goffinet F, et al. Pregnancy rates after in-vitro fertilization in cases of tubal infertility with and without hydrosalpinx: a meta-analysis of published comparative studies. Hum Reprod 1999; 14:1243–1249.
15. Capmas P, Suarthana E, Tulandi T. Management of Hydrosalpinx in the Era of Assisted Reproductive Technology: A Systematic Review and Meta-analysis. J Minim Invas Gynecol 2021; 28:418–441.
16. Bao H, Qu Q, Huang X, et al. Impact of hydrosalpinx fluid on early human embryos. Syst Biol Reprod Med 2017; 63:279–284.
17. Mukhurjee T, Copperman AB, McCaFrey C. Hydrosalpinx fluid has embryotoxic eFects on murine embryogenesis: a case for prophylactic salpingectomy. Fertil Steril 1996; 66:851–853.
18. Tay JI, Rutherford AJ, Killick SR, et al. Human tubal fluid: production, nutrient composition and response to adrenergic agents. Hum Reprod 1998; 70:492–499.
19. Koong MK, Jun JH, Song SJ, et al. A second look at the embryotoxicity of hydrosalpingeal fluid: an invitro assessment in a murine model. Hum Reprod 1998; 13:2852–2856.
20. Dickens CJ, Maguiness SD, Comer MT, et al. Human tubal fluid: formation and composition during vascular perfusion of the Fallopian tube. Hum Reprod 1995; 10:505–508.
21. Meyer WR, Castelbaum AJ, Somkuti S, et al. Hydrosalpinges adversely affect markers of endometrial receptivity. Hum. Reprod 1997; 12:1393–1398.
22. RCOG. National Collaborating Centre for Women's and Children's Health (UK) Fertility: Assessment and Treatment for People with Fertility Problems. London: Royal College of Obstetricians and Gynaecologists (UK); 2013.
23. Johnson N, van Voorst S, Sowter MC, et al. Surgical treatment for tubal disease in women due to undergo in vitro fertilisation. Cochrane Database Syst Rev 2010: CD002125.
24. Strandell A, Lindhard A, Waldenström U, Thorburn J, Janson PO, Hamberger L. Hydrosalpinx and IVF outcome: a prospective, randomized multicentre trial in Scandinavia on salpingectomy prior to IVF. Hum Reprod 1999; 14:2762–2769.

25. Johnson NP, Mak W, Sowter MC. Laparoscopic salpingectomy for women with hydrosalpinges enhances the success of IVF: a Cochrane review. Hum Reprod 2002; 17:543–548.
26. Sharif K, Kaufmann S, Sharma V. Heterotopic pregnancy obtained after in-vitro fertilization and embryo transfer following bilateral total salpingectomy: case report. Hum Reprod 1994; 9:1966–1967.
27. Gelbaya TA, Nardo LG, Fitzgerald CT, et al. Ovarian response to gonadotropins after laparoscopic salpingectomy or the division of fallopian tubes for hydrosalpinges. Fertil Steril 2006; 85:1464–1468.
28. Orvieto R, Saar-Ryss B, Morgante G, et al. Does salpingectomy affect the ipsilateral ovarian response to gonadotropin during in vitro fertilization-embryo transfer cycles? Fertil Steril 2011; 95:1842–1844.
29. Fan M, Ma L. Effect of salpingectomy on ovarian response to hyperstimulation during in vitro fertilization: a meta-analysis. Fertil Steril 2016; 106:322–329.e9.
30. Mizusawa Y, Matsumoto Y, Kokeguchi S, et al. A retrospective analysis of ovarian response to gonadotropins after laparoscopic unilateral or bilateral salpingectomy for hydrosalpinges. Health Sci Rep 2020; 3:e187.
31. Gomel V, Wang I. Laparoscopic surgery for infertility therapy. Curr Opin Obstet Gynecol 1994; 6:141–148.
32. Chu J, Harb HM, Gallos ID, et al. Salpingostomy in the treatment of hydrosalpinx: a systematic review and meta-analysis. Hum Reprod 2015; 30:1882–1895.
33. Bayrak A, Harp D, Saadat P, et al. Recurrence of hydrosalpinges after cuff neosalpingostomy in a poor prognosis population. J Assist Reprod Genet 2006; 23:285–288.
34. Melo P, Georgiou EX, Johnson N, et al. Surgical treatment for tubal disease in women due to undergo in vitro fertilisation (Review). Cochrane Database Syst Rev 2020.
35. LaCombe J, Ginsburg F. Adnexal torsion in a patient with hydrosalpinx who underwent tubal occlusion before in vitro fertilization. Fertil Steril 2003; 79:437–438.
36. McSwain H, Shaw C, Hall LD. Placement of the Essure permanent birth control device with fluoroscopic guidance: a novel method for tubal sterilization. J Vasc Interv Radiol 2005; 16:1007–1012.
37. McSwain H, Brodie MF. Fallopian tube occlusion, an alternative to tubal ligation. Tech Vasc Interv Radiol 2006; 9:24–29.
38. Yang X, Zhu L, Le F, et al. Proximal Fallopian Tubal Embolization by Interventional Radiology prior to Embryo Transfer in Infertile Patients with Hydrosalpinx: A Prospective Study of an Off-label Treatment. J Minim Invasive Gynecol 2020; 27:107–115.
39. Fouda UM, Elshaer HS, Youssef MA, et al. Extended doxycycline treatment versus salpingectomy in the management of patients with hydrosalpinx undergoing IVF-ET. J Ovarian Res 2020: 13:69.
40. Cohen A, Almog B, Tulandi T. Hydrosalpinx Sclerotherapy before In Vitro Fertilization: Systematic Review and Meta-analysis. J Minim Invasive Gynecol 2018; 25:600–607.
41. Volodarsky-Perel A, Buckett W, Tulandi T. Treatment of hydrosalpinx in relation to IVF outcome: a systematic review and meta-analysis. Reprod Biomed Online 2019; 39:413–432.

# Chapter 12

## Fertility preservation in patients with cancer: Recent advances and new insights

*Mausumi Das*

## INTRODUCTION

Survival rates among young cancer patients have improved considerably over the last few decades due to the development of more effective cancer treatments. Cancer survivors may face the possibility of infertility because of the disease itself or the necessary chemotherapy and radiotherapy treatment regimens. Many cancer patients are concerned about the possible impact of cancer therapies on their future chances of conception. The field of fertility preservation is expanding rapidly, driven by the need to provide safe, and effective fertility preservation options for young cancer patients. Advances in techniques such as oocyte and embryo cryopreservation and ovarian tissue cryopreservation with subsequent auto-transplantation or in vitro maturation (IVM) offer new hope to female cancer survivors of having their own children. Many male cancer sufferers can freeze sperm before potentially sterilising cancer treatment. Methods to restore fertility with cryopreserved testicular tissue are being developed. Emerging innovative technologies have provided a paradigm shift in our approach to fertility preservation in young cancer patients. Patients with cancer should be offered fertility preservation counselling as early as possible. Greater awareness of fertility preservation options and better service provision will help to optimise the reproductive health of cancer survivors. This review focuses on currently available strategies and recent advances in fertility preservation for cancer patients.

## INDICATIONS FOR FERTILITY PRESERVATION IN CANCER PATIENTS

Cancer treatments such as chemotherapy and radiotherapy may lead to loss of ovarian function, resulting in premature ovarian insufficiency and subsequent infertility. Female reproductive function may be affected by a reduction in the primordial follicle pool, endocrine dysfunction, or by anatomical or functional changes to the ovaries, uterus, cervix, or vagina [1]. The gonadotoxicity of various cancer treatments depends

**Mausumi Das** MD MRCOG MPH, Queen Charlotte and Hammersmith Hospitals, Imperial College Healthcare NHS Trust, and Chelsea and Westminster Hospital NHS Foundation Trust, London, UK
Email: mausumidas@nhs.net

on factors such as ovarian reserve, age of the patient at the time of treatment as well as the type, dosage, and duration of gonadotoxic therapy [2]. Male reproductive function may be affected by the cancer itself or the anticancer therapies, leading to impaired spermatogenesis, or endocrine, anatomical, or functional abnormalities [1]. Total body irradiation and high-dose alkylating therapy often used as conditioning regimens before bone marrow transplantation treatment for leukaemia, are associated with high risk of infertility [1].

Patients with cancer should be offered fertility preservation counselling as early as possible and should be referred for fertility preservation before the initiation of gonadotoxic treatment. The Childhood Cancer Survivor Study showed that childhood cancer survivors had an increased risk of infertility and an increased time to pregnancy compared with their siblings [3]. Chemotherapy with alkylating agents and increasing doses of uterine radiation were strongly associated with infertility [3]. Due to advances in cancer treatments, long-term survival is expected for 80% of children and adolescents diagnosed with cancer [4]. In view of the reproductive risks associated with cancer treatments, it is essential that cancer patients should be provided with rapid access to counselling and fertility preservation options [5].

# GONADOTOXIC EFFECTS OF COMMONLY USED ANTICANCER TREATMENTS

## Female patients

Chemotherapy has a direct apoptotic effect on the primordial follicles and can lead to ovarian atrophy. In addition, chemotherapeutic agents can also cause injury to blood vessels and focal ovarian cortical fibrosis [6]. Alkylating agents such as cyclophosphamide, ifosfamide, nitrosoureas, chlorambucil, melphalan, busulfan, and procarbazine, which are cell cycle non-specific agents, can cause single- and double-strand DNA breaks and can destroy resting primordial cells in addition to dividing cells [7–9]. Studies have demonstrated that women treated with increasing doses of alkylating agents are at greater risk of acute ovarian insufficiency and premature menopause [10]. Antineoplastic agents such as vincristine, methotrexate, and fluorouracil have been associated with a comparatively lower risk of premature ovarian insufficiency [8]. Although the doxorubicin, bleomycin, vincristine, and dacarbazine (ABVD) regimen used in the treatment of Hodgkin's disease has been reported to be less gonadotoxic compared to alkylating agents [11], the decrease in anti-Müllerian hormone (AMH) following treatment was found to be greater than that of the general population of that age group [12].

Radiotherapy can cause a significant reduction in the primordial follicle pool, leading to ovarian insufficiency. The effects of radiotherapy on the ovary are dose dependant. A dose of radiation of <2 Gy could destroy >50% of human primordial follicles [13]. Radiotherapy treatment is associated with premature ovarian insufficiency, reduced uterine vascularity, myometrial fibrosis, and endometrial impairment [13–15].

It has been proposed that when estimating the risk of post-treatment pre-mature ovarian insufficiency, the type and dose of the proposed gonadotoxic treatment as well as pre-treatment AMH levels, should be taken into consideration.

Endocrine treatments may delay time to pregnancy in women with hormone-sensitive breast cancer. The ATLAS (Adjuvant Tamoxifen: Longer Against Shorter) study reported that among women with oestrogen-receptor positive breast cancer, 10 years of treatment with tamoxifen provide greater protection against recurrence and mortality compared to 5 years of treatment [16]. As a result, many patients with breast cancer may need to further delay childbearing. Women may choose to pause adjuvant hormonal therapy to become pregnant, after discussing their individual risk of recurrence with their oncologist [20].

The effect of targeted agents such as monoclonal antibodies and immunotherapy on ovarian function is still unclear. So far, studies have not found any evidence of gonadotoxicity for the anti-human epidermal growth factor receptor 2 (HER2) agents trastuzumab and lapatinib. However, it has been suggested that an adverse effect on ovarian function in patients treated with bevacizumab cannot be excluded [1].

## Male patients

The gonadotoxic effect of cancer therapies on the spermatogonia depends on the type and dose of the chemotherapeutic agent or the radiotherapy dose. Spermatogonia and the germinal epithelium are most susceptible to the cytotoxic effects of alkylating agents, platinum compounds, and long-term hydroxyurea treatment [17]. Researchers have reported that treatment of testicular cancer with cisplatin and carboplatin regimens may lead to temporary azoospermia or oligospermia, with normospermia returning in 80% by 5 years [18]. High-dose chemotherapy, which may be required before a bone marrow transplant, usually results in irreversible germinal epithelium failure [18]. Chemotherapy with alkylating agents, testicular irradiation and surgery or radiation to the genitourinary organs or the hypothalamic-pituitary region are risk factors for impaired spermatogenesis, testosterone deficiency, and sexual dysfunction [17].

The germinal epithelium is also susceptible to the gonadotoxic effects of radiotherapy [17]. While doses of 2–3 Gy can affect spermatogonial stem cells (SSCs) and long-term azoospermia, doses of ≥ 6 Gy can deplete the SSC pool and lead to infertility [17]. Moreover, Leydig cell insufficiency and testosterone deficiency have been reported with doses of 20–24 Gy [17]. Cranial radiotherapy may also impact spermatogenesis by suppressing gonadotrophin release [1].

# CURRENT STRATEGIES FOR FERTILITY PRESERVATION IN FEMALE CANCER PATIENTS

## Embryo cryopreservation

Ovarian stimulation followed by surgical retrieval of oocytes, insemination, and embryo cryopreservation is currently the most well-established fertility preservation technique with proven feasibility and efficacy. This approach is suitable for post-pubertal females with adequate time for controlled ovarian stimulation and for those who have a male partner [5,19]. Patients should be counselled that both partners would need to consent to use the stored embryos in any future fertility treatment [20,21]. For embryos created with donor sperm, only the consent of the woman is required [20,21].

Embryos can be successfully cryopreserved by slow-freezing or vitrification. Vitrification of day-3 embryos or blastocysts has now become the method of choice for embryo cryopreservation. Evidence suggests that vitrification is associated with superior embryo cryosurvival rates when compared to slow-freezing, leading to improved clinical outcomes in cryopreserved cycles [22]. The age of the woman at the time of oocyte retrieval is a major determinant of the likelihood of live birth following the transfer of thawed cryopreserved embryos [5,23]. Limited data are available on live-births from cryopreserved embryos in cancer patients. Therefore, national and clinic-specific success rates following transfer of cryopreserved embryos in infertile and donor populations are mostly used for counselling purposes [5]. This may be further modified based on the patient's age and the number and quality of available embryos [5]. In the UK, the Human Fertilisation and Embryology Act allows storage of embryos and gametes for a maximum period of 55 years in situations where the patient is prematurely infertile or likely to become prematurely infertile [24].

## Oocyte cryopreservation

Oocyte cryopreservation following ovarian stimulation and egg retrieval is an effective strategy for fertility preservation that has increased in popularity over the last decade. The efficacy of oocyte cryopreservation has improved due to advances in cryopreservation techniques, such as oocyte vitrification, resulting in improved cryosurvival outcomes. Compared to slow-freezing, vitrification involves the use of high concentration of cryoprotectants and ultra-rapid cooling to prevent ice crystal formation [22,25]. Data suggest that clinical outcomes following oocyte vitrification and warming are superior to outcomes following slow-freezing and thawing [22]. Oocyte cryopreservation also gives women more reproductive autonomy and may be suitable for women who have no male partner [5,21]. An advantage of oocyte cryopreservation over embryo cryopreservation, is that partner consent is not required to use the stored oocytes in any future fertility treatment [20,21]. Women with a partner may be offered the option to cryopreserve unfertilised oocytes or split the retrieved oocytes with a view to both embryo and oocyte cryopreservation [21].

With improvements in cryopreservation techniques, pregnancy outcomes following oocyte cryopreservation in non-oncological patients have improved steadily. Some randomised controlled clinical trials (RCTs) of fresh versus vitrified/warmed oocytes in egg donation programmes, have reported that implantation and clinical pregnancy rates are comparable [5,26,27]. However, a retrospective study of Italian registry data suggested that implantation and pregnancy rates following oocyte cryopreservation may be lower compared with fresh or frozen embryos [28]. It has been estimated that at least 8–10 metaphase II oocytes should be vitrified to achieve reasonable success rates [29]. The authors found that in women ≤ 35 years old with cryopreserved oocytes for non-oncological reasons, the cumulative live birth rate (CLBR) increased from 15.4% with 5 oocytes to 40.8% with 8 oocytes, with an additional 8.4% gain per additional oocyte. However, the increase in the CLBR was slower in the ≥36-year-old age group [29].

There is a paucity of data on pregnancy and live birth rates from oocyte cryopreservation in cancer patients. A study reported a 35% CLBR in 80 cancer patients who returned to use their vitrified oocytes [30]. Age at vitrification and the number of available oocytes were associated with a higher probability of live birth [30]. There is a need for more data to determine if cancer patients have comparable clinical outcomes to those of elective fertility preservation patients [5]

## Ovarian stimulation for embryo or oocyte cryopreservation

Ovarian stimulation with gonadotrophins for embryo or oocyte cryopreservation is a well-established strategy for fertility preservation in patients with cancer. It is usually recommended if ovarian stimulation can be safely undertaken with a reasonable chance of oocyte retrieval and if there is enough time for the patient to undergo controlled ovarian stimulation and oocyte aspiration [5]. Ovarian stimulation with gonadotrophins, followed by oocyte aspiration for oocyte or embryo cryopreservation, takes approximately 2 weeks.

For ovarian stimulation in women seeking urgent fertility preservation, the gonadotrophin-releasing hormone (GnRH) antagonist protocol is recommended for its feasibility in urgent situations and shorter duration of treatment as compared with the GnRH agonist protocol [21]. Moreover, the GnRH antagonist protocol is associated with a lower risk of moderate and severe ovarian hyperstimulation syndrome (OHSS) compared with the long GnRH agonist protocol [31].

Although some researchers have proposed that response to ovarian stimulation and oocyte yields may be reduced in patients with cancer [32], other studies have not reported any impaired response to ovarian stimulation in cancer patients undergoing fertility preservation before gonadotoxic treatment [33–36]. In a study by Das et al. (2011) [33], in women with cancer who underwent controlled ovarian stimulation with the GnRH antagonist protocol, the total dose of gonadotrophins required for stimulation, duration of stimulation, number of mature oocytes retrieved as well as fertilisation rates did not differ from age-matched patients without cancer undergoing in vitro fertilisation (IVF) for male factor infertility. Similarly, Robertson et al. (2011) [34] did not observe a significant difference in the dose of gonadotrophins required for stimulation or in the number of oocytes retrieved in cancer patients compared with age-matched controls. In contrast, a meta-analysis concluded that the number of retrieved oocytes was significantly lower in cancer patients compared with age-matched patients without cancer [32]. However, it is worth noting that this study did not control for differences in ovarian stimulation protocols.

It has been suggested that breast cancer patients with *BRCA1* gene mutations may have a decreased ovarian reserve, as evidenced by lower serum AMH levels, compared with women without *BRCA* mutations and may experience earlier menopause [37–39]. There is growing evidence that BRCA genes may have an important role in the repair of double-stranded DNA breaks. Germline mutations in these genes may cause accelerated oocyte apoptosis and depletion, which may lead to a reduced response to ovarian stimulation [37]. Oktay et al. (2010) [40] reported that women with BRCA1 mutations had a reduced response to gonadotrophins and produced a lower number of oocytes compared with BRCA mutation-negative women. These findings should be considered when counselling women with BRCA mutations for fertility preservation.

## Random-start stimulation regimen

Conventionally, controlled ovarian stimulation for oocyte or embryo cryopreservation is started at the beginning of the follicular phase. This may lead to a significant delay in commencing cancer treatment, as cancer patients seeking fertility preservation may present at any stage during their menstrual cycle. This may result in patients foregoing fertility preservation treatments because of time constraints. Random-start ovarian stimulation protocols, which allow starting of ovarian stimulation regardless of the phase of menstrual cycle, provide significant advantages by decreasing the total time necessary for the controlled ovarian stimulation and oocyte retrieval [41]. Studies have shown that in random-start stimulation cycles, the number of total and mature oocytes retrieved, the oocyte maturity rate, and fertilisation rates are comparable to those in conventional early follicular phase-start ovarian stimulation cycles [41,42]. No difference was noted when comparing ovarian stimulation cycles in the late follicular or luteal phase [41–43]. Moreover, the presence of a corpus luteum or luteal phase progesterone levels did not have an adverse effect on the number of mature oocytes retrieved or fertilisation rates [42]. Antagonist protocols are recommended for random-start ovarian stimulation cycles [41].

Strategies to decrease the risk of OHSS may be especially important for cancer patients undergoing ovarian stimulation, as OHSS could potentially delay and complicate planned cancer treatment. Studies have shown that ovarian stimulation with GnRH antagonist protocols with GnRH agonists to trigger the final oocyte maturation may help to reduce the risk of OHSS [5,44,45].

To decrease the risk associated with ovarian stimulation in cancer patients with hormone-sensitive neoplasias such as oestrogen-sensitive breast cancer, the concurrent administration of aromatase inhibitors such as letrozole to reduce circulating oestrogen levels or tamoxifen as an oestrogen-receptor blocker during ovarian stimulation has been shown to be effective [46,47]. Reassuringly, it has been reported that ovarian stimulation with gonadotrophins and letrozole was unlikely to result in a significant increase in recurrence of breast cancer [48].

## Double ovarian stimulation regimen

Recently, new stimulation protocols consisting of double stimulations during both the follicular and luteal phases have been described, yielding higher oocyte retrieval rates within a short period of time. Kuang et al. (2014) [49] reported that two ovarian stimulations during the follicular and ensuing luteal phase in poor responder patients, provided more opportunities for retrieving oocytes. They found that the first and second stimulations resulted in a similar number of oocytes and embryos with comparable development potential. Ubaldi et al. (2016) [50] also confirmed that follicular and luteal phase stimulation provided a similar number of oocytes and embryos. These new approaches to ovarian stimulation are especially useful for cancer patients seeking fertility preservation, as they help to maximise the number of oocytes obtained, without delaying cancer treatment.

In cancer patients without an urgent need to commence treatment, the double stimulation or DuoStim protocol, involving two consecutive ovarian stimulation cycles and two oocyte retrievals can be considered to maximise the number of mature oocytes retrieved. However, long-term follow-up is required to assess the efficacy and safety of this approach [1].

## In vitro maturation of oocytes

In vitro maturation of oocytes is a viable option for urgent fertility preservation when patients do not have enough time to undergo ovarian stimulation before gonadotoxic cancer treatment or have contraindications to gonadotrophin stimulation due to hormone-sensitive tumours [51–55]. IVM involves the retrieval of immature oocytes in an unstimulated cycle followed by IVM and vitrification of the in vitro matured oocyte [51,52,55–57]. IVM avoids the exposure to increased oestrogen levels associated with controlled ovarian stimulation with gonadotrophins, thus avoiding the risk of stimulating hormone-sensitive tumours such as breast cancer. As oocytes can be retrieved at any time in the menstrual cycle, IVM may be a useful alternative when patients cannot delay chemotherapy, as the treatment can be completed within a short-time frame of 2–10 days [55]. Since IVM oocyte cryopreservation can be undertaken without any need for gonadotrophin stimulation, potential side effects such as OHSS can be avoided [55,58].

Several authors have described the application of IVM for urgent fertility preservation [51,54,59]. Creux et al. (2017) [54] evaluated the feasibility and efficacy of IVM when immature oocyte retrieval was performed in the early follicular, late follicular, or luteal phases in cancer patients undergoing urgent fertility preservation. The authors did not find any statistically significant difference in the number of oocytes retrieved, maturation rates after 48 hours of culture, fertilisation rates, or the total number of oocytes and embryos cryopreserved when immature oocyte retrieval was performed at various times in the menstrual cycle [54]. In women with malignancy undergoing IVM treatment for fertility preservation, the percentage of metaphase II oocytes matured in vitro was found to be similar to those of an age-matched infertile group, although, women with breast cancer had fewer numbers of retrieved oocytes than infertile controls [51].

Although strategies to increase the efficiency of IVM techniques have led to an improvement in pregnancy rates, the efficacy of current IVM procedures is still sub-optimal, resulting in lower reproductive potential, impaired embryo developmental competence and lower pregnancy and live birth rates compared with IVF procedures [54,55,58,60]. It has been suggested that the freezing and thawing processes could impair the efficiency of IVM cycles [55]. Researchers have also hypothesised that the spontaneous maturation of immature oocytes in vitro, results in a premature breakdown of oocyte-cumulus cell gap junctions, leading to a loss of cumulus cell metabolites, that are necessary to achieve successful fertilisation and embryo developmental competence [55,60]. Recently, various techniques have been introduced to improve IVM culture systems to mimic in vivo maturation processes, such as the introduction of 3D culture systems and adding growth factors to the culture medium [55].

Very few live births have been reported following IVM oocyte cryopreservation. Cohen et al. (2018) [61] reported five live births after vitrification and warming of oocytes matured in vitro in women diagnosed with polycystic ovary syndrome. Mayeur et al. (2021) [62] recently reported three live births in cancer patients who underwent fertility preservation using IVM techniques, two of which were from frozen oocytes and one following embryo cryopreservation. It has been reported that obstetric outcomes, including Apgar scores, growth restriction, and pregnancy complications are comparable in pregnancies conceived after IVF or IVM [63]. Moreover, current data do not suggest an increased incidence of congenital abnormalities following IVM procedures [64]. Long-term follow-up studies of children born following IVM procedures are required.

The IVM technique can also be combined with ovarian tissue cryobanking for urgent fertility preservation. Recovery of immature oocytes from antral follicles extracted from excised ovarian tissue, can be combined with IVM of oocytes followed by cryopreservation of either mature oocytes or embryos [65]. Segers et al. (2020) [66] recently reported three live births after ovarian tissue oocyte IVM, intra-cytoplasmic sperm injection (ICSI) and embryo transfer among patients who underwent unilateral oophorectomy for ovarian tissue cryopreservation.

IVM should be offered only by specialised centres with the necessary clinical and laboratory expertise. Further research to improve IVM techniques and vitrification/warming methods is necessary to improve the survival and embryo developmental competence of cryopreserved oocytes retrieved in IVM cycles [55]. This will help to improve the application of IVM procedures for fertility preservation in patients with cancer.

## Ovarian tissue cryopreservation

Ovarian tissue cryopreservation is a viable method of fertility preservation in patients undergoing gonadotoxic treatment where oocyte/embryo cryopreservation is not feasible or if there is inadequate time for ovarian stimulation and oocyte retrieval [5,21,66]. It is the only fertility preservation method available to prepubertal girls at risk of treatment-induced premature ovarian insufficiency, as ovarian stimulation is not a feasible option in this age group [5,67]. There is still a paucity of long-term data on the effectiveness, safety and reproductive outcomes following ovarian tissue cryopreservation [5]. While the procedure is still regarded as experimental in some countries, the European Society of Human Reproduction and Embryology (ESHRE) and the Practice Committee of the American Society for Reproductive Medicine have recommended that it may be offered to carefully selected patients [5,21].

Ovarian tissue cryopreservation can be performed at any time in the menstrual cycle and does not require gonadotrophin stimulation. It involves obtaining ovarian cortical tissue by laparotomy or laparoscopy, dissecting the ovarian tissue into fragments, and cryopreserving the tissue fragments [67]. The slow-freezing protocol is currently recommended as the standard procedure for ovarian tissue cryopreservation [21,67].

Ovarian tissue transplantation involves thawing of previously cryopreserved ovarian cortical tissue and surgically grafting the pieces back to patients [67]. To date, transplantation of previously cryopreserved ovarian tissue has led to the birth of over 180 healthy babies [1,5,68–71]. A recent meta-analysis reported a cumulative clinical and live birth plus on-going pregnancy rates of 57.5% and 37.7%, respectively, following ovarian tissue transplantation [72]. A prospective cohort study by Jadoul et al. (2017) [73] reported a 33% pregnancy rate among 545 patients who underwent ovarian cortex auto-transplantation. Age is a major determinant of the likelihood of pregnancy following ovarian tissue cryopreservation and transplantation [1]. It has been reported that endocrine function is generally restored between 12 and 20 weeks following transplantation and may last for up to 7 years [74].

Ovarian tissue cryopreservation and transplantation procedures carry a risk of reseeding tumour cells in cancer patients [5]. Indeed, autologous transplantation is contraindicated if there is a risk that cancer cells may be present in cryopreserved ovarian tissue [5]. Patients with haematological malignancies, such as leukaemia, often present unique challenges to fertility preservation counselling and management. They may have abnormal haematologic parameters, thus increasing the risk associated with surgical procedures. Moreover, if ovarian tissue cryopreservation is considered, there may be a risk of reseeding malignant cells with autologous transplantation [5]. Further research is therefore needed to confirm whether it can safely be undertaken in patients with leukaemia [5,75,76]. Recently, novel approaches have been described that include aspiration of immature oocytes from the excised ovarian cortical tissue followed by IVM of the immature oocytes [55]. As ovarian tissue cryopreservation and transplantation procedures can be technically challenging, they should be offered by specialised centres with the required surgical and laboratory expertise [5,21].

## Ovarian transposition

Transposition of the ovaries to sites away from the field of maximal radiation exposure to preserve ovarian function, may be considered in patients who are scheduled to undergo pelvic irradiation treatment for cancer [5,77]. This can be performed at the time of the initial cancer surgery or as a separate procedure [19,77–80]. However, the ovaries may not always be protected because of radiation scatter [19,79]. Although there is a paucity of long-term follow-up data, preservation of ovarian function has been reported in most studies [79,80]. It is recommended that the procedure should be performed as close to the time of radiation treatment because of the risk of remigration of the ovaries [19,79].

## Ovarian suppression with GnRH agonists

The use of GnRH agonists for ovarian protection during gonadotoxic chemotherapy remains controversial. Recent studies have demonstrated that temporary ovarian suppression with GnRH agonists during chemotherapy reduces the risk of ovarian insufficiency and improves the rate of spontaneous pregnancies in early breast cancer patients compared with those who did not receive this treatment [5,81]. The protective effect of GnRH agonist was not dependent on the hormone receptor status in breast cancer patients [82]. There was no evidence of benefit of concomitant GnRH agonist treatment in preserving ovarian function and fertility in patients with lymphoma undergoing chemotherapy [83]. It has been suggested that GnRH agonist may have a role in preventing excessive bleeding in patients with thrombocytopenia due to chemotherapy and stem-cell transplantation [84].

It is recommended that when established methods such as oocyte, embryo, or ovarian tissue cryopreservation are not feasible, GnRH agonists may be offered to breast cancer patients to lessen the likelihood of chemotherapy-induced premature ovarian insufficiency [5,19,81]. Further studies are required to establish the efficacy of this approach. Given the current lack of evidence of effectiveness and lack of long-term follow-up data, GnRH agonists are not recommended in place of proven fertility preservation methods [5].

## Fertility preserving options in patients with gynaecological cancers

The management of young women with localised gynaecological cancer can be challenging because of the desire to maintain reproductive function. Patients should be counselled regarding the indications and limitations of fertility sparing treatment for gynaecological malignancies [5]. For early-stage disease, fertility sparing surgical procedures that preserve reproductive potential, may be considered after careful consideration of the risks and benefits associated with each treatment option [85]. It has been suggested that radical trachelectomy should be restricted to stage IA2 to IB cervical cancer with diameter <2 cm and invasion <10 mm [19]. In women with borderline ovarian tumours, fertility sparing surgery is feasible, although there is an increased risk of disease recurrence. Most recurrent lesions following conservative surgery for borderline ovarian tumours were reported to be of a non-invasive nature, which did not seem to have an impact on subsequent survival [86]. Most pregnancies following fertility preserving surgery in patients with borderline ovarian tumours are spontaneous conceptions. However, ovarian stimulation and IVF are also options for women with early-stage borderline ovarian tumours [86]. Fortin et al. (2007) [87] reported a pregnancy rate of 40% in a series of 25 patients with borderline ovarian tumours who underwent ovarian stimulation or IVF for infertility, after conservative surgery. They observed four recurrences, including three in patients undergoing a cystectomy [87]. In a review of the literature, Denschlag et al. (2010) [88] reported that the risk of relapse of a borderline ovarian tumour after ovarian stimulation was 19.4%, although the relapses did not result in increased mortality. Cryopreservation of ovarian tissue has been recommended by some authors [89]. However, re-transplantation of the ovarian tissue may increase the risk of transplantation of borderline cells [90]. Conservative management of early-stage borderline ovarian tumours along with alternative therapeutic options to preserve fertility should be carefully evaluated by oncologists and fertility specialists [86]. A multi-disciplinary approach, including gynaecological oncologists, fertility specialists, as well as maternal fetal medicine specialists, is recommended to maximise reproductive potential. Patients may be offered egg or embryo cryopreservation before surgery. If a hysterectomy is planned, the patient should be counselled regarding surrogacy [5].

## Fertility preservation in female childhood cancer

Fertility preservation in children and adolescents requires a multi-disciplinary approach and close collaboration among oncologists, reproductive medicine specialists, paediatricians, and nursing staff. Post-pubertal girls under the age of 18 years as well as peri-pubertal girls may be suitable for ovarian stimulation for mature oocyte cryopreservation after careful counselling and informed consent [5]. IVM and ovarian tissue cryopreservation may also be considered in this age group [5,19]. Ovarian tissue cryopreservation is currently the only fertility preservation option in pre-pubertal girls [5,19,91].

# CURRENT STRATEGIES FOR MALE FERTILITY PRESERVATION

Male patients should be counselled about the risks of gonadotoxic chemotherapy or radiotherapy and the availability of fertility preservation options before starting cancer treatment [5]. Ideally, sperm banking should be undertaken before the commencement of any potentially gonadotoxic treatment. Men with cancer may have underlying impairment in semen parameters even before starting cancer treatment due to endocrine, autoimmune, or systemic effects [92–94]. Cryopreservation of sperm or testicular tissue should take place before starting gonadotoxic therapy because the sperm quality and DNA integrity may be affected even after a single treatment [19]. Hormonal therapy has not been demonstrated to be successful in preserving fertility in men following gonadotoxic treatment and is, therefore, not recommended [5].

## Cryopreservation of ejaculated sperm

Post-pubertal males should be offered sperm cryopreservation before starting gonadotoxic therapy. For men who are unable to ejaculate, several options can be considered such as the use of phosphodiesterase type 5 (PDE-5) inhibitors, vibratory stimulation, or electro-ejaculation [5]. In men who suffer from retrograde ejaculation, viable sperm can be collected from the urine following urinary alkalisation with or without instillation of sperm wash media into the bladder just prior to ejaculation [5].

## Cryopreservation of surgically extracted sperm

Surgical sperm extraction is an effective method for obtaining spermatozoa before gonadotoxic therapy in cancer patients who are unable to ejaculate or who have azoospermia or severe oligospermia [5,95]. Testicular tissue containing sperm can be cryopreserved.

Sperm can be isolated from the thawed tissue at a future date and used for assisted reproductive techniques such as IVF or ICSI to hopefully result in a pregnancy [5,94].

Onco-testicular sperm extraction after orchiectomy may provide viable sperm for cryopreservation before cytotoxic therapy in azoospermic or severely oligospermic patients with testicular cancer [95–97].

## Cryopreservation of testicular tissue in pre-pubertal boys

Fertility preservation poses a challenge in pre-pubertal males, as their reproductive systems have not begun spermatogenesis. Testicular tissue cryopreservation and the harvesting and banking of isolated SSCs have been proposed as viable methods of fertility preservation in pre-pubertal males and can be performed before starting gonadotoxic treatment [98–101]. If no sperm are recovered, immature testicular tissue can be cryopreserved. Testicular biopsy in pre-puberal boys is generally considered safe and was not found to have a significant impact on testicular growth or hormonal function [98,102–104]. However, for pre-pubertal boys, testicular tissue extraction for fertility preservation is still considered experimental and the Practice Committee of the American society for Reproductive Medicine has recommended that immature testicular tissue cryopreservation should only be offered to pre-pubertal patients, at significant risk of infertility due to the cancer or medical treatment, and in the context of a clinical trial [5]. The fertility potential of cryopreserved immature testicular tissue has yet to be proven for clinical use in humans and the technique is currently investigational [98]. Advances in the cryopreservation and activity of SSC may enable restoration of fertility in the future by auto-transplantation of a suspension of SSCs by injection into the testis to restore spermatogenesis or auto-transplantation of frozen-thawed testicular tissue grafts and IVM of SSCs [98,99]. However, autologous transplantation of cryopreserved testicular tissues may not be suitable for patients with leukaemia or testicular cancers due to the risk of re-seeding tumour cells [5]. Experimental procedures such as testicular tissue organ culture or xeno-grafting may allow spermatogenesis in vitro and can serve as a platform for future clinical applications [105,106].

## PREGNANCY OUTCOME IN CANCER SURVIVORS

Data from large population studies suggest that there is a reduction in the likelihood of pregnancy in cancer survivors. A retrospective cohort study of Scottish Cancer Registry records showed that cancer survivors achieved fewer pregnancies across all cancer types, compared to the general population. The chance of achieving a first pregnancy was also lower, especially in women with breast, cervical and brain/CNS cancers, and leukaemia [107]. Lambertini et al. (2020) [1] suggested that pregnancy rates following cancer treatment, depend on the type of cancer, with the lowest pregnancy rates reported for men with a history of acute leukaemia or non-Hodgkin's lymphoma and for women with a history of cervical or breast cancer.

Several researchers have reported a higher risk of pregnancy complications in childhood cancer survivors, including fetal loss, preterm delivery, low birth weight, hypertension, and post-partum haemorrhage [108,109]. In the US Childhood Cancer Survivor Study, Mueller et al. (2009) [110] found that infants born to childhood cancer survivors were more likely to be preterm or of low birth weight. The British Childhood Cancer Survivor study found that female survivors of childhood cancer treated with abdominal radiotherapy have a significantly higher risk of delivering premature and low-birth weight offspring [111]. Uterine and ovarian irradiation significantly increased the risk of stillbirth and neonatal death at doses greater than 10 Gy [112]. Abdomino-pelvic irradiation is associated with an increased risk of miscarriage, preterm birth, low birth weight, and placental abnormalities [113]. It has been hypothesised that this could be due to reduced uterine volume, impaired uterine distensibility, and injury to the endometrium and uterine vasculature. Close obstetric monitoring during pregnancy is therefore required for cancer survivors previously treated with pelvic or abdominal irradiation [113].

The timing of conception following chemotherapy appears to affect the risk of complications. Women who conceived >1 year after starting chemotherapy did not have any higher risks for preterm birth than women without a history of cancer [114,115]. Although a safe interval between completion of chemotherapy and oocyte or embryo cryopreservation has not been established [5], an interval of at least 1 year following completion of chemotherapy is generally recommended in cancer survivors [1]. In patients receiving tamoxifen, a gap of 3 months is recommended before conceiving [1]. For the anti-HER2 monoclonal antibody trastuzumab, a 7-month interval is recommended before trying for a pregnancy [1].

Reassuringly, studies have not found a significant increase in the risk of congenital malformations or genetic abnormalities in the offspring of cancer survivors [5,107,116]. The US Childhood Cancer Survivor Study, did not find any increased risk of malformations or infant death in children born to childhood cancer survivors, suggesting no increased germ cell mutagenicity [110]. Signorello et al. (2012) [116] also did not report an increased risk of congenital anomalies in infants born to women with a history of cancer and suggested that neither radiation nor exposure to alkylating agents was related to the risk of congenital abnormalities in children of cancer survivors. Likewise, a case-cohort study of 472 Danish survivors of childhood and adolescent cancer, did not find any significant association between genetic defects in children of cancer survivors with alkylating chemotherapy or radiotherapy doses to the gonads [117]. In contrast, a cohort study using Danish and Swedish national registries, reported a slightly increased risk of congenital anomalies among offspring of male cancer survivors when either cryopreserved sperm or fresh post-treatment sperm was used [1,118].

In terms of efficacy of assisted reproductive techniques following cancer treatment, studies have shown that the response to ovarian stimulation with gonadotrophins and number of oocytes retrieved is adversely affected by chemotherapy [52]. Moreover, the likelihood of a live birth after fertility treatment among women with prior cancer using autologous oocytes was significantly reduced compared with women without cancer [119]. However, in women using donor oocytes, live birth rates in cancer survivors were comparable to those of women without cancer [119]. Since the efficacy of fertility preservation procedures is significantly reduced after chemotherapy, early referral for fertility preservation before the initiation of gonadotoxic treatment is crucial.

## FERTILITY PRESERVATION SERVICE: RAPID ACCESS AND INTER-DISCIPLINARY APPROACH

Multi-disciplinary collaboration between oncologists and reproductive medicine specialists, and greater awareness and availability of fertility preservation services, is essential for providing effective and timely reproductive options for patients facing potentially gonadotoxic treatments. There should be an easily accessible referral pathway for healthcare providers to provide patients with counselling and rapid access to fertility preservation services. Oncologists should discuss the associated reproductive risks of intended cancer treatments with the patient and make urgent referrals to reproductive medicine specialists to discuss available fertility preservation options [5,21]. To counsel patients appropriately, several factors need to be considered, including pubertal status, partner status, underlying cancer pathology, planned treatment regimen, and urgency of treatment [1,5,21]. Better provision of information for patients and health care providers will aid decision making. Results of fertility outcomes in cancer patients should be recorded to enable effective pre-treatment counselling [120]. Clinics offering fertility preservation should have the expertise and facilities to undertake ovarian stimulation, oocyte, or embryo cryopreservation as well as sperm cryopreservation without delay. Effective communication among healthcare providers is crucial to determine the optimal method and timing of fertility preservation treatments, based on the type of cancer, and the planned treatment regimen.

## Key concepts for clinical practice

- Patients with cancer should be offered counselling as early as possible and should be referred for fertility preservation before starting gonadotoxic cancer treatment
- The gonadotoxicity of various cancer treatments depends on factors such as ovarian reserve, age of the patient, as well as the type, dosage, and duration of gonadotoxic therapy
- To counsel patients appropriately, factors such as pubertal status, partner status, underlying cancer pathology, planned treatment regimen, and urgency of treatment should be considered
- The efficacy of fertility preservation procedures is significantly reduced after gonadotoxic treatment. Early referral for fertility preservation before the initiation of gonadotoxic treatment is crucial
- Ovarian stimulation followed by surgical retrieval of oocytes and embryo cryopreservation is currently the most well-established fertility preservation technique with proven feasibility and efficacy
- Oocyte cryopreservation following ovarian stimulation and egg retrieval is an effective strategy for fertility preservation
- Ovarian stimulation with the GnRH antagonist protocol can shorten the duration of treatment and decrease the risk of OHSS
- Strategies to decrease the risk of OHSS include GnRH antagonist protocols with GnRH agonists to trigger the final oocyte maturation
- Random-start ovarian stimulation protocols, which allow starting of ovarian stimulation regardless of the phase of menstrual cycle, can decrease the total time necessary for controlled ovarian stimulation and oocyte retrieval
- In patients with hormone-sensitive neoplasias such as oestrogen-sensitive breast cancer, the concurrent administration of aromatase inhibitors like letrozole to decrease circulating oestrogen levels during ovarian stimulation, should be considered
- Ovarian tissue cryopreservation is a suitable method of fertility preservation if oocyte/embryo cryopreservation is not feasible or if there is insufficient time for ovarian stimulation and oocyte retrieval. It should only be offered by centres with the necessary surgical and laboratory expertise

- In vitro maturation of oocytes is a viable option for urgent fertility preservation when patients do not have enough time to undergo ovarian stimulation before gonadotoxic cancer treatment or have contraindications to gonadotrophin stimulation due to hormone-sensitive tumours. IVM can also be combined with ovarian tissue cryobanking for urgent fertility preservation
- Gonadotrophin-releasing hormone agonists are not recommended in place of proven fertility preservation methods. However, GnRH agonists may be offered to women with early breast cancer to decrease the risk of ovarian insufficiency due to chemotherapy
- Ovarian transposition may be offered to women scheduled to undergo pelvic irradiation
- Post-pubertal males should be offered sperm cryopreservation before starting gonadotoxic therapy
- Surgical sperm extraction is an effective method for obtaining spermatozoa before gonadotoxic therapy in cancer patients who are unable to ejaculate or who have azoospermia or severe oligospermia
- Testicular tissue cryopreservation and the harvesting and banking of isolated SSCs in pre-pubertal males are still considered experimental and should be undertaken only in the context of a clinical trial
- Hormonal therapy in men is not effective in preserving fertility and is not recommended
- Post-pubertal girls under the age of 18 years may be offered ovarian stimulation for oocyte cryopreservation after careful counselling. Fertility preservation in children and adolescents requires a multi-disciplinary approach and close collaboration among oncologists, reproductive medicine specialists, paediatricians, and nursing staff. For pre-pubertal children, the only options for fertility preservation are ovarian and testicular cryopreservation, which are still considered investigational procedures
- An interval of at least 1 year between completion of chemotherapy and oocyte/embryo cryopreservation is generally recommended in cancer survivors
- Abdomino-pelvic irradiation is associated with an increased risk of preterm birth, low birth weight, and placental abnormalities. Close obstetric monitoring during pregnancy is therefore required for cancer survivors previously treated with pelvic or abdominal irradiation
- An increased risk of congenital malformations or genetic abnormalities in the offspring of cancer survivors has not been reported
- There should be an easily accessible referral pathway for health care providers to provide patients with counselling and rapid access to fertility preservation services

## CONCLUSION

Patients with cancer should be offered counselling as early as possible and should be referred for fertility preservation before starting gonadotoxic cancer treatment. Fertility preservation requires a multi-disciplinary approach and close collaboration among oncologists and reproductive medicine specialists. There should be an easily accessible referral pathway for healthcare providers to provide patients with counselling and rapid access to fertility preservation services.

# REFERENCES

1. Lambertini M, Peccatori FA, Demeestere I, et al. Fertility preservation and post-treatment pregnancies in post-pubertal cancer patients: ESMO Clinical Practice Guidelines†. Ann Oncol 2020; 31:1664–1678.
2. Meirow D, Biederman H, Anderson RA, et al. Toxicity of chemotherapy and radiation on female reproduction. Clin Obstet Gynecol 2010; 53:727–739.
3. Barton SE, Najita JS, Ginsburg ES, et al. Infertility, infertility treatment, and achievement of pregnancy in female survivors of childhood cancer: a report from the Childhood Cancer Survivor Study cohort. Lancet Oncol 2013; 14:873–881.
4. Smith MA, Seibel NL, Altekruse SF, et al. Outcomes for children and adolescents with cancer: challenges for the twenty-first century. J Clin Oncol 2010; 28:2625–2634.
5. Practice Committee of the American Society for Reproductive Medicine. Fertility preservation in patients undergoing gonadotoxic therapy or gonadectomy: a committee opinion. Fertil Steril 2019; 112:1022–1033.
6. Meirow D, Dor J, Kaufman B, et al. Cortical fibrosis and blood-vessels damage in human ovaries exposed to chemotherapy. Potential mechanisms of ovarian injury. Hum Reprod 2007; 22:1626–1633.
7. Epstein RJ. Drug-induced DNA damage and tumor chemosensitivity. J Clin Oncol 1990; 8:2062–2084.
8. Lee SJ, Schover LR, Partridge AH, et al. American Society of Clinical Oncology recommendations on fertility preservation in cancer patients. J Clin Oncol 2006; 24:2917–2931.
9. Bedoschi G, Navarro PA, Oktay K. Chemotherapy-induced damage to ovary: mechanisms and clinical impact. Future Oncol 2016; 12:2333–2344.
10. Green DM, Sklar CA, Boice JD Jr, et al. Ovarian failure and reproductive outcomes after childhood cancer treatment: results from the Childhood Cancer Survivor Study. J Clin Oncol 2009; 27:2374–2381.
11. Hodgson DC, Pintilie M, Gitterman L, et al. Fertility among female hodgkin lymphoma survivors attempting pregnancy following ABVD chemotherapy. Hematol Oncol 2007; 25:11–15.
12. Policiano C, Subirá J, Aguilar A, et al. Impact of ABVD chemotherapy on ovarian reserve after fertility preservation in reproductive-aged women with Hodgkin lymphoma. J Assist Reprod Genet 2020; 37:1755–1761.
13. Wallace WH, Thomson AB, Kelsey TW. The radiosensitivity of the human oocyte. Hum Reprod 2003; 18:117–121.
14. Martinez F; International Society for Fertility Preservation–ESHRE–ASRM Expert Working Group. Update on fertility preservation from the Barcelona International Society for Fertility Preservation-ESHRE-ASRM 2015 expert meeting: indications, results and future perspectives. Fertil Steril 2017; 108:407–415.
15. Critchley HO, Wallace WH. Impact of cancer treatment on uterine function. J Natl Cancer Inst Monogr 2005; 64–68.
16. Davies C, Pan H, Godwin J, et al. Long-term effects of continuing adjuvant tamoxifen to 10 years versus stopping at 5 years after diagnosis of oestrogen receptor-positive breast cancer: ATLAS, a randomised trial. Lancet 2013; 381:805–816.
17. Kenney LB, Antal Z, Ginsberg JP, et al. Improving male reproductive health after childhood, adolescent, and young adult cancer: Progress and future directions for survivorship research. J Clin Oncol 2018; 36:2160–2168.
18. Howell SJ, Shalet SM. Testicular function following chemotherapy. Hum Reprod Update 2001; 7:363–369.
19. Oktay K, Harvey BE, Partridge AH, et al. Fertility Preservation in Patients With Cancer: ASCO Clinical Practice Guideline Update. J Clin Oncol 2018; 36:1994–2001.
20. Yasmin E, Balachandren N, Davies MC, et al. Fertility preservation for medical reasons in girls and women: British fertility society policy and practice guideline. Hum Fertil (Camb) 2018; 21:3–26.
21. Anderson RA, Amant F, Amant F, et al. ESHRE guideline: female fertility preservation. Hum Reprod Open 2020; 2020:hoaa052.
22. Rienzi L, Gracia C, Maggiulli R, et al. Oocyte, embryo and blastocyst cryopreservation in ART: systematic review and meta-analysis comparing slow-freezing versus vitrification to produce evidence for the development of global guidance. Hum Reprod Update 2017; 23:139–155.
23. Human Fertility and Embryology Authority. Fertility treatment 2018: trends and figures, 2020. [online] Available from https://www.hfea.gov.uk/docs/HFEA-Fertility-treatment-Trends-and-figures-2018.pdf [Last accessed May, 2022].
24. Human Fertilsation & Embryology authority. Egg freezing, 2022. [online] Available from: https://www.hfea.gov.uk/treatments/fertility-preservation/egg-freezing/ [Last accessed May, 2022].
25. Katayama KP, Stehlik J, Kuwayama M, et al. High survival rate of vitrified human oocytes results in clinical pregnancy. Fertil Steril 2003; 80:223–234.

26. Cobo A, Kuwayama M, Pérez S, et al. Comparison of concomitant outcome achieved with fresh and cryopreserved donor oocytes vitrified by the Cryotop method. Fertil Steril 2008; 89:1657–1664.

27. Cobo A, Meseguer M, Remohí J, et al. Use of cryo-banked oocytes in an ovum donation programme: a prospective, randomized, controlled, clinical trial. Hum Reprod 2010; 25:2239–2246.

28. Levi-Setti PE, Borini A, Patrizio P, et al. ART results with frozen oocytes: data from the Italian ART registry (2005-2013). J Assist Reprod Genet 2016; 33:123–128.

29. Cobo A, García-Velasco JA, Coello A, et al. Oocyte vitrification as an efficient option for elective fertility preservation. Fertil Steril 2016; 105:755–764.

30. Cobo A, García-Velasco J, Domingo J, et al. Elective and Onco-fertility preservation: factors related to IVF outcomes. Hum Reprod 2018; 33:2222–2231.

31. Al-Inany HG, Youssef MA, Ayeleke RO, et al. Gonadotrophin-releasing hormone antagonists for assisted reproductive technology. Cochrane Database Syst Rev 2016; 4:CD001750.

32. Friedler S, Koc O, Gidoni Y, et al. Ovarian response to stimulation for fertility preservation in women with malignant disease: a systematic review and meta-analysis. Fertil Steril 2012; 97:125–133.

33. Das M, Shehata F, Moria A, et al. Ovarian reserve, response to gonadotropins, and oocyte maturity in women with malignancy. Fertil Steril 2011; 96:122–125.

34. Robertson AD, Missmer SA, Ginsburg ES. Embryo yield after in vitro fertilization in women undergoing embryo banking for fertility preservation before chemotherapy. Fertil Steril 2011; 95:588–591.

35. Quinn MM, Cakmak H, Letourneau JM, et al. Response to ovarian stimulation is not impacted by a breast cancer diagnosis. Hum Reprod 2017; 32:568–574.

36. Tsampras N, Roberts SA, Gould D, et al. Ovarian response to controlled ovarian stimulation for fertility preservation before oncology treatment: A retrospective cohort of 157 patients. Eur J Cancer Care (Engl) 2018; 27:e12797.

37. Wang ET, Pisarska MD, Bresee C, et al. BRCA1 germline mutations may be associated with reduced ovarian reserve. Fertil Steril 2014; 102:1723–1728.

38. Phillips KA, Collins IM, Milne RL, et al. Anti-Müllerian hormone serum concentrations of women with germline BRCA1 or BRCA2 mutations. Hum Reprod 2016; 31:1126–1132.

39. Turan V, Oktay K. BRCA-related ATM-mediated DNA double-strand break repair and ovarian aging. Hum Reprod Update 2020; 26:43–57.

40. Oktay K, Kim JY, Barad D, et al. Association of BRCA1 mutations with occult primary ovarian insufficiency: a possible explanation for the link between infertility and breast/ovarian cancer risks. J Clin Oncol 2010 ; 28:240–244.

41. Cakmak H, Katz A, Cedars MI, et al. Effective method for emergency fertility preservation: random-start controlled ovarian stimulation. Fertil Steril 2013; 100:1673–1680.

42. Cakmak H, Rosen MP. Random-start ovarian stimulation in patients with cancer. Curr Opin Obstet Gynecol 2015;27:215–221.

43. von Wolff M, Capp E, Jauckus J, et al. Timing of ovarian stimulation in patients prior to gonadotoxic therapy: an analysis of 684 stimulations. Eur J Obstet Gynecol Reprod Biol 2016; 199:146–149.

44. Youssef MA, Van der Veen F, Al-Inany HG, et al. Gonadotropin-releasing hormone agonist versus HCG for oocyte triggering in antagonist-assisted reproductive technology. Cochrane Database Syst Rev 2014:CD008046.

45. Oktay K, Türkçüoğlu I, Rodriguez-Wallberg KA. GnRH agonist trigger for women with breast cancer undergoing fertility preservation by aromatase inhibitor/FSH stimulation. Reprod Biomed Online 2010; 20:783–788.

46. Reddy J, Oktay K. Ovarian stimulation and fertility preservation with the use of aromatase inhibitors in women with breast cancer. Fertil Steril 2012; 98:1363–1369.

47. Meirow D, Raanani H, Maman E, et al. Tamoxifen co-administration during controlled ovarian hyperstimulation for in vitro fertilization in breast cancer patients increases the safety of fertility-preservation treatment strategies. Fertil Steril 2014; 102:488–495.

48. Azim AA, Costantini-Ferrando M, Oktay K. Safety of fertility preservation by ovarian stimulation with letrozole and gonadotropins in patients with breast cancer: a prospective controlled study. J Clin Oncol 2008; 26:2630–2635.

49. Kuang Y, Chen Q, Hong Q, et al. Double stimulations during the follicular and luteal phases of poor responders in IVF/ICSI programmes (Shanghai protocol). Reprod Biomed Online 2014; 29:684–691.

50. Ubaldi FM, Capalbo A, Vaiarelli A, et al. Follicular versus luteal phase ovarian stimulation during the same menstrual cycle (DuoStim) in a reduced ovarian reserve population results in a similar euploid blastocyst formation rate: new insight in ovarian reserve exploitation. Fertil Steril 2016; 105:1488–1495.

51. Moria A, Das M, Shehata F, et al. Ovarian reserve and oocyte maturity in women with malignancy undergoing in vitro maturation treatment. Fertil Steril 2011; 95:1621–1623.

52. Das M, Shehata F, Son WY, et al. Ovarian reserve and response to IVF and in vitro maturation treatment following chemotherapy. Hum Reprod 2012; 27:2509–2514.

53. Berwanger AL, Finet A, El Hachem H, et al. New trends in female fertility preservation: in vitro maturation of oocytes. Future Oncol 2012; 8:1567–1573.

54. Creux H, Monnier P, Son WY, et al. Immature oocyte retrieval and in vitro oocyte maturation at different phases of the menstrual cycle in women with cancer who require urgent gonadotoxic treatment. Fertil Steril 2017; 107:198–204.

55. Son WY, Henderson S, Cohen Y, et al. Immature Oocyte for Fertility Preservation. Front Endocrinol (Lausanne) 2019; 10:464.

56. Son WY, Lee SY, Yoon SH, et al. Pregnancies and deliveries after transfer of human blastocysts derived from in vitro matured oocytes in in vitro maturation cycles. Fertil Steril 2007; 87:1491–1493.

57. Son WY, Tan SL. Laboratory and embryological aspects of hCG-primed in vitro maturation cycles for patients with polycystic ovaries. Hum Reprod Update 2010; 16:675–689.

58. Das M, Son WY, Buckett W, et al. In-vitro maturation versus IVF with GnRH antagonist for women with polycystic ovary syndrome: treatment outcome and rates of ovarian hyperstimulation syndrome. Reprod Biomed Online 2014; 29:545–551.

59. Abir R, Ben-Aharon I, Garor R, et al. Cryopreservation of in vitro matured oocytes in addition to ovarian tissue freezing for fertility preservation in paediatric female cancer patients before and after cancer therapy. Hum Reprod 2016; 31:750–762.

60. Albuz FK, Sasseville M, Lane M, et al. Simulated physiological oocyte maturation (SPOM): a novel in vitro maturation system that substantially improves embryo yield and pregnancy outcomes. Hum Reprod 2010; 25:2999–3011.

61. Cohen Y, St-Onge-St-Hilaire A, et al. Decreased pregnancy and live birth rates after vitrification of in vitro matured oocytes. J Assist Reprod Genet 2018; 35:1683–1689.

62. Mayeur A, Puy V, Windal V, et al. Live birth rate after use of cryopreserved oocytes or embryos at the time of cancer diagnosis in female survivors: a retrospective study of ten years of experience. J Assist Reprod Genet 2021; 38:1767–1775.

63. Buckett WM, Chian RC, Holzer H, et al. Obstetric outcomes and congenital abnormalities after in vitro maturation, in vitro fertilization, and intracytoplasmic sperm injection. Obstet Gynecol 2007; 110:885–891.

64. Shu-Chi M, Jiann-Loung H, Yu-Hung L, et al. Growth and development of children conceived by in-vitro maturation of human oocytes. Early Hum Dev 2006; 82:677–682.

65. Fadini R, Dal Canto M, Mignini Renzini M, et al. Embryo transfer following in vitro maturation and cryopreservation of oocytes recovered from antral follicles during conservative surgery for ovarian cancer. J Assist Reprod Genet 2012; 29:779–781.

66. Segers I, Bardhi E, Mateizel I, et al. Live births following fertility preservation using in-vitro maturation of ovarian tissue oocytes. Hum Reprod 2020; 35:2026–2036.

67. Dolmans MM, Manavella DD. Recent advances in fertility preservation. J Obstet Gynaecol Res 2019; 45:266–279.

68. Ernst E, Bergholdt S, Jørgensen JS, et al. The first woman to give birth to two children following transplantation of frozen/thawed ovarian tissue. Hum Reprod 2010; 25:1280–1281.

69. Donnez J, Dolmans MM, Pellicer A, Restoration of ovarian activity and pregnancy after transplantation of cryopreserved ovarian tissue: a review of 60 cases of reimplantation. Fertil Steril 2013; 99:1503–1513.

70. Donnez J, Dolmans MM. Fertility Preservation in Women. N Engl J Med 2017; 377:1657–1665.

71. Lotz L, Dittrich R, Hoffmann I, et al. Ovarian Tissue Transplantation: Experience From Germany and Worldwide Efficacy. Clin Med Insights Reprod Health 2019; 13:1179558119867357.

72. Pacheco F, Oktay K. Current success and efficiency of autologous ovarian transplantation: A meta-analysis. Reprod Sci 2017; 24:1111–1120.

73. Jadoul P, Guilmain A, Squifflet J, et al. Efficacy of ovarian tissue cryopreservation for fertility preservation: lessons learned from 545 cases. Hum Reprod 2017; 32:1046–1054.

74. Kim SS. Assessment of long term endocrine function after transplantation of frozen-thawed human ovarian tissue to the heterotopic site: 10 year longitudinal follow-up study. J Assist Reprod Genet 2012; 29:489–493.

75. Dolmans MM, Marinescu C, Saussoy P, et al. Reimplantation of cryopreserved ovarian tissue from patients with acute lymphoblastic leukemia is potentially unsafe. Blood 2010; 116:2908–2914.

76.  Rosendahl M, Andersen MT, Ralfkiær E, et al. Evidence of residual disease in cryopreserved ovarian cortex from female patients with leukemia. Fertil Steril 2010; 94:2186–2190.
77.  Tulandi T, Al-Took S. Laparoscopic ovarian suspension before irradiation. Fertil Steril 1998; 70:381–383.
78.  Bisharah M, Tulandi T. Laparoscopic preservation of ovarian function: an underused procedure. Am J Obstet Gynecol 2003; 188:367–370.
79.  Irtan S, Orbach D, Helfre S, et al. Ovarian transposition in prepubescent and adolescent girls with cancer. Lancet Oncol 2013; 14:e601–608.
80.  Laios A, Duarte Portela S, Papadopoulou A, et al. Ovarian transposition and cervical cancer. Best Pract Res Clin Obstet Gynaecol 2021; 75:37–53.
81.  Lambertini M, Moore HCF, Leonard RCF, et al. Gonadotropin-releasing hormone agonists during chemotherapy for preservation of ovarian function and fertility in premenopausal patients with early breast cancer: A systematic review and meta-analysis of individual patient-level data. J Clin Oncol 2018; 36:1981–1990.
82.  Lambertini M, Boni L, Michelotti A, et al. Ovarian suppression with triptorelin during adjuvant breast cancer chemotherapy and long-term ovarian function, pregnancies, and disease-free survival: A randomized clinical trial. JAMA 2015; 314:2632–2640.
83.  Demeestere I, Brice P, Peccatori FA, et al. No evidence for the benefit of gonadotropin-releasing hormone agonist in preserving ovarian function and fertility in lymphoma survivors treated with chemotherapy: Final long-term report of a prospective randomized trial. J Clin Oncol 2016; 34:2568–2574.
84.  Meirow D, Rabinovici J, Katz D, et al. Prevention of severe menorrhagia in oncology patients with treatment-induced thrombocytopenia by luteinizing hormone-releasing hormone agonist and depo-medroxyprogesterone acetate. Cancer 2006; 107:1634–1641.
85.  Eskander RN, Randall LM, Berman ML, et al. Fertility preserving options in patients with gynecologic malignancies. Am J Obstet Gynecol 2011; 205:103–110.
86.  Daraï E, Fauvet R, Uzan C, et al. Fertility and borderline ovarian tumor: a systematic review of conservative management, risk of recurrence and alternative options. Hum Reprod Update 2013; 19:151–166.
87.  Fortin A, Morice P, Thoury A, et al. Impact of infertility drugs after treatment of borderline ovarian tumors: results of a retrospective multicenter study. Fertil Steril 2007; 87:591–596.
88.  Denschlag D, von Wolff M, Amant F, et al. Clinical recommendation on fertility preservation in borderline ovarian neoplasm: ovarian stimulation and oocyte retrieval after conservative surgery. Gynecol Obstet Invest 2010; 70:160–165.
89.  Fain-Kahn V, Poirot C, Uzan C, et al. Feasibility of ovarian cryopreservation in borderline ovarian tumours. Hum Reprod 2009; 24:850–855.
90.  von Wolff M, Montag M, Dittrich R, et al. Fertility preservation in women—a practical guide to preservation techniques and therapeutic strategies in breast cancer, Hodgkin's lymphoma and borderline ovarian tumours by the fertility preservation network FertiPROTEKT. Arch Gynecol Obstet 2011; 284:427–435.
91.  Anderson RA, Mitchell RT, Kelsey TW, et al. Cancer treatment and gonadal function: experimental and established strategies for fertility preservation in children and young adults. Lancet Diabetes Endocrinol 2015; 3:556–567.
92.  Meirow D, Schenker JG. Cancer and male infertility. Hum Reprod 1995; 10:2017–2022.
93.  Katz DJ, Kolon TF, Feldman DR, et al. Fertility preservation strategies for male patients with cancer. Nat Rev Urol 2013; 10:463–472.
94.  Agarwal A, Ong C, Durairajanayagam D. Contemporary and future insights into fertility preservation in male cancer patients. Transl Androl Urol 2014; 3:27–40.
95.  Furuhashi K, Ishikawa T, Hashimoto H, et al. Onco-testicular sperm extraction: testicular sperm extraction in azoospermic and very severely oligozoospermic cancer patients. Andrologia 2013; 45:107–110.
96.  Schrader M, Müller M, Sofikitis N, et al. "Onco-tese": testicular sperm extraction in azoospermic cancer patients before chemotherapy-new guidelines? Urology 2003; 61:421–425.
97.  Carrasquillo R, Sávio LF, Venkatramani V, et al. Using microscope for onco-testicular sperm extraction for bilateral testis tumors. Fertil Steril 2018; 109:745.
98.  Picton HM, Wyns C, Anderson RA, et al. A European perspective on testicular tissue cryopreservation for fertility preservation in prepubertal and adolescent boys. Hum Reprod 2015; 30:2463–2475.
99.  Onofre J, Baert Y, Faes K, et al. Cryopreservation of testicular tissue or testicular cell suspensions: a pivotal step in fertility preservation. Hum Reprod Update 2016; 22:744–761.
100. Johnson EK, Finlayson C, Rowell EE, et al. Fertility Preservation for Pediatric Patients: Current State and Future Possibilities. J Urol 2017; 198:186–194.

101. Goossens E, Jahnukainen K, Mitchell RT, et al. Fertility preservation in boys: recent developments and new insights †. Hum Reprod Open 2020; 2020:hoaa016.
102. Ginsberg JP, Carlson CA, Lin K, et al. An experimental protocol for fertility preservation in prepubertal boys recently diagnosed with cancer: A report of acceptability and safety. Hum Reprod 2010; 25:37–41.
103. Wyns C, Curaba M, Petit S, et al. Management of fertility preservation in prepubertal patients: 5 years' experience at the Catholic University of Louvain. Hum Reprod 2011; 26:737–747.
104. Uijldert M, Meißner A, de Melker AA, et al. Development of the testis in pre-pubertal boys with cancer after biopsy for fertility preservation. Hum Reprod 2017; 32:2366–2372.
105. Kita K, Watanabe T, Ohsaka K, et al. Production of functional spermatids from mouse germline stem cells in ectopically reconstituted seminiferous tubules. Biol Reprod 2007; 76:211–217.
106. Sato T, Katagiri K, Gohbara A, et al. In vitro production of functional sperm in cultured neonatal mouse testes. Nature 2011; 471:504–507.
107. Anderson RA, Brewster DH, Wood R, et al. The impact of cancer on subsequent chance of pregnancy: a population-based analysis. Hum Reprod 2018; 33:1281–1290.
108. Clark H, Kurinczuk JJ, Lee AJ, et al. Obstetric outcomes in cancer survivors. Obstet Gynecol 2007; 110:849–854.
109. Hudson MM. Reproductive outcomes for survivors of childhood cancer. Obstet Gynecol 2010; 116:1171–1183.
110. Mueller BA, Chow EJ, Kamineni A, et al. Pregnancy outcomes in female childhood and adolescent cancer survivors: a linked cancer-birth registry analysis. Arch Pediatr Adolesc Med 2009; 163:879–886.
111. Reulen RC, Bright CJ, Winter DL, et al. Pregnancy and labor complications in female survivors of childhood cancer: The British Childhood Cancer Survivor Study. J Natl Cancer Inst 2017; 109:djx056.
112. Signorello LB, Mulvihill JJ, Green DM, et al. Stillbirth and neonatal death in relation to radiation exposure before conception: a retrospective cohort study. Lancet 2010; 376:624–630.
113. Wo JY, Viswanathan AN. Impact of radiotherapy on fertility, pregnancy, and neonatal outcomes in female cancer patients. Int J Radiat Oncol Biol Phys 2009; 73:1304–1312.
114. Hartnett KP, Mertens AC, Kramer MR, et al. Pregnancy after cancer: Does timing of conception affect infant health? Cancer 2018; 124:4401–4407.
115. Buonomo B, Brunello A, Noli S, et al. Tamoxifen Exposure during Pregnancy: A Systematic Review and Three More Cases. Breast Care (Basel) 2020; 15:148–156.
116. Signorello LB, Mulvihill JJ, Green DM, et al. Congenital anomalies in the children of cancer survivors: a report from the childhood cancer survivor study. J Clin Oncol 2012; 30:239–245.
117. Winther JF, Olsen JH, Wu H, et al. Genetic disease in the children of Danish survivors of childhood and adolescent cancer. J Clin Oncol 2012; 30:27–33.
118. Ståhl O, Boyd HA, Giwercman A, et al. Risk of birth abnormalities in the offspring of men with a history of cancer: a cohort study using Danish and Swedish national registries. J Natl Cancer Inst 2011; 103:398–406.
119. Luke B, Brown MB, Missmer SA, et al. Assisted reproductive technology use and outcomes among women with a history of cancer. Hum Reprod 2016; 31:183–189.
120. Lavery S, Tsiligiannis S, Carby A. Reproductive options for female cancer patients: balancing hope and realistic expectation. Curr Opin Oncol 2014; 26:501–507.

# Chapter 13

# A guide to diagnosing and managing the menopause

*Imogen Shaw, Neepa Thacker, Nicholas Panay*

## INTRODUCTION

Menopause occurs when a woman's ovarian activity diminishes, resulting in the final menstrual period, at an average age of 51 years in the UK [1]. It is determined retrospectively after a woman has experienced 12 months of amenorrhoea.

By 2030, it is estimated that 1.2 billion women will be menopausal worldwide, and around 85% will have experienced a menopause-related symptom.

Menopausal symptoms can significantly affect a woman's professional and personal life, including family relationships, so it is vital that these women are provided with an individualised assessment of their menopausal symptoms, up to date advice, and support by healthcare professionals.

## PRESENTATION

Virtually all women experience menstrual irregularities and hormonal fluctuations in the peri-menopausal phase. Up to 80% of women develop hot flushes, but only 20–30% seek medical advice [2], despite their symptoms lasting an average of 7 years [3].

Menstrual cycles may initially shorten due to luteal phase deficiencies, and then tend to lengthen to 1–2 months, progressing to several months of amenorrhoea, when women may experience increasing menopausal symptoms. These may temporarily abate with the revival of a few more normal cycles but will become more constant through the month as the ovaries struggle to maintain an adequate oestrogen output.

Women can experience sleep disturbances even in the absence of hot flushes and usually notice erratic and non-refreshing sleep rather than difficulty falling asleep.

**Imogen Shaw** MA, MB Bchir, DRCOG, MRCGP, PG DIP Gynaecology, GPwSI in Gynaecology, Menopause Specialist and Private GP; Co-author of NICE Menopause Guideline 2015, London, UK
Email: imogenshaw@nhs.net

**Neepa Thacker** MBBS BSc MRCGP DRCOG DCH DFRSH MEd, GPwSI in Menopause/Women's Health, Chelsea and Westminster Hospital, London, UK
Email: neepa.thacker@nhs.net

**Nicholas Panay** BSc FRCOG MFSRH, Menopause and PMS Centre, Queen Charlotte's and Chelsea Hospital, and Chelsea and Westminster Hospital; Professor of Practice, Imperial College London; Co-author of NICE menopause guideline 2015, London, UK
Email: nickpanay@msn.com

Mood symptoms such as irritability, anger, anxiety, fluctuating mood swings or low mood, tearfulness, lack of motivation or cognitive difficulties (poor concentration, memory and lack of mental sharpness) are common. A new diagnosis of depression is more common during the menopausal transition, especially in women with a history of previous depression or mood disorders.

Women with a history of migraines, especially hormone-related, may find an increase in the frequency and duration of migraines through the menopausal transition, which are triggered by fluctuating oestrogen levels. Many women find their migraines improve or even cease once through the menopausal transition.

Mastalgia can occur in the early menopausal transition but tends to diminish as serum oestradiol levels reduce.

Joint aches and muscular pains are also commonly reported.

Sensitive questions regarding vaginal dryness, dyspareunia, libido and urinary symptoms such as overactive bladder, recurrent UTIs and incontinence should not be forgotten, as these are symptoms that women do not always volunteer without enquiring.

**Table 13.1** illustrates the most common symptoms experienced by women transitioning through the menopause [4].

## DIAGNOSIS

Menopause is a clinical diagnosis for women between 45 and 55 years. Serum follicle-stimulating hormone (FSH) measurement in women over 45 years is not necessary as levels fluctuate widely during the menopausal transition, unless they have atypical symptoms [5].

In women taking hormones rendering them amenorrhoeic (e.g. low dose POP and IUS), and women who have had a hysterectomy or endometrial ablation, where the menopause cannot be diagnosed by alteration in bleeding patterns, two serum FSH levels 4–6 weeks apart can be measured.

For women aged between 40 and 45 years with peri-menopausal symptoms, serum beta-human chorionic gonadotropin ($\beta$-hCG), prolactin, TSH and FSH measurements should be considered, depending on the clinical scenario, as oestradiol levels may be inadequate despite regular menstrual cycles.

Women under the age of 40 years presenting with symptoms suggestive of premature ovarian insufficiency should have two serum FSH measurements 4–6 weeks apart, with referral to a gynaecologist or endocrinologist for further evaluation.

| Table 13.1 Prevalence of menopausal symptoms in women mean age 54 years [4] ||
|---|---|
| Symptoms | Percentage % |
| Flushes | 40 |
| Night sweats | 17 |
| Insomnia | 16 |
| Vaginal dryness | 13 |
| Mood disorders | 12 |
| Weight increase | 12 |
| Major depression | 7 |

It is vital that the diagnoses of early menopause (40–45 years) or premature ovarian insufficiency (under 40 years) are not overlooked as both are associated with an excess risk of cardiovascular disease (CVD), osteoporosis, and impaired cognitive function. This is negated by appropriate doses of hormone replacement therapy (HRT) up till at least 50 years [6].

## MANAGEMENT (FIGURE 13.1)

Menopausal management should be tailored to the individual woman. A thorough medical and family history is necessary to formulate a personalised overall risk profile for the woman and ensure that she has no contraindications to HRT.

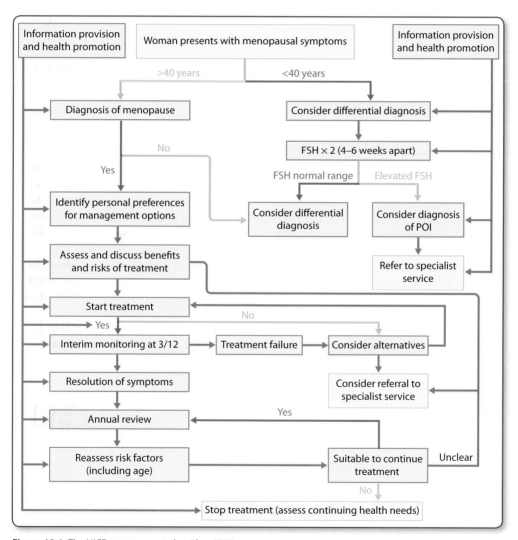

**Figure 13.1** The NICE management algorithm 2015.

FSH, follicle-stimulating hormone; NICE, National Institute for Health and Care Excellence; POI, premature ovarian insufficiency.

A personal or family history of breast or hormonally-sensitive cancers, early ischaemic heart disease, osteoporosis, migraine, and venous thromboembolism (VTE) should be noted, as this will influence a woman's risk profile.

National Institute for Health and Care Excellence (NICE) recommends that those with a strong family history of VTE or thrombophilia (e.g. Factor V Leiden) should be referred to a haematologist for further assessment before initiating HRT. NICE also suggests that women at high risk of breast cancer should be referred to a menopause specialist for further assessment.

Smoking status, weekly alcohol consumption and exercise levels should be discussed as the part of a woman's risk assessment and also provides an excellent opportunity for lifestyle advice.

Contraceptive needs should be ascertained as all women should be using some form of contraception for a year after their last menstrual period if over 50 years, and for 2 years if under 50.

A note of blood pressure and body mass index (BMI) should be recorded, but no other examination or additional tests are required unless clinically indicated.

## Conservative management

Lifestyle modification can be effective for those women with mild symptoms that do not interfere significantly with their life or when HRT is contraindicated. Behavioural measures should be recommended, such as wearing lightweight clothing, using fans, regular exercise, ensuring adequate sleep and avoiding triggers (e.g. spicy foods, caffeine and stress).

Many women use complementary and alternative therapies for their menopausal symptoms. The safety and efficacy of most of these treatments are not well studied, as they are not subjected to the same regulatory scrutiny as licenced pharmacological products. Hence, some alternative therapies may interact with other medications and/or cause potential adverse effects. If herbal treatments are chosen, patients should look for the Traditional Herbal Remedy (THR) Certification Mark validating strength and quality, although this again does not guarantee efficacy and safety [7].

Cognitive-behavioural therapy can help in improving mood and has a modest effect on menopause-associated insomnia [8].

## Non-hormonal therapies

There are various non-hormonal treatments that a woman may choose to help with her menopausal symptoms.

There is randomised control trial (RCT) evidence for a modest effect of antidepressant medications such as selective serotonin reuptake inhibitors (SSRIs, e.g. paroxetine, escitalopram, citalopram) or serotonin and norepinephrine reuptake inhibitors ( (SNRIs, e.g. venlafaxine) on vasomotor and psychological symptoms. Paroxetine and fluoxetine have been shown to interact with and reduce the efficacy of Tamoxifen, so should be avoided concomitantly. Other medications that have shown some benefit include Gabapentin, Oxybutynin and Clonidine [8].

Genitourinary (GU) symptoms due to vulvovaginal atrophy can be treated with non-hormonal vaginal moisturisers used every 3–4 days (e.g. Replens or Yes), together with additional lubricants as required. These should match the osmolality and pH of natural vaginal secretions as closely as possible [9].

Other non-hormonal treatments of GU symptoms include the oral selective oestrogen receptor modulator (SERM) Ospemifene, which has positive effects on the vaginal epithelium and bone density.

Laser treatment to the vagina has been shown in small studies to regenerate the vaginal mucosa, increase collagen and restore glycogen content. The studies were mainly industry generated by the laser companies. A recent Australian RCT has shown that treatment with fractional carbon dioxide laser versus sham (control) treatment did not find any significant difference in vaginal symptoms between the groups after 12 months [10]. More research is required to confirm the benefits and any adverse events.

## Pharmacological therapy: Current evidence

### Cardiovascular disease

The 2002 Women's Health Initiative (WHI) study recruited women with an average age of 63 years. Therefore, research results cannot be appropriately applied to calculate the risks and benefits of HRT in women starting treatment early in the menopausal transition. The WHI study was a large RCT that demonstrated an unfavourable risk:benefit profile of HRT in women [11]. The increased risk of cardiovascular events was seen in the 60–69 years and 70–79 years age groups; this was mainly attributed to the arterial and venous pro-thrombotic effects of relatively high dose conjugated oestrogens and medroxyprogesterone acetate (MPA) on women with likely pre-existing CVD [11].

More recent trials have demonstrated the safety of HRT in healthy women within 10 years of the menopause or younger than 60 years.

Kronos Early Estrogen Prevention Study (KEEPS) was a 4-year, randomised, double-blind, placebo-controlled trial in 727 women ages 45–54 years.[12] This study reported that women given oral conjugated oestrogen (0.45 mg daily) or transdermal oestradiol (50 µg daily) combined with cyclical monthly oral progesterone, showed reduced menopausal symptoms, and improvement of some markers of CVD (increased HDL; decreased LDL with oral oestrogen; decreased insulin resistance with transdermal oestrogen). However, it was found that HRT had no effect on surrogate markers of atherosclerosis progression (coronary artery calcium and carotid intima-medial thickness) when compared with placebo. The authors suggest that the lack of protective effect seen could be due to the young age and low-risk profile of participants, and the short duration of the trial[12].

In the Early versus Late Intervention Trial with Estradiol (ELITE) trial, 643 post-menopausal women were randomised into two study arms according to the time that had elapsed since their menopause; either under 6 years (early) or over 10 years (late) [13]. They received either oral 17beta-oestradiol 1 mg daily with progesterone 45 mg vaginal gel sequentially for 10 days per month for non-hysterectomised women, or a placebo for a median of 5 years. Progression of subclinical atherosclerosis (measured as coronary artery intima-media thickness) was slower than placebo in the early intervention group, however, rates of progression were similar to placebo in the late intervention group [13].

The 2015 Cochrane review found that treatment with HRT in a population who were < 10 years post menopause or were under 60 years old, demonstrated an all-cause mortality benefit [relative risk (RR) 0.70; 95% confidence interval (CI) 0.52–0.95] and CVD benefit (death from cardiovascular causes and non-fatal myocardial infarction) (RR 0.52; 95% CI 0.29–0.96) compared to placebo. There was a statistically non-significant increased risk of stroke (RR 1.37; 95% CI 0.80–2.34). There was, however, strong evidence of increased risk of VTE (RR 1.74; 95% CI 1.11–2.73) in the HRT group compared to placebo [14].

A comprehensive search of RCTs focussing on mortality associated with HRT replacement in younger and older post-menopausal women showed that the odds ratios (OR) for total mortality associated with HRT was 0.98 (95% CI 0.87–1.12). HRT reduced mortality in the younger age group (OR 0.61; CI 0.39–0.95), but not in the older age group (OR 1.03; CI 0.90–1.18). For all ages combined, HRT did not significantly affect the risk for cardiovascular or cancer mortality, but reduced mortality from other causes (OR 0.67; CI 0.51–0.88) [15].

National Institute for Health and Care Excellence 2015 guidance stated that HRT does not increase the incidence of CVD or affect cardiovascular mortality rates when commenced in women under 60 years of age [16]. NICE advises that HRT should primarily be used for symptom control and not for the management of chronic disease, and that treatment should be tailored to the individual woman and involve counselling regarding the risks and benefits of any potential treatments recommended. This guidance is still recommended by most menopause experts [16].

The age of menopause is known to contribute to cardiovascular risk. This was further evaluated in the InterLACE consortium (International collaboration for a Life-course Approach to reproductive health and Chronic disease Events) which provided pooled data from more than 200,000 postmenopausal women. This study showed that for every year earlier that a woman experienced menopause, there was an associated increased CVD risk of 3% compared with a natural menopause, and a 5% increase with a surgically induced menopause. Therefore, women should be encouraged to take HRT up till at least 51 years for CVD protection [17].

## Breast cancer

National Institute for Health and Care Excellence states HRT with oestrogen alone is associated with little or no increased risk of breast cancer. Combined HRT (oestrogen and progesterone) can be associated with an increased risk of breast cancer related to treatment duration, which reduces after stopping treatment [16].

A re-analysis of the WHI study showed that the increased risk of breast cancer associated with combined HRT did not reach statistical significance in women who had not previously used HRT (**Box 13.1**) [18].

A meta-analysis of published and unpublished observational studies by the Oxford epidemiology group published in the Lancet in 2019 found a greater risk of breast cancer than was previously thought [19].

---

### Box 13.1 WHI study-incidence of breast cancer [18]

Incidence of breast cancer quoted from the WHI study was:

- Background risk of 3 breast cancers/1,000 women per year (6% risk over 20 years)
- Oestrogen-only HRT was associated with (−0.5 fewer cases) 2.5 breast cancers/1,000 women per year (5% risk over 20 years)
- HRT with oestrogen and progesterone was associated with (0.8 additional cases) 3.8 breast cancers/1,000 women per year (7.6% risk over 20 years)

HRT, hormone replacement therapy; WHI, Women's Health Initiative.

This suggests that the risk of breast cancer increases with the duration of use of HRT and that women who have taken HRT for over 1 year remain at increased risk of breast cancer for >10 years after stopping HRT [19].

Although healthcare professionals need to be aware of these results, as stated in the commentary published by the International Menopause Society, most of the cases for this meta-analysis were derived from the methodologically flawed Million Women study, so they require careful interpretation [20].

However, both publications agree that combined HRT does carry a greater risk than oestrogen alone, which may be attributable to the type of progestogen used.

There are now four more recent studies (two from France, one from the UK and one from Finland) reporting no or lower risk of breast cancer with dydrogesterone and micronised progesterone compared to synthetic progestogens over 5 years.

The E3N French cohort study reported that 5 years of combined HRT with micronised progesterone or dydrogesterone was not associated with any increased risk of breast cancer (RR 0.9; 95% CI 0.7–1.2). In contrast, synthetic progestogens were associated with a significantly increased risk (RR 1.4; 95% CI 1.2–1.7).

In a follow-up of the same cohort, it was reported that with an increased duration of use (mean use 8.7 years), the risk increased even with micronised progesterone and dydrogesterone (RR 1.31; 95% CI 1.15–1.48), however, still less than with synthetic progestins (RR 2.02; 95% CI 1.86–2.26) [21].

The International Menopause Society published a systematic literature review on the impact of micronised progesterone on the mammary gland [22].

Their recommendations on HRT regimens containing micronised progesterone were:
- Oestrogens combined with oral or vaginal (off-label use) micronised progesterone do not increase breast cancer risk for up to 5 years of treatment duration
- There is limited evidence that oestrogens combined with oral micronised progesterone applied for >5 years are associated with an increased breast cancer risk
- Combined HRT counselling should include breast cancer risk – regardless of the progestogen chosen [22]

The Lancet meta-analysis [19] did not examine other risks and benefits that also need to be weighed up in a woman's decision to take HRT (**Box 13.2**). For example the increased risk of breast cancer associated with HRT is less than the increased risk associated with obesity or from regular alcohol consumption. Mortality figures were also not analysed. These have been further examined in systematic reviews, showing that starting HRT close to the menopause may reduce all-cause and cardiac mortality, with no increase in breast cancer mortality [23].

---

### Box 13.2 The Lancet meta-analysis findings [19]

With a background breast cancer risk of 6.3%, HRT for 5 years from age 50 years would be associated with an increased incidence of breast cancer for women between 50 and 69 years of age:

- Using oestrogen and daily progestogen risk increased from 6.3 to 8.3%: A 2% increased risk over 20 years
- Using oestrogen and intermittent progestogen, risk increased to 7.7%: A 1.4% increased risk over 20 years
- Using oestrogen only, risk increased to 6.8%: A 0.5% increased risk over 20 years

| Table 13.2 HRT and other lifestyle risk factors for breast cancer | | |
|---|---|---|
| Lifestyle risk factors | | Absolute excess risk per 1,000 women over 5 years aged 50–59 |
| Post-menopausal obesity | Overweight* vs. healthy weight | +4 |
| | Obese# vs. healthy weight | +10 |
| Alcohol | 4–6 units/day | +8 |
| | ≥6 units/day | +11 |
| Unopposed oestrogen use for 5 years | WHI study 2020 | -6 |
| | NICE menopause 2015 | +3 |
| | CGHFBC 2019 | +3 |
| Combined HRT use for 5 years | WHI study 2020 | +8 |
| | NICE menopause 2015 | +9 |
| | CGHFBC 2019 | +10 |

*Body mass index (BMI) >25
#BMI >30
CGHFBC, Collaborative Group on Hormonal Factors in Breast Cancer; HRT, hormone replacement therapy; NICE, National Institute for Health and Care; WHI, Women's Health Initiative.

The risks and benefits of HRT before and after a breast cancer diagnosis have been succinctly summarised in a British Menopause Society (BMS) consensus statement 2020 (**Table 13.2**) [24]:

- In women with a low underlying risk of breast cancer (i.e. most of the population), the benefits of HRT for up to 5 years' use for symptom relief will exceed potential harm:
  - Unopposed oestrogen is associated with no or little change in risk, but this may be influenced by the age at HRT initiation
  - There is no evidence of a dosage effect with oestrogen
  - Vaginal oestrogen is not associated with an increased risk
  - Combined HRT can be associated with an increased risk, which appears duration-dependent
  - Whilst risk with continuous combined HRT (ccHRT) may be greater than that with sequential HRT, the difference in risk is small and may be offset by protection against endometrial cancer
  - Avoidance of synthetic progestogens in combined preparations may minimise risk
  - Risk is limited to lean women
  - The risk associated with HRT (including past users) is less than other lifestyle risk factors for breast cancer
  - In women with primary ovarian insufficiency (POI), years of HRT exposure should be counted from the age of 50 years
  - Communicating risk in terms of absolute excess risk with framing minimises misinterpretation
- In women at high risk or breast cancer survivors:
  - There is no additive effect of HRT exposure in women at elevated personal risk due to a family history or high-risk benign breast condition
  - If the use of HRT or vaginal oestrogen is considered, this should only be for managing oestrogen deficiency symptoms after discussion with the woman's breast specialist team
  - Vaginal oestrogens can be used in women taking Tamoxifen, but they should be avoided in those women taking aromatase inhibitors

## Osteoporosis

Lifestyle measures should be encouraged to preserve bone density after the menopause, including adequate calcium and vitamin D intake, regular exercise, smoking cessation, and keeping alcohol use within the recommended limits of under 14 units per week.

Daily calcium requirement is 1,200 mg; this should be ideally obtained from dietary intake alone. Women with inadequate dietary intake should supplement their diet with 500–1,000 mg/day of calcium and a vitamin D supplement of around 1,000 IU daily.

In women, the annual rates of bone mineral density (BMD) loss appear to be highest between the year prior to, and 2 years after the final menstrual period, with usual rates of bone loss of 0.5–1.5% per year. However, a small percentage of women are "rapid bone losers" who may lose as much as 3–5% of their bone mass per year.

A woman's future fracture risk can be assessed using algorithms such as the FRAX tool (www.shef.ac.uk/FRAX) which calculates a 10-year probability of hip fracture or major osteoporotic fracture. The accuracy can be enhanced by the addition of a DEXA scan result, giving the woman's current bone mineral density.

Oestrogen, taken by oral or transdermal routes, has been shown to decrease bone resorption and thereby increase spinal BMD by 3–6% after 2 years, with smaller increases in hip BMD. Lower-dose preparations (0.3 mg of conjugated equine oestrogens; 25 µg oestradiol patch, or 0.5 mg of 17beta-oestradiol) are sufficient to protect most women from bone loss, though the effect is dose-related.

There is good evidence from RCTs (such as the WHI [11]) that HRT not only increases BMD but also reduces the risk of both spine, hip and other osteoporotic fractures, even in women at low risk as well as in those with established osteoporosis.

Oestrogen is still felt to be the best option for the prevention of bone loss in women aged < 60 years or within 10 years of their last menstrual period, especially those with POI.

In older women, no longer having menopausal symptoms, whose risk:benefit profile no longer favours using HRT, bone protection can be achieved with other non-hormonal treatments such as bisphosphonates, denosumab and teriparatide [25].

## Venous thromboembolism

Data from the WHI trials showed that HRT caused approximately a two-fold increase in VTE risk in the combined HRT group compared with placebo (HR 2.06; 95% CI 1.6–2.7), from 1.7 per 1,000 person-years in the placebo group to 3.5 per 1000 person-years in the HRT groups [26]. A smaller increase was also seen with unopposed conjugated equine oestrogen treatment when compared with placebo (HR 1.32; 95% CI 0.99–1.75) [27].

A similar two-fold increase in VTE risk with combined HRT was noted in the HERS trial (Heart and Estrogen/Progestin Replacement Study) [28] and a Cochrane review [29].

The type of oral oestrogen used appears to affect VTE, with conjugated oestrogens showing a greater risk than oestradiol. The ESTHER study found that transdermal oestrogens do not share the increased VTE risk seen with oral oestrogens, showing odds ratios for VTE with oral oestrogen of 4.2 (95% CI 1.5–11.6) or transdermal oestrogen of 0.9 (95% CI 0.4–2.1), compared with nonusers.

The ESTHER study also observed that the type of progestogen is significant, with micronised progesterone having a lower VTE risk compared with older progestogens [30].

## Stroke

In the WHI study, a 31% increase in ischaemic stroke risk was seen with combined oestrogen and progestogen use compared with placebo (HR 1.31; 95% CI 1.02–1.68), and in the oestrogen only arm (HR 1.39; 95% CI 1.1–1.77).

An excess risk was seen in all age groups, but due to the low baseline risk for stroke in women in their 50s, there was an extremely low absolute excess risk of stroke in women ages 50–59 years (0.15 on HRT vs. 0.13 placebo cases per 100 women per year, which did not reach statistical significance) [31].

Stroke risk appears to be lower with transdermal compared with oral oestrogen preparations [32].

## Dementia

The Women's Health Initiative Memory Study (WHIMS), a large RCT involving older post-menopausal women given placebo or a conjugated equine oestrogen with or without medroxyprogesterone, showed an increased risk of dementia in both treatment arms. However, the results were not statistically significant for oestrogen-only users [33,34].

A Finnish observational study based on national registries found decreased risks of dementia with long-term oestrogen use but no associations with long-term combined oestrogen-progestogen use [35].

Two nested case-control studies using the UK GP database looked at 118,501 women aged over 55 years with a primary diagnosis of dementia between 1998 and 2020, compared with matched controls. Overall, no increased risks of developing dementia associated with HRT were observed. A decreased risk of dementia was found among women younger than 80 years who had been taking oestrogen-only therapy for 10 years or more (OR 0.85; 95% CI 0.76–0.94). Increased risks of specifically developing Alzheimer's disease were found among women who had used oestrogen-progestogen therapy for 5–9 years (OR 1.11; CI 1.04–1.20, +5 cases per 10,000 woman-years) and for 10 years or more (OR 1.19; CI 1.06–1.33, +7 extra cases per 10,000 woman-years) [36].

The data so far have not shown increased risks of dementia in younger women taking HRT but have shown that starting HRT over 65 years is associated with an increased risk of dementia. The sub-group of women using oestrogen and progestogen longer term did find an increased risk of Alzheimer's dementia. These studies need to be considered when prescribing HRT for older women or continuing longer-term treatment.

## Hormone replacement regimens

Any woman with a uterus, even post-endometrial ablation, must have progestogenic opposition with oestrogen replacement to maintain a thin endometrium and prevent endometrial hyperplasia/cancer. Older HRT formulations have synthetic progestogens, which increase breast cancer risk and have more progestogenic side effects. Using newer and body identical progesterone or body similar progestogens (such as dydrogesterone) may have advantages including better tolerability, lower breast cancer and VTE risks [37].

If less than a year has elapsed since a woman's last menstrual period, a cyclical preparation should be prescribed, giving 14 days of a progestogen per month, which will then induce a monthly bleed. Combined preparations consisting of 1 or 2 mg of oral 17 beta-oestradiol, or a transdermal oestradiol patch releasing 50 μg oestradiol daily, together with 14 days of a progestogen are available.

If other strengths of oestradiol are required, they need to be prescribed with separate progestogens such as micronised progesterone 200 mg or MPA 5 mg daily for 12–14 days per month.

Once a woman is menopausal (1 year post her last period) or has been on cyclical HRT for around 3 years, she can be started on, or switched to a ccHRT preparation containing a single daily dose of progestogen through the month, on which she should remain bleed free.

These are again available as combined oral preparations with 1 or 2 mg of oestradiol or 50 µg of transdermal oestradiol. If other strengths of oestradiol are required a separate progestogen as 100 mg of micronised progesterone or 2.5 mg of MPA daily can be prescribed. The contemporary approach is to start with lower doses, such as transdermal oestradiol 25–37.5 µg or oral oestradiol 0.5–1 mg daily and titrate up to relieve symptoms. Lower doses are associated with less vaginal bleeding, breast tenderness, fewer effects on coagulation and inflammatory markers, and a lower risk of stroke and VTE than standard-dose therapy.

Younger women with POI or after bilateral oophorectomy often require higher doses (e.g. 2 mg of oral oestradiol or 100 µg of transdermal oestradiol as a patch or gel).

Breakthrough bleeding is not unusual in the first 3 months of ccHRT, but if this continues, and depending on clinical suspicion, it should be investigated by ultrasound and, if indicated, by hysteroscopy and biopsy.

Tibolone is a practical option when ccHRT stimulates breakthrough bleeding or breast tenderness in post-menopausal women. It has weak oestrogenic, progestogenic, and testosterone-like effects. It is the only preparation licenced in the UK for low libido.

Any woman who has had a hysterectomy can have oestrogen-only HRT in the form of patches, gel, spray or tablets. These all have a similar risk of breast cancer. Lower dose transdermal oestrogen preparations of 50 µg or less do not increase the risk of VTE and hence are the preferred choice for women with an increased background VTE risk, such as those with thrombophilia (e.g. Factor V Leiden) or obesity (BMI > 30) [38].

A transdermal preparation with careful dose titration is recommended for women with migraines because of their potentially increased stroke risk and to avoid precipitating migraines.

Systemic HRT will alleviate GU symptoms for most women, e.g. vaginal dryness or pain on intercourse due to vulvovaginal atrophy. For women either not wishing to take systemic preparations or who only experience GU symptoms, low-dose vaginal oestrogen preparations or Prasterone (local oestrogen and testosterone) can be very effective and be used long-term without a progestogen. Women on systemic HRT who have persistent symptoms of vulvovaginal atrophy can also use additional local oestrogen if required without fear of overdose.

Testosterone levels in women decline gradually through adult life and tend to be in the lower end of the normal range by 50 years. However, in women physiological testosterone levels do not correlate with libido, as this is composed of multiple factors including physical and psychological health and quality of relationships.

Ninety nine percent of circulating testosterone is bound to sex hormone-binding globulin (SHBG). Therefore, any increase in SHBG concentration, as occurs with the addition of oral oestrogen prescriptions, will decrease the circulating levels of free testosterone. This may benefit women with androgenic problems such as acne and hirsutism but may not help libido.

The only evidence-based indication for testosterone replacement in women is currently for the treatment of postmenopausal women who have been diagnosed as having hypoactive sexual desire disorder (HSDD). Testosterone replacement in women has not yet been proven to have any significant effect on the musculo-skeletal system, mood, well-being or cognition. There is evidence that physiological doses of testosterone replacement can have a beneficial effect on sexual function, as seen in the Intrinsa patch studies which showed of an average of one additional satisfying sexual event per month, and increases in sexual desire, arousal, and orgasmic function [39].

As there are currently no licenced testosterone preparations for women in the UK, treatment is usually commenced by a specialist. Male testosterone gels are prescribed off-licence for women at a tenth of the male dose, to maintain blood levels within a female physiological range. Blood testosterone levels then need to be measured at 3 months, then 6 monthly thereafter. Side effects, such as excess hair growth, are uncommon when the correct female dose is used [40].

Women under 50 years require contraceptive cover for 2 years after their last period, and women above 50 years require an additional year of protection.

A levonorgestrel-releasing intrauterine system (LNG-IUS) is an effective way to provide both contraception and endometrial protection when systemic oestrogen is prescribed. Data from the Finnish Cancer Registry suggest that LNG-IUS use may carry a similar risk of breast cancer to other oral progestogens [41].

A 20 µg or oestradiol containing combined oral contraceptive pill (e.g. Qlaira or Zoely) are good options for low-risk women under 50 years, as they provide oestrogen supplementation in addition to contraception.

Patients should be reviewed at 3 months after HRT initiation to assess any persistent symptoms or medication problems. Bleeding patterns from sequential HRT usually settle after 3 months.

Side effects from oestrogen can include abdominal bloating, mastalgia, breast enlargement, headaches, nausea, leg cramps, fluid retention, and dyspepsia.

Progestogenic side effects include acne, mood disturbance, fluid retention, headaches, lower abdominal or back pain, and mastalgia. Progestogen intolerance can be minimised through the use of vaginal progesterone, reduced dose or duration of progestogen/ progesterone, a LNG-IUS or Tibolone.

Weight gain is common around the menopause and not usually attributed to HRT.

Once stabilised, a patient should be reviewed at least yearly but reminded to consult promptly should she discover new red flag symptoms, breast discomfort or lump, or any unscheduled bleeding (**Box 13.3**).

No additional smears or mammograms are considered necessary for women on HRT, but they should continue with the national breast screening programme every 3 years.

## Referral

Women with persistent symptoms despite HRT in primary care can be referred to local menopause services for specialist advice.

Women with complex medical histories should be referred for specialist consultant care that may require a coordinated approach involving other health professionals such as psychologists, haematologists or oncologists.

A 2020 summary of the BMS and the Women's Health Concern's recommendations on HRT in menopausal women can be found on their website [42].

> ### Box 13.3 Red flag symptoms requiring HRT assessment
>
> Patients should be alerted to report these symptoms to assess the requirement to stop HRT. Incidence of breast cancer quoted from the WHI study was:
>
> - Chest pain
> - Sudden breathlessness
> - Haemoptysis
> - Calf pain or swelling
> - New liver dysfunction
> - Uncontrolled hypertension (above 160/95)
> - Symptoms suggestive of a cerebrovascular event (CVA/TIA)
> - New-onset breast discomfort/lump
> - Unscheduled vaginal bleeding after being stabilised on treatment
>
> CVA, cerebrovascular accidents; HRT, hormone replacement therapy; TIA, transient ischaemic attack.

## KEY MESSAGES

- Menopause is a clinical diagnosis, so FSH levels are not usually needed
- Take a good history to explore a women's most problematic symptoms and their expectations of treatment
- Discuss a woman's potential personal risks and benefits referring to the current evidence to help to negotiate an individualised treatment plan
- Use cyclical HRT if women still have periods, swapping to a bleed free regimen within 3 years
- Transdermal HRT avoids the VTE risks associated with oral HRT
- Taper off HRT use as symptoms abate, guided by the woman's views
- Provide annual reviews of women taking HRT to reassess their risk profile and ensure they maintain symptom control

Websites for further menopause information and support groups for patients:

- www.thebms.org.uk
- www.womens-health-concern.org
- https://www.menopausematters.co.uk
- https://www.daisynetwork.org

## COMPETING INTERESTS

Professor Nick Panay has acted in an advisory capacity and lectured for a number of pharmaceutical companies including Abbott, Besins, Lawley, Mylan, Novo Nordisk, SeCur, Shionogi, Theramex and Viatris.

## REFERENCES

1. Gold, EB. The Timing of the Age at Which Natural Menopause. Obstet Gynecol Clin North Am 2011; 38:425–440.
2. Gold EB, Colvin A, Avis N, et al. Longitudinal analysis of the association between vasomotor symptoms and race/ethnicity across the menopausal transition: study of women's health across the nation. Am J Public Health 2006; 96:1226–1235.

3.    Avis NE, Crawford SL, Greendale G, et al. Study of Women's Health across the Nation. Duration of menopausal vasomotor symptoms over the menopause transition. JAMA Intern Med 2015; 175:531–539.
4.    Sussman M, Trocio J, Best C, et al. Prevalence of menopausal symptoms among mid-life women: findings from electronic medical records. BMC Womens Health 2015; 15:58.
5.    Randolph JF Jr, Crawford S, Dennerstein L, et al. The value of follicle-stimulating hormone concentration and clinical findings as markers of the late menopausal transition. J Clin Endocrinol Metab 2006; 91:3034–3040.
6.    Panay N, Anderson RA, Nappi RE, et al. Premature ovarian insufficiency: an International Menopause Society White Paper. Climacteric 2020; 23:426–446.
7.    Gov.uk. Guidance: Apply for a traditional herbal registration. [online ] Available from: https://www.gov.uk/guidance/apply-for-a-traditional-herbal-registration-thr. [Last Accessed May, 2022]
8.    Woyka J. Consensus statement for non-hormonal-based treatments for menopausal symptoms. Post Reprod Health 2017;23:71–75.
9.    Edwards D, Panay N. Treating vulvovaginal atrophy/genitourinary syndrome of menopause: how important is vaginal lubricant and moisturiser composition? Climacteric 2016; 19:151–161.
10.   Li FG, Maheux-Lacroix S, Deans R, et al. Effect of Fractional Carbon Dioxide Laser vs Sham Treatment on Symptom Severity in Women With Postmenopausal Vaginal Symptoms: A Randomised Clinical Trial. JAMA 2021; 326:1381–1389.
11.   Rossouw JE, Anderson GL, Prentice RL, et al. Risks and benefits of Estrogen plus progestin in healthy postmenopausal women: principal results From the Women's Health Initiative randomised controlled trial. Writing Group for the Women's Health Initiative Investigators. JAMA 2002; 288:321.
12.   Harman, SM, Brinton, EA, Cedars, M, et al. KEEPS: The Kronos Early Estrogen Prevention Study. Climacteric 2005; 8:3–12.
13.   Hodis HN, Mack WJ, Shoupe D, et al. Testing the Menopausal Hormone Therapy Timing Hypothesis: The Early versus Late Intervention Trial with Estradiol. Circulation 2014; 130:A13283.
14.   Boardman HMP, Hartley L, Eisinga A, et al. Hormone therapy for preventing cardiovascular disease in postmenopausal women. Cochrane Database of Syst Rev 2015; 3:CD002229.
15.   Salpeter SR, Walsh JME, Greyber E, et al. Mortality associated with hormone replacement therapy in younger and older women: a meta-analysis. J Gen Intern Med 2004; 19:791–804.
16.   NICE. Menopause: diagnosis and management (NICE guideline [NG23]). London: NICE; 2019.
17.   Zhu D, Chung H-F, Dobson AJ, et al. Type of menopause, age of menopause and variations in the risk of incident cardiovascular disease: pooled analysis of individual data from 10 international studies. Hum Reprod 2020; 35:1933–1943.
18.   Anderson GL, Chlebowski RT, Rossouw JE, et al. Prior hormone therapy and breast cancer risk in the Women's Health Initiative randomised trial of Estrogen plus progestin. Maturitas 2006; 55:103–115.
19.   Collaborative Group on Hormonal Factors in Breast Cancer. Type and timing of menopausal hormone therapy and breast cancer risk: individual participant meta-analysis of the worldwide epidemiological evidence. Lancet 2019; 394:1159–1168.
20.   Stevenson JC, Farmer RDT. HRT and breast cancer: a million women ride again. Climacteric 2020; 23226–228.
21.   Fournier A, Berrino F, Clavel-Chapelon F. Unequal risks for breast cancer associated with different hormone replacement therapies: results from the E3N cohort study. Breast Cancer Res Treat 2008; 107:103.
22.   Stute P, Wildt L, Neulen J. The impact of micronised progesterone on breast cancer risk: a systematic review. Climacteric 2018; 21:111–122.
23.   Judy M, Chinchilli VM, Foy AJ. A systematic review and meta-regression analysis to examine the 'timing hypothesis' of hormone replacement therapy on mortality, coronary heart disease, and stroke. Int J Cardiol Heart Vasc 2019; 22:123–131.
24.   Marsden J, Pedder H. The risks and benefits of hormone replacement therapy before and after a breast cancer diagnosis. Post Reprod Health 2020; 26:126–135.
25.   Jansen JP, Bergman GJ, Huels J, et al. The efficacy of bisphosphonates in the prevention of vertebral, hip, and nonverterbal-non hip fractures in osteoporosis: a network meta-analysis. Semin Arthritis Rheum 2011; 40:275–284.
26.   Cushman M, Kuller LH, Prentice R, et al. Estrogen plus progestin and risk of venous thrombosis. Women's Health Initiative Investigators. JAMA 2004; 292:1573.
27.   Curb JD, Prentice RL, Bray PF, et al. Venous thrombosis and conjugated equine Estrogen in women without a uterus. Arch Intern Med 2006; 166:772.
28.   Hulley S, Grady D, Bush T, et al. Randomised trial of Estrogen plus progestin for secondary prevention of coronary heart disease in postmenopausal women. Heart and Estrogen/progestin Replacement Study (HERS) Research Group. JAMA 1998; 280:605.

29. Marjoribanks J, Farquhar C, Roberts H, et al. Long-term hormone therapy for perimenopausal and postmenopausal women. Cochrane Database Syst Rev 2017; 1:CD004143.
30. Canonico M, Oger E, Plu-Bureau G, et al. Hormone therapy and venous thromboembolism among postmenopausal women: impact of the route of estrogen administration and progestogens: the ESTHER study. Circulation 2007; 115:840.
31. Wassertheil-Smoller S, Hendrix SL, Limacher M, et al. WHI Investigators. Effect of Estrogen plus progestin on stroke in postmenopausal women: the Women's Health Initiative: a randomised trial. JAMA 2003; 289:2673.
32. Renoux C, Dell'aniello S, Garbe E, et al. Transdermal and oral hormone replacement therapy and the risk of stroke: a nested case-control study. BMJ 2010; 340:c2519.
33. Shumaker SA, Legault C, Kuller L, et al, Women's Health Initiative Memory Study. Conjugated equine estrogens and incidence of probable dementia and mild cognitive impairment in postmenopausal women: Women's Health Initiative Memory Study. JAMA 2004; 291:2947–2958.
34. Shumaker SA, Legault C, Rapp SR, et al, WHIMS Investigators. Estrogen plus progestin and the incidence of dementia and mild cognitive impairment in postmenopausal women: the Women's Health Initiative Memory Study: a randomised controlled trial. JAMA 2003; 289:2651–2662.
35. Imtiaz B, Taipale H, Tanskanen A, et al. Risk of Alzheimer›s disease among users of postmenopausal hormone therapy: a nationwide case-control study. Maturitas 2017; 98:7–13.
36. Vinogradova Y, Dening T, Hippisley-Cox J, et al. Use of menopausal hormone therapy and risk of dementia: nested case-control studies using Q Research and CPRD databases. BMJ 2021; 375:n2182.
37. Panay N. Medical Advisory Council of the British Menopause Society. BMS - Consensus statement: Bioidentical HRT. Post Reprod Health 2019; 25:61–63.
38. Vinogradova Y, Coupland C, Hippisley-Cox J. Use of hormone replacement therapy and risk of venous thromboembolism: nested case-control studies using the Q Research and CPRD databases. BMJ 2019; 364:k4810.
39. Davis SR, Baber R, Panay N, et al. Global Consensus Position Statement on the Use of Testosterone Therapy for Women. Climacteric 2019; 22:429–434.
40. Panay N, BMS Tools for Clinicians. Testosterone replacement in menopause. BMS 2019; 25:40–42.
41. Soini T, Hurskainen R, Grénman S, et al. Levonorgestrel-releasing intrauterine system and the risk of breast cancer: A nationwide cohort study Acta Oncologica 2016; 55:188–192.
42. Hamoda H, Panay N, Pedder H, et al. The British Menopause Society and Women's Health Concern 2020 recommendations on hormone replacement therapy in menopausal women. Post Reprod Health 2020; 26:181–209.

# Chapter 14

# Surgical management of stress urinary incontinence

*Visha Tailor, Vik Khullar*

## INTRODUCTION

Surgery for stress urinary incontinence can be carried out after conservative measures if they have not improved symptoms to satisfaction. The lifetime risk for a woman to undergo stress urinary incontinence surgery is 13.6% [1]. The ages at which the risk is highest is 46 (annual risks of 3.8/100 women) and 70 years (3.9/1,000 women) [1]. Surgery for stress urinary incontinence is usually the most effective way to cure symptoms with up to 90% cure rate depending on the procedure choice.

The aim of surgical management of stress urinary incontinence can be to augment urethral closure or to provide support to the bladder neck. Historically, there have been many described methods for treating stress urinary incontinence; however, some methods have exposed themselves as having limited supporting evidence of their use. Anterior colporrhaphy, needle suspension, paravaginal defect repair, porcine dermis sling, and the Marshall–Marchetti–Krantz procedure should no longer be carried out to treat stress urinary incontinence [2].

It is important for women to be engaged in the surgical treatment decision making process. When identifying which surgical procedure to proceed with the risks and benefits of each procedure option needs to be outlined to the woman. The final choice of intervention should take into consideration individual choice, symptoms, degree of bother, and patient goals and expectations. Many medical bodies and establishments have provided decision aids and developed standardised patient information sheets to help guide this pre-operative counselling.

Whilst it is an established concept that the best outcomes for stress urinary incontinence surgery is following the primary procedure, the long-term outcomes of any procedure are not 100% for objective and subjective cure rates. To monitor surgical outcomes, complications, and improve standards of patient care, it is therefore recommended that women are discussed within a multi-disciplinary team meeting, be included in a national

**Visha Tailor** BSc MBBS MRCOG, Subspeciality Trainee in Urogynaecology, Imperial College NHS Trust, London, UK
Email: vishatailor@nhs.net

**Vik Khullar** BSc MBBS FRCOG MD, Professor of Urogynaecology, Imperial College NHS Trust, London, UK
Email: vik.khullar@imerial.ac.uk

registry of surgery and have preferably face-to-face follow-up within 6 months of their surgery [2].

# COLPOSUSPENSION

The colposuspension procedure was first described by Burch in 1961. This was a widely adopted procedure that was hailed as the gold-standard surgical approach to treating stress urinary incontinence for many years until the introduction of mid-urethral sling procedures. Successful outcomes following colposuspension are reported in 85–90% [3] at 1 year and 70% of women at 20 years [4,5].

The colposuspension procedure was initially described with an open surgical approach carried out under general anaesthesia. Modern practice has seen its evolution and adaption to include laparoscopic and robotic colposuspension. The aim of this operation is to elevate the bladder neck and bladder base. Two or three bilateral non-absorbable or long-term absorbable sutures between the paravaginal fascia and the ipsilateral iliopectineal ligament, also known as Cooper's ligament, are made. Following placement of these sutures, a cystoscopy can be carried out to identify any bladder injury.

It is common practice to place a drain in the space of Retzius and a suprapubic catheter to complete the procedure. The use of a suprapubic catheter can reduce the risk of impaired post-operative voiding and significant bacteriuria compared with a transurethral catheter but may have increased risks of complications such as haematuria, urinary leak, catheter blockage, and spontaneous expulsion [6–8]. Insertion of a drain can be considered to clear serous fluid from the space of Retzius, facilitate identification of a previously unidentified bladder injury, and to reduce the risk of haematoma formation, however, drain placement may increase the risk of post-operative infections and longer hospital stay [9,10].

Short-term complications of the procedure include bladder and urethral intra-operative entry, haemorrhage particularly from peri-vesical venous vessels, infection, and post-operative voiding difficulties. Suture placement beneath the bladder neck can lead to an increase risk of post-operative voiding difficulties [11]. Longer term risks included the unmasking or development of de novo detrusor overactivity (14–17%), posterior vaginal wall prolapse (14–49%), vault or cervical prolapse (42%), dyspareunia (2–5%), recurrent UTI (4.5%), and erosion of non-absorbable sutures [3–5,12].

It is common practice for a posterior vaginal wall repair to be concomitantly carried out if there is significant posterior vaginal wall prolapse. It has been suggested to avoid a colposuspension if there is a fixed immobile urethra and if bladder neck elevation will be restricted by scarring in the retropubic space from previous surgery [11].

## Laparoscopic colposuspension

Laparoscopic colposuspension can be pursued by surgeons with laparoscopy expertise. The short-term subjective and objective success rates to 18 months are comparable to open colposuspension [13]. However, there is inconsistent and currently limited evidence to otherwise conclude that the laparoscopic colposuspension has superior efficacy and safety to an open colposuspension [2].

The advantages of a laparoscopic approach include reduced risk of haemorrhage, reduced post-operative pain, shorter length of hospitalisation, and a faster recovery to normal activity. These are offset by longer operating times and possible increased bladder injury [13].

## MID-URETHRAL SLING PROCEDURES

This procedure was first described by Ulmsten and Petros in 1995 to restore the pubo-urethral ligament and the sub-urethral vaginal hammock to treat stress urinary incontinence [14]. It has since gained popularity in its use having similar cure rates as the colposuspension procedure with improved recovery and less likely to require repeat continence surgery [14–16]. It is particularly effective for women with urethral hypermobility [17].

This procedure typically uses a strip of synthetic type 1 macro-porous polypropylene mesh that is inserted transvaginally to lie under the mid-urethra. Curved trocars are used to pass the mesh tape retropubically emerging on the abdomen immediately above the pubic symphysis 2 cm either side of the midline (**Figure 14.1**). A rigid catheter guide is used to facilitate contralateral displacement of the bladder, bladder neck, and urethra away from the tip of the trocar as it passes through the retropubic space. The free ends of the mesh tape are not fixed so that they remain tension free [18]. This represents what is commonly known as a tension free vaginal tape (TVT) procedure.

The mid-urethral sling procedures have been influenced by manufacturing companies who have developed insertion kits and instruments to facilitate ease and variations of this procedure. There are several adaptations of the TVT surgical method including insertion of a mid-urethral sling with a retropubic top-down (abdomen to vagina) approach, transobturator approach (medial-to-lateral or lateral-to-medial insertion) the use of a single incision, and modifications to the mesh to include self-fixing tips and mini-slings (**Figure 14.1**). A transobturator approach may be discussed particularly if the women have had previous pelvic surgery. There is some evidence to recommend avoidance of the 'top-down' retropubic approach as the outcomes are less efficacious, however, which

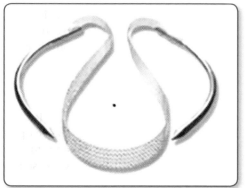

**Figure 14.1** Reproduced with permission from Ethicon: Retro-pubic synthetic sling system to insert the tension free mesh sling using the curved trochar to guide the mesh sling into position.

approach is the best is not definitively known and the surgeon should carry out the approach that is most familiar to them [19].

Mid-urethral sling procedures were originally developed to be carried out as an office procedure with local anaesthesia but can also be completed with general anaesthetic and regional anaesthesia. The procedure can also be combined with anterior colporrhaphy if concomitant anterior vaginal wall prolapse is present.

Short-term risks of the procedure include urinary tract infection, bleeding and bladder, or bowel perforation (~5%). Longer term there is a risk of voiding dysfunction, incomplete bladder emptying, de novo or unmasking of detrusor activity (5.3%), mesh extrusion or erosion (2–6%), groin pain, and dyspareunia [12,20–22]. The transobturator approach to mid-urethral sling insertion is associated with a reduced risk of voiding dysfunction, bladder injury (0.6% vs. 4.5%), blood loss, and major vascular injury. However, this method is associated with a higher risk of groin pain (6.4% vs. 1.3%) and need for a secondary incontinence surgery [21].

Overall subjective cure rates at 1 years are reported as 71–97% and 51–88% after 5 years for TVT [21]. Long-term treatment success has been reported in 82% of women after 13 years with 67.5% patient satisfaction [23]. The transobturator approach for mid-urethral sling insertion has similar outcomes of 71% treatment success at 9 years [20].

Since the first United States Food and Drug Administration (USFDA) warning regarding the use of mesh for vaginal prolapse and incontinence surgery in 2008, there has been growing concern over the continued use of transvaginal mesh. This has attracted widely publicised controversy which has led to suspension or severely restricted use of vaginal mesh procedures for prolapse together with mesh mid-urethral sling procedures until further review in many countries. Following mesh complications, women may require further surgery with partial resection or complete removal of the mesh sling (1.1% at 9 years) [24]. Such procedures should be undertaken in a tertiary referral centre with the support of a specialist multi-disciplinary team to manage this complication.

The negative publicity relating to mesh complications may sway a woman away from having this procedure if this remains an available surgical treatment. Clear counselling and guidance should be provided to the patient regarding the benefits, risks, and long-term risks of the procedure. If minimal or no long-term data is available, (e.g. for single incision mesh kits), the relative immaturity of the procedure should also be discussed due to the paucity of safety and efficacy information.

## Future considerations

The material used for this procedure may impact outcomes and the long-term risk of mesh extrusion. Biological meshes, commonly porcine small intestinal mucosa graft products have been trialled. The data of outcomes remains inconclusive, with porcine slings more likely to lead to repeat surgery [2]. They are therefore not currently recommended for routine use. Similarly, there is limited data for the use of cadaveric allograft materials. There has been research to develop an optimal mesh or scaffold to support vaginal prolapse surgery utilising light weight polypropylene mesh, composite meshes, and biological meshes. Success with these platforms may see further evolution of the mid-urethral sling procedure.

# AUTOLOGOUS FASCIAL PUBOVAGINAL SLING

This procedure involves the placement of autologous rectus fascia or tensor fascia lata beneath the urethra to form a sling. The use of native tissue to create a sub-urethral sling was first described by Price in 1933 [25]. Over time, as with the previously described surgeries, the method of harvesting and using a native tissue fascial sling has developed and remains commonly practiced as described by McGuire and Lytton in 1978 [26]. Having once been usurped in the 1990s by the use of mesh mid-urethral sling procedures, the current concerns surrounding mesh use have encouraged a resurgence in popularity of the autologous fascial pubo-vaginal sling to treat stress urinary incontinence.

The procedure is carried out under general anaesthesia and requires two incisions, either a low transverse abdominal incision or lateral thigh incision to access the fascia and a second midline anterior vaginal incision. Use of the tensor fascia lata may be preferable for high BMI patients or if women have had previous abdominal surgery. An 8–10 cm strip of fascia 1 cm wide is harvested. Prolene or a slow-absorbing suture is sewn at each end to create a 'sling on a string'. Each string arm of the sling is tunnelled trans-vaginally retropubically following a plane of dissection to create a sub-urethral sling. This is facilitated by the use of two clamps (e.g. long Rogers clamp) or with curved trochars (**Figure 14.2**) to elevate and support the bladder neck and proximal urethra. The sling sutures are delivered through the rectus fascia immediately above the pubic symphysis. The two string ends are tied to keep the sling tension free on the rectus sheath shelf. A cystoscopy can be carried out after sling placement to ensure no bladder injury has been created. The rectus sheath window from the sling harvesting is closed, often with a synthetic absorbable monofilament polydioxanone (PDS) suture. Post-operatively a trans-urethral or suprapubic catheter is placed.

Long-term treatment success has been reported for 85–92% of women up to 15 years following autologous fascial pubovaginal sling insertion [19]. However, the procedure carries a risk of long-term voiding dysfunction for 5–10% of women requiring regular self-catheterisation. It is therefore good practice to teach clean intermittent self-catheterisation pre-operatively.

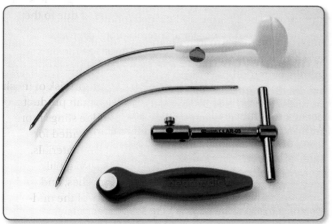

**Figure 14.2** Reproduced with permission from Neomedic and supplied by JUNE Medical. Reusable needle passers and handles designed for positioning of autologous fascial slings.

Additional risks include a 5–10% risk of intra-operative bladder injury, wound infection, 10% risk of transient post-operative urine retention, 10% risk of worsening or developing overactive bladder symptoms, 10% risk of symptom recurrence, abdominal hernia, slow voiding, groin pain, and dyspareunia [27].

The success and complication profile between the described surgical methods differ. Compared with colposuspension, autologous fascial pubo-vaginal sling insertion may be more effective at treating stress urinary incontinence with a lower risk of requiring a secondary continence procedure [12,19]. It is considered as effective as mid-urethral mesh slings. However, autologous fascial sling insertion is associated with a higher risk of developing voiding dysfunction, the need to self-catheterise, urinary tract infection, wound infection, and overactive bladder symptoms [12,27,28]. In comparison, synthetic mesh insertion has a shorter recovery time but increased rates of mesh exposure [28].

# URETHRAL BULKING PROCEDURES

This procedure dates back to the early 1900s with the description of peri-urethral injections of paraffin and sodium morrhuate to stimulate inflammation or sclerosis to treat stress urinary incontinence [29,30]. Today, urethral bulking procedures remain a popular choice for the management of stress urinary incontinence due to their minimally invasive approach and lower overall complication rate.

Urethral bulking can be considered if the above mentioned procedures are not suitable or acceptable to the woman [2] as the procedure is considered to be less effective. The procedure is approved for treating stress urinary incontinence due to intrinsic sphincter deficiency.

The intention of the procedure is to 'bulk' the bladder neck 1 cm distal form the bladder neck or mid-urethra to improve urethral coaptation. Currently, the most popular approach to urethral bulking is urethrocystoscopy and trans urethral injection (**Figure 14.3**). Alternatively, a trans cutaneous approach with peri-urethral injections can be carried out but this may carry a higher risk of post-procedural urinary retention and slightly lower patient satisfaction [31]. Various products are available, often supplied as single use kits to facilitate ease of use as an office procedure with local anaesthetic. Alternatively regional or general anaesthetic can also be provided.

The woman is positioned in lithotomy to be cleaned and draped following which local anaesthetic and antibiotics can be administered as per local microbiology protocols. For transurethral injection, the bulking agent is typically injected at three to four sites commonly at the 2, 6, and 10 o'clock positions until the created bleb reaches the midline of the urethra (**Figure 14.4**) [32].

Many bulking agents have been tested including collagen (Contigen), polytetrafluoroethylene (Teflon paste), silicone beads, carbon beads (Durasphere), calcium hydroxylapatite (Coaptite), and autologous fat to name a few. Current practice more often favours the use of a polyacrylamide hydrogel (FDA approved Bulkamid) or polydimethylsiloxane silicone particles (FDA approved Macroplastique). However, the optimal bulking agent remains elusive, and there is currently insufficient evidence to conclude that one bulking agent is more efficacious than another.

Urethral bulking has an overall complication rate of 32% [33]. Many are transient complications and can vary depending on the bulking agent used [33]. Common complications include transient urinary retention, urinary tract infection (3.5%), dysuria,

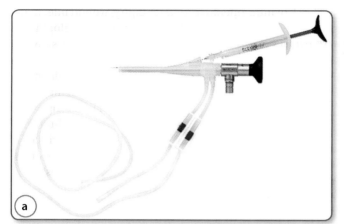

**Figure 14.3** Reproduced with permission from Contura Ltd. Urethrocystoscope with sheath to facilitate urethral bulking.

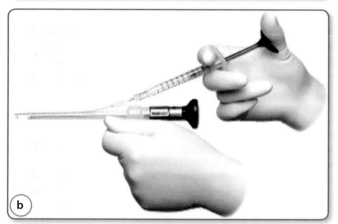

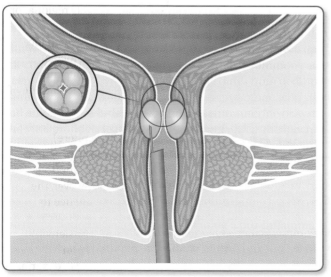

**Figure 14.4** Reproduced with permission from Contura Ltd. Transurethral injection of a bulking agent 1 cm distal from the bladder neck to improve urethral coaptation. 3–4 circumferential injections are made to create a bleb that occludes the urethral opening.

| Table 14.1 Cure and improvement outcomes over time for urethral bulking with Bulkamid [35,51–55 ] and Macroplastique [34,56–58 ] | | | | | |
|---|---|---|---|---|---|
| | 12 months | 18–24 Months | ~3 years | 5 years | 7 years |
| Bulkamid | 66–83% | 64% | 82% | 74% | 65% |
| Macroplastique | 44–79% | 64–84% | - | 47–80% | - |

Note: Further long-term and good quality evidence is required to draw conclusions on the optimal and most efficacious product for urethral bulking.

voiding dysfunction (up to 15%), and overactive bladder symptoms (7–21%) [31,34,35]. Rarer reported complications of urethral bulking agents include sterile and non-sterile peri-urethral abscess formation [36,37], migration of injection particles and urethral diverticula [36]. Macroplastique in particular can be associated with transient haematuria (45%) and dysuria (47%) [31]. Contigen (glutaraldehyde cross-linked bovine collagen) was previously commonly used with much reported data, however, it has been removed from the market in 2011 due to its association with hypersensitivity reactions.

It is not unusual for approximately a third of women to have repeat urethral bulking treatment [34,38] to improve efficacy after the first injection. Over time the treatment efficacy can be lost (**Table 14.1**) with 19% of women at 7 years reported to receive a secondary continence surgery [35,38].

## Experimental agents

There remains a need to develop an optimised bulking agent that is biocompatible, inducing minimal inflammatory reaction on injection, retains volume, and resists migration to preserve durability of outcomes. Research with autologous fat and autologous muscle stem cells have been trialled. However, reported pulmonary embolism and patient death have halted further development of peri-urethral autologous fat injection for this purpose [39,40].

The use of autologous fat or muscle-derived stem cells has been considered to encourage sphincteric regeneration. This requires further research but initial studies demonstrate mixed treatment success of 25–79% at 12 months [30,41,42] and only 29% success at 24 months with no adverse events reported [43]. Human umbilical cord blood stem cells have also been studied with less efficacious results of 36% subjective improvement and 27% no improvement at 12 months [30]. The use of stem cells as a urethral bulking agent is not yet recommended outside of investigative protocols.

## SURGICAL MANAGEMENT AFTER FAILED PRIMARY SURGERY

After a failed primary stress urinary incontinence surgery, women may wish to have a second procedure carried out. There is currently limited and heterogeneous available evidence to provide guide further management of recurrent stress urinary incontinence. At present, there are no formal recommendations for which secondary operation should follow each primary procedure carried out and further studies are required to provide

| Table 14.2 Some of the reported risks of primary procedure failure and reported outcomes following secondary continence procedure. Given the significant level of heterogeneity of procedures and circumstances, it is difficult to draw clear conclusions from existing data | | | | | |
|---|---|---|---|---|---|
| | Colposuspension | TVT | TOT | AFS | Bulking |
| % Undergoing repeat procedure following this primary surgery | 3.4–12% 5 years [22,59,60] | 2.3–6% at 5 years [23,61] 3.2–0.2% ≥ 9 years [24,61,62] | 9% 5 years [60] 8% at 9 years [20] | 2–6% 5 years [59,60] 0% 10 years [62] | 44% 5 years [60] 19% 7 years [35] |
| % of cure and or improvement following this as a secondary procedure | 71% at 4 years [63] | 76% at 21 months [64] | 62% at 9 years [65] | 69% cure 14 months [66] 65% success at 5 years [67] | 25% after MUS at 1 year [68] 61% at 5 years [35] |

evidenced-based guidance [15]. Therefore women seeking further treatment should be discussed in a multi-disciplinary team meeting. Members of the multidisciplinary team would ideally include a urogynaecologist, a urologist with expertise in female urology, a continence nurse specialist, a pelvic floor physiotherapist, a colorectal surgeon, pain specialist, and a radiologist [2].

Options for a secondary stress urinary incontinence procedure include the previously discussed options; however, most procedures are less efficacious as a secondary procedure (**Table 14.2**).

# ARTIFICIAL URINARY SPHINCTER

An artificial urinary sphincter (AUS) is more commonly used in men and recommended in women if previous continence surgery has failed. An artificial sphincter device is implanted to allow the patient to void through the urethra. An AUS has three components: (1) a urethral cuff placed just below the bladder neck, (2) a pump placed within the labia, and (3) a fluid filled reservoir placed in the lower abdomen (**Figure 14.15**). The procedure is carried out under general anaesthesia in a one stage or two stage procedure. The AUS is ready to use 6 weeks after insertion. The cuff remains in an inflated state to provide continence. When voiding is desired the pump is utilised to empty the water in the cuff to the reservoir. The cuff gradually refills to re-established a closed urethral sphincter and maintain continence. 70% of women are continent following this procedure, however, there are associated risks to consider [44].

Risks of artificial urethral sphincter insertion include post-operative haematuria and pain, infection around the device, migration of the sphincter components, mechanical failure leading to removal of the device (6–15%), urinary tract infection, overactive bladder symptoms, voiding dysfunction, and the need to self-catheterise [12,44].

Care must be taken, should the patient require catheterisation so prevent damage to the urethral sphincter and device. Currently, there is only limited evidence for its use in women [45], however, there is demand for its further research and device development.

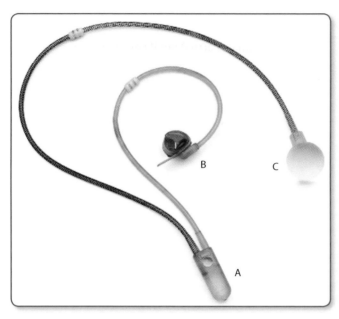

**Figure 14.5** Reproduced from Boston Scientific. Example of an artificial urethral sphincter (AMS 800) with three components: (A) a pump, (B) urethral cuff, and (C) a fluid filled reservoir.

# CONSIDERATIONS

Women of child bearing age with stress urinary incontinence should consider surgical treatment ideally after they have completed their family. After a continence procedure, pregnancy is thought to increase the risk of symptom reoccurrence independent of the mode of delivery [19,46]. 5–22% following caesarean delivery and 20–30% following vaginal delivery develop recurrent stress urinary incontinence symptoms. No significant difference in the mode of delivery to the risk of recurrence has been identified [46,47]. There is also a risk of urinary retention during pregnancy with the need to carry out clean intermittent self-catheterisation and associated risk of urinary tract infections [47].

Pre-operatively patient factors should be optimised such as good diabetic control and BMI optimisation. Women with diabetes are at higher risk of mesh erosion and obese women may not have as efficacious outcomes as normal BMI women [12,19].

Efficacy of surgical procedures may be affected by age. For example the outcomes of mesh mid-urethral sling procedures with a retropubic or trans-obturator application appear to as efficacious in women > 65 years, however, outcomes may not be as long-lasting [12,48,49]. Further research to understand the impact of age to specific procedures is needed.

It is not uncommon for women to present with concomitant vaginal prolapse. Colposuspension, mid-urethral mesh sling, or autologous fascial sling procedures can be carried out in tandem with prolapse surgery [12,19]. Combined TVT and anterior colporrhaphy demonstrate a higher risk of cure in the short term, however, adverse events such as short-term voiding dysfunction and prolonged post-operative catheterisation are more common post-operatively [50]. The long-term outcomes for concomitant colposuspension or autologous fascial sling procedures with prolapse surgery are less well documented [12].

# CONCLUSION

Surgery for stress urinary incontinence (SUI) can be carried out if conservative measures have not improved symptoms to satisfaction.

Procedures including a colposuspension, autologous fascial pubovaginal sling insertion or urethral bulking procedure are widely practiced to treat SUI. There are differing risks associated with each procedure.

The insertion of a synthetic mesh mid-urethral sling has good surgical outcomes but is associated with specific mesh complications and subsequently banned from use in some countries.

It is important for women to be engaged in the surgical treatment decision making process. It is appropriate to have a choice of treatment modalities to accommodate the varying presentation of symptoms, acceptability of risks and baseline demographics of the woman.

The use of a surgery registry can be used to monitor surgical outcomes, complications, and improve standards of patient care.

The success rate of any surgical procedure to treat stress urinary incontinence is highest when it is carried out as the primary surgery.

Further research is needed to provide guidance on the optimal secondary procedure if needed, to develop an optimal surgical scaffold for sling procedures or further development into an efficacious urethral bulking agent.

# REFERENCES

1. Wu JM, Matthews CA, Conover MM, et al. Lifetime Risk of Stress Urinary Incontinence or Pelvic Organ Prolapse Surgery. Obstet Gynecol 2014; 123:1201–1206.
2. NICE. (2019) Urinary incontinence and pelvic organ prolapse in women: management (NG123). [online] Available from: www.nice.org.uk/guidance/ng123 [Last accessed May, 2022]
3. Lapitan MCM, Cody JD, Mashayekhi A. Open retropubic colposuspension for urinary incontinence in women. Cochrane Database Syst Rev 2017; 2017:CD002912.
4. Alcalay M, Stanton SL, Monga A. Burch colposuspension: a 10-20 year follow up. Br J Obstet Gynaecol 1995; 102:740–745.
5. BSUG. Colposuspension for Stress Urinary Incontinence, 2018. [online] Available from: https://bsug.org.uk/budcms/includes/kcfinder/upload/files/Colposuspension Apr 2018.pdf [Last accessed May, 2022].
6. Andersen JT, Heisterberg L, Hebjørn S, et al. Suprapubic versus transurethral bladder drainage after colposuspension/vaginal repair. Acta Obstet Gynecol Scand 1985; 64:139–143.
7. Healy EF, Walsh CA, Cotter AM, et al. Suprapubic compared with transurethral bladder catheterization for gynecologic surgery. Obstet Gynecol 2012; 120:678–687.
8. Li M, Yao L, Han C, et al. The incidence of urinary tract infection of different routes of catheterization following gynecologic surgery: a systematic review and meta-analysis of randomized controlled trials Int Urogynecol J 2019; 30:523–535.
9. Benedetti-Panici P, Maneschi F, Cutillo G, et al. A randomized study comparing retroperitoneal drainage with no drainage after lymphadenectomy in gynecologic malignancies. Gynecol Oncol 1997; 65:478–482.
10. Ghezzi F, Franchi M, Buttarelli M, et al. The use of suction drains at Burch colposuspension and postoperative infectious morbidity. Arch Gynecol Obstet 2003; 268:41–44.
11. Richmond DH. Operations for urinary incontinence. In: Lopes T, Spirtos N, Monaghan RJ (Eds). Bonney's Gynaecological Surgery, 11th Edition. United States: Wiley-Blackwell; 2011.
12. Burkhard FC, Bosch JL, Cruz F, et al. Urinary Incontinence in Adults [Internet]. Eur Assoc Urol 2020:100.
13. Freites J, Stewart F, Omar MI, et al. Laparoscopic colposuspension for urinary incontinence in women, 2019. [online] Available from: https://www.cochranelibrary.com/cdsr/doi/10.1002/14651858.CD002239.pub4/full [Last accessed May, 2022].

14. Ulmsten U, Petros P. Intravaginal slingplasty (IVS): An ambulatory surgical procedure for treatment of female urinary incontinence. Scand J Urol Nephrol 1995; 29:75–82.

15. Bakali E, Johnson E, Buckley BS, et al. Interventions for treating recurrent stress urinary incontinence after failed minimally invasive synthetic midurethral tape surgery in women. Cochrane Database Syst Rev 019; 2019:CD009407.

16. Saraswat L, Rehman H, Omar MI, et al. Traditional suburethral sling operations for urinary incontinence in women. Cochrane Database Syst Rev 2020; 2021:CD001754.

17. Wlaźlak E, Viereck V, Kociszewski J, et al. Role of intrinsic sphincter deficiency with and without urethral hypomobility on the outcome of tape insertion. Neurourol Urodyn 2017; 36:1910–1916.

18. Ethicon. (2019). GYNECARE TVT™ Sling Retropubic System [Internet]. Gynecare TVT Instuctions for use. [online] Available from: https://www.jnjmedicaldevices.com/en-US/product/gynecare-tvt-sling [Last accessed May, 2022].

19. Kobashi KC, Albo ME, Dmochowski RR, et al. Surgical Treatment of Female Stress Urinary Incontinence: AUA/SUFU Guideline. J Urol 2017; 198:875–883.

20. Karmakar D, Mostafa A, Abdel-Fattah M. Long-term outcomes of transobturator tapes in women with stress urinary incontinence: E-TOT randomised controlled trial. BJOG 2017; 124:973–981.

21. Ford AA, Rogerson L, Cody JD, et al. Mid-urethral sling operations for stress urinary incontinence in women. Cochrane Database Syst Rev 2017.

22. Ward K, Hilton P. Tension-free vaginal tape versus colposuspension for primary urodynamic stress incontinence: 5-year follow up. BJOG 2007; 115:226–233.

23. Song PH, Kwon DH, Ko YH, et al. The long-term outcomes of the tension-free vaginal tape procedure for treatment of female stress urinary incontinence: Data from minimum 13 years of follow-up. Low Urin Tract Symptoms 2017; 9:10–14.

24. Berger AA, Tan-Kim J, Menefee SA. Long-term risk of reoperation after synthetic mesh midurethral sling surgery for stress urinary incontinence. Obstet Gynecol 2019; 134:1047–1055.

25. Price P. Plastic operations for incontinence of urine and of feces. Arch Surg 1933; 26:1043.

26. Mcguire EJ, Lytton B. Pubovaginal sling procedure for stress incontinence. J Urol 1978; 119:82–84.

27. BSUG. Autologous fascial sling to treat stress urinary incontinence, 2018. [online] Available from: https://bsug.org.uk/budcms/includes/kcfinder/upload/files/Autologous fascial sling BSUG Mar 2018-2.pdf [Last accessed May, 2022].

28. Plagakis S, Tse V. The autologous pubovaginal fascial sling: An update in 2019. Low Urin Tract Symptoms 2020; 12:2–7.

29. Murless BC. The Injection Treatment of Stress Incontinence. BJOG 1938; 45:67–73.

30. Hillary CJ, Roman S, MacNeil S, et al. Regenerative medicine and injection therapies in stress urinary incontinence. Nat Rev Urol 2020; 17:151–161.

31. Kirchin V, Page T, Keegan PE, et al. Urethral injection therapy for urinary incontinence in women. Cochrane Database Syst Rev 2017; 2017: CD003881.

32. Contura. Bulkamid standard operating procedure, 2018. [online] Available from: https://bulkamid.com/wp-content/uploads/2019/03/BULK_2018_041.2_SOP_12.04.18.pdf [Last accessed May, 2022].

33. De Vries AM, Wadhwa H, Huang J, et al. Complications of urethral bulking agents for stress urinary incontinence: An extensive review including case reports. Female Pelvic Med Reconstr Surg 2018; 24:392–398.

34. Ghoniem GM, Miller CJ. A systematic review and meta-analysis of Macroplastique for treating female stress urinary incontinence. Int Urogynecol J 2013; 24:27–36.

35. Brosche T, Kuhn A, Lobodasch K, et al. Seven-year efficacy and safety outcomes of Bulkamid for the treatment of stress urinary incontinence. Neurourol Urodyn 2021; 40:502–508.

36. Kumar D, Kaufman MR, Dmochowski RR. Case reports: Periurethral bulking agents and presumed urethral diverticula. Int Urogynecol J 2011; 22:1039–1043.

37. Gopinath D, Smith ARB, Reid FM. Periurethral abscess following polyacrylamide hydrogel (Bulkamid ®) for stress urinary incontinence. Int Urogynecol J 2012; 23:1645–1648.

38. McGowan S, Campbell P, Dolan L. The use of urethral bulking agents in the treatment of stress urinary incontinence. Obstet Gynaecol 2020; 22:137–146.

39. Currie I, Drutz HP, Deck J, et al. Adipose tissue and lipid droplet embolism following periurethral injection of autologous fat: Case report and review of the literature. Int Urogynecol J 1997; 8:377–380.

40. Lee PE, Kung RC, Drutz HP. Periurethral autologous fat injection as treatment for female stress urinary incontinence: A randomized double-blind controlled trial. J Urol 2001; 165:153–158.

41. Mitterberger M, Marksteiner R, Margreiter E, et al. Autologous myoblasts and fibroblasts for female stress incontinence: a 1-year follow-up in 123 patients. BJU Int 2007; 100:1081–1085.

42. Sèbe P, Doucet C, Cornu JN, et al. Intrasphincteric injections of autologous muscular cells in women with refractory stress urinary incontinence: A prospective study. Int Urogynecol J 2011; 22:183–189.

43. Sharifiaghdas F, Zohrabi F, Moghadasali R, et al. Autologous Muscle-derived Cell Injection for Treatment of Female Stress Urinary Incontinence: A Single-Arm Clinical Trial with 24-months Follow-Up. Urol J 2019; 16:482–487.

44. British Association of urological surgeons. Insertion of an artificial urinary sphincter (AUS) in women, 2020. [online] Available from: https://www.baus.org.uk/_userfiles/pages/files/Patients/Leaflets/AUS female.pdf [Last accessed May, 2022].

45. Lipp A, Shaw C, Glavind K. Mechanical devices for urinary incontinence in women. In: Lipp A (Ed). Cochrane Database Syst Rev 2011.

46. Bergman I, Westergren Söderberg M, Lundqvist A, et al. Associations between childbirth and urinary incontinence after midurethral sling surgery. Obstet Gynecol 2018; 131:297–303.

47. Pollard ME, Morrisroe S, Anger JT. Outcomes of pregnancy following surgery for stress urinary incontinence: A systematic review. J Urol 2012; 187:1966–1970.

48. Franzen K, Andersson G, Odeberg J, et al. Surgery for urinary incontinence in women 65 years and older: a systematic review. Int Urogynecol J 2015; 26:1095–1102.

49. Ahn SH, Park YJ, Kong MK, et al. Impact of age on outcomes of midurethral sling procedures in women. Int Urogynecol J 2020; 31:785–789.

50. van der Ploeg J, van der Steen A, Oude Rengerink K, et al. Prolapse surgery with or without stress incontinence surgery for pelvic organ prolapse: a systematic review and meta-analysis of randomised trials. BJOG 2014; 121:537–547.

51. Toozs-Hobson P, Al-Singary W, Fynes M, et al. Two-year follow-up of an open-label multicenter study of polyacrylamide hydrogel (Bulkamid®) for female stress and stress-predominant mixed incontinence. Int Urogynecol J 2012; 23:1373–1378.

52. Pai A, Al-Singary W. Durability, safety and efficacy of polyacrylamide hydrogel (Bulkamid(®)) in the management of stress and mixed urinary incontinence: three year follow up outcomes. Cent Eur J Urol 2015; 68:428–433.

53. Boennelycke M, Christensen L, Nielsen LF, et al. Fresh muscle fiber fragments on a scaffold in rats–a new concept in urogynecology? Am J Obstet Gynecol 2011; 205:235.

54. Lose G, Sørensen HC, Axelsen SM, et al. An open multicenter study of polyacrylamide hydrogel (Bulkamid) for female stress and mixed urinary incontinence. Int Urogynecol J 2010; 21:1471–1477.

55. Sokol ER, Karram MM, Dmochowski R. Efficacy and safety of polyacrylamide hydrogel for the treatment of female stress incontinence: a randomized, prospective, multicenter North American study. J Urol 2014; 192:843–849.

56. Ghoniem G, Corcos J, Comiter C, et al. Durability of urethral bulking agent injection for female stress urinary incontinence: 2-year multicenter study results. J Urol 2010;183:1444–1449.

57. Tamanini JTN, D'Ancona CAL, Netto NR. Macroplastique implantation system for female stress urinary incontinence: Long-term follow-up. J Endourol 2006; 20:1082–1086.

58. Serati M, Soligo M, Braga A, et al. Efficacy and safety of polydimethylsiloxane injection (Macroplastique ®) for the treatment of female stress urinary incontinence: results of a series of 85 patients with ≥3 years of follow-up. BJU Int 2019; 123:353–359.

59. Brubaker L, Richter HE, Norton PA, et al. 5-Year continence rates, satisfaction and adverse events of burch urethropexy and fascial sling surgery for urinary incontinence. J Urol 2012; 187:1324–1330.

60. Foss Hansen M, Lose G, Kesmodel US, et al. Reoperation for urinary incontinence: a nationwide cohort study, 1998–2007. Am J Obstet Gynecol 2016; 214:263.

61. Gurol-Urganci I, Geary RS, Mamza JB, et al. Long-term rate of mesh sling removal following midurethral mesh sling insertion among women with stress urinary incontinence. JAMA 2018; 320:1659.

62. Khan ZA, Nambiar A, Morley R, et al. Long-term follow-up of a multicentre randomised controlled trial comparing tension-free vaginal tape, xenograft and autologous fascial slings for the treatment of stress urinary incontinence in women. BJU Int 2015; 115:968–977.

63. Thakar R, Stanton S, Prodigalidad L, et al. Secondary colposuspension: results of a prospective study from a tertiary referral centre. BJOG 2002; 109:1115–1120.

64. Meyer F, Hermieu JF, Boyd A, et al. Repeat mid-urethral sling for recurrent female stress urinary incontinence. Int Urogynecol J 2013; 24:817–22.

65. Abdel-Fattah M, Cao G, Mostafa A. Long-term outcomes of transobturator tension-free vaginal tapes as secondary continence procedures. World J Urol 2017; 35:1141–1148.

66. Milose JC, Sharp KM, He C, et al. Success of autologous pubovaginal sling after failed synthetic mid urethral sling. J Urol 2015; 193:916–920.
67. Sharifiaghdas F, Mahmoudnejad N, Honarkar Ramezani M, et al. Salvage autologous fascial sling after failed anti-incontinence surgeries: Long term follow up. Urol J 2019; 16:193–197.
68. Zivanovic I, Rautenberg O, Lobodasch K, et al. Urethral bulking for recurrent stress urinary incontinence after midurethral sling failure. Neurourol Urodyn 2017; 36:722–726.

# Chapter 15

# Early cervical cancer: Update on detection and treatment

*Sabrina Piedimonte, Shannon Salvador*

## EPIDEMIOLOGY

Cervical cancer is fourth most common cancer in women, with 530,000 new cases per year, and highest prevalence in underdeveloped countries [1]. Southeast Asia, Latin America and Sub-Saharan Africa represent two-thirds of the prevalent cases [1]. The 5-year survival rate was recently estimated to be 64.5% and decreases with increasing age (82.3% under 40 and 52.4% >50) [2]. It is projected that by the year 2030, the global burden of cervical cancer will rise by 2% [3]. However, the World Health Organization has committed, with its members, to eliminate cervical cancer by 2030 through a global strategy involving human papillomavirus (HPV) vaccination, high-performance screening and effective treatment of women with cervical disease. HPV-16 and HPV-18 alone cause approximately 70% of cervical cancers [4], with an additional 20% being attributed to types 31/33/45/52/58. Although cytology screening has been monumental in diagnosing pre-invasive disease, it may detect only 50–60% of high-grade lesions. In recent years, there has been immense progress in cervical cancer, including HPV vaccination, new International Federation of Gynecology and Obstetrics (FIGO) staging, sentinel lymph node dissection and a transition back to abdominal radical hysterectomy (RH). This chapter will summarise updates in detection and treatment for invasive cervical cancer.

## DETECTION

### Clinical presentation

Microinvasive cervical cancer is generally asymptomatic and presents as a pre-invasive lesion identified at colposcopy through biopsy and subsequently treated with a Loop electrosurgical excision procedure (LEEP) procedure. In a study including 12,714 LEEP specimens, the incidence of invasive cancer was 5.98%; 0.24% of low-grade squamous

**Sabrina Piedimonte** MDCM MSc, Gynecologic Oncology Fellow, University of Toronto, Toronto, Canada
Email: sabrina.piedimonte@uhn.ca

**Shannon Salvador** MD MSc, Gynecologic Oncologist, Jewish General Hospital, Assistant Professor, McGill University, Montreal, Quebec, Canada
Email: shannon.salvador@mcgill.ca

intraepithelial lesion (LSIL), 6.37% of high-grade squamous intraepithelial lesion (HSIL) and 24.31% of adenocarcinoma in-situ (AIS) diagnosed by punch biopsy were further confirmed as having cervical cancer on LEEP [5]. The horizontal extent and depth of invasion is often reported in the LEEP specimen and is added to the final hysterectomy specimen for prognostic and adjuvant treatment purposes [6].

In patients who have not undergone routine cervical cytology, common presentations of cervical cancer include pain, bleeding, and hydronephrosis. *Abnormal vaginal bleeding* is the most common presenting symptom of invasive cancer and classically described by patients as 'post-coital bleeding', but may also be intermenstrual or postmenopausal [7]. This is due to the tumour becoming friable and possibly necrotic. Some patients present with vaginal discharge that may be watery, mucoid, or purulent and malodorous but this is non-specific and may be mistaken for normal discharge or vaginitis [8]. The classic triad of advanced cervical cancer is *pain, leg oedema, and weight loss* [9], but may also present as a vesico-vaginal or recto-vaginal fistula.

On physical examination, which used to be the mainstay of staging, a speculum examination may reveal an exophytic, ulcerative or polypoid lesion, but most commonly will be microscopic and only detected on biopsy. A vaginal rectal examination must always be performed including examination of the vaginal fornices, the rectovaginal space and the parametria. The vagina is also inspected on speculum examination, but significant vaginal involvement often obscures the primary cervical lesion.

## New FIGO 2018 staging

Previous iterations of the FIGO staging were focussed on clinical diagnosis to allow for low resource countries and settings to provide timely access to care and to be able to compare outcomes based on stage across the world. In previous FIGO staging reviews, stage I included all tumours confined to the cervix (FIGO 1950 and 1971), later sub-dividing stage I into IA (preclinical invasive carcinoma) and IB (FIGO 1974) [10]. In 1985, FIGO divided stage IA into IA1 (minimal microscopically evident stromal invasion) and IA2 (measurable lesions detected microscopically, depth of invasion ≤5 mm and horizontal spread ≤7 mm). This sub-staging was based on the increasing association between tumour size and worse prognosis. In 1994, further expansion of the subcategory was to define stage IA1 as stromal invasion ≤3 mm and horizontal spread ≤7 mm and stage IA2 as stromal invasion >3 mm to ≤5 mm and horizontal spread ≤7 mm. Specifically, 'bulky' stage IB was considered an important prognostic factor in stage I disease with a 90% survival for patients with stage IB in comparison to 50–60% for IB 'bulky' tumours [10]. Therefore, stage IB was divided into IB1 (≤4 cm) and IB2 (>4 cm) and that was the last updated FIGO staging prior to 2018 [11].

The most recent revision to the FIGO staging system for cervical cancer was done in 2018 based on prognostic and clinicopathological factors. This reflects a shift from clinical staging and allows for imaging modalities to describe the size and extent of tumours, including computed tomography (CT), positron emission tomography-CT (PET-CT) and magnetic resonance imaging (MRI). The new guidelines reflect the following changes:

1. To allow the use of imaging and/or pathological assessment of the cervical tumour to designate size and extent for stage I and II
2. To allow lymph node assessment by imaging or pathologic findings. A positive lymph node is designated as a IIIc whereas lymph nodes were not included in previous staging models

A summary of the changes is shown in **Table 15.1**.

**Table 15.1 Summary of changes between the FIGO 2009 and FIGO 2018 staging**

| Stage | | 2009 FIGO definition | 2018 FIGO definition |
|---|---|---|---|
| IA | | Confined to cervix | Confined to cervix |
| | | ≤5 mm deep, ≤7 mm wide | ≤5 mm deep (removal of width criteria) |
| | IA1 | ≤3 mm deep | ≤3 mm deep |
| | IA2 | >3 mm and <5 mm deep | > 3 mm deep and <5 mm deep |
| IB | | >5 mm | >5 mm |
| | IBI | ≤4 cm maximum tumour diameter | ≤2 cm maximum diameter |
| | IB2 | >4 cm tumour diameter | >2 cm and ≤4 cm maximum diameter |
| | IB3 | | >4 cm maximum diameter |
| II | | Unchanged from previous | |
| III | | Lower vaginal, pelvic sidewall and ureter | Lower vaginal, pelvic sidewall and ureter and lymph nodes |
| | IIIA | Lower one-third of vagina | Lower one-third of vagina |
| | IIIB | Pelvic sidewall | Pelvic sidewall |
| | IIIC | | IIIC1: Pelvic lymph nodes<br>IIIC2: Para-aortic lymph nodes |
| IV | | Unchanged from previous | |
| FIGO, International Federation of Gynecology and Obstetrics. | | | |

For the complete FIGO 2018 staging chart, please see the open access journal: https://obgyn.onlinelibrary.wiley.com/doi/full/10.1002/ijgo.12749 [12].

# Stage I

## Stage IA
In the new FIGO guidelines, the description of stage IA no longer includes the lateral extent of the tumour.
- IA1: Measured stromal invasion <3.0 mm
- IA2: Measured stromal invasion ≥3.0 mm and <5.0 mm

This change is to reflect the excellent prognosis of microinvasive cervical cancer and those amenable to a conservative approach (conisation, trachelectomy) rather than a radical hysterectomy (RH). The lateral spread of tumour is no longer included in the microscopic stage IA to reduce the chance of artefactual error [13]. Stage IA disease can be staged only at histopathologic analysis as these tumours are not visible on MRI [14].

## Stage IB
Invasive carcinoma with a measured deepest invasion ≥5.0 mm that is limited to the cervix.
- IB1: Invasive carcinoma ≥5.0 mm depth of invasion and <2.0 cm in greatest dimension
- IB2: Invasive carcinoma ≥2.0 cm and <4.0 cm in greatest dimension
- IB3: Invasive carcinoma ≥4.0 cm in greatest dimension

The new staging adds a third sub-classification of stage IB that is reflective of the significantly lower recurrence rates in patients with stage I tumours <2.0 cm versus tumours 2.0–4.0 cm in greatest dimension. Based on evidence from randomised clinical trials (RCTs), population-based studies and recent propensity matched retrospective studies, tumours >2 cm have had poorer progression free (PFS) and overall survival (OS) when performed by minimally invasive surgery (MIS) [15–19]. In addition, Matsuo et al found that patients with tumours <2 cm had a two-fold increase in survival as compared to larger tumours based on an analysis of the Surveillance, Epidemiology, and End Results (SEER) database [20]. Therefore, more accurate preoperative determination of tumour size is important and may impact staging, treatment planning, and survival. The size of the tumour has traditionally been measured clinically, but this is often subjective and may change between the initial assessment and the time of the surgery. It is estimated that when comparing clinical stage, based on physical examination and final pathology, the concordance diminishes as stage increases: 85.4%, 77.4%, 35.3%, and 20.5% for stage IB1, IB2, IIA, and IIB, respectively [10]. Vaginal involvement and larger tumour diameter are considered the main causes of inaccurate staging. Adequate estimation of tumour size is critical to guide appropriate treatment selection and determine if patients are good candidates for surgical management (conservative or radical) versus primary chemoradiation. Increasing tumour size is also an important prognostic factor and is associated with poorer survival and other clinicopathologic features such as parametrial or lymphovascular invasion. The 5-year survival rate declines from 91.6% (95% CI 90.4–92.6%) for patients with tumours ≤2 cm to 83.3% (95% CI 81.8–84.8%) for tumours >2 to ≤4 cm, and 76.1% (95% CI 74.3–77.8%) for >4 cm tumours [21]. A retrospective review of patients with stage IBI found that primary tumour size >2 cm predicts parametrial invasion ($p < 0.01$) with 13% parametrial involvement (PMI) in patients with tumours >2 cm and 1.3% in those with tumours <2 cm [22].

It is also important to note that while lymphovascular space invasion (LVSI) is a known risk factor for parametrial involvement and lymph node metastasis [23,24], the presence of LVSI does not change the stage but should still be used as a prognostic factor and guide adjuvant treatment decisions. Yan et al retrospectively reviewed patients with early-stage cervical cancer (stage IB-IIA) and identified that the incidence of LVSI was positively associated with the depth of stromal invasion ($p = 0.009$) and lymph node metastasis ($p < 0.001$). LVSI was also found to be an independent factor that affects OS ($p = 0.009$) and PFS ($p = 0.006$) in patients with early-stage cervical cancer [25]. However, in this study patients with LVSI were more likely to receive adjuvant treatment. In addition, a meta-analysis showed that LVSI increased the risk of parametrial involvement more than seven times [26]. Another study found that the presence of LVSI in the conisation specimen was predictive of 51.2% of patients meeting intermediate/high risk criteria on final hysterectomy specimen; compared to only 9.5% without LVSI [27]. Therefore LVSI, though not used for staging purposes, is associated with parametrial invasion and lymph node metastasis and may guide adjuvant treatment decisions.

The extension of tumour into the uterine corpus also does not alter the stage but may impact adjuvant treatment [28]. It is a negative prognostic factor and associated with 53.8% 5-year survival as compared to 92% in patients without uterine extension. In 301 radical hysterectomy specimens, uterine extension was present in 7.8% in stage IB, 25.5% in stage IIA, and 38.2% in stage IIB [29].

## Stage II

The definitions for stage II tumours remain unchanged and include tumours that have extended beyond the uterus into the vagina and parametrium but not to the lower third of the vagina and not reaching the pelvic wall. However, the size of the lesion can now be measured clinically, on imaging, or pathology.

- IIA1: Invasive carcinoma <4.0 cm in greatest dimension
- IIA2: Invasive carcinoma ≥4.0 cm in greatest dimension
- IIB: With parametrial invasion

The use of imaging for assessment of parametrial involvement can be challenging. MRI may perform better than CT imaging for evaluation of parametrium [30]. False-negative and false-positive results have been reported as infection or stretching of the upper vagina due to larger tumour size can confound the results [12].

Colposcopy may be used to assess the extent of vaginal involvement. Examination under anaesthesia may be useful to improve the accuracy of clinical assessment where imaging facilities are lacking.

### Predictors of parametrial involvement

In a retrospective study of 127 women clinically staged to be IB1-IIA2 based on the 2009 FIGO staging, 37 (29.1%) had parametrial involvement determined by surgical pathology [31]. On univariate analysis, endophytic clinical presentation, larger tumour size, LVSI, pathological vaginal invasion, and uterine body involvement were significantly different among the groups with and without parametrial involvement. In multivariate analysis, endophytic tumour (OR 11.34; 95% CI 1.34–95.85; $p = 0.02$) and larger tumour size (OR 32.31; 95% CI 2.46–423.83; $p = 0.008$) were the independent risk factors for PMI. Threshold of 31 mm in tumour size predicted PMI with 71% sensitivity and 75% specificity. 18 patients had a tumour size >30 mm and endophytic presentation; 14 (77.7%) of these had PMI.

## Stage III

- Stage IIIA: Extension to the lower third of the vagina
- Stage IIIB: Extension to the pelvic side wall and/or hydronephrosis or a non-functioning kidney
- Stage IIIC:
  - Stage IIIC1: Pelvic lymph nodes
  - Stage IIIC2: Para-aortic lymph nodes*

The novelty in the FIGO 2018 staging is the inclusion of lymph node status as stage IIIC. This change reflects the fact that presence of pelvic or para-aortic lymph node metastases has poorer survival compared to those who do not have lymph node metastases [32,33]. Lymph nodes can be identified by imaging and then subjected to biopsy to confirm a diagnosis and guide treatment decisions. Imaging can include CT, MRI and PET-CT. The sensitivity of these modalities for detecting nodal metastasis varies from 60% to 88%, with specificity as high as 97%. Alternatively, surgical assessment of lymph nodes by either full pelvic and para-aortic dissection or sentinel lymph node dissection may also be done. Any tumour that would previously be stage I or II with positive lymph nodes is upstaged to a IIIC in the current FIGO staging system to more accurately predict prognosis.

Based on the FIGO guidelines, surgico-pathologic assessment of lymph nodes is the gold standard, in centres where there is access to the required surgical skills and may include sentinel lymph node assessment or full pelvic or para-aortic lymph node dissection.

---

*Can include radiological or pathologic determination of stage.

However, since 85% of cases presently occur in low-resource settings, imaging may be used to assess the status of the lymph nodes to prevent delays in initiation of treatment where access to such advanced surgical techniques might be limited.

One study done after the introduction of the FIGO 2018 guidelines found a significant difference in prognosis when previous stages were upstaged to stage IIIC because of lymph node status. Patients that were upstaged had a significantly worse OS ($p = 0.008$) than patients whose stage did not change. Similar observations were made within sub-stages, when node-positive IB or IIB tumours were upstaged to IIIC [34].

### Presence of isolated tumour cells or micro-metastases

Metastases in lymph nodes are graded as isolated tumour cells (<0.2 mm), micro-metastases (0.2–2.0 mm), or macro-metastases (>2.0 mm). Presence of isolated tumour cells or micro-metastases signifies low volume metastasis and their implication in prognosis and treatment recommendations is unclear. A discussion on isolated tumour cells and micro-metastasis will be done in a different section of this chapter.

## Stage IV

- Stage IVA: Spread to adjacent organs
- Stage IVB: Spread to distant organs

There has been no change to stage IV disease in the new FIGO guidelines. Evaluation of the bladder and rectum by cystoscopy and proctosigmoidoscopy, respectively, is recommended if the patient is symptomatic [12]. Cystoscopy should be considered in cases with a barrel-shaped endocervical growth, extension of growth to the anterior vaginal wall. Histological confirmation should be done to assign the case to stage IV.

### Involvement of ovary

Involvement of the ovary has been reported in <1% of cases of squamous cell carcinoma (SCC) and in <5% of cases of non-squamous cell carcinoma in early-stage cervical cancer. Since it is often associated with the presence of other risk factors, there is limited data on its impact on survival as an independent risk factor and ovarian involvement does not change the stage.

## Validation of the FIGO system

The new FIGO 2018 system has been validated to determine whether the change in staging has led to more accurate predictions of recurrence and survival. Using the National Cancer Database of the American College of Surgeons, a total of 62,212 women with cervical cancer diagnosed between 2004 and 2015 were identified [21]. The 5-year survival in the FIGO 2018 grading scheme was 91.6% (95% CI 90.4–92.6%) for stage IB1 tumours, 83.3% (95% CI 81.8–84.8%) for stage IB2 tumours, and 76.1% (95% CI 74.3–77.8%) for IB3 lesions. In contrast, for women with stage III tumours, a higher FIGO stage was not necessarily associated with worse 5-year survival: stage IIIA (40.7%; 95 CI 37.1–44.3%), stage IIIB (41.4%; 95% CI 39.9–42.9%), stage IIIC1 (positive pelvic nodes) was 60.8% (95% CI 58.7–62.8%) and stage IIIC2 37.5% (95% CI 33.3–41.7%) [21]. Based on this population study, the new FIGO staging system improves predictive accuracy in stage IB, however still does not address the differences in survival due to positive lymph node involvement – possibly due to the previous under-reporting of isolated tumour cells, micro-metastasis and the introduction of sentinel lymph node dissection (SLND) which are discussed in another section of this chapter.

Another study by Matsuo et al confirmed these findings and the validation of the 2018 FIGO staging based on the SEER database between 1998 and 2014 [20]. On multivariable analysis, stage IB2 disease was independently associated with double the risk of cervical cancer mortality compared to stage IB1 disease (adjusted HR 1.98; 95% CI 1.62–2.41; $p < 0.001$). In the stage III cohort ($n = 11,733$), stage IIIC1 was independently associated with improved cause-specific survival compared to stage IIIB disease (adjusted HR 0.79; 95% CI 0.74–0.85; $p < 0.001$).

Data from 662 cervical cancer patients (stages IB and IIA) with surgical risk factors treated at Zhejiang Cancer Hospital between 2008 and 2011 were retrospectively reviewed to determine the prognostic significance of the FIGO 2018 staging [25]. Univariate log-rank test and multivariate Cox regression models were adopted to evaluate the relationship between 2018 FIGO stage and survival [32]. On re-staging of patients, 17.3%, 44.5%, 25.4%, and 37.1% of the patients with FIGO 2009 stage IB1, IB2, IIA1, and IIA2, respectively, were upgraded to FIGO 2018 stage IIIC1, and 2.1%, 3.0%, 3.1%, and 2.1% patients, respectively, were upgraded to stage IIIC2. The 5-year OS of patients with FIGO 2018 stage IB1, IB2, IB3, IIA1, IIA2, IIIC1, and IIIC2 were 95.3%, 95.1%, 90.4%, 92.4%, 86.4%, 81.9%, and 56.3%, respectively. The 5-year PFS rates were 94.0%, 91.0%, 88.5%, 91.4%, 86.4%, 79.5%, and 43.8%, respectively. Therefore the 2018 FIGO staging system for cervical cancer predicted the prognosis of patients with risk factors after radical surgery in that the survival for stage IIA1 patients was better than stage IB3 patients. Stage IIIC1 patients had worse survival depending on the number of positive lymph nodes.

In summary, the new FIGO 2018 guidelines add a more precise staging system reflecting improved imaging modalities, understanding of tumour size as a prognostic factor, incorporation of lymph node dissection and positive nodes as another prognostic factor. This staging system has been validated prospectively and more accurately classifies cervical cancer into prognostic groups based on survival.

## Detection methods

### Cytology

Cervical cytology is routinely used for screening of precancerous lesions in the asymptomatic population. When a clinically sizable mass is found, cytology results will be indeterminate, and a biopsy is preferred. Thus, any visible tumour or ulceration requires punch biopsy or diagnostic LEEP for histologic confirmation. A firm or expanded cervix should also undergo biopsy and endocervical curettage (ECC) as there may be a lesion in the endocervix. Invasive carcinoma on cytology may be seen as malignant cells in a background of debris, blood and inflammatory cells. It may sometimes be possible to differentiate squamous and glandular cells. The false negative rate on cytology for invasive cancer is 50%.

### Human papillomavirus testing

In recent years, co-testing with HPV has been introduced and may increase the detection rate of precancerous lesions. In the United States, HPV testing has been used to triage atypical squamous cells of undetermined significance (ASCUS) cytology in women >30. Co-testing is now accepted as a screening alternative and may be done every 5 years after a negative test, as opposed to 3 years for cytology only. In the ATHENA trial, HPV co-testing was superior to cytology alone for detecting CIN3+ over 3 years. In addition, HPV testing alone could detect 64% of CIN3+ and was the first study to support HPV testing alone [35]. Based on the Kaiser Permanente trial of 1,262,713 women undergoing HPV testing, Demarco et al reported that among HPV-negative women, 5-year risks for CIN 3+ were 0.10% for Negative for Intraepithelial Lesion or Malignancy (NILM), 0.44% for ASCUS, 1.8% for LSIL, 3.0% for ASC-H and 29% for HSIL+ cytology [36]. For HPV-positive women, 5-year risks were 4.0% for NILM, 6.8% for ASC-US, 6.1% for LSIL, 28% for ASC-H, and 50% for HSIL+ cytology [36]. HPV testing may also be used to space out subsequent testing. After 2 negative co-testing results, rates of invasive cervical cancer in a US-based cohort were very low (0.003%; 95% CI 0.002–0.006%) and equal at 3- and 5-year screening intervals [37].

## Colposcopy

Abnormalities seen on cytology are referred to colposcopy according to the American Society of Colposcopy and Cervical Pathology (ASCCP) guidelines [38]. Any clinically suspicious lesion should have immediate punch biopsy. The biopsy should be taken from the most suspicious area, with care to avoid any necrotic areas [8]. When there are no clinical lesions seen, colposcopic-guided biopsies should be performed. Diagnostic LEEP is necessary if malignancy is suspected but is not found with directed cervical biopsies (for instance, some patients with high-grade cervical intraepithelial neoplasia, inadequate colposcopy, and in patients with an endocervical curettage positive for moderate to severe dysplasia) [8] or in cases where the histology and the cytology are discordant.

## Cystoscopy

The new FIGO staging guidelines recommend cystoscopy if the patient is symptomatic, in cases with a barrel-shaped endocervical growth and extension into the anterior vaginal wall [12]. In a study of 100 patients, cystoscopy identified eight patients with bladder invasion including 1 stage IIIA, 2 stage IIIB, and 5 stage IV [39]. All patients had CT indication of possible invasion. There were two false positives on CT proven by cystoscopic biopsy. Both the sensitivity and the negative predictive value of CT for bladder invasion were 100%. In another study, the sensitivity, specificity, positive predictive value, negative predictive value, and accuracy of the CT scan for bladder invasion were 100%, 92%, 40%, 100%, and 92%, respectively [40]. Of 305 cases, 14% had evidence of bladder invasion on CT among which 40% were histologically proven by cystoscopy. In light of these results, cystoscopy may be indicated in cases where CT identifies invasion into the bladder but should not be used routinely in absence of suspicion of bladder invasion [39,41].

## Proctosigmoidoscopy

Proctosigmoidoscopy is only recommended if the patient is symptomatic [12]. In one study of 103 patients, proctoscopy failed to reveal metastatic cervical adenocarcinoma and thus not done routinely in absence of clinical suspicion of rectal invasion as confirmed by other studies [42,43].

## Imaging studies

In most high-income countries, pre-treatment imaging to assess tumour size, involvement of adjacent structures and nodal disease has become standard of care. According to the National Comprehensive Cancer Network (NCCN) guidelines 2.0, pelvic MRI, chest radiography and/or chest/abdominal/pelvic CT, or whole-body PET-CT in the primary diagnostic work-up is recommended to assess local tumour extent and metastatic spread and the choice of imaging modality depends on what element is being assessed [44]. The following section will review the pre-treatment imaging modalities and its role in the work up of cervical cancer.

## Magnetic resonance imaging (Figure 15.1)

It has typically been viewed as the imaging modality of choice for cervical cancer as it can accurately detect the size of the tumour, involvement of the parametrium and/or adjacent structures (bladder, rectum) in addition to lymph node metastasis, which has been recently added to the staging system [30]. The high soft tissue contrast resolution of MRI makes it the preferred modality in local staging of cervical cancer [35]. In a multi-centre study, the overall accuracy of staging increased from 61% to 81.4% after combining clinical

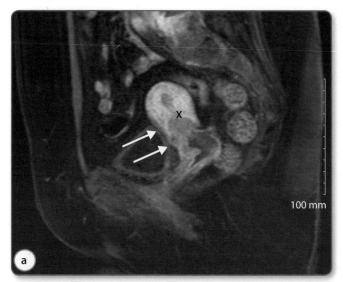

**Figure 15.1** (a) A 86-year-old woman presenting with vaginal bleeding and a cervical mass. Sagittal T1-weighted gadolinium study of the pelvis shows extension of the tumour into the lower uterine segment (callipers) while maintaining the fat plane between the tumour and the bladder (arrows). (b) The sagittal T2-weighted MRI shows the extension of the tumour into the vaginal wall anteriorly (arrow).

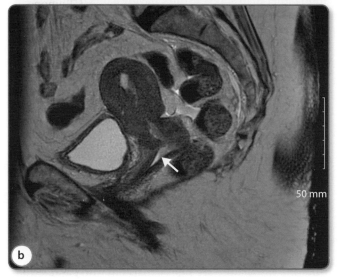

findings with MRI [45]. Clinical staging particularly underestimates tumour size if there is endocervical tumour growth (endogenous type). This section will review MRI technique and performance on tumour size, parametrial invasion and adjacent structures.

## MRI technique
The standard MRI protocol for imaging of the pelvis for cervical cancer includes axial T1-weighted fast spin-echo (FSE) images with a large field of view to evaluate the entire pelvis and upper abdomen for lymphadenopathy and bone marrow abnormalities; high-resolution T2-weighted FSE images in the axial and sagittal planes to evaluate the primary tumour; and dynamic fat-saturated contrast-enhanced 3-dimensional (3D) dynamic T1-weighted images (small field of view) in the sagittal planes to evaluate the extent of myometrial and cervical involvement [30]. High-resolution T2-weighted FSE sequences perpendicular to the long-axis of the uterine corpus are favoured for evaluation of the primary tumour and parametrial invasion [46]. Thin-section 3-mm to 5-mm oblique axial T2-weighted images provide great detail of the cervix and are able to assess parametrial invasion more accurately than the axial T2-weighted images.

Gadolinium contrast may help visualise small tumours and can make it easier to evaluate urinary bladder or vaginal invasion [30]. The tumour extent, including involvement of the lower uterine segment, fistulae, as well as recurrent tumour after therapy, are better defined with contrast. Some authors also argue that contrast enhanced MRI is of utmost value for small lesions, in patients with post-cervical cancer treatment and surgical planning in fertility sparing treatment in addition to distinguishing between an endometrial and cervical primary [46]. In one review, the sensitivity, specificity and accuracy of conventional MRI on tumour size >4 cm was 81%, 95%, 93% respectively, for deep stromal invasion: 89%, 88% and 88%, for parametrial invasion: 40–74%, 77–98%, 70–97% and for lymph node metastasis 37–60%, 92–93% respectively and will be reviewed individually in the next sections of this chapter [47].

## Size of tumour
Determining the size of tumour is crucial in treatment planning as size over 4 cm upstages to IB3 and warrants chemoradiation rather than surgery. Thus, having a precise imaging modality in addition to clinical examination is necessary. Pre-treatment MRI has been found to have good tumour size agreement with post-surgical pathologic findings (agreement 0.855; 95% CI 0.76–0.91) but the performance on assessing size post-treatment is less reliable (agreement 0.503; 95% CI 0.42–0.58). For fertility sparing, MRI has high accuracy in providing distance of the tumour free margin to the internal os, which is important for treatment planning [48]. Recently, a deep learning neural network was used to detect cervical cancer based on T2 weighted images; the neural network model created based on a set of 177 cervical cancer patients and 241 non-patients had a sensitivity of 88%, specificity of 93% and accuracy of 91% while the blinded radiologists had a 78.3–86.7% sensitivity, 91.7–95% specificity, and accuracy of 86.7–89.2% [49]. This shows how machine learning may evolve to more accurately detect cervical tumours in pre-treatment planning.

## Parametrial involvement
Magnetic resonance imaging has a high negative predictive value (94–100%) for parametrial invasion, but the sensitivity is low and varies between 38% and 100% [50]. Disruption of the stromal ring, obliteration of peri-uterine fat planes, encasement of the ureters, and involvement of peri-uterine vasculature are signs consistent with parametrial

invasion. An additional diffusion weighted imaging (DWI) sequence may also add to the precision in evaluation of parametrial involvement, increasing the sensitivity and specificity (82% and 97%, respectively) compared with MRI without DWI sequences (72% and 91%, respectively) [51]. One meta-analysis has shown that MRI is significantly more sensitive in the assessment of parametrial invasion than clinical examination under anaesthesia [42]. However, accurate depiction of PMI on MRI relies on adequately planned images perpendicular to the long axis of the cervix; it can be over or underestimated. In a retrospective study of 1,347 patients with stage IB1–IIA2 cervical cancer who underwent radical hysterectomy, 10.2% had pathological parametrial invasion [43]. Maximal tumour diameter (OR 2; $p$ <0.001) and MRI presence of PMI (OR 7.0; $p$ <0.001) were predictive of pathologic risk factors. However, if patients had low risk factors including maximal tumour diameter <2.5 cm and no PMI on MRI, then the rate of pathologic PMI decreased to 1.3%. Other studies also confirm the higher risk of parametrial involvement with increasing tumour size [22,52,53]. The use of MRI for determination of size is of utmost importance with the new FIGO staging as IB2 and IB3 tumours are less amenable to a surgical approach and more likely require chemoradiation.

## Adjacent structures (vagina/bladder/rectum)

For detection of vaginal disease, MRI accuracy has been reported as 86–93% and is defined as the replacement of low signal intensity of the vaginal tissue by high-signal-intensity tumour [54]. Large exophytic tumours extending into the vaginal canal often limit evaluation of the vaginal wall but can be improved using endo-vaginal gel. In addition, loss of the normal low T2-weighted signal intensity of the vaginal wall that is contiguous with the primary cervical tumour mass is indicative of vaginal involvement [7]. When a tumour extends from the cervix into the vagina but does not invade it, a rim of high T2-weighted signal intensity surrounding the mass improves the radiologist's confidence that the vagina is not involved. The vaginal wall should be depicted in its entirety in at least two orthogonal planes. Assessment of involvement of the upper two-thirds of the vagina is often overestimated at MRI especially in the vaginal fornices. Local extension of tumour to the bladder can be evaluated using MRI with a sensitivity of 83% and specificity of 100% [46]. Mucosal invasion of the bladder must be present for the tumour to be classified as stage IV disease, as there is significantly worse prognosis compared to serosal or muscular invasion only [55]. Superficial involvement including, loss of the normal fat plane between the cervix and the bladder or rectum, or the tumour breaches the normal low T2-weighted signal intensity of the bladder or bowel serosa but does not invade into the lumen is not included as stage IV but should still be reported on MRI [56]. MRI findings that suggest bladder invasion include nodular and irregular bladder wall, tumour protruding into the bladder lumen, and high signal intensity of the anterior aspect of the posterior wall of the bladder on T2-weighted images [57]. Suspected bladder or rectal involvement should be confirmed by biopsy with cystoscopy or proctoscopy before assigning stage IVA [13]. Presence of a vesico-vaginal fistula is diagnostic for bladder wall invasion. Rectal invasion by cervical cancer is less common than bladder invasion but carries a worse prognosis [46].

## Lymph node involvement

The specificity of MRI for metastatic lymph nodes (LNs) in cervical cancer has been reported to be 71–100%, but the sensitivity remains low (38–56%) [58]. One explanation is possibly the presence of micro-metastases that are too small to be seen on MRI. The use of lymph node specific contrast agent based on ultrasmall particles of iron oxide (USPIO) has been shown to dramatically improve the diagnostic performance of MRI for the detection of metastatic lymph nodes in uterine cancer with reported sensitivity of 91–100%, specificity of 87–94% and accuracy of 88–95% [47]. To date however, PET-CT more accurately detects nodal metastasis and thus MRI is not commonly used for this purpose.

### MRI as criteria for less invasive surgery

One study used MRI criteria for no residual disease on post conisation MRI to determine whether patients with stage IB1 had low risk of parametrial involvement and thus could undergo a simple hysterectomy [59]. They retrospectively analysed 125 stage IB1 patients who had an MRI followed by a radical hysterectomy. Patients were classified into two groups: MRI invisible tumour and MRI visible tumour. The rate of parametrial involvement in this population was 5.6%; the MRI criteria identified 59.2% of candidates for less radical surgery, among which only one had pathologic criteria of parametrial involvement. Patients with MRI visible tumours also had significantly lower PFS, all patients with MRI invisible tumour were alive at 100 months follow-up compared to 80% in MRI visible tumours.

## Positron emission tomography-computed tomography (Figure 15.2)

Positron emission tomography-computed tomography simultaneously combines two imaging techniques, to visualise both morphologic and metabolic tumour characteristics, thus allowing definition of structural and functional data in fused images [47]. The most commonly used radiotracer is fluorodeoxyglucose (18-FDG), which is a glucose analogue that accumulates in malignant tissue. PET has limited spatial resolution and thus is not commonly used for assessment of primary cervical tumour. For the detection of pelvic lymph node metastases, FDG PET-CT yields a slightly lower diagnostic performance than sentinel node biopsy but performs better than MRI, CT and US and is therefore the non-invasive modality of choice for patients at high risk of metastatic disease [10,60,61]. The reported sensitivities and specificities of FDG PET-CT in the detection of lymph node metastases are 72–75% and 93–100% respectively [60,62].

The metabolic activity within the primary tumour, as measured by maximum standardised uptake value ($SUV_{max}$), has been shown in many studies to be a prognostic indicator in patients with cervical cancer [63]. Yagi et al found that patients with higher $SUV_{max}$ tumours have lower OS and PFS. These higher $SUV_{max}$ tumours are also associated with LN metastases, advanced stage, LVSI, and larger tumours [64]. Using ROC curves, the optimal cut-off values of the $SUV_{max}$ for predicting tumour sizes of ≥20 mm and ≥40 mm were 4.71 and 9.66, respectively, with relatively high sensitivity and specificity, and there was a significant correlation between the $SUV_{max}$ and tumour size. In addition, multivariate analysis demonstrated that a high $SUV_{max}$ in the primary tumour was an independent prognostic factor for impaired PFS (HR 3.947; $p = 0.011$) among the variables including FIGO stage, LN metastasis, LVSI, tumour size and histological subtype. Similarly, a high $SUV_{max}$ was an independent factor for predicting impaired PFS when analysed in stage IB patients alone (HR 4.851; $p = 0.026$) [64]. Yang and colleagues found that PET-CT better evaluates the depth of cervical stromal invasion than conventional methods using $SUV_{max} = 7.83$ or MTV = 8.76 mL and may allow for better treatment planning [65].

Most importantly, PET-CT is the best modality for detection of distant metastatic disease. In a the ACRIN 6671/GOG 0233 multi-centre trial, FDG PET-CT had high specificity (98%), positive predictive value (79%) and sensitivity of 55% for detecting distant

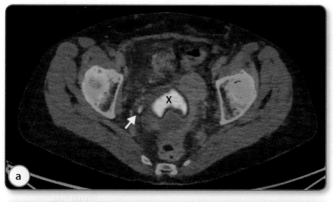

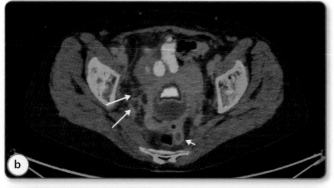

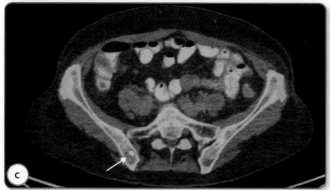

**Figure 15.2** (a) PET scan uptake within a primary cervical cancer (callipers) in a 65-year-old woman which was identified to be a 2.4 × 2.0 × 2.3 cm tumour on the MRI. However, the PET shows extension into the right parametrial space (arrowhead). (b) The PET scan goes on to show further involvement of the pelvic lymph nodes (arrows) and a meso-rectal node (arrowhead). The MRI did not identify the presence of any suspicious pelvic lymph nodes. (c) Bone metastases were also identified with FDG uptake in the right iliac bone posteriorly (arrow).

metastases (non-regional lymph nodes, lesions in the peritoneum, bone, liver, and lung) in patients with locoregional advanced cervical cancer [66]. In addition, unexpected distant metastases were diagnosed in 14% of patients with locoregional advanced cervical cancer [66]. Thus, the use of FDG PET-CT, particularly in high-risk cervical cancer patients, would potentially benefit patients by enabling more tailored therapy, reducing the unnecessary need for aggressive procedures in patients not eligible for curative therapy [47].

For locally advanced cervical cancer, a randomised control trial was done to assess performance of PET-CT; patients were randomised 2:1 to either PET-CT in addition to a CT scan [67]. Patients in the PET-CT group (39.3%) received more extensive radiation treatment or palliative treatment compared with the CT group, (39.3% vs. 25.0%; OR 2.05; 95% CI 0.96–4.37; $p = 0.06$). More patients in the PET-CT group (21.4%) received extended field radiotherapy to para-aortic nodes and 14 (12.5%) to common iliac nodes compared with 8 (14.3%) and 3 (5.4%), respectively, in the CT group (OR 1.64; 95% CI). Therefore, in locally advanced cervical cancer, PET-CT allowed detection and treatment of nodal disease that would otherwise have been missed with traditional CT. One recent study assessed PET-CT and SLN for detection of lymph node metastasis, the study included 36 patients of which 28 had pre-operative PET: the sensitivity, specificity, positive predictive value, negative predictive value (NPV), and accuracy of $^{18}$F-FDG PET/CT were 40.0%, 78.3%, 28.6%, 85.7%, and 71.4%, respectively [68]. In addition, PET-CT was able to prompt a change in treatment in one-third of patients by altering treatment or a radiation therapy plan in those already scheduled for radiation therapy.

Therefore, PET-CT and particularly the SUV has a role in pre-operative planning of early localised cervical cancer and can identify metastatic disease in high-risk patients. Current recommendations for pre-operative use are in patients with stage IB1 disease or greater who are eligible for surgical treatment and in patients with stage II–IVA disease to help assess for nodal and distant metastatic disease [44,69]. There is a minimal role of PET-CT for early cervical cancer amenable to surgery, as the risk of LN metastasis is so low and micro-metastasis would be too small to pick up with PET. One of the pitfalls of PET-CT is that physiologic FDG uptake within the bladder, ureters, or bowel may mask sites of disease or be mistaken for pathologic uptake. The ovaries and endometrium may demonstrate physiologic FDG uptake during ovulation and menstruation, thus mimicking disease [56].

## Computed tomography

It is the least commonly used imaging modality in cervical cancer. The poor ability of detecting soft tissue contrast is a limitation in evaluation of early cervical cancer; 50% of cervical cancers are isodense to the adjacent stroma and cannot be properly delineated [46,70]. When a tumour can be visualised, it is usually an ill-defined hypodense lesion within the cervix. However, CT has very low sensitivity for detecting small tumours and varies between 32% and 80% [71]. The accuracy of detection of cervical tumours with CT is not commonly reported in the literature as it is much lower than MRI and PET-CT [72]. For parametrial invasion, accuracy is estimated to be at 55%, which is less than with MRI, but in studies including early stage disease, accuracy can be as high as 94%, similar to MRI [72,73]. For lymph node detection, a size cut-off between 0.8 and 1.0 cm is usually required and detection is improved with the presence of necrosis, but performance is lower than PET/CT. In addition, detection of micro-metastasis and isolated tumour cells would not be feasible with CT [74]. Other studies report that in locally advanced cervical cancer or in early-stage disease with suspicious lymph nodes on pelvic MRI or transvaginal/transrectal ultrasound, contrast-enhanced CT of the thorax, abdomen, and pelvis is widely employed as primary diagnostic work-up for the detection of LN metastases and distant spread [47]. Aside from its use in depicting suspicious lymph nodes, contrast material–enhanced CT plays an important role in depicting stage IIIB–IVB disease, with 92% accuracy for ureteric, pelvic sidewall, bladder, and rectal involvement and depiction of distant metastases [75]. There is significant overlap between the performance of PET-CT and conventional CT in the detection of nodal disease and therefore the new ESGO-ESTRO-ESP guideline recommends CT or PET-CT for assessment of nodal and distant disease in locally advanced cervical cancer, whereas PET-CT is preferred in patients eligible for chemoradiotherapy with curative intent [69].

## Enhanced recovery after surgery protocols

Another important aspect of locally advanced cervical cancer management is the implementation of Enhanced Recovery after Surgery (ERAS) protocol in patients that are surgical candidates. Given the important change in management favouring laparotomy, the value of ERAS protocols is further heightened to improve postoperative outcomes, increase return to baseline function and decrease length of stay (LOS) compared to historical cohorts undergoing abdominal radical hysterectomy (ARH). Pre-operatively, patients need to be counselled about ERAS, encouraged for smoking cessation, weight loss if possible, diabetes control and correction of anaemia [76]. Oral intake should be tolerated up to 4 hours pre-operatively with fluids up to 2 hours; some centres advocate for carb-loading. In addition, pre-operative analgesia and anti-emetic may be given in the holding bay prior to surgery to improve postoperative outcomes.

# TREATMENT

## Management algorithms (Table 15.2)

### Stage IA1 microinvasive (<3 mm depth, no LVSI), non-fertility sparing

If margins from the initial cone biopsy and endocervical curettage are negative, stage IA1 tumours can be treated with cone biopsy or extra-fascial hysterectomy. The new NCCN guidelines recommend cone biopsy for stage IA1 without LVSI [77]. If the margins are negative and the patient is inoperable due to other medical issues, observation is recommended. Extra-fascial hysterectomy is warranted for operable patients. If there are positive margins on cone biopsy, either repeat the cone biopsy to evaluate the depth of invasion or extra-fascial/modified RH and pelvic lymph node (PLN) assessment.

This group of patients has <5% risk of LN metastases or relapse and has been managed by surgical techniques ranging from cold knife conisation to RH with a near 100% rate of disease control [78]. Postsurgical confirmation of LVSI in a conisation specimen may be an indication for definitive hysterectomy, completion parametrectomy and lymphadenectomy [68]. However, *LVSI is very uncommon in stage IA1.*

For non-operable stage IA1, intracavitary brachytherapy offers a 97% disease control rate and may be a good option.

### Stage IA1 microinvasive (<3 mm depth, no LVSI) fertility sparing

For stage IA1 without LVSI, a cone biopsy with negative margins is preferable. If the margins of the cone biopsy are positive, the cone can be repeated or a trachelectomy can be performed [77].

### Stage IA1 with LVSI and stage IA2, non-fertility sparing

Patients with stage IA and LVSI have a 5–13% risk of pelvic lymph node metastasis. The risk of parametrial involvement is low, especially with a negative sentinel lymph node but has been reported up to 11% in some studies [59]. Parametrial invasion remains a surgical planning concern in stage IA2 patients, as even limited parametrial invasion confers a 43% risk for nodal metastases. Some question the need for a complete RH and suggest a simple hysterectomy could be adequate treatment for these patients. An analysis of the SEER database on 1,567 patients revealed no difference in survival between local excision, simple hysterectomy and RH. For stage IA1, survival was 96.6%, 98.4% and 96.5% following

| **Table 15.2 Summary of new NCCN guidelines 2020** | | | |
|---|---|---|---|
| Stage | Treatment goal | Primary treatment | After surgical findings |
| Stage IA1 no LVSI | Non-fertility sparing | Cone:<br>Negative margins:<br>• Inoperable-observe<br>• Operable-extrafascial hysterectomy<br>Positive margins:<br>• Repeat cone or<br>• Extrafascial or modified radical trachelectomy if margins + carcinoma | Node/-margin/-parametrium:<br>• Observation<br>versus<br>• Pelvic EBRT ± chemoradiotherapy if Sedlis criteria |
| | Fertility sparing | Cone biopsy with negative margins | +nodes/+margin/+parametrium:<br>1. EBRT + chemotherapy ± vaginal brachytherapy |
| Stage 1A1 LVSI and stage IA2 | Non fertility sparing | Modified RH+ PLND<br>OR<br>Pelvic EBRT or brachytherapy | |
| | Fertility sparing | • Cone with negative margins + margins – repeat cone or do trachelectomy + PLND<br>or<br>• Radical trachelectomy + PLND | +Para-aortic node: No distant metastases: EBRT, chemotherapy, brachytherapy<br>Distant metastases: Systemic chemotherapy + individualised EBRT |
| Stage IB1/IB2 | Non fertility sparing | • Radical hysterectomy + PLND ± PaLND<br>• Pelvic EBRT + brachytherapy ± concurrent chemo | |
| | Fertility sparing | Radical trachelectomy + PLND + PaLND | |
| Stage IB3/IIA2 | Non-fertility sparing | • Definitive pelvic EBRT + concurrent chemotherapy + brachytherapy<br>• Radical hysterectomy + PLND ± para-aortic node<br>• Pelvic EBRT + concurrent chemotherapy +brachytherapy + adjuvant hysterectomy | |
| | Fertility sparing | Not recommended | |

EBRT, external beam radiation therapy; LVSI, lymphovascular space invasion; NCCN, National Comprehensive Cancer Network; PaLND, para-aortic lymph node dissection; PLND, pelvic lymph node dissection.

excision, hysterectomy and radical hysterectomy, respectively. For stage IA2, survival rates were 100%, 96.9% and 99.4%, respectively [79]. Another large study including 842 patients with clinical stage IA1/2 and IB1 cervical cancer were reviewed to determine parametrial involvement [80]. Thirty-three patients (4%) had pathologic invasion, eight in those with positive lymph nodes and 25 in those that had malignant cells in the parametrial tissue. Parametrial invasion was associated with older age (42 vs. 40 years; $p < 0.04$), larger tumour size (2.2 cm vs. 1.8 cm; $p < 0.04$), higher incidence of LVSI (85% vs. 45%; $p = 0.0004$), tumour grades 2 and 3 (95% vs. 65%; $p = 0.001$), greater depth of invasion (18.0 mm vs. 5.0 mm; $p < 0.001$), and pelvic lymph node metastases (44% vs. 5%; $p < 0.0001$). The incidence of parametrial involvement in patients with tumour size <2 cm, negative pelvic lymph nodes, and depth of invasion ≤10 mm was 0.6%, suggesting a possibility of less radical hysterectomy in these select patients. Currently, the NCCN recommends modified RH and PLN assessment or pelvic external beam radiation therapy (EBRT) and brachytherapy as a middle ground for these patients.

## Stage IA1 with LVSI and stage IA2 fertility sparing

Cone biopsy or radical trachelectomy may be considered in fertility sparing options in addition to pelvic lymph node dissection (PLND). If the margins of the cone biopsy are positive, a repeat cone is indicated: if the margins are again positive then an immediate RH and PLND are indicated. If the repeat cone margins are negative, RH but should be delayed 6 weeks to allow tissue reactions to subside [77].

Radical trachelectomy may be a fertility-sparing surgical option but must be completed with a lymph node assessment to exclude nodal metastasis. If no nodal metastases are identified, a trachelectomy is performed, the uterus and vagina are connected and a cerclage is placed. This is reserved for young women with tumours <4 cm.

## Stage IB1/IB2/IIA1

The non-fertility sparing treatment options include:
- RH, PLND, ± para-aortic lymph node dissection (PaLND) and consideration of sentinel lymph node dissection (SLND)
- Pelvic EBRT, brachytherapy ± concurrent chemotherapy

The survival outcomes between radical primary surgery or radiation are similar: 83–92% for surgery and 83–91% after primary radiation [81]. Therefore, the decision relies on patient factors including age, tumour features and clinical patterns of recurrence.

## Stage IB1 lesion <2 cm/IB2

These are the ideal candidates for RH +P LND, ± PaLND. Surgical treatment is curative and guides adjuvant treatment if the lymph nodes are positive. The 5-year survival after surgery ranges from 83% to 92%.
- If the lymph nodes are found to be positive at the time of the surgery, there needs to be a discussion as to proceeding with surgery versus aborting and providing primary chemoradiation. The operative risk is higher than the benefit as the patient will require postoperative radiation and local control can be achieved through primary chemoradiation. However, the dose and toxicity of adjuvant radiation is less than for primary chemoradiation and may be beneficial in a young, sexually active patient. Disadvantages of a completion hysterectomy include delays in starting chemoradiotherapy, increased morbidity and duplication of treatment providing local control. In addition, an in-situ uterus allows access for intracavitary brachytherapy. In the Landoni trial, patients with stage IB-IIA were randomised to primary surgery or radiation; in patients with tumours <4 cm, the 5-year DFS was 80% with surgery and 82% with primary radiation, therefore consideration for the least morbid procedure should be made given no difference in survival [81]
- Postoperative surgical specimen stage IB1 node negative but intermediate risk factors based on Sedlis criteria (**Table 15.3**): Adjuvant radiotherapy given to patients who have two out of the three of the Sedlis criteria prevents pelvic relapse [82]. This is based on evidence from the following trial: patients with node negative but high-risk features (more than one-third deep stromal invasion, capillary LVSI, and tumour diameter of 4 cm) were randomised to receive adjuvant pelvic radiation (RT) or observation alone. The RT arm showed a 46% reduction in risk of recurrence [hazard ratio (HR) 0.54; 90% CI 0.35–0.81; $p = 0.007$] and a statistically significant reduction in risk of progression or death (HR 0.58; 90% CI 0.40–0.85; $p = 0.009$). Only 8.8% of patients receiving RT recurred

### Table 15.3 Sedlis Criteria

| LVSI | Stromal Invasion | Tumour size |
|------|------------------|-------------|
| + | Deep 1/3 | Any |
| + | Middle 1/3 | ≥ 2 cm |
| + | Superficial 1/3 | ≥5 cm |
| − | Middle or deep 1/3 | ≥4 cm |

LVSI, lymphovascular space invasion.

compared to 44.0% in the observation arm, supporting the benefit of adjuvant radiation in patients meeting these pathologic criteria [82]

- Postoperative stage IB1 with high-risk features: Indications for adding concurrent chemotherapy to adjuvant radiation include positive lymph nodes, parametrial invasion, or positive surgical margins (Peter's Criteria). Oncologic outcomes are improved in patients receiving concurrent chemoradiation ± vaginal brachytherapy. This is based on a randomised control trial comparing radiation only versus chemoradiation in patients with stage IA2, IB, and IIA initially treated with radical hysterectomy and pelvic lymphadenectomy, and who had positive pelvic lymph nodes and/or positive margins and/or microscopic involvement of the parametrium [83]. The survival was improved in patients receiving concomitant chemotherapy and radiation. The HR for PFS and OS in the RT only arm versus the RT + chemotherapy arm are 2.01 ($p = 0.003$) and 1.96 ($p = 0.007$), respectively. The projected PFS and OS at 4 years was 63% and 71% with RT and 80% and 81% with RT + chemotherapy [84]. A sub-analysis of this study found that the absolute improvement in 5-year survival for adjuvant chemotherapy in patients with tumours 2 cm was only 5% (77% vs. 82%), while for those with tumours >2 cm was 19% (58% vs. 77%) [85]. Similarly, the absolute 5-year survival benefit was less among patients with one nodal metastasis (79% vs. 83%) than when at least two nodes were positive (55% vs. 75%)

d. If the para-aortic nodes are positive, imaging should be done for metastatic disease including a PET-CT scan. If the imaging is negative for distant metastases, extended field EBRT and concurrent platinum containing chemotherapy and brachytherapy should be done. If there are possible distant metastases on imaging, a biopsy is suggested to prove involvement and systemic therapy ± individualised EBRT may be necessary

## Fertility sparing for stage IB1/IB2: Radical trachelectomy and pelvic lymph node dissection and para-aortic lymph node dissection (consider SLND)

Fertility sparing surgery has only been studied in patients with tumours <2 cm. Small cell, neuroendocrine and adenoma malignum are not suitable for fertility sparing treatment given the aggressive nature of these histologic subtypes. For adequate candidates, the fertility sparing approach is radical trachelectomy, PLND ± PaLND, with consideration of SLND.

One prospective trial, the CONTESSA study is currently enrolling patients with FIGO stage IB2 tumours 2–4 cm and desire for fertility sparing treatment to receive neoadjuvant chemotherapy for 3 cycles followed by radical trachelectomy, with plan to complete accrual of 90 patients by 2022 [86].

## Stage IB3 and IIA2

For patients with tumours >4 cm, the 5-year disease-free survival was 57% after radiation and 63% after surgery in the Landoni trial [81].
There are three options for these patients [77]:
1. Definitive pelvic EBRT + concurrent chemotherapy + brachytherapy
2. RH, PLND ± PaLND and tailored adjuvant radiation
3. Pelvic EBRT+ concurrent chemotherapy + brachytherapy + adjuvant hysterectomy

## Primary chemoradiation for stage IB3

This is the preferred treatment which leads to increased survival but increased morbidity. There is a correlation between tumour size and outcome: 10-year DFS of 90% in stage IB <2 cm, 76% 2–4 cm, 61% 4.1–5 cm, and 47% >5 cm. Bulky tumours require aggressive radiation and lead to high complication rates (mostly fistulas).

## Primary radical hysterectomy + postoperative tailored radiation

Older patients tolerate radical surgery better than radiation.
Advantages of primary surgery include:
- Accurate staging
- *Resection of bulky nodes:* Improves prognosis
- *Removal of primary cancer:* Avoids determining whether there it is viable residual disease
- Preservation of ovarian function

The risk of adjuvant chemoradiation will be elevated and the patient will have to be counselled in terms of the complications for each procedure and the side effects of radiotherapy.

Primary surgery is treatment of choice in patients with acute or chronic pelvic inflammatory disease or issues making primary radiation difficult.

## Neoadjuvant chemoradiation followed by adjuvant hysterectomy

The role of adjuvant hysterectomy after chemoradiation is unclear and is complicated by increased fibrosis from radiation and is not often used. Neoadjuvant chemotherapy may be considered an option but did not gain widespread use and is not an option in the NCCN guidelines. However, in patients with cervical cancer diagnosed during pregnancy, neoadjuvant chemotherapy is the treatment of choice in the second and third trimesters with completion radical caesarean hysterectomy at fetal lung maturity, generally at 34 weeks [7].

## Technical aspects of cervical cancer treatment

### Cone biopsy

Cervical conisation can be performed using 'cold-knife conisation' or LEEP. These procedures are reserved for treatment of stage IA1/LVSI with a desire for fertility sparing techniques and in cases of adenocarcinoma in-situ. It is also used for diagnostic purposes when determining which further treatment strategies will be needed in the initial diagnosis of a cervical cancer. Cold knife conisation is less commonly performed and mostly reserved for cases involving the endocervix or adenocarcinoma in situ, since this requires operating room resources with regional or general anaesthesia and has widely been replaced with LEEP. In a cold knife conisation, stay sutures are generally placed at the 3 o'and 9 o'clock positions at the cervicovaginal junction but this can be the surgeon's preference. These sutures can be used to help and create traction on the cervix and decrease bleeding. Injection of 5–10 mL of a premixed solution of local anaesthesia and epinephrine at a concentration of 1:100,000 is done into the stroma of the ectocervix circumferentially around the os. Using a #11 blade, the cone can be gradually developed and carved around the lesion to the necessary dimensions. Care should be taken to maintain the integrity of the specimen and avoid fragmentation, which may make pathologic assessment of margins more challenging. A suture should be placed at the 12 O'clock position of the specimen to help with pathologic orientation. Following the cone, the remaining endocervical canal is curetted with a Kevorkian curette. The stay sutures can be used to tie a piece of oxidised cellulose in place which the patient should be warned will pass about 1–2 weeks following the procedure. Alternatively, haemostasis can be achieved with Bovie cautery at 40 W ball electrode and Monsel's paste.

In a LEEP procedure, bipolar electrocautery is used with a cautery tip wire loop that is in a circular shape of different sizes, allowing tailoring of the procedure to the cervical mass. The LEEP can be done in a properly equipped colposcopy clinic under local anaesthesia.

## Radical hysterectomy

It consists of en-bloc excision of the uterus and cervix with the parametrium which includes the round, broad, cardinal, and utero-sacral ligaments and the upper one-third to one-half of the vagina. The procedure requires thorough knowledge of pelvic anatomy, meticulous attention, and careful technique to allow dissection of the ureters and mobilisation of both bladder and rectum from the vagina in areas that are prone to bleeding due to increased tumour vascularity; particularly within the vasculature of the pelvic side walls and the venous plexuses at the lateral corners of the bladder where excessive blood loss may be encountered.

## Types of hysterectomy EORTC-GCG classification

1. *Extra-fascial or simple hysterectomy:* In a simple hysterectomy, the uterine arteries are transected just hugging the cervix, the utero-sacral and cardinal ligaments are taken at this level too. No parametrial tissue is obtained. The ureter is identified but a complete ureterolysis is not carried out. This procedure is warranted for adenocarcinoma in situ, pre-invasive squamous cancer and microinvasive IA1. In another commonly used classification, Querleu and Morrow, this is a type A hysterectomy

2. *Type II modified RH (**Figure 15.3**):* The uterine artery is transected where it crosses the ureter. The cardinal ligament is transected at the medial ½ and the proximal uterosacral is transected. The advantage of a modified RH is to remove as much parametrial tissue while maintaining perfusion to the distal ureter and bladder. The ureters are freed from their paracervical position but are not dissected out of the pubo-vesical ligament in the Wertheim classification, while the EORTC-GCG classification has the ureters dissected to their entry into the bladder. The uterine artery is ligated medially to the ureter as it lies in 'the tunnel'. The utero-sacral ligaments are transected midway between the uterus and the sacral attachment. The medial halves of both cardinal ligaments are removed, as is the upper 1–2 cm of the vagina. A type II modified RH is acceptable for cases of microinvasive carcinomas and in postradiation recurrences limited to the cervix. This is very similar to the type B, Querleu and Morrow classification, in which the ureters are unroofed and dissected laterally so that the paracervical tissue can be transected at

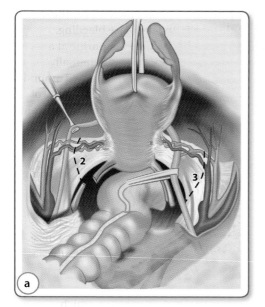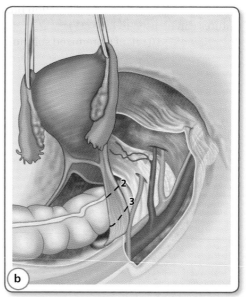

**Figure 15.3** Boundaries of a radical hysterectomy. (a) Dotted lines to identify a type II and a type III transection of the cardinal ligament. (b) Dotted lines to identify a type II and type III transection of the uterosacral ligament.

the level of the ureteral tunnel. Type B1 does not remove the lateral paracervical lymph nodes while type B2 does

3. *Type III RH (**Figure 15.3**):* This is the most common procedure for stage IB tumours. This consists of a wide excision of the parametrial and paravaginal tissue. The uterine artery is dissected and ligated at the source of the superior vesical artery/internal iliac artery. When the ureter is dissected off the pubo-vesical ligament (between the lower end of the ureter and the superior vesical artery), care must be taken to preserve the ligament in order to provide additional blood supply to the distal ureter and lower the risk of fistula formation by preserving the superior vesical artery. The utero-sacral ligaments are transected at the sacrum and the cardinal ligament is transected at the pelvic sidewall. The upper one-third of the vagina is excised. The Querleu and Morrow classification relates this as a type C hysterectomy but further divides the technique into C1 as nerve sparing and C2 as not

4. *Type IV extended RH:* This consists of the complete removal of the peri-ureteral tissue. The ureter is completely dissected from vesico-uterine peritoneum, the superior vesical artery is sacrificed and three-fourths of the vagina is excised. This procedure is used primarily for more extensive anterior central recurrences when preservation of the bladder is seemingly still possible. The type D hysterectomy of the Querleu and Morrow classification completely exposes the roots of the sciatic nerve with resection of the entire paracervix at the pelvic sidewall

## Surgical steps of radical hysterectomy (Box 15.1)

1. *Position (**Figure 15.4**):* The optimal position for a radical hysterectomy is the dorsal lithotomy with bilateral pneumatic compression devices given the length of the procedure

## Box 15.1: Summary of steps for radical hysterectomy

1. *Position:* Dorsal lithotomy
2. *Cervical infiltration:* 4 cc of patent blue, or Tc99 or Indocyanine green at 3 o' and 9 o'clock
3. *Incision:* Use Maylard, Cherney or Midline to provide enough access
4. Opening of para-vesicle and para-rectal spaces:
   - Paravesical space boundaries:
     - *Medial:* Obliterated umbilical
     - *Lateral:* Obturator internus muscle
     - *Posterior:* Cardinal
     - *Anterior:* Pubic symphysis
   - Pararectal space boundaries:
     - *Medial:* Rectum/ureter
     - *Lateral:* Hypogastric artery
     - *Anterior:* Cardinal ligament
     - *Posterior:* Sacrum

   Tissue in between is the parametrium, palpated for any tumour
5. Sentinel lymph node dissection
   - If nodes are positive consider aborting procedure versus completing radical hysterectomy and adjuvant radiation
6. Full pelvic lymph node dissection in cases of clinically enlarged nodes or failure of SLN mapping
7. Bladder dissection
8. Ureteric Dissection off broad ligament
9. *Ligation of uterine:* At origin at superior vesical or hypogastric in type III or C or point where it crosses ureter in type B, mobilised by traction
10. Unroofing ureteric tunnel to vesico-uterine ligament:
    - *Roof of tunnel:* Anterior vesico-uterine ligament
    - Mobilise ureter off peritoneal attachment
    - Mobilise off side of uterus to expose posterior or caudal vesico-uterine ligament
11. *Posterior dissection:*
    - Incise peritoneum across pouch of Douglas
    - Identify recto-vaginal space
    - Take rectum off post vagina and utero-sacral using sharp and blunt dissection
    - Utero-sacral ligament transected at posterior attachment
12. *Lateral dissection:*
    - Divide utero-sacrals
    - Cardinals clamped at pelvic sidewall in type III or medial half in type B2 more clamps to reach vagina
    - Clamp IP at this stage if removing ovary
13. Vaginal Dissection:
    - Length of vagina to be removed depends on nature of primary lesion and colposcopic findings
    - If no vaginal intraepithelial neoplasia, remove 1.5 cm enter vagina anteriorly and transect circumferentially
    - Suture angles

2. *Cervical infiltration in sentinel lymph node mapping (**Figure 15.5**):* The cervix is infiltrated with 4 cc of methylene blue, Tc99 and/or Indocyanine green at 3 o'clock and 9 o'clock (do this about 15 minutes before procedure) if a sentinel lymph node dissection is planned. The 3 o'clock and 9 o'clock position is the optimal position for mapping

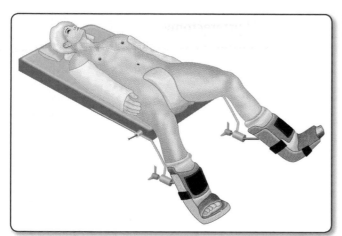

**Figure 15.4** Position: Modified dorsal lithotomy.

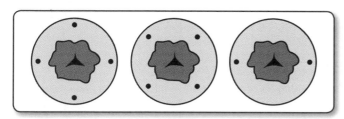

**Figure 15.5** Sentinel lymph node tracer injection.

3. *Incision (**Figure 15.6**):* A Maylard, Cherney or midline incision are used to provide sufficient access and visualisation. A retractor such as a Bookwalter is set up to allow adequate visualisation and may be moved in the event a para-aortic lymphadenectomy will be performed (**Figure 15.7**)

4. *Opening of spaces (**Figure 15.8**):* Begin by accessing the retroperitoneum with an incision parallel to the infundibulo-pelvic ligament. Alternatively, the round ligament may be grasped, ligated and divided close to the pelvic sidewall prior to starting the development of the retroperitoneal spaces. If the plan is to abort the procedure in the event of positive lymph nodes as determined by the frozen section, then the round ligament should be left intact. The spaces can be developed with blunt dissection using a finger, scissors, or clamp. Identify ureter as it crosses pelvic brim:
   - Paravesical* space boundaries
     - *Medial:* Superior vesical artery
     - *Lateral:* Obturator internus muscle
     - *Posterior:* Cardinal
     - *Anterior:* Pubic symphysis
   - Pararectal* space boundaries:
     - *Medial:* Rectum/ureter
     - *Lateral:* Hypogastric artery

---

*The space in between the paravesical space and the pararectal space is the 'parametria' – the surgeon's fingers may be placed into these spaces to feel the parametria and determine if there is any tumour present causing the procedure to be aborted.

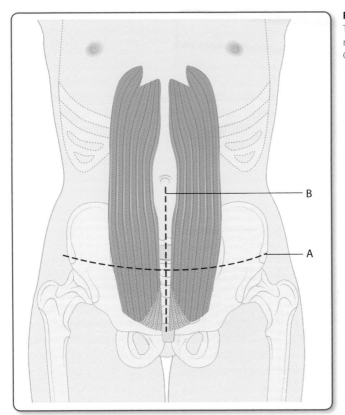

**Figure 15.6** Abdominal incision. The preferred incision types for a radical hysterectomy are a midline, Cherney or Maylard.

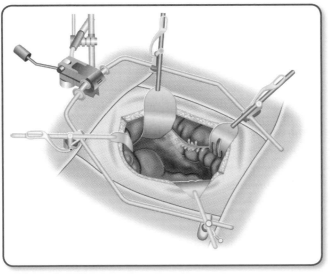

**Figure 15.7** Placement of the retractor blades.

- *Anterior:* Cardinal ligament
- *Posterior:* Sacrum

5. *Uterine artery ligation (**Figure 15.9**):* Once the avascular spaces are open, the uterine artery is exposed for ligation. The surgical steps include dissection from its origin, which

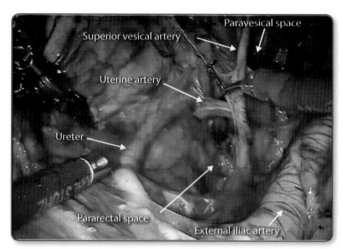

Superior vesical artery

Paravesical space

Uterine artery

Ureter

Pararectal space

External iliac artery

**Figure 15.8** Opening of avascular spaces. Intraoperative representation of the para-vesical and para-rectal spaces dissected following a pelvic lymphadenectomy.

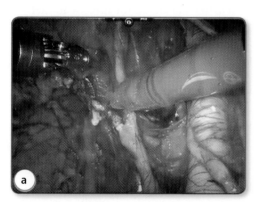

a

**Figure 15.9** Ligation of uterine artery. (a) Ligation of uterine artery at source of internal iliac with two hemoclips placed. (b) The uterine artery can be clipped or suture ligated and then transected at the source of the internal iliac (c) Illustration of uterine artery after it has been transected.

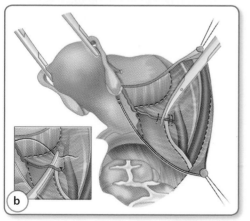

b

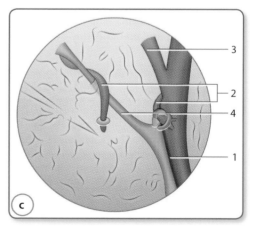

c

is the anterior division of internal iliac artery, following the uterine artery to where the ureter crosses underneath and continue to follow the artery to show its course toward the lateral aspect of the uterus within the parametrial tissue. Ligate the uterine artery at the source of the internal iliac for a type III radical hysterectomy or at the crossing of the ureter in a type II. Ligating the uterine at the source allows complete parametrial removal. Acceptable ways of uterine artery ligation include suturing, hemoclip, stapling device, bipolar coagulator. In addition, the uterine artery may arise from the internal iliac artery prior to its division or it may have common origins with the inferior vesical, middle rectal, internal pudendal, or vaginal arteries therefore is important to dissect it completely and mostly, to identify the ureter again prior to ligation

6. *Bladder dissection (**Figure 15.10**):* After developing the avascular spaces of the pelvis and transecting the round ligament, the vesico-uterine peritoneum is incised to mobilise the bladder off the uterus and away from the cervix and the top one-third of the vagina. This step can be done with electro-cautery or scissors, however blunt dissection is discouraged as there is an increased risk of fistula. For RH, it is important to continue this dissection at least 2–3 cm down the upper vagina. This allows for assessment of possible tumour extension anteriorly toward the bladder. Once the dissection is complete, the vesico-uterine peritoneum and bladder may be elevated and pushed away from the uterus cervix and vagina

7. *Unroofing the ureteric tunnel (**Figure 15.11**):* The cut end of the uterine artery is lifted and any tissue adherent to the ureter is removed to free the ureter. The ureteric tunnel is developed with sharp and blunt dissection using a right-angled clamp and sutures as needed. Unroofing the ureter off the vesico-uterine ligament allows complete mobilisation of the parametrium toward the specimen and the parametrial tissue remains attached to the cervix. The ureter proceeds through the parametrium and the lateral parametrial tissue must be brought over the ureter and toward the uterus in a type C hysterectomy. This dissection is difficult, and care should be taken as there are many small vessels which should be ligated with sutures and hemoclips. Significant blood loss can occur during this part of the procedure. It is important to avoid electrocautery as this may devascularise the ureter and cause some degree of unwanted ureteric injury

8. *Posterior dissection (**Figure 15.12**):* The posterior dissection requires an incision in the peritoneum across the pouch of Douglas followed by identification of the rectovaginal space. Using sharp and blunt dissection, the rectum can be mobilised off the posterior vagina and uterosacral ligaments. The rectum is then retracted posteriorly toward the sacrum and medially toward the opposite side of the pelvis that is currently being

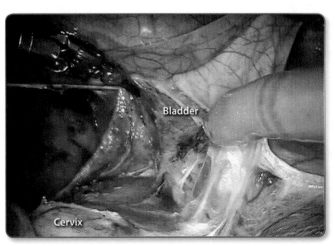

**Figure 15.10** Dissection of vesico-uterine peritoneum and bladder.

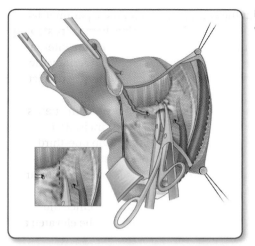

**Figure 15.11** Unroofing the ureteric tunnel. Dissection of vesico-uterine peritoneum to unroof the ureter.

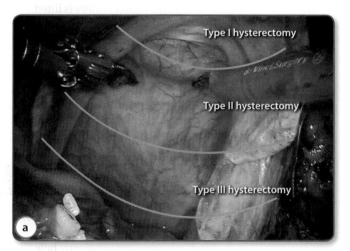

Type I hysterectomy

Type II hysterectomy

Type III hysterectomy

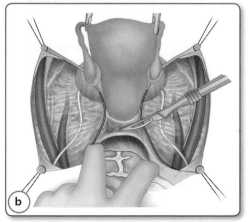

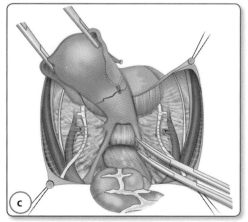

**Figure 15.12** Posterior dissection: (a) Posterior delineation of the types of hysterectomies and incision for appropriate posterior dissection. (b) Dissection of rectum off uterus and opening of recto-vaginal space. (c) Transection of utero-sacral ligaments.

dissected. The ureter is mobilised from the medial aspect of the broad ligament and separated from the uterosacral ligament which can be transected with stapling devices, clamps, suture ligatures, or cautery. The uterosacral ligaments are transected close to their distal attachments in a Class III hysterectomy. In a Class II hysterectomy, the uterosacral ligaments would be transected more proximally about midway between the cervix and the sacrum

9. *Lateral dissection (Figure 15.13):* The cardinal ligaments are clamped at the pelvic sidewall in type III hysterectomy or approximately 2 cm lateral to the cervix in a type II hysterectomy. To preserve the autonomic nerves of the parasympathetic plexus, paracervical tissue is taken above the deep uterine vein. If the ovaries are to be preserved, the utero-ovarian ligament can be transected and the fallopian tubes dissected from the ovaries to be included in the surgical specimen. In cases requiring oophorectomy, the infundibulo-pelvic ligament can be divided at this time

10. *Vaginal dissection (Figure 15.14):* The length of vagina to be removed depends on the nature of primary lesion and colposcopic findings. The presence of vaginal intraepithelial neoplasia may require >1–2 cm of removal. The vagina is entered anteriorly and transected circumferentially. The closure of the angles can be done in a standard fashion but consideration can be made for suturing the vaginal angle to paravaginal tissue and uterosacral ligament to avoid vault prolapse

## Nerve sparing radical hysterectomy

From the superior hypogastric plexus, two hypogastric nerves have sympathetic fibres that run in a small plexus beneath the ureter and are responsible for bladder compliance, urinary continence and smooth muscle contractions [88]. The hypogastric nerves fuse with parasympathetic fibres of pelvic splanchnic nerves from S2, S3, and S4 nerves roots of the sacral plexus. The parasympathetic fibres are responsible for vaginal lubrication and genital swelling during sexual arousal, detrusor contractility and various rectal functions. The procedure involves two steps:

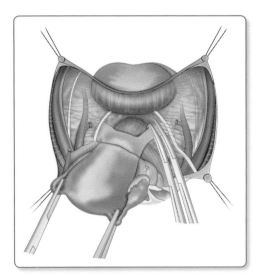

**Figure 15.13** Lateral dissection and division of cardinal ligaments.

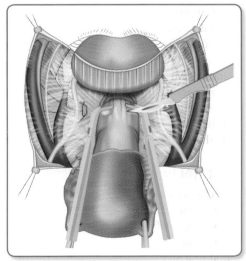

**Figure 15.14** Vaginal dissection.

1. Dissection of utero-sacrals
2. Dissection of parametrium

The hypogastric nerve is found running 1–2 cm dorsal to the ureter in the peritoneal leaf. Once the hypogastric nerve is identified, it is dissected from the peritoneal leaf in a similar manner to the ureter and then lateralised as the utero-sacral ligaments are clamped and cut.

A nerve sparing radical hysterectomy is done in a more conservation (type B) type of radical hysterectomy. Landoni et al randomised patients to type II versus type III radical hysterectomy from stage IB to IIA and found no difference in recurrence rate (24% vs. 26%) or deaths (18% vs. 20%) but a significantly higher morbidity with a type III (13% vs. 28%) suggesting the possibility of less radical surgery in select IB tumours [87].

## Pelvic lymph nodes (Figure 15.15)

If sentinel lymph node mapping is being done, radiotracers or dyes can take up to 15–30 minutes to map and may be performed after the development of the avascular spaces or at the completion of the hysterectomy.

A full pelvic and possible para-aortic lymph node dissection are necessary if pre-operatively or intra-operatively enlarged lymph nodes are identified, failure of SLN mapping on the ipsilateral side, or SLN mapping technology or skills are not available.

- *Boundaries:* The boundaries for the dissection are the common iliac bifurcation cephalad, the deep iliac circumflex vein caudad, the psoas muscle lateral, the ureter medial, and the obturator nerve dorsally. These structures and the surrounding spaces must be identified and dissected to proceed safely
- *External iliac vessels:* The lymph nodes are grasped, lifted off the vessels and dissected off the psoas muscle laterally and the vessels below. Surgical clips may be applied where the vessels are feeding the nodes. The dissection begins at the bifurcation of the iliac vessels and extends to where the deep iliac circumflex vein is identified. The lymphatics overlying the external iliac vein are dissected from lateral to medial. This nodal bundle can be removed and identified as the external iliac vessel lymph nodes
- *Obturator space:* The external iliac vessels can be retracted medially away from the psoas muscle and the obturator fossa becomes accessible. The advantage to medial retraction of the vessels is that haemostatic control can be performed by identifying small vessels that enter the obturator nodal bundle from the pelvic sidewall. The obturator nerve can often be identified behind the nodal bundle through medial traction of the vessels and the nerve can be dissected from the back of the bundle. With lateral traction of the vessels, the obturator nodal bundle can now be elevated from the space and the distal attachments divided. As the bundle is retracted medially, the remaining lymphatic attachments can be divided until the cephalad attachments to the internal iliac vessel are reached. Great care must be taken to divide the last connections of the bundle to the surrounding tissue at this point to avoid injury to the vessel

## Sentinel lymph node dissection (Figure 15.16)

The prevalence of lymph nodal involvement in early-stage cervical cancer is estimated to be approximately 15–20% [88] and can be determined by surgical pelvic lymph node dissection. When a pathologic frozen section assessment is performed during the surgery to determine cancer involvement of the lymphatic system, the decision to abort the remaining procedure and continue treatment with primary chemoradiation can be done whereas discovery of involvement of the pelvic lymph nodes on final surgical specimen

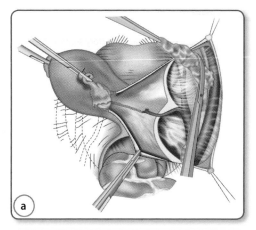

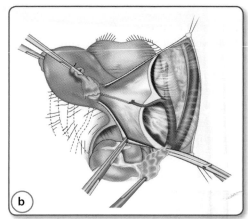

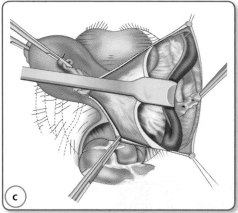

**Figure 15.15** Pelvic lymphadenectomy. (a and b) Pelvic lymphadenectomy over external iliac arteries. (c) Exposure of obturator fossa by retracting external iliac vessels medially.

guides adjuvant treatment. However, a complete pelvic lymph node dissection can lead to a significant amount of morbidity and may not be needed in all early-stage cervical cancers. Given the new FIGO staging and poorer prognosis in patients with lymph node involvement (stage IIIC), SLND is an alternative for surgical staging without the morbidity associated with a complete lymphadenectomy. SLND also detects lymph nodes in areas that would not otherwise be detected by routine lymphadenectomy. In addition, ultra-staging of sentinel lymph nodes has added significant value to detect nodal positivity when submitting a lower number of lymph nodes. This section will review the landmark trials (AGO and SENTICOL study series) in sentinel lymph node dissection in cervical cancer.

## AGO study

The AGO study was a prospective multi-centre validation study of sentinel lymph node dissection in cervical cancer [89]. Patients underwent SLND with technetium, patent blue or both followed by systematic pelvic and, if indicated, para-aortic node dissection. The detection rate of pelvic sentinel nodes was 88.6% (95% CI 85.8–91.1%) and was significantly higher for the combination of technetium and patent blue (93.5%; 95% CI 90.3–96.0%). Of the 106 patients with pelvic lymph node metastases, 82 had pelvic sentinel node metastases. The overall sensitivity was 77.4% (95% CI 68.2–85.0%), which was lower

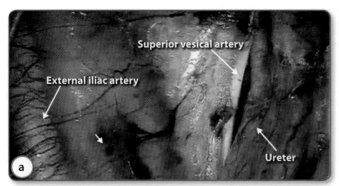

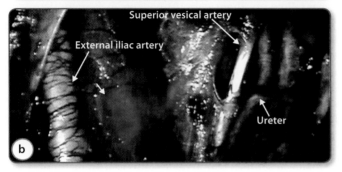

**Figure 15.16** Sentinel lymph node mapping. (a) Arrowhead indicates external iliac artery sentinel lymph node identified with blue dye. (b) Sentinel lymph node identified with ICG-green.

than the predefined non-inferiority margin of 90% ($p < 0.001$). Sensitivity in women with tumours <20 mm (90.9%), with bilateral detection (87.2%), or with both substances applied (80.3%) was higher compared with the total population. Several criticisms of this study included the lack of ultrastaging, no definition of surgeon volume/experience, injection of radiocolloid dye one day prior to surgery, and inclusion of >4 cm tumours in 43% of cases possibly leading to a lower mapping rate.

## SENTICOL-I trial

The SENTICOL-I trial was a prospective multi-centre study done to determine the sensitivity and negative predictive value (NPV) of SLN biopsy, using histologic examination of all nodes from the pelvic and/or para-aortic lymphadenectomy specimens as the reference standard [90]. As a validation study, all patients had SLN followed by complete lymphadenectomy. The study determined that combined radio-isotope and blue dye mapping detected at least one SLN in 136 patients (97.8%; 95% CI 93.8–99.6%), 23 had true-positive results and two who had false-negative results. The sensitivity was 92.0% (23 of 25; 95% CI 74.0–99.0%) and negative predictive value was 98.2% for node metastasis detection. No false-negative results were observed in the 104 patients (76.5%) in whom SLN were identified bilaterally. SLND was most reliable when detected bilaterally and a recent sub-analysis reported that the NPV of bilateral SLN detection was actually 100% [91].

A sub-analysis of the SENTICOL-I trial included 139 patients undergoing lymphoscintigraphy and sentinel lymph node dissection [92]. Lymphoscintigraphy, consisting of injecting radio-active dye one day pre-operative followed by imaging had an 87.8% lymph node detection rate while intraoperative lymph node mapping rate was

97.8%, respectively. Agreement between lymphoscintigraphy and SLN mapping was low for the number of SLNs ($\kappa$ = 0.23; –0.04; 0.49) and bilateral SLNs ($\kappa$ = 0.36; 0.2; 0.52). Although time consuming, lymphoscintigraphy did identify non-sentinel node involvement which was able to guide surgical exploration.

## SENTICOL II

The SENTICOL II study was a prospective randomised multi-centre study between March 2009 and July 2012, including 206 patients with stage IA-IIA1 cervical cancer. The protocol included frozen section of SLN; those with negative frozen section assessment underwent randomisation between a full PLND and SLND only to determine the accuracy of SLN frozen section. The primary endpoints of the study included pre- and postoperative morbidity, quality of life, and 3-year follow-up. There were 101 patients in the complete LND group and 105 patients in the SLND group. There were no false negative cases in the SLN group. There was more morbidity in the complete LND group (51.5% vs. 31.4%, $p$ = 0.0046) and significantly lower quality of life. There was no difference in 3-year PFS between both groups (92.0% in SLND arm and 94.4% in SLND + PLND arm) [93].

Based on SENTICOL I and SENTICOL II, factors associated with lower bilateral sentinel mapping rates were age $\geq$70 years [adjusted OR 0.02; 95% CI (0.001–0.28); $p$ = 0.004], tumour size > 20 mm [adjusted OR 0.46; 95% CI (0.21–0.99); $p$ = 0.048] and BMI > 30 kg/m$^2$ (adjusted OR 0.28; 95% CI 0.12–0.65; $p$ = 0.003) [94]. High volume centres were associated with improved bilateral lymph node mapping (adjusted OR 8.05; 95% CI 2.06–31.50; $p$ = 0.003). Further sub-analysis looking at sentinel lymph node status as a predictor of PMI found that among 114 patients with tumours <20 mm on pre-operative MRI and negative SLN after ultra-staging, only one patient had parametrial involvement (0.9%) [94]. Parametrial involvement was significantly associated with tumour size $\geq$ 20 mm on pre-operative MRI (adjusted OR 9.30; 95% CI 1.71–50.57; $p$ = 0.01) and micro-metastatic or macro-metastatic SLN (adjusted OR 8.98; 95% CI 1.59–50.84; $p$ = 0.01). Therefore, the use of MRI and sentinel biopsy together could identify a lower risk group of stage IB1 patients who may be candidates for a simple rather than radical hysterectomy.

A recent systematic review found that the pooled detection rate of sentinel node mapping was 89.2% (95% CI 86.3–91.6) [88]. Sentinel node detection and sensitivity are related to the mapping material; lower detection rates with blue dye alone and highest in the combined tracer/blue dye method, although the combined methods may be a risk factor for anaphylactic reactions. Several factors leading to poorer uptake include: inappropriate injection, lower volume of injected dye, and longer time since injection (50 vs. 30 min) [91]. Diluted blue dye and superficial injection were associated with higher success. Fluorescent dyes and infrared had low detection rates while carbon nanoparticles had a good detection rate in one study and could show promise in the future. There is a suggestion that for fertility sparing procedures, SLND can help predict parametrial involvement as patients with negative sentinel nodes have no parametrial involvement, but the identification of parametrial sentinel nodes may be limited by the proximity to the injection site [95]. Intra-operative frozen section would be of importance to determine which patients are amenable to a primary surgical approach and which would benefit from chemoradiation. However, based on the systematic review, the pooled sensitivity of intraoperative frozen section assessment of the sentinel lymph nodes was low (60%) due to the inability to detect micro-metastasis and isolated tumour cells and thus require immunohistochemistry on final analysis. When immunohistochemistry was used, the pooled sensitivity was 91.5% as compared to 88.6% without. Bilateral lymph node detection was found in younger patients, smaller tumours and when blue dye was used. Unilateral uptake may be due to nodal involvement on the detection failure side, but in this meta-analysis the pooled side-specific sensitivity was 96.9%. Cormier et al described a contralateral side-specific pelvic lymph node dissection and en-bloc parametrectomy in all cases where unilateral uptake occurred and reported a 87.5% patient-based sensitivity and 92.6% side-specific sensitivity with this method [96]. With the addition of parametrectomy, the sensitivity increased to 100% without any false negative results. Another literature review including 47 studies and 4,130 patients determined a set of criteria in patients in which SLND could safely replace PLND [97]. The diagnostic accuracy of SLND was highest when the following criteria were met as prerequisites: bilateral SLN detection, no suspicious lymph nodes on pre-operative imaging or during surgery, and a primary tumour diameter of <40 mm [estimated sensitivity of 99.6%; (95% CI 98–100%) and 99.9% NPV]. These criteria reduce the residual risk of occult metastases to 0.08% (1/1,257). In addition, bilateral sentinel node detection and ultra-staging were deemed safer and superior compared to unilateral detection, frozen section, and H&E analysis.

Criteria for SLND over full PLND:
1. Stage IA2, IB1, IIA primary tumour size < 40 mm
2. No suspicious pre- and intra-operative lymph nodes
3. Bilateral negative SLNs on frozen section
4. Ultra-staging on sentinel nodes

Patients with previous conisation have traditionally had less uptake of SLND tracers, however a recent report indicates a detection rate of 91% [88]. Patients with neoadjuvant radiation or chemotherapy also have a lower detection rate, likely due to the altered lymphatic channels. Pooled sentinel node detection rate in these patients was low (73.8%), however, pooled sensitivity was high (94.7%). tumour size (>2 cm) and stage (>IB2) were associated with low detection rate and sensitivity. The reason for failure of lymphatic mapping in large or locally advanced tumours is the higher possibility of lymph nodal involvement and LVSI, inhibiting lymphatic flow. There is also a high false negative rate in patients with large tumours due to the lymphovascular space being completely replaced with tumour [96]. In these patients, careful consideration of a full lymphadenectomy may be necessary.

Very few studies have examined the effect of SLND on survival. One large retrospective study from 1984 to 2005 compared PFS and immediate peri-operative outcomes in 1188 node negative patients; 1078 underwent full bilateral PLND and 110 underwent bilateral SLND [98]. There was no difference in 2 years and 5 years PFS (95% vs. 97% and 92% vs. 93% respectively), tumour size, histology, depth of invasion, intra-operative complications or short-term morbidity. Full PLND was associated with increased surgical time (2.8 hours vs. 2.0 hours, $p < 0.001$), blood loss (500 mL vs. 100 mL; $p < 0.001$), transfusion (23% vs. 0%; $p < 0.001$) and postoperative infection (11% vs. 0%; $p = 0.001$).

There are two currently on-going prospective studies to evaluate survival outcomes after SLND. The SENTICOL III trial is an international, multi-centre randomised control trial to assess 3-year survival and patient reported outcomes (quality of life) in sentinel lymph node dissection versus complete lymphadenectomy and is recruiting patients with stages IA1/LVI+ to IIA1. The accrual is set until 2021 with last follow-up in 2026 and plans to recruit 950 patients [99]. The SENTIX trial is a prospective multi-centre trial to determine the non-inferiority of SLN to systematic pelvic lymphadenectomy [100]. The primary endpoint is recurrence rate; the secondary endpoint is the prevalence of lower-leg lymphoedema and symptomatic pelvic lymphocele. The final analysis of PFS is set to be in 2021 based on a sample size of 300 patients treated per protocol and a non-inferiority margin of 5% (90% power; $p = 0.05$) for recurrence rate.

## Isolated tumour cells and micro-metastasis

Another important finding from the SENTICOL studies was the impact of ultra-staging. Based on a sub-analysis of the SENTICOL I study, 139 patients with stage IA1 and LVSI, stage IA2, and IB1 were included among which 13 experienced recurrences [101]; 11 in node negative patients and two in patients with positive sentinel lymph nodes; one patient had macro-metastasis and one patient had micro-metastasis. No patient with isolated tumour cells (ITCs) experienced a recurrence. Combining both the SENTICOL I and SENTICOL II studies, 24 patients (7.5%) had low-volume metastasis [102]. Risk factors associated with the low-volume metastasis included higher stage ($p = 0.02$) and stromal invasion ($p = 0.01$) at a cut-off of 8 mm. In multivariate analysis, the higher stage ($p = 0.02$) and the LVSI ($p = 0.02$) were significantly associated with micro-metastases and isolated tumour cells. Patients with low-volume metastasis had similar disease-free survival (DFS) (92.7%) to node-negative patients (93.6%); this was not affected by adjuvant treatment. In another analysis of the 313 patients from 2005 to 2012 in both SENTICOL studies, metastatic SLN was diagnosed in 52 patients (16.6%). Macro-metastases, micro-metastases and ITCs were found in 27, 12 and 13 patients respectively. Ultra-staging significantly increased the positive SLN rate from 7% to 16.6% ($p < 0.0001$). Frozen section identified 23 SLNs with macro-metastases in 20 patients and five SLNs with micro-metastases in two patients, while no ITCs were identified on frozen section. Subsequent ultra-staging of these negative SLNs found macro-metastases, micro-metastases and isolated tumour cells in additional 7, 11 and 17 SLNs respectively. The sensitivity and the negative predictive value of frozen section were 42.3% and 89.7% respectively. The false negative rate increased with increasing tumour size $\geq 20$ mm (OR 4.46; 95% CI 1.45–13.66; $p = 0.01$) and preoperative brachytherapy (OR 4.47; 95% CI 1.37–14.63; $p = 0.01$). High volume centres had a lower false negative rate (OR 0.09; 95% CI 0.02–0.51; $p = 0.01$).

## Radical trachelectomy (Figures 15.17 to 15.19)

The steps of a radical trachelectomy for fertility sparing surgery are the same as a radical hysterectomy but the cervix is transected off the uterus at the level of the isthmus. The uterus is then sutured to the vaginal vault and an abdominal cerclage is placed. Based on the technical aspects of the procedure, consideration should be made at this step to ligate the uterine artery or preserve.

## Open versus minimally invasive surgery

The first radical hysterectomy which was described by Wertheim in the 1890s and subsequently re-popularised by Meigs in the 1950s. Traditional laparotomy for radical hysterectomy has been associated with excellent 5-year survival in well selected patients but has increased risk of substantial long-term morbidity. The extensive dissections with close proximity to the ureter and great vessels required correct identification and ligation of the uterine artery and the utero-sacral ligaments which can damage pelvic nerves and leads to lower urinary dysfunction, sexual dysfunction, and colorectal motility disorders [103]. There was also a high incidence of peri-operative mortality [100]. This led to the introduction of minimally invasive techniques to improve peri-operative outcomes. The first laparoscopic radical hysterectomy was reported by Nezhat in 1996 followed by the first robotic hysterectomy by Sert in 2006 [104,105]. Since 2008, there has been a shift in practice favouring MIS radical hysterectomy, with

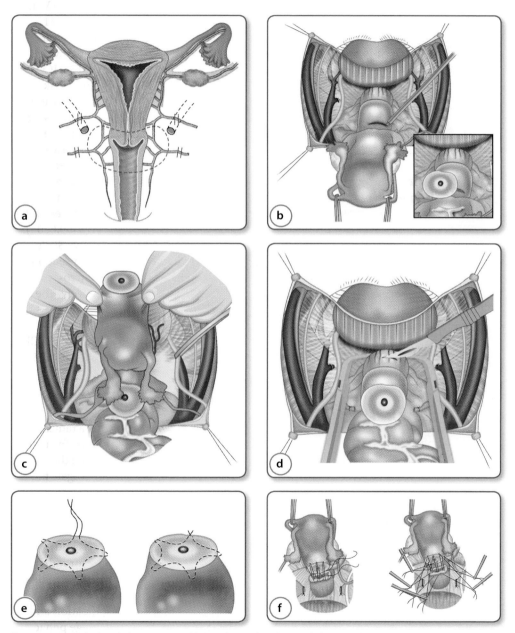

**Figure 15.17** Radical trachelectomy steps. (a) Boundaries of a radical trachelectomy. (b) Uterocervicojunction incision. (c) Eversion of the uterus. (d) Colpotomy. (e) Cerclage placement. (f) Re-attachment of uterus to vagina.

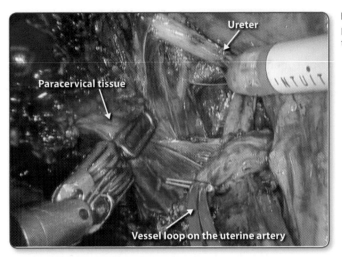

**Figure 15.18** Resection of paracervical tissue after the uterus transected from cervix.

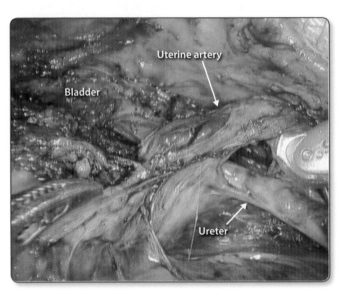

**Figure 15.19** Preservation of the uterine artery at radical trachelectomy.

a steep decline in ARH and rise of robotics as preferred MIS approach, while adoption of laparoscopy was significantly lower and reached a plateau (**Figure 15.20**) [106]. This highlights a trend favouring robotic radical hysterectomy (RRH) in the US in the first 7 years of MIS adoption; 75% of gynaecologic oncologists surveyed by the Society of Gynecologic Oncology (SGO) in 2015 performed trachelectomies and RH for cervical cancer with robotics rather than laparoscopy [107]. A case-control study comparing 210 RRH and 140 laparoscopic radical hysterectomies (LRH) showed no difference in outcomes between laparoscopy and robotics. In addition, few studies have compared laparoscopy to robotics since both offer minimally invasive benefits and therefore, the choice relies on surgeon's preference, institutional availability and properly selected patients [106]. One explanation for the low adoption of LRH in the US may be the commonly cited limitations including 2D visualisation, limited range of motion with

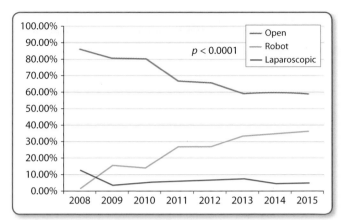

**Figure 15.20** Trends in adoption of radical hysterectomy in the US between 2008 and 2015 using the National inpatient sample. *Source:* With permission from Piedimonte S, Czuzoj-Shulman N, Gotlieb W, et al. Robotic Radical Hysterectomy for Cervical Cancer: A Population-Based Study of Adoption and Immediate Postoperative Outcomes in the United States. J Minim Invas Gynecol 2019; 26:551–557.

straight instruments and poor surgeon ergonomics. LRH cases are usually performed by experienced gynaecologic surgeons with excellence and ease in laparoscopy. On the other hand, robotics has a rapid learning curve, estimated to be between 9 and 20 cases [108], with increased proficiency with practice on a virtual simulator and may be adopted by a wider range of gynaecologic oncologists [109]. **Table 15.4** summarises the retrospective studies performed comparing RRH, ARH and LRH, reporting on short-term and long-term oncologic outcomes.

A meta-analysis including 17 studies by Jin et al has shown superior outcomes of RRH to ARH. Patients treated with RRH and LRH had lower estimated blood loss and a shorter length of stay than ORH but longer operative times. RRH patients had less postoperative complications compared to LRH patients (OR 0.42; 95% CI 0.20–0.87), while LRH patients had a lower incidence of postoperative complications compared to ARH patients (OR 0.53; 95% CI 0.37–0.75). Cluster analysis also supported improved clinical outcomes for RRH, however this study did not report on oncologic outcomes [110]. When comparing LRH to RRH, Zhou et al performed a meta-analysis including 15 studies and 1,161 patients with cervical cancer, of which 468 (40.31%) underwent RRH and 693 (59.69%) underwent LRH [111]. Only six studies reported on recurrence and found no significant difference between RRH and LRH (OR 0.91; 95% CI 0.36–2.31; $p = 0.84$) and no significant difference in DFS (OR 1.90; 95% CI 0.38–9.44; $p = 0.43$: test of heterogeneity, $p = 0.96$; I2 = 0%). The above studies were all retrospective and thus of limited quality and the main objective was to demonstrate the feasibility, safety and superior short-term outcomes of MIS radical hysterectomy. There was minimal reporting of oncologic outcomes and these studies cannot appropriately adjust for confounding factors. Based on this data and the wide adoption of robotic surgery, most centres continued to perform MIS for cervical cancer. In 2018, the first multi-centre randomised control trial aiming to prove non-inferiority of MIS RH was published and shockingly demonstrated a significantly worse OS and PFS for MIS radical hysterectomy, leading to an abrupt shift in practice back to ARH and modification of the NCCN guidelines and ESGO guidelines [77]. The change in practice is based on the following landmark trials.

## Laparoscopic approach to cervical cancer trial

The Laparoscopic Approach to Cervical Cancer (LACC) trial was the first multi-centre randomised control trial comparing minimally invasive radical hysterectomy to

Table 15.4 Robotic versus Open studies in the pre-LACC era. *Continues on pages 275–276*

| | Country | Dates | Study type | Study groups | Eligibility | Results |
|---|---|---|---|---|---|---|
| Magrina [165] (2008) | US | 2003–2006 | Retrospective | RRH 27 LRH 31 ARH 35 | Stage IA2–IB2 cervical cancer | No differences in intra- or postoperative complications among the three groups, at 31.1 months no recurrences in either group |
| Boggess (2008) | USA | 2005–2007 | Retrospective | RRH 51 ARH 49 | Stage IA1 to IIA cervical cancer | Lower EBL, shorter LOS, less complications 7.8% RAH, 16.3%. ORH, ($p = .35$). No report on survival |
| Nezhat [166] (2008) | | 2000–2008 | Retrospective | RRH 13 LRH 30 | Stages IA1 to IIA cervical cancer, <4 cm tumour or, uterine size < 12 cm, | No statistical differences in OR time (323 min vs. 318 min), EBL (157 mL vs. 200 mL), or LOS (2.7 days vs. 3.8 days) |
| Cantrell [167] (2010) | US | 2005–2008 | Retrospective | RRH 63 ARH 64 | Stage IA1–IIB cervical cancer. Endometrial carcinoma and metastatic diseases were excluded. | RRH: 94% PFS and OS at 36 months ARH: 89% PFS and 93% OS |
| Halliday [168] (2010) | Canada | 2003–2009 | Retrospective | RRH 16 ARH 24 | Stage IA1 with LVSI on cone biopsy to IIA cervical cancer. Candidates for radical trachelectomy and women with positive sentinel LNs were excluded | RRH: longer OR time (351 min vs. 283 min $p = 0.0001$), lower EBL (106 mL vs. 546 mL $p < 0.0001$), lower complications (19% vs. 63% $p = 0.003$). Shorter LOS (1.9 days vs. 7.2 days, $p < 0.0001$) |
| Soliman [169] (2010) | USA | January 2007–November 2010 | Prospective | RRH 34 LRH 31 ARH 3 | Stage IA1– IB2/IIA | • Shorter OR time, ARH vs. LRH and RRH (265 vs. 338 vs. 328 min, $p = 0.002$)<br>• Lower EBL in LRH and RRH vs. RAH (100 vs. 100 vs. 350 mL, $p < 0.001$)<br>• Higher conversion rates in LRH (16%) vs. RRH (3%).<br>• Shorter LOS in RRH (1 day) vs. LRH or RAH (2 vs. 4 days, $p < 0.01$) |
| Wright [170] (2012) | US | 2006–2010 | Prospective | 1,610 ARH 217 LRH and 67 RRH | Patients in the Premier prospective database undergoing radical hysterectomy using ICD codes | Most patients in ARH Perioperative complications: 15.8% ARH, 9.2% LRH and 13.4% RRH ($p = 0.04$) |
| Hoogendam [171] (2014) | Netherlands | 2008 and 2013 | Retrospective | 104 RRH | High-risk stage IA1-2 and IB1/IIA | PFS 81.4 and OS 88.7% |

## Table 15.4 Continued.

| | Country | Dates | Study type | Study groups | Eligibility | Results |
|---|---|---|---|---|---|---|
| Segaert et al. (2015) [172] | Belgium | 2007–2014 | Prospective | RRH 109 | | 2 years and 5 years OS: 96% and 89%<br>5-year DFS per stage : 100% stage IA and 75% for IB1 |
| Kim 2015 | South Korea | January 2008 to May 2013 | Retrospective 3:1 case matched | LRH 23<br>RRH 69 | Stage IAI- IIA cervical cancer | RRH: longer OR time (317 min vs. 236 min; $p < 0.001$), lower EBL (200 vs. 350; $p = 0.036$). No difference in intraoperative and postoperative complications (4.3% for RRH vs. 1.45% for LRH; $p = 0.439$)<br>RRH recurrence: 8.7% LRH recurrence 10.1%<br>3-year RFS: 91.3% RRH group and 89.9% in the LRH group ($p = 0.778$) |
| Sert et al. (2016) [173] | US Norway | 2005–2011 | Retrospective, multi-institutional | ARH 232<br>RRH 254 | Stage IA1 to IB1 cervical carcinoma. Exclusion: tumour > 4 cm, uterine size 12 cm, history of radiotherapy, pregnancy, metastatic disease, pelvic or aortic LNs N 2 cm, histologically positive LNs were excluded | Lower EBL, transfusion LOS for RRH vs. ARH Longer OR time for RRH than ORH similar postoperative complications, less intra-operative complications (4% vs. 10%, $p = 0.004$) no significant difference in recurrence and death at 39 months ($p = 1.00$ and $p = 0.48$, respectively) |
| Wang [174] (2016) | China | | Retrospective case matched | LRH 203<br>ARH 203 | Stage IA2 to IIA2 cervical cancer | Similar 5-year RFS (91.3% LRH vs. 90.4% ARH, $p = 0.83$) and OS (93.2% LRH vs. 92.1% ARH, $p = 0.94$) and pattern of recurrence ($p = 0.63$)<br>LRH: Shorter OR time, less blood loss, shorter LOS |
| Zanagnolo [2016] | Spain | 2006–2014 | Retrospective | RRH ($n = 203$)<br>ARH ($n = 104$) | | 5-year PFS 89% ORH, 90% RRH, ( $p = 0.986$)<br>5-year OS: 98% ORH, 97% RRH, ( $p = 0.644$) |
| Gallotta [175] (2017) | Italy | 2010–2016 | Retrospective case matched | 210 RRH (cases)<br>110 LRH controls) | Stage Ia2-1B2 cervical cancer | PFS 88.0% RRH, 84.0% LRH, ($p = 0.87$). Central and/or lateral pelvic disease: Most common site of relapse<br>3-year OS: 90.8% in RRH vs. 94.0% LRH. No difference between RRH and LRH |
| Shah [176] (2017) | USA | 2001–2012 | Retrospective | 109 RRH<br>202 ARH | Stage IA1–1B2, including squamous, adenocarcinoma and adenosquamous | Shorter (LOS) in RRH (42.7 vs. 112.6 hours, $p < 0.001$), lower EBL; 105.9 vs. 482.6 mL, $p < 0.001$). More complications ARH (23.4% vs. 9.2% RRH ($p = 0.002$)<br>Similar recurrence rate (10.1% vs. 10.4%, $p = 0.730$). RRH not a predictor of PFS ($p = 0.230$) or OS ($p = 0.85$) |

## Table 15.4 Continued.

| | Country | Dates | Study type | Study groups | Eligibility | Results |
|---|---|---|---|---|---|---|
| Shazly [177] (2015) | USA | Database inception–February 2014 | Meta-analysis | 1013 RRH 710 LRH 2290 ARH | Stages IA1-IIA cervical cancer | less EBL, shorter LOS, less fever and blood transfusion, and wound complications for RRH versus ARH and wound-related complications no difference between RRH and LRH |
| Corrado [178] (2018) | Italy | January 2001–December 2016 | Retrospective | 101 ARH 152 LRH 88 RRH | Stage IA1 to IIA1 cervical cancer, no evidence of LN or distant metastasis | No difference between LRH, ARH in LOS, intraoperative and postoperative complications No difference in oncologic outcomes ARH and RRH |

ARH, abdominal radical hysterectomy; LACC, Laparoscopic Approach to Cervical Cancer; LRH, laparoscopic radical hysterectomy; OS, overall survival; PFS, progression free survival; RRH, robotic radical hysterectomy.

laparotomy [15]. Patients with stage IA1 (with LVI), IA2 (stromal invasion, 3–5 mm in depth and <7 mm in width), or IB1 (tumour size of ≤4 cm in the greatest dimension without nodal involvement), histologic subtype of squamous-cell carcinoma, adenocarcinoma, or adeno-squamous carcinoma were randomised to undergo either ARH or MIS RH. The study was powered to test the hypothesis of non-inferiority of MIS to ARH after 4.5 years of follow-up and included 33 centres worldwide between 2008 and 2017. In this study, 319 patients underwent MIS RH and 312 ARH. The disease-free survival at 4.5 years of follow-up was 86% for MIS compared to 96% for laparotomy. The HR for recurrence or death in MIS 4.39 after adjusting for age, body mass index, stage of disease, lymphovascular invasion, lymph node involvement, and ECOG performance-status score. Results are consistent between the robotic and laparoscopy group based on a sensitivity analysis included in the study supplement. There was also a lower OS at 3 years: 93.8% MIS versus 99.0% open. Most of the recurrences occurred in the vaginal vault and were more common in the open group (43% vs. 15%). Tumour sizes were similar between both groups (43% open vs. 42% MIS were > 2 cm) with a similar proportion of tumours >2 cm among the recurrences in both groups. Of the recurrences, all but one was stage IB1, and 11 did not receive adjuvant therapy following surgery; one patient with stage 1A1 has positive LVSI. This is the first prospective trial to demonstrate worse oncologic outcomes in MIS RH at a time where the adoption of MIS approaches was increasing.

Shortly after this trial, a population-based study using the SEER database included 2,461 women with stage IA2 or IB1 undergoing radical hysterectomy (1,225 MIS, 1,236 open) and also showed worse survival with MIS, confirmed by sensitivity analysis and sub-analysis. The 4-year mortality was 9.1% among women who underwent MIS radical hysterectomy 5.3% among those who underwent ARH (HR 1.65; 95% CI 1.22–2.22; $p = 0.002$), corresponding to a 65% higher risk of mortality after propensity score matching based on surgical approach [16]. When adjusting for adjuvant treatment, all-cause mortality remained higher in the MIS group (HR 1.62; 95% CI 1.20–2.19). They also adjusted for robotic versus laparoscopy, tumour size >2, and for histology and found similar survival results among multiple sensitivity analysis. In exploratory subgroup analyses, RRH was associated to a higher risk of death than ARH (HR 1.61; 95% CI 1.18-2.21), as was LRH (HR 1.50; 95% CI 0.97–2.31). In addition, comparing to a time prior to the adoption of MIS, the 4-year relative survival rate was stable following radical hysterectomy (annual percentage change 0.3%; 95% CI –0.1 to 0.6) while a decline of 0.8% was observed after the introduction of MIS.

The secondary objective of the LACC trial to compare adverse events (AE) of MIS versus ARH was recently published and found no significant difference between both approaches [112]. There were similar rates of intraoperative grade 2 complications (12% MIS vs. 10% ARH) and 54% grade 2 postoperative AE in MIS and 48% open ($p = 0.14$). There was a curiously high rate of AE: 71% in the robotic surgery group and 57% of the laparoscopy group. However, the LACC trial was not powered or designed to detect differences between robotic and laparoscopic surgery especially given that there were only 41 cases performed robotically in the trial across the 33 sites. Also, the trial design collected and reported all adverse events and not just clinically relevant adverse events; therefore, the reported rates may lack clinical significance. There were more vault complications in the MIS group (4% vs. 0.8%; $p = 0.1$), whereas more patients in the open group had wound complications (6% vs. 1.4%; $p = 0.04$) and cardiac complications (4% vs. 0.7%; $p = 0.02$).

The LACC trial and the National Cancer Database study have called into question the safety of minimally invasive radical hysterectomy for early-stage surgical cancer as it is founded on a well-designed multi-centre randomised control trials in addition to a supporting population-based study. Multiple counterarguments and a search for explanations following these two trials have arisen: recruitment sites for the LACC trial were mostly in smaller countries, comments on surgeon skill, use of a uterine manipulator, larger size of tumours, laparoscopy versus robotic, non-standardised use of adjuvant treatment, closure of the vaginal vault, among others. This has stimulated countries and centres to look at their own data and determine whether these findings were applicable and look deeper at factors truly affecting survival.

A large international multi-centre retrospective study including patients undergoing RH for stage IA1 (LVSI+), IA2, and IB1 squamous, adenocarcinoma, or adenosquamous carcinoma was performed between January 1, 2010 and December 31, 2017 [113]. There were 815 patients included, with 255 undergoing ARH (29.1%) and 560 undergoing MIS RH (70.9%). In the ARH group, 19 (7.5%) recurrences occurred while 51 (9.1%) recurrences occurred in the MIS group ($p = 0.43$). MIS was independently associated with an increased hazard of recurrence (adjusted HR 1.88; 95% CI 1.04–3.25). Other factors independently associated with an increased hazard of recurrence included tumour size, grade, and adjuvant radiation. There was no difference in OS in the unadjusted analysis (HR 1.14; 95% CI 0.61–2.11) or after risk adjustment (adjusted HR 1.01; 95% CI 0.5–2.2). In patients with tumours < 2 cm, 2/82 (2.4%) recurred in the ARH group and 16/182 (8.8%) in the MIS RH group ($p = 0.058$). A propensity matched analysis showed an increased risk of recurrence in the MIS group (HR 2.83; 95% CI 1.1–7.18), corresponding to 7/159 (4.4%) in the open RH group and 18/156 (11.5%) in the minimally invasive RH group ($p = 0.019$).

In Europe, the SUCCOR trial was a multi-centre European retrospective cohort study including 1,272 patients that underwent ARH or MIS RH for stage IB1 cervical cancer (FIGO 2009) from January 2013 to December 2014. They reported double the risk of recurrence (HR 2.07; 95% CI 1.35–3.15; $p = 0.001$) and death (HR 2.45; 95% CI 1.30–4.60; $p = 0.005$) for MIS compared to ARH [84]. In addition, the use of the uterine manipulator accounted for 2.76 times the risk of recurrence. Another study looking specifically at the effect of the uterine manipulator on risk of recurrence evaluated 224 patients undergoing MIS RH in two different high-volume centres; 115 had surgery with the use of an intra-uterine manipulator while 109 did not [114]. Patients without uterine manipulator were more likely to have residual disease in the hysterectomy specimen ($p < 0.001$), positive LVSI ($p = 0.02$), positive margins ($p = 0.008$), and positive lymph node metastasis ($p = 0.003$). PFS at 5 years was 80% in the no intra-uterine manipulator group and 94% in the intra-uterine manipulator group but after controlling for confounding factors [residual disease at hysterectomy, tumour size and high-risk pathologic criteria (positive margins, parametria or lymph nodes)]. The use of an intra-uterine manipulator was not significantly associated with worse PFS (HR 0.4; 95% CI 0.2–1.0; $p = 0.05$). Tumour size was the only factor associated with PFS (HR 2.1; 95% CI 1.5–3.0, for every 10 mm increase, $p < 0.001$).

In Canada, a population based retrospective cohort study from 2006 to 2017 evaluated 958 women undergoing RH (MIS 475; ARH 483). The 5-year mortality was 12.5% for MIS and 5.4% for ARH with a 16.2% risk of recurrence compared to 8.4% in open [115]. This study adjusted for patient factors and surgeon volume yet still reported an adjusted HR of 2.2 for death and 1.97 for recurrence in stage IB patients treated with MIS compared to ARH. This difference was not observed in stage IA patients. This finding shed light on the selection criteria for surgical approach; stage IB includes a wide range of patients with deep stromal invasion without a visible mass to a 2-cm mass based on subjective physician evaluation. In addition, all these studies included the old FIGO staging and may have been more likely to operate on 'bulky' stage IB cancers [116].

In addition, such as the LACC trial, most MIS surgeries in this study were performed by laparoscopy (89.6%), which has been consistently reported to be more technically challenging. A propensity matched analysis between January 1990 and December 2018 comparing laparoscopy and open radical hysterectomy in a multi-centre European study also demonstrated a higher recurrence risk in laparoscopy patients [116]. Patients undergoing laparoscopic radical hysterectomy had shorter PFS than patients undergoing ARH (HR 1.98; 95% CI 1.32–2.97; $p = 0.005$). Laparoscopic patients were more likely to develop intrapelvic recurrences (74% vs. 34%; $p < 0.001$) and peritoneal carcinomatosis (17% vs. 1%; $p = 0.005$) compared to open patients.

A study based on the Korean nationwide database analysed 6,335 patients undergoing RH: 3,235 ARH and 3,100 LRH [103]. Patients were compared using propensity score matching based on patient characteristics (age at operation, year of diagnosis, insurance status, comorbidities, and the extent of lymphadenectomy), hospital characteristics (hospital location, hospital region, and hospital size), and two-way interaction terms in order to compare similar patients in each group. Adoption of laparoscopy increased from 46.1% in 2011 to 51.8% in 2014 and patients were more likely to undergo laparoscopy if they were younger and in a metropolitan centre. The LRH group had less complications, shorter hospital stay and less cost, and was also associated to improved survival compared to ARH (HR 0.74; 95% CI 0.64–0.85).

In the Netherlands, a nationwide multi-centre retrospective study was performed using the country's Netherlands Cancer Registry, a population-based registry with coverage of all newly diagnosed malignancies in the Netherlands since 1989 [18]. They included patients with newly diagnosed cervical cancer between 2010 and 2017 who underwent RH at one of their specialised cancer centres for stage IA2 with LVSI, IB1 and IIA1; adenocarcinoma, SCC or adenosquamous carcinoma. Patients receiving neoadjuvant chemotherapy and chemoradiation were excluded. There were 740 patients in the ARH group and 369 in the LRH group; 59% of these patients had tumours over 2 cm, and more commonly in the ARH group 66% vs. 44%, $p < 0.01$). Full cohort unadjusted analysis showed a lower 5-year DFS (82.8% vs. 91.0%) and 5-year OS (91.1% vs. 95.2%) in ARH compared with LRH. Patients with tumours less than 2 cm showed a 5-year DFS of 91.4% and 96.0% in the ARH and LRH group. Five-year OS was 96.4% and 98.5% respectively. In tumours over 2 cm, DFS was 85.0% and 82.5% in the ARH and LRH group, respectively and 5-year OS was 94.2% and 92.8%. Therefore, based on this population study in seven specialised gynaecologic oncology centres, there was no difference in survival between ARH and MIS RH.

There have recently been three systematic reviews and meta-analyses published pooling the outcomes of ARH versus MIS RH [117–119]. The one reported by Nitecki et al included only 15 high quality studies only (Newcastle Ottawa Grade >7) and those adjusting for confounders, meant to represent the strongest data [117]. Among 9,499 patients who underwent RH, 49% ($n = 4,684$) had MIS of whom 57% ($n = 2,675$) received RRH. There were 530 recurrences and 451 deaths reported. A random effects model was done to pool the results of all studies. The pooled hazard of recurrence or death was 71% higher among patients who underwent MIS RH compared to ARH (HR 1.71; 95% CI 1.36–2.15; $p < 0.001$), with some degree of heterogeneity (I2 = 30.6%; $p = 0.05$). The pooled results of 13 studies that reported confounder adjusted HRs for all-cause mortality including 8,751 patients demonstrated that MIS RH was associated with a 56% higher hazard of death compared with ARH (HR 1.56; 95% CI 1.16–2.11; $p = 0.004$), with low to moderate heterogeneity (I2 = 41.6%; $p = 0.06$). There was no statistically significant association between the prevalence of RRH and magnitude of the association between MIS RH and the risk of recurrence or death [2.0% increase in the HR for each 10-percentage point increase in prevalence of robot-assisted surgery (95% CI –3.4% to 7.7%)] or risk of all-cause mortality. In a stratified analysis, MIS RH was associated with an increased risk of recurrence or death in studies in which robot-assisted laparoscopy predominated (HR 1.88; 95% CI 1.36–2.60) and in those in which traditional laparoscopy predominated (HR 1.54; 95% CI 1.10–2.16).

Another review by Smith et al included 50 cohort studies and 1 RCT, analysing 22,593 women with cervical cancer; among these studies 41 were included in a quantitative analysis [118]. The odds of PFS for MIS RH were worse than ARH (OR 1.54; 95% CI 1.24–1.94, 14 studies). In studies with longer follow-up, the odds of PFS were progressively worse with MIS RH (HR 1.48 for 36+ months, 95% CI 1.21–1.82, 10 studies; HR 1.69 for 48+ months, 95% CI 1.26–2.27, 5 studies; and HR 2.020 for 60+ months, 95% CI 1.36–3.001; 3 studies). However, for OS, there was no statistically significant difference between MIS and ARH (OR 0.94; 95% CI 0.66–1.35, 14 studies). A third meta-analysis included 28 studies and 18,961 patients [119]. Patients with FIGO 2009 stage < IIB who underwent MIS had a lower rate of OS (HR 1.43; 95% CI 1.06–1.92; $p = 0.019$) and PFS (HR 1.50; 95% CI 1.21–1.85; $p < 0.001$) than those who underwent open surgery. Eight studies provided OS and 10 studies provided PFS of tumours <2 cm, and the pooled results indicated no statistically significant difference in OS (HR 1.07; 95% CI 0.65–1.76; $p = 0.801$) and PFS (HR 1.20; 95% CI 0.65–2.19, $p = 0.559$) between the MIS RH group and ARH group (**Figure 15.6**). The studies were subjected however to a large amount of heterogeneity, and thus the strongest evidence remains from the RCT and National Cancer Database study. These studies highlight the need for objective selection criteria for MIS based on clinicopathological factors in the post LACC era; selection criteria may include absence LVSI, tumours <2 cm. Further studies are needed to address not only the decision-making process but prognostic factors and predictors of recurrence.

## In specialised centres for robotics

In a small retrospective study from a Canadian high-volume centre in robotics, the recurrence was 7% for RRH (4 out of 74 cases) versus 17% for ARH (5 out of 24 cases) but did not include any LRH cases [120]. There was no difference in grade, stage, histologic subtype, tumour size, or vaginal margin involvement. There was a lower rate of complications (13% vs. 50%; $p < 0.001$) and shorter LOS in RRH (1 day vs. 7 days; $p < 0.001$) compared to ARH. Though this study was limited by a small sample size, it highlights improved outcomes in a specialised academic centre in robotics.

Similarly, in a high-volume robotic centre, a retrospective cohort study was performed at Memorial Sloan Kettering from 2007 to 2017, patients with stage IA1 with LVSI, IA2, or IB1 cervical carcinoma were analysed by treatment modality to compare oncologic and perioperative outcomes [121]. There were 117 MIS cases of which 90.6% were robotic and 79 ARH cases both groups were similar in terms of baseline characteristics. Surgical approach was decided at the physician's discretion. There was no difference in FIGO substage, histologic subtype, clinical tumour size, pathologic tumour size, positive margins, presence of LVSI, or the size of parametrial resection between both groups. In addition, the rate of MIS increased at their institution from 13% in 2007 when the robotic platform was first introduced to 60–80% in recent years The MIS group had more cases with no residual tumour in the hysterectomy specimen (24.8% vs. 10.1%; $p = 0.01$). None of the cases without residual tumour had recurrences. There was more node positivity in the ARH group (53.2% vs. 33.3%; $p = 0.006$). There was no difference in disease free survival or disease specific survival [87% vs. 86.6%; $p = 0.92$ and 96.5% vs. 93.9% ($p = 0.93$)] between MIS and ARH respectively. The 5-year OS rates were 96.5% and 87.4%, respectively ($p = 0.15$). In addition, all the recurrences were in FIGO stage IB1 cases with residual tumour in the hysterectomy specimen. The recurrences were equal between locoregional and distant sites but the ARH group most often had recurrences in retroperitoneal nodes. The sites of first recurrence were vaginal cuff (16.7% vs. 12.5%), pelvis (8.3% vs. 0%), extra-abdominal (liver, lung, bone; 33.3% vs. 12.5%), and multiple sites (8.3% vs. 25%), respectively ($p = 0.35$). It is important to point out that 83% of patients in the ARH group received adjuvant treatment as compared to 33% in the RRH group. Based on this study, MIS was not associated with worse survival in a high-volume robotic cancer centre and in highly selected lower risk patients.

A retrospective multi-centre study including 40 centres in mainland China between January 2004 and December 2016 was performed using a national database and evaluating oncological outcomes of 10,314 cervical cancer patients with stage IA1 LVI+ to IIA2 undergoing RRH ($n = 1,048$) or ARH ($n = 9,266$) and evaluated the 3-year OS between both groups [19]. Patients in the RRH group were more likely to have LVSI than those in the ARH group, and patients in the ARH group were more likely to have large tumour size and deep stromal invasion than those in the RRH group. On multivariable analysis, RRH was associated with lower 3-year PFS (HR 1.20; 95% CI 1.09–1.52; $p = 0.035$) but not OS (HR 1.23; 95% CI 0.89–1.70; $p = 0.206$). After propensity score matching based on clinic-pathologic features (age, FIGO stage, histology, tumour size, depth of stromal invasion, LVSI, lymph node metastasis, surgical margin invasion, parametrial tumour involvement, and postoperative adjuvant treatment), patients who underwent RRH had a significantly decreased 3-year OS compared to those who underwent ARH (94.4% vs. 97.8%; $p = 0.002$). However, in patients with tumours <2 cm, RRH was not associated with decreased 3-year OS (HR 1.69; 95% CI 0.423–6.734; $p = 0.458$), once again highlighting important selection criteria for MIS.

In the UK, Patel et al reported the outcomes of 90 robotic radical hysterectomies for stage IB1 cervical cancer [17]. The 5-year OS was 98%, but this information was only available for 30% of the cohort. Women with tumours <2 cm had a 98.3% OS compared to 83.4% for tumour size >2 cm. In addition, those without LVSI had 100% 5-year survival, irrespective of tumour size. Therefore, this study suggests worse prognosis in larger tumours and those with LVSI, albeit a small sample size, and emphasises the need for selection criteria for MIS. The overall 5-year survival for death from disease only was 92.8%. OS by tumour size alone showed that women with tumours <2 cm had a 98.3% 5-year survival compared to 83.4% for tumour size >2 cm. Irrespective of tumour size, those that had no evidence of LVSI had a 100% 5-year survival. The overall 5-year survival for death from disease only was 92.8%. OS by tumour size alone showed that women with tumours <2 cm had a 98.3% 5-year survival compared to 83.4% for tumour size >2 cm. Irrespective of tumour size, those that had no evidence of LVSI had a 100% 5-year survival.

The outcomes of RRH have yet to be elucidated prospectively and will be the subject of the currently enrolling RACC (Robot-assisted Approach to Cervical Cancer) trial. This is a multi-centre randomised prospective trial to compare RRH to laparotomy. The trial began enrolling in 2019 and plans to close to accrual in 2027, testing the hypothesis that RRH is non-inferior to laparotomy with regards to PFS with fewer postoperative complications and improved patient reported outcomes. This study is enrolling women over 18 with cervical cancer FIGO (2018) stages IB1, IB2, and IIA1 squamous, adenocarcinoma, or adenosquamous subtypes [122]. This is also the first study to include patient reported outcomes as a measure.

## Minimally invasive surgery versus open in fertility sparing surgery

When considering fertility sparing surgery in cervical cancer, the tumour is typically < 2 cm in size and requires pathologic evidence of negative lymph nodes. The evidence presented against MIS in cervical cancer is strongest for patients with tumours >2 cm and/or LSVI, while those with microinvasive disease need to be counselled about the potential risks of MIS but can still be offered the procedure based on national and international guidelines. For fertility sparing surgery, there is no similar evidence with regards to adverse oncologic outcomes in MIS fertility sparing trachelectomies. Viera et al reported outcomes of short-term morbidity between 48 ART (abdominal radical trachelectomy) and 42 MIS patients [123]. The MIS group had significantly lower EBL and LOS, but no differences in complication rate were reported (30% MIS vs. 31% ART). The pregnancy rate was higher in the ART group when compared to the MIS group (51% vs. 28%; $p$ = 0.018). During the follow-up period, there was one recurrence in the ART group and none in the MIS group, but the follow-up time was shorter [25 months (range, 10–69) vs. 66 months (range, 11–147)].

Bentivengna et al performed a systematic review on all patients undergoing radical trachelectomy between January 1987 and February 2016, including 159 studies and 3,098 patients of which 21 papers reported outcomes of laparoscopic radical trachelectomy (LRT), and 13 on robotic radical trachelectomy (RRT) [124]. In a sub-analysis of LRT based a on a review of trachelectomies, 238 patients underwent LRT reported in 18 series; 55 patients had stage IA disease, two stage IB2, one stage IIA, and all others stage IB1 disease, 42 patients had stage IB1 tumours >2 cm among the 12 studies reporting tumour size. All except four teams preserved the uterine artery, and four also used nerve-sparing surgery. Among these patients, 15 (6%) of 238 patients had recurrent disease, of whom seven (17%) were among the 42 with stage IB1 tumours. A second sub-analysis of robotic trachelectomy (RRT) patients included 89 patients reported in nine series reported after 2008. This review could not yet report the oncologic outcomes of RRT.

There is currently an on-going prospective multi-centre randomised trial [International radical Trachelectomy Assessment (IRTA) study] evaluating long-term outcomes of MIS trachelectomies in patients with stage IA2-IB1 <2 cm. The primary endpoint is disease-free survival measured as the time from surgery until recurrence or death due to disease and will be compared between patients who underwent open versus minimally invasive radical trachelectomy. A projected 535 patients will be included; 256 open and 279 minimally invasive radical trachelectomy. Assuming that the 4.5-year disease-free survival rate for patients who underwent open surgery is 95.0%, 80% power will be needed to detect a 0.44 HR using $\alpha$ level 0.10, corresponding to an 89.0% disease-free survival rate at 4.5 years in the minimally invasive group.

In summary, the recent updates with the first RCT in the surgical management of early cervical cancer stage IA2-IIB2 favour an abdominal approach to radical hysterectomy, with significantly longer PFS and OS and confirmed by multiple retrospective population-based, propensity matched studies. Patients with tumour size <2 cm and absence of LVSI may be amenable to a minimally invasive approach but should be counselled adequately based on national and international guidelines. The long-term oncologic results for fertility sparing MIS radical trachelectomies are still on-going and patients should be treated as per the current recommended guidelines.

## Regionalisation of care

There is evidence that regionalisation of care for radical hysterectomy has an impact on outcomes based on low, mid and high-volume centres. In a retrospective multi-centre study comparing low-volume (<32 cases), mid-volume (32–104 cases), and high-volume (105 cases), women in high-volume centres had a decreased risk of recurrence (adjusted HR 0.69; 95% CI 0.58–0.82; $p < 0.001$) and all-cause mortality (adjusted HR 0.73; 95% CI 0.59–0.90; $p = 0.003$) compared with those in mid-volume centres [125]. The difference was mostly in local recurrence (adjusted HR 0.62; 95% CI 0.49–0.78; $p < 0.001$) but not distant recurrence (adjusted HR 0.85; 95% CI 0.67–1.06; $p = 0.142$) compared with those in mid-volume centres. After propensity score matching, treatment at a high-volume centre was an independent risk factor for decreased recurrence (adjusted HR 0.69; 95% CI 0.57–0.84; $p < 0.001$) and all-cause mortality (adjusted HR 0.75; 95% CI 0.59–0.95). A population-based cohort study comparing RRH and ARH for cervical cancer stage IA1-IB, was done using the Swedish Quality Register of Gynecologic Cancer, which captures all women in Sweden treated at only seven specialised centres to which cervical cancer patients are centralised. Among 864 women included, (236 had ARH and 628 had RRH. The 5-year OS was 92% and 94% and DFS was 84% and 88% for ARH and RRH respectively. Using propensity score analysis and matched cohorts of 232 women in each surgical group, no significant differences were seen in survival: 5-year OS of 92% in both groups (HR 1.00; 95% CI 0.50–2.01), emphasising the possible advantage of centralisation of care for cervical cancer.

However, a recent analysis of the National Cancer Database failed to show any difference in survival between low volume and high-volume centres in the United States [126]. One of the possible explanations may be that the incidence of cervical cancer in the United States is lower than other countries, with even lower numbers for surgically treated cervical cancer; a high-volume centre had between 6 and 20 MIS RH per year which may be <1 per year per gynaecologic oncology surgeon. Although patients treated at high volume centres were 11.4% more likely to receive guideline-compliant surgery (67.8% vs. 56.4%; $p = 0.001$), there was no difference in 5-year survival, 90-day survival and all-cause mortality across volume quartiles. The 5-year survival was 90.5% in high volume centres, 89.5% in medium-high, 92.2% in medium-low, and 91.8% in low volume centres. Thirty-day mortality was significantly lower at high volume centres (0 deaths in 880 patients) versus low volume centres (1 in 1,058 patients, $p = 0.02$).

# RADICAL HYSTERECTOMY COMPLICATIONS

## Intraoperative complications

The radical hysterectomy, especially by laparotomy, can be a highly morbid procedure and all patients should be managed with an ERAS protocol to reduce the complication risk [77]. The estimated blood loss is between 500 mL and 1,500 mL for an open radical hysterectomy [91]. Potential intraoperative complications include injury to pelvic vessels, ureter, bladder, rectum and obturator nerve. The most important aspect of intraoperative complication is immediate recognition and repair with the most appropriate surgical team to avoid long-term complications.

## POSTOPERATIVE COMPLICATIONS

Postoperative complications are more frequently seen in patients over 60 years old and in patients undergoing a type III radical hysterectomy but some of these complications can be avoided by following an ERAS protocol for gynaecologic oncology [76]. Postoperatively, ERAS protocols are evidence-based guidelines for recovery and include timely removal of drains, early initiation of oral intake, increased ambulation and adequate pain and nausea control. This may now serve to improve outcomes of abdominal radical hysterectomy as compared to historical cohorts and attempt to limit length of stay and earlier return to baseline function.

Urinary tract infection is the most common complication related to prolonged catheterisation [83]. Bladder dysfunction including incontinence and urinary retention is cited up to 80%, but usually resolves at 12 months [127]. Fever is another common complication and may be related to atelectasis, UTI, wound infection, or DVT which are commonly misdiagnosed. Prolonged ileus may occur from ascites related to pelvic lymphadenectomy. Venous thromboembolism is common but often underdiagnosed and patients should be considered for prophylactic anticoagulation following the surgery for 28 days [76]. Utero-vaginal and vesico-vaginal complications are very rare. Based on a study of 2,548 patients undergoing ARH from 2008 to 2015 using the NIS database, the overall rate of any complications after ARH was 21.8% and 18% for robotic RH; ileus (9.1%), fever (4.1%) and wound infections (1.8%) were the most commonly reported postoperative complications [103]. Wenzel et al reported on 472 patients undergoing RH between 2015 and 2017; the overall short-term complication rate was 35% [128]. The most common complication was urinary retention requiring re-catheterisation [15%]. In univariable analysis, ARH (OR 3.42; 95% CI 1.73–6.76), chronic pulmonary disease (OR 3.14; 95% CI 1.45–6.79), vascular disease (OR 1.90; 95% CI 1.07–3.38), and medical centre (OR 2.83; 95% CI 1.18–6.77) emerged as independent predictors of the occurrence of complications. A large study using a Chinese database included 18,447 patients and found that LRH was associated to more ureteral injury (OR 3.83; 95% CI 2.11–6.95), bowel injury (OR 14.83; 95% CI 1.32–167.25), vascular injury (OR 3.37; 95% CI 1.18–9.62), postoperative vesico-vaginal fistula (OR 4.16; 95% CI 2.08–8.32), ureterovaginal fistula (OR 4.16; 95% CI 2.08–8.32), recto-vaginal fistula (OR 8.04; 95% CI 1.63–39.53) as compared to ARH, while ARH has more bowel obstructions [129].

### Recommended removal of foleys catheter

One study found that after nerve sparing RH, the median duration for postoperative bladder catheterisation was 3.5 (range 3–5) days. Within the 5th postoperative day, 82.7% had a PVR urine volume < 100 mL. No patients had PVR more than 100 mL more than 10 days after the operation with no need for self-catheterisation. One series reported on 97 patients undergoing type II or III RRH; 46 (47.4%) had Foley removal prior to discharge, and a mean LOS of 1.1 ± 0.41 days. Among these, 27 (58.6%) were able to spontaneously void and did not require replacement of a Foley; none were readmitted or brought to the office for Foley reinsertion [130]. Another small study comparing early versus delayed Foley removal in 47 versus 48 patients respectively found no significant difference in rates of Foley reinsertion, median PVR or urinary tract infections.

## Bowel dysfunction

Patients undergoing radical hysterectomy are also at risk for short term bowel issues including constipation, incomplete emptying, and faecal incontinence, which may be due to partial denervation of the bowel but resolve within 2 years of surgery.

## Late complications

The sympathetic and parasympathetic nerves to the bladder and rectum are often disrupted during radical hysterectomy as they run in the inferior portion of the cardinal and uterosacral ligaments and are most often divided during the division of the parametrium and uterosacral ligaments. Secondary to transection of the hypogastric nerve, prolonged bladder dysfunction may occur. Denervation results in detrusor hypertonicity [127]. Neurogenic bladder is characterised by decreased bladder capacity, detrusor underactivity and diminished bladder sensation, which causes voiding dysfunction and may require catheterisation [131]. Voiding by the clock with the aid of abdominal muscles and occasionally self-catheterisation may help to restore bladder function. In one series, the rate of bladder dysfunction was 21%, but varied among different surgeons from 0-44%. Stress urinary incontinence develops in approximately 30% of women who have undergone radical hysterectomy(129). The common cystometric abnormalities found are hypertonic bladder with elevated urethral pressure. Patients with a hypotonic bladder have a worse prognosis. In a study comparing long-term bladder dysfunction in nerve sparing radical hysterectomy to conventional radical hysterectomy, the rates of long-term urinary frequency were 14.1% versus 33.5%, urinary incontinence 36.5% versus 54.5% , urinary retention 23.5% versus 38.9% and straining to void 10.6% versus 40.7% , respectively ($p < 0.05$ for all) [132]. Manchana et al reported that up to 15% of patients experienced voiding dysfunction and required urethral catheterisation for >30 days, with 3% requiring catheterisation for >6 months [133]. In addition, Komatsu et al found that urological intervention was required in 45 patients (54.2%), and self-urethral catheterisation was performed in 41 (49.3%) patients. Patients with prolonged catheterisation were at higher risk of elevated creatinine function at 2 years [131].

Sexual dysfunction is common and may be in the range of 55%. The issues can be insufficient lubrication, reduced genital swelling at arousal, reduced vaginal length, elasticity and dyspareunia, all related to the shortening of the vagina required for RH (1.5–2 cm). Damage to the autonomic nerves, resulting in difficulties in achieving sexual arousal and orgasm is also reported [134]. One study by Jensen et al found that among the 173 early-stage cervical cancer patients treated by surgery compared with age-matched healthy controls, significant short-term sexual difficulties including dyspareunia, orgasmic problems, and vaginal shortness were found up to 6 months postoperatively, whereas significant lack of sexual desire and lack of lubrication persisted 2 years postoperatively [134]. Most patients who were sexually active before their cancer diagnosis were sexually active again 12 months after surgery (91%). In addition, the extent of RH may be associated with rates of sexual dysfunction. A type II modified RH is associated with less sexual dysfunction compared to a type III based on an EORTC quality of life survey distributed to 105 patients undergoing radical hysterectomy. Survey scores related to sexual function were significantly lower in patients undergoing type II versus type III radical hysterectomy 8.33 and 26.94 ($p = 0.0035$) [135].

Lymphoedema is undoubtedly a burdensome complication of complete pelvic lymphadenectomy in the range of 20% but has recently been mitigated by the introduction of the SLND [136]. Supra-femoral lymph node dissection and adjuvant radiation are risk factors for postoperative lymphoedema development [136]. Another study found that omitting lymphadenectomy of deep circumflex nodes decreased the lymphoedema rate from 32% to 8% [53]. Based on a systematic review of patients with stage IA2-IB1 undergoing less radical surgery for cervical cancer (simple hysterectomy only), lymphoedema developed in 24% of the 2,662 women included while lymphocysts were reported in 22% of patients [137].

In summary, short-term and long-term complications may be reduced with an ERAS protocol and by selection of patients for a less radical hysterectomy, nerve-sparing techniques and sentinel lymph node dissection compared to a complete lymphadenectomy. Currently with the standard of care being laparotomy for >2 cm tumours, we must accept this level of complication to preserve oncologic outcomes.

## PROGNOSTIC FACTORS

### Status of the lymph nodes

Lymph node positivity is the most important prognostic factor in cervical cancer [138–140]. Prognosis is also dependent on the number of nodes and size of metastasis (isolated tumour cells, micro-metastasis, macro-metastasis). Patients who were upstaged in the new FIGO staging system due to node positivity had a significantly worse OS ($p = 0.008$; HR 2.32; 95% CI 1.22–4.40) than patients whose stage did not change [34]. Similar observations were made within sub-stages when node-positive IB or IIB tumours were upstaged to IIIC (HR 2.20; 95% CI 1.02–4.76; $p = 0.040$). In 261 patients with FIGO stage IA-IIB tumours undergoing radical hysterectomy and pelvic lymphadenectomy, 86 patients (33.0%) had lymph node metastases; 73 patients had pelvic lymph node metastases only and 13 patients had both pelvic and para-aortic lymph node metastases. Pelvic lymph nodes were most likely in the external iliac artery region [141]. Presence of lymph node metastases was significantly associated with preoperative FIGO stage ($p = 0.001$) and final pathological tumour stage ($p < 0.001$), status of resection margin ($p = 0.002$) and LVSI ($p < 0.001$). In 970 patients with at least FIGO IB cervical cancer, pre-operative status of the lymph node had prognostic significance in patients with stage IB1/IIA (HR for PFS 2.10, $p = 0.001$; HR for OS 1.99; $p = 0.005$) [142]. The significance decreased or disappeared with advancing stages. Similarly, the prognostic significance of the pre-treatment lymph node metastasis decreased with increasing age, parametrial involvement or LVSI [142]. However, one issue with this study is that the sensitivity, specificity, positive predictive value, and negative predictive value were quite low and reported to be 44.3%, 87.0%, 44.0%, and 85.7%, respectively. In addition, the number of nodes may have an adverse effect on survival as one study found a strong correlation between the number of metastatic LNs and lymph node ratio ($r = 0.83$, $p < 0.01$) [143]. The 5-year OS was 73%. The OS curves among the pelvic LNR groups significantly differed: the 5-year OS rates of the low, intermediate, and high pelvic LNR groups were 83%, 66%, and 17% ($p < 0.01$), respectively. Based on the SENTICOL trials, patients with low-volume metastasis (including micro-metastasis and isolated tumour cells) had similar

DFS (92.7%) to node-negative patients (93.6%). The addition of adjuvant treatment in presence of low-volume metastasis did not modify the DFS, therefore there is unlikely benefit of adjuvant treatment in patients with micro-metastasis and isolated tumour cells [101,102]. This is different to other studies found in the literature. In the largest retrospective series to date which included 645 patients, Cibula et al observed the same prognosis in patients with positive LNs for micro-metastasis and macro-metastasis in terms of OS [144]. In this study, OS was significantly reduced in patients with macro-metastasis and micro-metastasis; the HR for OS was 6.85 for macro-metastasis (95% CI 2.59–18.05) and 6.86 for micro-metastasis (95% CI 2.09–22.61) respectively. Other small retrospective studies also show worse prognosis for micro-metastasis. There is very limited data related to ITCs; in both the SENTICOL and small retrospective studies, ITCs were not significantly associated with worse prognosis. Nonetheless, prognosis related to micro-metastasis and ITCs remains controversial, especially for ITCs where limited data is available and these did not change adjuvant management.

## Size of tumour

Matsuo et al found that patients with tumours <2 cm had a two-fold increase in survival as compared to larger tumours based on an analysis of the SEER database [15]. The 5-year survival rate declines from 91.6% (95% CI 90.4–92.6%) for patients with tumours ≤2 cm to 83.3% (95% CI 81.8–84.8%) for tumours >2 to ≤4 cm, and 76.1% (95% CI 74.3–77.8%) for >4 cm tumours [16]. In another study of 13,735 cases from the SEER database between 1997 and 2005, Wagner et al found a significant survival difference in stage I patients with tumours 2–4 cm (HR 3.26; 95% CI 2.64–4.04) and >4 cm (HR 6.65; 95% CI 5.45–8.12), compared to patients with <2 cm tumours [145]. One study combined HPV DNA status and tumour size to develop a novel predictive marker. Multivariate analysis showed that the HPV DNA, tumour size, and stage were independent prognostic factors for OS and distant metastasis-free survival [146]. The authors choose tumour size and HPV DNA as the risk stratification factors to build a new prediction model which can better predict OS for locally advanced cervical cancer than FIGO stage.

## Depth of stromal invasion

The degree of stromal invasion has been found to be an independent predictor of prognosis in stage IB cervical cancer [147]. To better understand this finding, a study of 3,298 cervical cancer patients with FIGO (2009) stage IB-IIA were reviewed and included only if there was postoperative histological confirmation of deep stromal invasion (middle or deep one-third of stromal invasion, full-thickness and outer full-thickness invasion) [148]. Patients with full- and outer-full-thickness invasion exhibited significantly higher recurrence rates compared to inner full-thickness group. The 5-year OS rate for patients with inner third, full thickness and outer thickness invasion was 89.9%, 79.5% and 60.2%, respectively, and a statistically significant difference was also found ($p < 0.001$). OS was independently associated with the depth of deep stromal invasion.

## Lymphovascular space invasion

In a retrospective analysis of 193 patients undergoing ARH for stage IB or II cervical cancer, LVSI was associated with a significantly worse prognosis [149]. The 5-year OS was 97% in patients without LVSI compared with 78% for patients with LVSI ($p < 0.0001$). LVSI correlated significantly with tumour stage, nodal status and the location of positive nodes. Even in lower risk tumours less than 2 cm and without isthmic involvement, OS was significantly reduced with the presence of LVSI (100% in 55 patients without LVSI compared with 92% in 34 patients with LVSI ($p < 0.05$); three-fourths patients with recurrence had positive LVSI. On multivariable analysis, LVSI and nodal involvement were poor prognostic factors (RR of death 5.7 for LVSI, 4.9 for pelvic nodes and 17.1 para-aortic nodes). Another study had a 45% rate of LVSI of which 53% were treated with adjuvant radiation; in these patients no difference in survival was seen (89.8% vs. 91.5%), possibly due to the benefit of adjuvant treatment in most of the patients [150]. Using the NCDB, 3,239 patients with stage IA1 and 1,049 patients with stage IA2 carcinoma of the cervix were identified. LVSI was found in 10.5% of patients with stage IA1 disease and 18.8% of stage IA2 [151]. Positive nodes were found in 7.8% of patients with LVSI versus 1% of patients without in stage IA1 and 14.6% versus 1.7% in IA2 ($p < 0.001$). In a univariable analysis, the HR for death associated with LVSI was 1.05 (95% CI 0.45–2.45) for women with stage IA1 tumours and 2.36 (95% CI 1.04–5.33) for those with IA2 neoplasms; thus the effect on survival is more pronounced in patients with stage IA2 disease.

## Parametrial involvement

Patients with tumours ≤2 cm without LVSI are less likely to have PI, unless lymph node metastasis or deep stromal invasion is present [152]. Therefore, it may be questioned in this population whether parametrectomy is beneficial [81,153,154]. One study including 842 patients with stage IA, IB found that PI was associated to older age, larger tumour, LVSI, depth of invasion and pelvic LN metastasis. In patients with tumour size <2 cm, negative nodes and <10 mm depth of invasion, the rate of PI was 0.6% [80]. In another study of 647 patients using the machine learning support vector algorithm, parametrial involvement was an independent risk fact for OS (HR 3.871; 95% CI 1.375–10.9) [155]. In another study, 16 patients with stage IB1 tumours and PI were older (55.9 ± 9.5 vs. 49.0 ± 9.9 years, $p = 0.005$), and had deeper cervical stromal invasion (9.59 ± 4.87 vs. 7.47 ± 5.48 mm, $p = 0.048$), larger tumour size (2.32 ± 1.15 vs. 1.74 ± 1.14 cm, $p = 0.043$,), higher incidences of LVSI (87.5% vs. 28.8%, $p < 0.001$), and greater lymph node metastasis (68.8% vs. 10.8%,) than the 260 patients without PI. The highest prediction accuracy of survival using the support vector machine algorithm was 94.3% when combining only LN status and parametrial involvement, while inclusion of five risk factors (stage, LN status, PI, tumour size, depth of invasion) had only 69% predictability. In a retrospective study of 749 patients with stage I–IV cervical cancer, pelvic nodal metastasis ($p = 0.018$), parametrial invasion ($p = 0.015$), and presence of disease in the surgical margin ($p = 0.011$) were all independent prognostic factors for OS [156]. The 5-year OS rate was 54.3% for patients with metastasis to the parametrium including all stages. One study found that 763 surgically treated cervical cancer patients (10%) had pathologic evidence of tumour in the parametria [157]. Fifty percent of PI found postoperatively was due to continuous extension of the primary process into the parametria. In the other 50%, the parametrial tumour was separate from the primary process. The discontinuous group was associated with LN positivity 79% of the time. The OS was 48 months in the continuous group and 46 months in the discontinuous group.

## Histologic subtype

The survival of patients with tumour extending to the parametrium or pelvic lymph node(s) is adversely affected by histology of pure adenocarcinoma [158]. In a study of 318 patients with stage IB-IIB, adenocarcinoma/adenosquamous (AC/ASC) carcinoma was found to be an adverse independent prognostic factor for cervical cancer patients treated by RH and postoperative RT (2.675, $p < 0.01$) [159]. The 5-year RFS for squamous carcinoma (SCC) and AC/ASC were 83.4% and 66.5%, respectively. In a study including 5,181 patients, 5-year RFS was 85.1%, 78.2%, and 72.3% for SCC, adenocarcinoma, and adenosquamous carcinoma, respectively ($p < 0.001$) [160]. The 5-year OS was 89.7%, 83.1%, and 79.6%, respectively ($p < 0.001$). In multivariable analysis, AC/AASC were independent prognostic factors for worse RFS; comparing for adenocarcinoma versus SCC, the HR was 2.594 (95% CI 2.030–3.316, $p < 0.001$) and comparing adenosquamous carcinoma to SCC, the HR was 2.105 (95% CI 1.517–2.920); $p < 0.001$. There was a higher OS for AC versus SCC [HR 2.976 (95% CI 2.226–3.977), $p < 0.001$] and for ASC compared to SCC [HR 2.295 (95% CI 1.579–3.338), $p < 0.001$]. In one study of patients with non-squamous or AC subtypes, the 5-year PFS and OS were 61.2% and 67.6%, compared to 90.1% and 88.3%, respectively, for the squamous or adenocarcinoma group [161].

## Status of vaginal margin

In a review of 1,223 patients with stage IA2, IB or IIA cervical cancer undergoing radical hysterectomy, 4% of patients had positive or close vaginal margins, including tumours within 0.5 cm from the vaginal margin. The 5-year survival was significantly improved when adjuvant radiotherapy was added (81.3% vs. 28.6%, $p < 0.05$) [162,163]. Among 119 patients undergoing radical hysterectomy for stage IA2-IIA, 63% of patients had close surgical margins <5 mm with a recurrence rate of 24%, compared to 9% in patients without close margin [164]. A surgical margin of ≤2 mm was significantly associated with an increased risk of overall recurrence (36% vs. 9%; $p = 0.009$) as well as locoregional recurrence (22% vs. 4%; $p = 0.0034$).

# CONCLUSION

Even though cervical cancer currently ranks as the fourth most common cancer in women, the development and distribution of effective HPV vaccines will cause this rate to decrease in the future. Early-stage cervical cancers will be harder to identify through the current screening methods and the radical surgeries described in this chapter required to treat these early-stage cancers will become even more localized to subspeciality centers. It will be important for physicians desiring to treat this population, seek out the training required for these procedures and ensure they maintain the skills needed especially in fertility sparing situations.

# REFERENCES

1.   de Martel C, Plummer M, Vignat J, et al. Worldwide burden of cancer attributable to HPV by site, country and HPV type. Int J Can 2017; 141:664–670.
2.   Razzaghi H, Saraiya M, Thompson TD, et al. Five-year relative survival for human papillomavirus-associated cancer sites. Cancer 2018; 124:203–211.
3.   Forman D, de Martel C, Lacey CJ, t al. Global burden of human papillomavirus and related diseases. Vaccine 2012; 30:F12–F23.
4.   Bosch FX, Munoz N. The viral etiology of cervical cancer. Virus Res 2002; 89:183–190.
5.   Cong Q, Song Y, Wang Q, et al. A Large Retrospective Study of 12714 Cases of LEEP Conization Focusing on Cervical Cancer that Colposcopy-Directed Biopsy Failed to Detect. BioMed Res Int 2018; 2018:5138232.
6.   PathologyOutlines.com. (2021). Cervix General Staging (Parra-Herran C). [online] Available from https://www.pathologyoutlines.com/topic/cervixstaging.html. [Last Accessed May, 2022].

7.   Berek JS, Hacker NF. Berek & Hacker's Gynecologic Oncology, 6th edition. Philadelphia: Wolters Kluwer; 2015.

8.   UptoDate. (2021). Invasive cervical cancer: Epidemiology, risk factors, clinical manifestations, and diagnosis 2021 (Frumovitz M). [online] Available from: https://www-uptodate-com.proxy3.library. mcgill.ca/contents/invasive-cervical-cancer-epidemiology-risk-factors-clinical-manifestations-and-diagnosis?search=symptoms%20cervical%20cancer&sectionRank=1&usage_type=default&anchor=H6&source=machineLearning&selectedTitle=1~150&display_rank=1#H6. [Last Accessed May, 2022].

9.   Saia D. Clinical Gynecologic Oncology. New York: Elsevier; 2017.

10.  Salvo G, Odetto D, Saez Perrotta MC, et al. Measurement of tumor size in early cervical cancer: an ever-evolving paradigm. Int J Gynecol Can 2020; 30:1215–1223.

11.  FIGO staging for carcinoma of the vulva, cervix, and corpus uteri. Int J Gynaecol Obstet 2014; 125:97–98.

12.  Bhatla N, Berek JS, Cuello Fredes M. Revised FIGO staging for carcinoma of the cervix uteri. Int J Gynaecol Obstet 2019; 145:129.

13.  Bhatla N, Aoki D, Sharma DN, et al. Cancer of the cervix uteri. Int J Gynaecol Obstet 2018;143:22.

14.  Nicolet V, Carignan L, Bourdon F, et al. MR imaging of cervical carcinoma: a practical staging approach. Radiographics 2000; 20:1539–1549.

15.  Ramirez PT, Frumovitz M, Pareja R, et al. Minimally Invasive versus Abdominal Radical Hysterectomy for Cervical Cancer. N Engl J Med 2018: 30380365.

16.  Melamed A, Margul DA-O, Chen L, et al. Survival after Minimally Invasive Radical Hysterectomy for Early-Stage Cervical Cancer. N Engl J Med 2018; 379:1905–1914.

17.  Patel H, Madhuri K, Rockell T, et al. Robotic radical hysterectomy for stage 1B1 cervical cancer: A case series of survival outcomes from a leading UK cancer centre. Int J Med Robot 2020; 16:e2116.

18.  Wenzel HHB, Smolders RGV, Beltman JJ, et al. Survival of patients with early-stage cervical cancer after abdominal or laparoscopic radical hysterectomy: a nationwide cohort study and literature review. Eur J Can 2020; 133:14–21.

19.  Chen B, Ji M, Li P, et al. Comparison between robot-assisted radical hysterectomy and abdominal radical hysterectomy for cervical cancer: A multicentre retrospective study. Gynecol Oncol 2020; 157:429–436.

20.  Matsuo K, Machida H, Mandelbaum RS, et al. Validation of the 2018 FIGO cervical cancer staging system. Gynecol Oncol 2019; 152:87.

21.  Wright JD, Matsuo K, Huang Y, et al. Prognostic Performance of the 2018 International Federation of Gynecology and Obstetrics Cervical Cancer Staging Guidelines. Obstet Gynecol 2019; 134:49–57.

22.  Kato T, Takashima A, Kasamatsu T, et al. Clinical tumor diameter and prognosis of patients with FIGO stage IB1 cervical cancer (JCOG0806-A). Gynecol Oncol 2015; 137:34–39.

23.  Gulseren V, Kocaer M, Gungorduk O, et al. Preoperative predictors of pelvic and para-aortic lymph node metastases in cervical cancer. J Can Res Ther 2019; 15:1231–1234.

24.  Lee KB, Lee JM, Park CY, et al. Lymph node metastasis and lymph vascular space invasion in microinvasive squamous cell carcinoma of the uterine cervix. Int J Gynecol Can 2006; 16:1184–1187.

25.  Yan W, Qiu S, Ding Y, et al. Prognostic value of lymphovascular space invasion in patients with early stage cervical cancer in Jilin, China: A retrospective study. Medicine 2019; 98:e17301.

26.  Ma C, Zhang Y, Li R, et al. Risk of parametrial invasion in women with early stage cervical cancer: a meta-analysis. Arch Gynecol Obstet 2018; 297:573–580.

27.  Hutchcraft ML, Smith B, McLaughlin EM, et al. Conization pathologic features as a predictor of intermediate and high risk features on radical hysterectomy specimens in early stage cervical cancer. Gynecol Oncol 2019; 153:255–258.

28.  Horn LC, Brambs CE, Opitz S, et al. The 2019 FIGO classification for cervical carcinoma-what's new? Der Pathologe 2019; 40:629–635.

29.  Noguchi H, Shiozawa I, Kitahara T, et al. Uterine body invasion of carcinoma of the uterine cervix as seen from surgical specimens. Gynecol Oncol 1988; 30:173–182.

30.  Bhosale P, Peungjesada S, Devine C, et al. Role of Magnetic Resonance Imaging as an Adjunct to Clinical Staging in Cervical Carcinoma. J Comp Assist Tomogr 2010; 34:855–864.

31.  Canaz E, Ozyurek ES, Erdem B, et al. Preoperatively Assessable Clinical and Pathological Risk Factors for Parametrial Involvement in Surgically Treated FIGO Stage IB-IIA Cervical Cancer. Int J Gynecol Can 2017; 27:1722–1728.

32.  Martimbeau PW, Kjorstad KE, Iversen T. Stage IB carcinoma of the cervix, the Norwegian Radium hospital. II. Results when pelvic nodes are involved. Obstet Gynecol 1982; 60:215–218.

33.  Stehman FB, Bundy BN, DiSaia PJ, et al. Carcinoma of the cervix treated with radiation therapy. Part I. A multi-variate analysis of prognostic variables in the Gynecologic Oncology Group. Cancer 1991; 67:2776.

34. de Gregorio A, Widschwendter P, Ebner F, et al. Influence of the New FIGO Classification for Cervical Cancer on Patient Survival: A Retrospective Analysis of 265 Histologically Confirmed Cases with FIGO Stages IA to IIB. Oncology 2020; 98:91–97.

35. Wright TC, Stoler MH, Behrens CM, et al. Primary cervical cancer screening with human papillomavirus: end of study results from the ATHENA study using HPV as the first-line screening test. Gynecol Oncol 2015; 136:189–197.

36. Demarco M, Lorey TS, Fetterman B, et al. Risks of CIN 2+, CIN 3+, and Cancer by Cytology and Human Papillomavirus Status: The Foundation of Risk-Based Cervical Screening Guidelines. J Low Genit Tract Dis 2017; 21:261–267.

37. Castle PE, Kinney WK, Xue X, et al. Effect of Several Negative Rounds of Human Papillomavirus and Cytology Co-testing on Safety Against Cervical Cancer: An Observational Cohort Study. Ann Int Med 2018; 168:20–29.

38. Perkins RB, Guido RS, Castle PE, et al. 2019 ASCCP Risk-Based Management Consensus Guidelines for Abnormal Cervical Cancer Screening Tests and Cancer Precursors. J Low Genit Tract Dis 2020; 24:102–131.

39. Liang CC, Tseng CJ, Soong YK. The usefulness of cystoscopy in the staging of cervical cancer. Gynecol Oncol 2000; 76:200–203.

40. Sharma DN, Thulkar S, Goyal S, et al. Revisiting the role of computerized tomographic scan and cystoscopy for detecting bladder invasion in the revised FIGO staging system for carcinoma of the uterine cervix. Int J Gynecol Can 2010; 20:368–372.

41. Boivin D, Grégoire M. Place of cystoscopy in the staging of cervical cancer. Progres en urologie 2003; 13: 1351–1353.

42. Massad LS, Calvello C, Gilkey SH, et al. Assessing disease extent in women with bulky or clinically evident metastatic cervical cancer: yield of pretreatment studies. Gynecol Oncol 2000; 76:383–387.

43. Jeong BK, Huh SJ, Choi DH, et al. Indications for endoscopy according to the revised FIGO staging for cervical cancer after MRI and CT scanning. J Gynecol Oncol 2012; 23:80–85.

44. Koh WJ, Abu-Rustum NR, Bean S. Cervical cancer, version 3.2019, NCCN clinical practice guidelines in oncology. J Natl Compr Canc Netw 2019; 17:64.

45. Zhang W, Chen C, Liu P. Impact of pelvic MRI in routine clinical practice on staging of IB1-IIA2 cervical cancer. Cancer Manag Res 2019; 11:3603.

46. Mansoori B, Khatri G, Rivera-Colón G, et al. Multimodality Imaging of Uterine Cervical Malignancies. Am J Roentgenol 2020; 215:292–304.

47. Haldorsen IS, Lura N, Blaakær J, et al. What Is the Role of Imaging at Primary Diagnostic Work-Up in Uterine Cervical Cancer? Curr Oncol Rep 2019; 21:77.

48. Cheng J, Hou Y, Li J, et al. Agreement Between Magnetic Resonance Imaging and Pathologic Findings in the Tumor Size Evaluation Before and After Neoadjuvant Chemotherapy Treatment: A Prospective Study. Int J Gynecol Can 2017; 27:1472–1479.

49. Urushibara A, Saida T, Mori K, et al. Diagnosing uterine cervical cancer on a single T2-weighted image: Comparison between deep learning versus radiologists. Eur J Radiol 2020; 135:109471.

50. Shweel MA, Abdel-Gawad EA, Abdel-Gawad EA, et al. Uterine cervical malignancy: diagnostic accuracy of MRI with histopathologic correlation. J Clin Imaging Sci 2012; 2:42.

51. Woo S, Suh CH, Kim SY, et al. Magnetic resonance imaging for detection of parametrial invasion in cervical cancer: an updated systematic review and meta-analysis of the literature between 2012 and 2016. Eur Radiol 2018; 28:530.

52. Kamimori T, Sakamoto K, Fujiwara K, et al. Parametrial involvement in FIGO stage IB1 cervical carcinoma diagnostic impact of tumor diameter in preoperative magnetic resonance imaging. Int J Gynecol Can 2011; 21:349–354.

53. Yamazaki H, Todo Y, Takeshita S, et al. Relationship between removal of circumflex iliac nodes distal to the external iliac nodes and postoperative lower-extremity lymphedema in uterine cervical cancer. Gynecol Oncol 2015; 139:295–299.

54. Sala E, Wakely S, Senior E, et al. MRI of Malignant Neoplasms of the Uterine Corpus and Cervix. Am J Roentgenol 2007; 188:1577–1587.

55. Nam H, Huh SJ, Park W. Prognostic significance of MRI-detected bladder muscle and/or serosal invasion in patients with cervical cancer treated with radiotherapy. Br J Radiol 2010; 83:868.

56. Salib MY, Russell JHB, Stewart VR, et al. 2018 FIGO Staging Classification for Cervical Cancer: Added Benefits of Imaging. Radiographics 2020; 40:1807–1822.

57. Kim SH, Han MC. Invasion of the urinary bladder by uterine cervical carcinoma: evaluation with MR imaging. AJR 1997; 168:393.

58.  Choi HJ, Ju W, Myung SK, et al. Diagnostic performance of computer tomography, magnetic resonance imaging, and positron emission tomography or positron emission tomography/computer tomography for detection of metastatic lymph nodes in patients with cervical cancer: meta-analysis. Can Sci 2010; 101:1471–1479.
59.  Lee JY, Youm J, Kim JW, et al. Identifying a low-risk group for parametrial involvement in microscopic Stage IB1 cervical cancer using criteria from ongoing studies and a new MRI criterion. BMC Can 2015; 15:167.
60.  Papadia A, Gasparri ML, Genoud S, et al. The combination of preoperative PET/CT and sentinel lymph node biopsy in the surgical management of early-stage cervical cancer. J Can Res Clin Oncol 2017; 143:2275–2281.
61.  Selman TJ, Mann C, Zamora J, et al. Diagnostic accuracy of tests for lymph node status in primary cervical cancer: a systematic review and meta-analysis. Can Med Assoc 2008; 178:855–862.
62.  Kang S, Kim SK, Chung DC, et al. Diagnostic value of (18)F-FDG PET for evaluation of paraaortic nodal metastasis in patients with cervical carcinoma: a metaanalysis. J Nuc Med 2010; 51:360–367.
63.  Viswanathan C, Faria S, Devine C, et al. [18F]-2-Fluoro-2-Deoxy-D-glucose-PET Assessment of Cervical Cancer. PET Clin 2018; 13:165–177.
64.  Yagi S, Yahata T, Mabuchi Y, et al. Primary tumor SUV(max) on preoperative FDG-PET/CT is a prognostic indicator in stage IA2-IIB cervical cancer patients treated with radical hysterectomy. Mole Clin Oncol 2016; 5:216–222.
65.  Yang Z, Xu W, Ma Y, et al. (18)F-FDG PET/CT can correct the clinical stages and predict pathological parameters before operation in cervical cancer. Eur J Radiol 2016; 85:877–884.
66.  Gee MS, Atri M, Bandos AI, et al. Identification of Distant Metastatic Disease in Uterine Cervical and Endometrial Cancers with FDG PET/CT: Analysis from the ACRIN 6671/GOG 0233 Multicenter Trial. Radiology 2018; 287:176–184.
67.  Elit LM, Fyles AW, Gu CS, et al. Effect of Positron Emission Tomography Imaging in Women With Locally Advanced Cervical Cancer: A Randomized Clinical Trial. JAMA Netw Open 2018; 1:e182081.
68.  Reyneke F, Snyman LC, Lawal I, et al. Diagnostic value of sentinel lymph node scintigraphy and 2-[(18) F]-fluoro-2-deoxy-D-glucose positron emission tomography/computed tomography in the detection of metastatic lymph nodes in patients with early-stage cervical cancer. World J Nucl Med 2020; 19:240–245.
69.  Cibula D, Pötter R, Planchamp F, et al. The European Society of Gynaecological Oncology/European Society for Radiotherapy and Oncology/European Society of Pathology Guidelines for the Management of Patients With Cervical Cancer. Int J Gynecol Cancer 2018; 28:641–655.
70.  Scheidler J, Heuck AF. Imaging of cancer of the cervix. Radiol Clin North Am 2002; 40:577–590.
71.  Bourgioti C, Chatoupis K, Moulopoulos LA. Current imaging strategies for the evaluation of uterine cervical cancer. World J Radiol 2016; 8:342–354.
72.  Tsili AC, Tsangou V, Koliopoulos G, et al. Early-stage cervical carcinoma: the role of multidetector CT in correlation with histopathological findings. J Obstet Gynaecol 2013; 33:882–887.
73.  Yang WT, Lam WW, Yu MY, et al. Comparison of dynamic helical CT and dynamic MR imaging in the evaluation of pelvic lymph nodes in cervical carcinoma. AJR Am J Roentgenol 2000; 175:759–766.
74.  Liu B, Gao S, Li S. A comprehensive comparison of CT, MRI, positron emission tomography or positron emission tomography/CT, and diffusion weighted imaging-MRI for detecting the lymph nodes metastases in patients with cervical cancer: a meta-analysis based on 67 studies. Gynecol Obstet Invest 2017; 82:209–222.
75.  Pannu HK, Corl FM, Fishman EK. CT evaluation of cervical cancer: spectrum of disease. Radiographics 2001; 21:1155–1168.
76.  Nelson G, Bakkum-Gamez J, Kalogera E, et al. Guidelines for perioperative care in gynecologic/oncology: Enhanced Recovery After Surgery (ERAS) Society recommendations-2019 update. Int J Gynecol Cancer 2019; 29:651–668.
77.  Abu-Rustum NR, Yashar CM, Bean S, et al. NCCN Guidelines Insights: Cervical Cancer, Version 1.2020. J Natl Compr Canc Netw 2020; 18:660–666.
78.  Chi D, Berchuck A, Dizon D, et al. Principles and Practice of Gynecologic Oncology, 7th edition. Philadelphia: Lippincott Williams & Wilkins; 2017.
79.  Bean LM, Ward KK, Plaxe SC, et al. Survival of women with microinvasive adenocarcinoma of the cervix is not improved by radical surgery. Am J Obstet Gynecol 2017; 217:332.e1–332.e6.
80.  Covens A, Rosen B, Murphy J, et al. How important is removal of the parametrium at surgery for carcinoma of the cervix? Gynecol Oncol 2002; 84:145–149.
81.  Landoni F, Maneo A, Colombo A, et al. Randomised study of radical surgery versus radiotherapy for stage Ib-IIa cervical cancer. Lancet 1997; 350:535–540.

82. Rotman M, Sedlis A, Piedmonte MR, et al. A phase III randomized trial of postoperative pelvic irradiation in Stage IB cervical carcinoma with poor prognostic features: follow-up of a gynecologic oncology group study. Int J Radiat Oncol Biol Phys 2006; 65:169–176.

83. Peters 3rd WA, , Liu PY, Barrett 2nd RJ, et al. Concurrent chemotherapy and pelvic radiation therapy compared with pelvic radiation therapy alone as adjuvant therapy after radical surgery in high-risk early-stage cancer of the cervix. J Clin Oncol 2000; 18:1606–1613.

84. Chiva L, Zanagnolo V, Querleu D, et al. SUCCOR study: an international European cohort observational study comparing minimally invasive surgery versus open abdominal radical hysterectomy in patients with stage IB1 cervical cancer. Int J Gynecol Cancer 2020; 30:1269–1277.

85. Monk BJ, Wang J, Im S, et al. Rethinking the use of radiation and chemotherapy after radical hysterectomy: a clinical-pathologic analysis of a Gynecologic Oncology Group/Southwest Oncology Group/Radiation Therapy Oncology Group trial. Gynecol Oncol 2005; 96:721–728.

86. Plante M, van Trommel N, Lheureux S, et al. FIGO 2018 stage IB2 (2-4 cm) Cervical cancer treated with Neo-adjuvant chemotherapy followed by fertility Sparing Surgery (CONTESSA); Neo-Adjuvant Chemotherapy and Conservative Surgery in Cervical Cancer to Preserve Fertility (NEOCON-F). A PMHC, DGOG, GCIG/CCRN and multicenter study. Int J Gynecol 2019; 29:969–975.

87. Landoni F, Maneo A, Cormio G, et al. Class II versus class III radical hysterectomy in stage IB-IIA cervical cancer: a prospective randomized study. Gynecol Oncol 2001; 80:3–12.

88. Kadkhodayan S, Hasanzadeh M, Treglia G, et al. Sentinel node biopsy for lymph nodal staging of uterine cervix cancer: A systematic review and meta-analysis of the pertinent literature. Eur J Surg Oncol 2015; 41:1–20.

89. Altgassen C, Hertel H, Brandstädt A, et al. Multicenter validation study of the sentinel lymph node concept in cervical cancer: AGO Study Group. J Clin Oncol 2008; 26:2943–2951.

90. Lécuru F, Mathevet P, Querleu D, et al. Bilateral Negative Sentinel Nodes Accurately Predict Absence of Lymph Node Metastasis in Early Cervical Cancer: Results of the SENTICOL Study. J Clin Oncol 2011; 29:1686–1691.

91. Mathevet P, Guani B, Ciobanu A, et al. Histopathologic Validation of the Sentinel Node Technique for Early-Stage Cervical Cancer Patients. Ann Surg Oncol 2021; 28:3629–3635.

92. Bats AS, Frati A, Mathevet P, et al. Contribution of lymphoscintigraphy to intraoperative sentinel lymph node detection in early cervical cancer: Analysis of the prospective multicenter SENTICOL cohort. Gynecol Oncol 2015; 137:264–269.

93. Bentley J. Colposcopic management of abnormal cervical cytology and histology. J Obstet Gynaecol Can 2012; 34:1188–1202.

94. Balaya V, Bresset A, Guani B, et al. Pre-operative surgical algorithm: sentinel lymph node biopsy as predictor of parametrial involvement in early-stage cervical cancer. Int J Gynecol Cancer 2020; 30:1317–1325.

95. Strnad P, Robova H, Skapa P, et al. A prospective study of sentinel lymph node status and parametrial involvement in patients with small tumour volume cervical cancer. Gynecol Oncol 2008; 109:280–284.

96. Cormier B, Diaz JP, Shih K, et al. Establishing a sentinel lymph node mapping algorithm for the treatment of early cervical cancer. Gynecol Oncol 2011; 122:275–280.

97. Tax C, Rovers MM, de Graaf C, et al. The sentinel node procedure in early stage cervical cancer, taking the next step; a diagnostic review. Gynecol Oncol 2015; 139:559–567.

98. Lennox GK, Covens A. Can sentinel lymph node biopsy replace pelvic lymphadenectomy for early cervical cancer? Gynecol Oncol 2017; 144:16–20.

99. Lecuru FR, McCormack M, Hillemanns P, et al. SENTICOL III: an international validation study of sentinel node biopsy in early cervical cancer. A GINECO, ENGOT, GCIG and multicenter study. Int J Gynecol Cancer 2019; 29:829–834.

100. Cibula D, Dusek J, Jarkovsky J, et al. A prospective multicenter trial on sentinel lymph node biopsy in patients with early-stage cervical cancer (SENTIX). Int J Gynecol Cancer 2019; 29:212–215.

101. Guani B, Dorez M, Magaud L, et al. Impact of micrometastasis or isolated tumor cells on recurrence and survival in patients with early cervical cancer: SENTICOL Trial. Int J Gynecol Cancer 2019; 29:447–452.

102. Guani B, Balaya V, Magaud L, et al. The Clinical Impact of Low-Volume Lymph Nodal Metastases in Early-Stage Cervical Cancer: The Senticol 1 and Senticol 2 Trials. Cancers (Basel) 2020; 12:1061.

103. Kim JH, Kim K, Park SJ, et al. Comparative Effectiveness of Abdominal versus Laparoscopic Radical Hysterectomy for Cervical Cancer in the Postdissemination Era. Cancer Res Treat 2019; 51:788–796.

104. Nezhat CR, Burrell MO, Nezhat FR, et al. Laparoscopic radical hysterectomy with paraaortic and pelvic node dissection. Am J Obstet Gynecol 1992; 166:864–865.

105. Sert BM, Abeler VM. Robotic-assisted laparoscopic radical hysterectomy (Piver type III) with pelvic node dissection--case report. Eur J Gynaecol Oncol 2006; 27:531–533.

106. Piedimonte S, Czuzoj-Shulman N, Gotlieb W, et al. Robotic Radical Hysterectomy for Cervical Cancer: A Population-Based Study of Adoption and Immediate Postoperative Outcomes in the United States. J Minim Invasive Gynecol 2019; 26:551–557.
107. Conrad LB, Ramirez PT, Burke W, et al. Role of Minimally Invasive Surgery in Gynecologic Oncology: An Updated Survey of Members of the Society of Gynecologic Oncology. Int J Gynecol Cancer 2015; 25:1121–1127.
108. Boggess JF, Gehrig PA, Cantrell L, et al. A case-control study of robot-assisted type III radical hysterectomy with pelvic lymph node dissection compared with open radical hysterectomy. Am J Obstet Gynecol 2008; 199:357.e1–7.
109. Rajanbabu A, Drudi L, Lau S, et al. Virtual reality surgical simulators-a prerequisite for robotic surgery. Indian J Surg Oncol 2014; 5:125–127.
110. Jin YM, Liu SS, Chen J, et al. Robotic radical hysterectomy is superior to laparoscopic radical hysterectomy and open radical hysterectomy in the treatment of cervical cancer. PloS one. 2018; 13:e0193033.
111. Zhou J, Xiong BH, Ma L, et al. Robotic vs laparoscopic radical hysterectomy for cervical cancer: a meta-analysis. Int J Med Robot 2016; 12:145–154.
112. Obermair A, Asher R, Pareja R, et al. Incidence of adverse events in minimally invasive vs open radical hysterectomy in early cervical cancer: results of a randomized controlled trial. Am J Obstet Gynecol 2020; 222:249.e1–249.e10.
113. Uppal S, Gehrig PA, Peng K, et al. Recurrence Rates in Patients With Cervical Cancer Treated With Abdominal Versus Minimally Invasive Radical Hysterectomy: A Multi-Institutional Retrospective Review Study. J Clin Oncol 2020; 38:1030–1040.
114. Nica A, Kim SR, Gien LT, et al. Survival after minimally invasive surgery in early cervical cancer: is the intra-uterine manipulator to blame? Int J Gynecol Cancer 2020; 30:1864–1870.
115. Cusimano MC, Baxter NN, Gien LT, et al. Impact of surgical approach on oncologic outcomes in women undergoing radical hysterectomy for cervical cancer. Am J Obstet Gynecol 2019; 221: 619.e1–619.e24.
116. Bogani G, Ghezzi F, Chiva L, et al. Patterns of recurrence after laparoscopic versus open abdominal radical hysterectomy in patients with cervical cancer: a propensity-matched analysis. Int J Gynecol Cancer 2020; 30:987–992.
117. Nitecki R, Ramirez PT, Frumovitz M, et al. Survival After Minimally Invasive vs Open Radical Hysterectomy for Early-Stage Cervical Cancer: A Systematic Review and Meta-analysis. JAMA Oncol 2020; 6:1019–1027.
118. Smith AJB, Jones TN, Miao D, et al. Minimally Invasive Radical Hysterectomy for Cervical Cancer: A Systematic Review and Meta-analysis. J Minim Invasive Gynecol 2021; 28:544–555.e7.
119. Wang Y, Li B, Ren F, et al. Survival After Minimally Invasive vs. Open Radical Hysterectomy for Cervical Cancer: A Meta-Analysis. Front. Oncol 2020; 10:1236.
120. Matanes E, Abitbol J, Kessous R, et al. Oncologic and Surgical Outcomes of Robotic Versus Open Radical Hysterectomy for Cervical Cancer. J Obstet Gynaecol Can 2019; 41:450–458.
121. Brandt B, Sioulas V, Basaran D, et al. Minimally invasive surgery versus laparotomy for radical hysterectomy in the management of early-stage cervical cancer: Survival outcomes. Gynecol Oncol 2020; 156:591–597.
122. Falconer H, Palsdottir K, Stalberg K, et al. Robot-assisted approach to cervical cancer (RACC): an international multi-center, open-label randomized controlled trial. Int J Gynecol Cancer 2019; 29:1072–1076.
123. Vieira MA, Rendón GJ, Munsell M, et al. Radical trachelectomy in early-stage cervical cancer: A comparison of laparotomy and minimally invasive surgery. Gynecol Oncol 2015; 138:585–589.
124. Bentivegna E, Gouy S, Maulard A, et al. Oncological outcomes after fertility-sparing surgery for cervical cancer: a systematic review. Lancet Oncol 2016; 17:e240–e253.
125. Matsuo K, Shimada M, Yamaguchi S, et al. Association of Radical Hysterectomy Surgical Volume and Survival for Early-Stage Cervical Cancer. Obstet Gynecol 2019; 133:1086–1098.
126. Aviki EM, Chen L, Dessources K, et al. Impact of hospital volume on surgical management and outcomes for early-stage cervical cancer. Gynecol Oncol 2020; 157:508–513.
127. UptoDate. Radical Hysterectomy (Mann WJ), 2021. [online] Available from https://www.uptodate.com/contents/radical-hysterectomy [Last Accessed May, 2022].
128. Wenzel HHB, Kruitwagen RFPM, Nijman HW, et al. Short-term surgical complications after radical hysterectomy-A nationwide cohort study. Acta Obstet Gynecol Scand 2020; 99:925–932.
129. Liang C, Liu P, Cui Z, et al. Effect of laparoscopic versus abdominal radical hysterectomy on major surgical complications in women with stage IA-IIB cervical cancer in China, 2004-2015. Gynecol Oncol 2020; 156:115–123.
130. Fitzsimmons CK, Stephens AJ, Ahmad S, et al. Timing of postoperative Foley catheter removal from robotic-assisted radical hysterectomy in patients with early-stage cervical cancer. Gynecol Oncol 2019; 154:157.

131. Komatsu H, Oishi T, Osaku D, et al. Long-term evaluation of renal function and neurogenic bladder following radical hysterectomy in patients with uterine cervical cancer. J Obstet Gynaecol Res 2020; 46:2108–2114.

132. Wenwen W, Bin L, Jing Z, et al. [Evaluation of postoperative bladder function and prognosis after modified nerve sparing radical hysterectomy]. Zhonghua fu chan ke za zhi. 2014; 49:341–347.

133. Manchana T, Sirisabya N, Lertkhachonsuk R, et al. Long term complications after radical hysterectomy with pelvic lymphadenectomy. J Med Assoc Thai 2009; 92:451–456.

134. Jensen PT, Groenvold M, Klee MC, et al. Early-stage cervical carcinoma, radical hysterectomy, and sexual function. A longitudinal study. Cancer 2004; 100:97–106.

135. Plotti F, Nelaj E, Sansone M, et al. Sexual function after modified radical hysterectomy (Piver II/Type B) vs. classic radical hysterectomy (Piver III/Type C2) for early stage cervical cancer. A prospective study. J Sex Med 2012; 9:909–917.

136. Ohba Y, Todo Y, Kobayashi N, et al. Risk factors for lower-limb lymphedema after surgery for cervical cancer. Int J Clin Oncol 2011; 16:238–243.

137. Wu J, Logue T, Kaplan SJ, et al. Less-radical Surgery for Early Stage Cervical Cancer: A Systematic Review. Am J Obstet Gynecol 2021: 224:348–358.e5.

138. Allam M, Feely C, Millan D, et al. Depth of cervical stromal invasion as a prognostic factor after radical surgery for early stage cervical cancer. Gynecol Oncol 2004; 93:637–641.

139. Delomenie M, Bonsang-Kitzis H, Bats AS, et al. The clinical implication of lymph nodes micrometastases and isolated tumor cells in patients with cervical cancer: A systematic review. Eur J Obstet Gynecol Reprod Biol 2019; 241:71–76.

140. Yu Q, Lou XM, He Y. Prediction of local recurrence in cervical cancer by a Cox model comprised of lymph node status, lymph-vascular space invasion, and intratumoral Th17 cell-infiltration. Med Oncol 2014; 31:795.

141. Widschwendter P, Janni W, Scholz C, et al. Prognostic factors for and pattern of lymph-node involvement in patients with operable cervical cancer. Arch Gynecol Obstet 2019; 300:1709–1718.

142. Jeong SY, Park H, Kim MS, et al. Pretreatment Lymph Node Metastasis as a Prognostic Significance in Cervical Cancer: Comparison between Disease Status. Cancer Res Treat 2020; 52:516–523.

143. Joo JH, Kim YS, Nam JH. Prognostic significance of lymph node ratio in node-positive cervical cancer patients. Medicine (Baltimore) 2018; 97:e11711.

144. Cibula D, Abu-Rustum NR, Dusek L, et al. Prognostic significance of low volume sentinel lymph node disease in early-stage cervical cancer. Gynecol Oncol 2012; 124:496–501.

145. Wagner AE, Pappas L, Ghia AJ, et al. Impact of tumor size on survival in cancer of the cervix and validation of stage IIA1 and IIA2 subdivisions. Gynecol Oncol 2013; 129:517–521.

146. Huang Y, He Q, Xu K, et al. A new marker based on risk stratification of human papillomavirus DNA and tumor size to predict survival of locally advanced cervical cancer. Int J Gynecol Cancer 2019; 29:459–465.

147. Chittithaworn S, Hanprasertpong J, Tungsinmunkong K, et al. Association between prognostic factors and disease-free survival of cervical cancer stage IB1 patients undergoing radical hysterectomy. Asian Pac J Cancer Prev 2007; 8:530–534.

148. Zhu J, Cao L, Wen H, et al. The clinical and prognostic implication of deep stromal invasion in cervical cancer patients undergoing radical hysterectomy. J Cancer 2020; 11:7368–7377.

149. Morice P, Piovesan P, Rey A, et al. Prognostic value of lymphovascular space invasion determined with hematoxylin-eosin staining in early stage cervical carcinoma: results of a multivariate analysis. Ann Oncol 2003; 14:1511–1517.

150. Weyl A, Illac C, Lusque A, et al. Prognostic value of lymphovascular space invasion in early-stage cervical cancer. Int J Gynecol Cancer 2020; 30:1493–1499.

151. Margolis B, Cagle-Colon K, Chen L, et al. Prognostic significance of lymphovascular space invasion for stage IA1 and IA2 cervical cancer. Int J Gynecol Cancer 2020; 30:735–743.

152. Baiocchi G, de Brot L, Faloppa CC, et al. Is parametrectomy always necessary in early-stage cervical cancer? Gynecol Oncol 2017; 146:16–19.

153. Vanichtantikul A, Tantbirojn P, Manchana T. Parametrial involvement in women with low-risk, early-stage cervical cancer. Eur J Cancer Care (Engl) 2017; 26.

154. Klat J, Sevcik L, Simetka O, et al. What is the risk for parametrial involvement in women with early-stage cervical cancer with tumour <20 mm and with negative sentinel lymph nodes? Aust N Z J Obstet Gynaecol 2012; 52:540–544.

155. Xie L, Chu R, Wang K, et al. Prognostic Assessment of Cervical Cancer Patients by Clinical Staging and Surgical-Pathological Factor: A Support Vector Machine-Based Approach. Front Oncol 2020; 10:1353.

156. Teke F, Yöney A, Teke M, et al. Evaluation of outcome and prognostic factors in 739 patients with uterine cervix carcinoma: a single institution experience. Contemp Oncol (Pozn) 2015; 19:130–136.
157. van den Tillaart SAHM, Trimbos JBMZ, Dreef EJ, et al. Patterns of parametrial involvement in radical hysterectomy specimens of cervical cancer patients. Int J Gynecol Pathol 2011; 30:185–192.
158. Takeda N, Sakuragi N, Takeda M, et al. Multivariate analysis of histopathologic prognostic factors for invasive cervical cancer treated with radical hysterectomy and systematic retroperitoneal lymphadenectomy. Acta Obstet Gynecol Scand 2002; 81:1144–1151.
159. Huang YT, Wang CC, Tsai CS, et al. Clinical behaviors and outcomes for adenocarcinoma or adenosquamous carcinoma of cervix treated by radical hysterectomy and adjuvant radiotherapy or chemoradiotherapy. Int J Radiat Oncol Biol Phys 2012; 84:420–427.
160. Cao L, Wen H, Feng Z, et al. Distinctive clinicopathologic characteristics and prognosis for different histologic subtypes of early cervical cancer. Int J Gynecol Cancer 2019; 29:1244–1251.
161. Agarwal S, Schmeler KM, Ramirez PT, et al. Outcomes of patients undergoing radical hysterectomy for cervical cancer of high-risk histological subtypes. Int J Gynecol Cancer 2011; 21:123–127.
162. Averette HE, Nguyen HN, Donato DM, et al. Radical hysterectomy for invasive cervical cancer. A 25-year prospective experience with the Miami technique. Cancer 1993; 71:1422–1437.
163. Estape RE, Angioli R, Madrigal M, et al. Close vaginal margins as a prognostic factor after radical hysterectomy. Gynecol Oncol 1998; 68:229–232.
164. McCann GA, Taege SK, Boutsicaris CE, et al. The impact of close surgical margins after radical hysterectomy for early-stage cervical cancer. Gynecol Oncol 2013; 128:44–48.
165. Magrina JF, Kho RM, Weaver AL, et al. Robotic radical hysterectomy: comparison with laparoscopy and laparotomy. Gynecol Oncol 2008; 109:86–91.
166. Nezhat FR, Datta MS, Liu C, et al. Robotic radical hysterectomy versus total laparoscopic radical hysterectomy with pelvic lymphadenectomy for treatment of early cervical cancer. JSLS 2008; 12:227–237.
167. Cantrell LA, Mendivil A, Gehrig PA, et al. Survival outcomes for women undergoing type III robotic radical hysterectomy for cervical cancer: a 3-year experience. Gynecol Oncol 2010; 117:260–265.
168. Halliday D, Lau S, Vaknin Z, et al. Robotic radical hysterectomy: comparison of outcomes and cost. J robotic surg 2010; 4:211–216.
169. Soliman PT, Frumovitz M, Sun CC, et al. Radical hysterectomy: a comparison of surgical approaches after adoption of robotic surgery in gynecologic oncology. Gynecol Oncol 2011; 123:333–336.
170. Wright JD, Herzog TJ, Neugut AI, et al. Comparative effectiveness of minimally invasive and abdominal radical hysterectomy for cervical cancer. Gynecol Oncol 2012; 127:11–17.
171. Hoogendam JP, Verheijen RH, Wegner I, et al. Oncological outcome and long-term complications in robot-assisted radical surgery for early stage cervical cancer: an observational cohort study. BJOG 2014; 121:1538–1545.
172. Segaert A, Traen K, Van Trappen P, et al. Robot-Assisted Radical Hysterectomy in Cervical Carcinoma: The Belgian Experience. Int J Gynecol Cancer 2015; 25:1690–1696.
173. Sert BM, Boggess JF, Ahmad S, et al. Robot-assisted versus open radical hysterectomy: A multi-institutional experience for early-stage cervical cancer. Eur J Surg Oncol 2016; 42:513–522.
174. Wang W, Chu HJ, Shang CL, et al. Long-Term Oncological Outcomes After Laparoscopic Versus Abdominal Radical Hysterectomy in Stage IA2 to IIA2 Cervical Cancer: A Matched Cohort Study. Int J Gynecol Cancer 2016; 26:1264–1273.
175. Gallotta V, Conte C, Federico A, et al. Robotic versus laparoscopic radical hysterectomy in early cervical cancer: A case matched control study. Eur J Surg Oncol 2018; 44:754–759.
176. Shah CA, Beck T, Liao JB, et al. Surgical and oncologic outcomes after robotic radical hysterectomy as compared to open radical hysterectomy in the treatment of early cervical cancer. J Gynecol Oncol 2017; 28:e82.
177. Shazly SA, Murad MH, Dowdy SC, et al. Robotic radical hysterectomy in early stage cervical cancer: A systematic review and meta-analysis. Gynecol Oncol 2015; 138:457–471.
178. Corrado G, Cutillo G, Saltari M, et al. Surgical and Oncological Outcome of Robotic Surgery Compared With Laparoscopic and Abdominal Surgery in the Management of Locally Advanced Cervical Cancer After Neoadjuvant Chemotherapy. Int J Gynecol Cancer 2016; 26:539–546.

# Chapter 16

## Targeted therapy for ovarian cancers: PARP inhibitors, anti-angiogenics and immunotherapy

*David L Phelps, Laura A Tookman, Sadaf Ghaem-Maghami*

## INTRODUCTION

Ovarian cancer is newly diagnosed in over 300,000 women per year worldwide and results in 200,000 annual deaths [1]. For the purposes of this book chapter, discussion here refers to epithelial ovarian cancer (EOC), which is the most common type of ovarian cancer. Historically EOC has been managed with a "one size fits all' approach, however, it is now recognised that there are distinct pathological subtypes which behave and respond to treatment differently. Surgery and chemotherapy are the mainstay of treatment for advanced stage [International Federation of Gynaecology and Obstetrics (FIGO) stage II to IV] EOC, with both treatment modalities significantly improving prognosis. Cytoreductive surgery aims to remove as much tumour burden as possible either before or mid-chemotherapy. Platinum-based chemotherapy (e.g. carboplatin, cisplatin) is DNA alkylating and is the most commonly used in combination with taxane-based chemotherapy (e.g. paclitaxel, docetaxel), directed at the cellular cytoskeleton. Combination treatment with both agents yields superior prognosis when compared to platinum monotherapy [2]. These systemic anti-cancer treatments, while effective, have a host of off-target effects causing considerable morbidity. They do not target patient- or tumour-specific biology and cannot be regarded as targeted therapy. Despite maximal therapy at diagnosis, most patients with advanced EOC will relapse and ultimately their disease will become resistant to chemotherapy treatment. This chapter will discuss some of the recent advances in targeted treatment for EOC. It will focus on treatments that (as of the date of writing) are now approved and regarded as *standard of care*.

**David L Phelps** BM PhD MRCOG, Consultant Surgeon in Gynaecological Oncology, University Hospitals Southampton, Honorary Clinical Lecturer, Imperial College London, UK
Email: d.phelps@imperial.ac.uk

**Laura A Tookman** MBBS PhD MRCP, Consultant Medical Oncologist, Imperial College Healthcare; Honorary Clinical Senior Lecturer, Imperial College London, UK
Email: laura.tookman1@nhs.net

**Sadaf Ghaem-Maghami** MBBS PhD MRCOG, Honorary Consultant Surgeon in Gynaecological Oncology, Imperial College Healthcare; Chair of Gynaecological Oncology, Imperial College London, UK
Email: s.ghaem-maghami@imperial.ac.uk

Targeted therapy for EOC relies on the discovery of tumour-specific cellular pathways or genetic alterations that can be exploited by drugs. Increasingly, medical conditions can be treated by targeted therapies. Monoclonal antibody therapy, for example, uses modified antibodies, to target cancer cells by modifying cellular pathways, induce apoptosis or deliver cytotoxic agents to tumour cells. These mechanisms are designed to be purposeful and to effect change at specific molecular targets that have direct and/or indirect anti-cancer consequences. To date, the most successful monoclonal antibody treatment for EOC is bevacizumab. This targets vascular endothelial growth factor A (VEGF-A) to inhibit neo-angiogenesis and therefore tumour growth.

Specific somatic genetic mutations, and resultant pathway changes, in tumours have been targeted with the advent of poly-adenosine-di-phosphate ribose polymerase (PARP) inhibitors. PARP is an enzyme instrumental in repairing DNA damage in cells. PARP's inhibition, in susceptible cancer cells, results in accumulation of toxic unrepaired DNA damage, ultimately resulting in cell death. PARP inhibitors (PARPi) were thought to be particularly useful in EOC treatment as around 15% of EOC patients carry germ line or somatic BRCA mutations ($BRCA^{mut}$), with up to 20% $BRCA^{mut}$ in high-grade serous subtypes [3,4]. BRCA1 and BRCA2 genes are broadly accepted as tumour suppressor genes and they play important roles in DNA repair mechanisms [5]. The mutation of these genes, results in dysregulation of the genes and therefore, DNA repair mechanisms resulting in increased rates of breast and ovarian cancers in women with BRCA mutations. Specifically, the DNA repair mechanism dysregulated in mutated BRCA is homologous recombination of double strand DNA (dsDNA) break repair. However, homologous recombination deficiency (HRD) is not exclusively caused by BRCA mutations and up to 50% of women with high-grade EOC have deficient homologous recombination without BRCA mutation [6].

Immunotherapy in EOC has been extensively investigated as a potential approach for treatment. Immunotherapeutic treatments have been a resounding success for many cancer types, particularly melanoma but these treatments have unfortunately not led to such dramatic treatment responses in EOC. Immunotherapy, therefore, remains an emerging concept in EOC treatment but has been investigated with several trials. EOC appears to be an immunoreactive tumour, especially as an association has been shown between the number of tumour infiltrating lymphocytes and prognosis [7]. Tumour infiltrating lymphocyte manipulation has shown promise with inhibition of EOC progression in preclinical and clinical studies [8].

## ANTI-ANGIOGENICS

Creation of a vascular supply (angiogenesis) is essential for the tumour growth and spread. This provides the rationale for the development of agents that target this pathway. Targeting angiogenesis can be achieved through inhibition of circulating pro-angiogenic factors such as VEGF or by targeting receptors (e.g. VEGF receptors) and downstream signalling of the pathways involved in angiogenesis. Among the various anti-angiogenic drugs, bevacizumab, a humanised anti-VEGF-A monoclonal antibody, is the most widely studied in EOC [9].

Bevacizumab was first approved for use in combination with chemotherapy in recurrent EOC. Initially, the benefit of bevacizumab was shown in the platinum resistant setting with an improved progression free survival (PFS) from 3.4 to 6.7 months [HR 0.48, 95%

confidence interval (CI) 0.38–0.60; $p < 0.001$] [10]. Subsequently, an improvement in PFS was seen with the use of bevacizumab in addition to chemotherapy in the platinum sensitive setting [11,12] and also in those who previously received bevacizumab in the first line setting [13]. The addition of bevacizumab to chemotherapy in relapsed EOC has failed to consistently show a significant overall survival (OS) benefit and is not currently available in England on the NHS for use in relapsed ovarian cancer.

Administration of bevacizumab in combination with standard chemotherapy (carboplatin and paclitaxel) followed by maintenance therapy in the front-line setting has demonstrated improved PFS [14,15] and has European Medicines Agency (EMA) and United States Food and Drug Administration (FDA) approval for use in this setting. An OS benefit was, however, only identified with the use of bevacizumab in the subgroup of patients at high risk of progression (e.g. those with FIGO stage IV disease and those with residual disease following surgery) [14,15]. In view of these results, bevacizumab treatment is available in England through the Cancer Drug Fund for high-risk patients in combination with chemotherapy followed by maintenance treatment (for a total of 18 cycles) [16]. Bevacizumab is not, however, patient- or tumour-specific and there are no predictive biomarkers to support its use. Side effects of treatment include risk of bowel perforation, hypertension, thrombosis and proteinuria.

Other multitargeted agents against the angiogenic pathway such as pazopanib [an oral protein kinase inhibitor of VEGFR and platelet-derived growth factor receptor (PDGFR)] [17], nintedanib [a potent inhibitor of VEGFR, fibroblast growth factor receptor (FGFR), and PDGFR] [18], trebananib (angiopeptin-1 and -2 inhibitor) [19] and cediranib (VEGF receptor 1-3 inhibitor) [20] have been investigated in various settings in EOC. Despite demonstrating clinical activity none have yet been approved for use in ovarian cancer.

Combining antiangiogenic drugs (including bevacizumab) with other targeted agents such as PARPis (see later) is yielding positive results in certain groups of patients and trials are ongoing [21].

# PARP INHIBITORS

Poly-adenosine-di-phosphate ribose polymerase inhibitors have arguably been the most exciting discovery in recent years in the field of targeted therapy for EOC. They are generally well-tolerated, have an acceptable side-effect profile, are administered orally and have been associated with remarkable improvements in PFS.

The first PARPi to be approved in the UK was olaparib (in 2016) for patients with recurrent high-stage EOC in tumours that have a *BRCA* mutation (either germ line or somatic) that had at least partially responded to platinum-based chemotherapy [22,23]. SOLO2 demonstrated the benefits of olaparib in the recurrent EOC setting, finding that PFS was significantly prolonged for the first and second relapse when used in the platinum-sensitive relapse timeframe in women with *BRCA1/2$^{mut}$*. The survival effects were impressive with a 70% reduced risk of progression (HR 0.30, 95% CI 0.22–0.41; $p$ <0.0001; median PFS 19.1 vs. 5.5 months) [23]. Subsequent analysis of OS revealed a 12.9 months advantage when using olaparib for platinum-sensitive, relapsed, *BRCA1/2$^{mut}$*, compared to placebo [median OS 51.7 months vs. 38.8 months, HR 0.74 (95% CI 0.54–1.00); $p = 0.054$].[23] While statistical significance was not met, the authors conclude that this likely represents a clinically meaningful survival advantage [24]. Currently, in the relapsed setting, olaparib is recommended for patients with a BRCA mutation in whom disease has recurred after three or more cycles of platinum based chemotherapy and can also be accessed on the NHS through the cancer drug fund for those in response to platinum based chemotherapy [25].

Phase III clinical trials of two further PARPis; niraparib [NOVA (26)] and rucaparib [ARIEL3 (27)] subsequently showed PFS benefit when administered in the maintenance setting to those in response to platinum based chemotherapy. Benefit was shown in patients regardless of whether they harboured a $BRCA^{mut}$ or whether the tumours had HRD. Both drugs are currently available via the Cancer Drug Fund for treatment in this setting in the UK. Whilst patients positive for HRD have the best prolongation of survival under PARP treatment, PARPis have now been approved by the FDA and EMA for use in all women with platinum-sensitive relapsed high-stage EOC, irrespective of their BRCA or HRD status [28]. Strong data exist for PFS, but good quality data are currently lacking for OS. This remains the subject of on-going trial data collection and longer follow up is required for the OS data to mature [29].

The SOLO1 trial in 2018 was an international, randomised, double-blind, phase III trial to evaluate the efficacy of the PARPi olaparib as maintenance therapy in patients with newly diagnosed EOC [30]. It was limited to FIGO stage III and IV patients with $BRCA1/2^{mut}$ (germline or somatic) who had achieved a partial (PR) or complete response (CR) to platinum-based chemotherapy [30]. Randomisation was to either placebo treatment or olaparib and 391 patients were recruited (260 to olaparib and 131 to placebo). The addition of olaparib as a maintenance therapy post first-line chemotherapy resulted in a significantly reduced risk of disease progression or death: 70% lower when compared to placebo (HR for disease progression or death 0.30; 95% CI 0.23–0.41; $p$ <0.001) [30]. The use of niraparib in the first-line setting has shown benefit with advanced EOC regardless of BRCA or HRD status [31]. Both olaparib (for those with $BRCA^{mut}$) and niraparib (regardless of mutation status) are approved and available within the NHS via the Cancer Drug Fund for use as maintenance treatment in the first-line setting in patients who have achieved CR or PR to platinum-based treatment.

With the successes of PARPi addition in primary and recurrent disease, the PAOLA-1 trial investigated the effect of combination treatment with PARPi and the anti-angiogenic bevacizumab [21] PAOLA-1 randomised 806 patients in whom response was seen with first-line platinum and taxane-based chemotherapy plus bevacizumab. Olaparib was added in 537 women and a further 269 received placebo. After 22.9 months of median follow-up, PFS was 22.1 months in the bevacizumab-olaparib arm and 16.6 in the bevacizumab-placebo arm [21]. In patients with HRD positive tumours, including $BRCA1/2^{mut}$, the effect was even more pronounced with PFS improving from 17.7 months (bevacizumab + placebo) to 37.2 months (bevacizumab + olaparib) (HR 0.33; 95% CI 0.25–0.45) [21]. The National Institute for Clinical Excellence (NICE) in the UK subsequently recommended the use of olaparib in combination with bevacizumab in the first-line maintenance setting for those with a $BRCA1/2^{mut}$ or those tumours that demonstrated HRD on an appropriate assay [21,29].

# IMMUNOTHERAPY

In the past 20 years, there have been major advances in cancer immunotherapy, significantly changing the treatment of various types of cancer. Immune checkpoint inhibitors, including cytotoxic T-lymphocyte associated protein 4 (CTLA-4) and programmed cell death protein 1 (PD-1)/programmed cell death ligand 1 (PD-L1) inhibitors, which reverse the signals from the immunosuppressive tumour microenvironment have been investigated and used in the treatment of cancers. In addition, there has been much progress in use of oncolytic viruses, cancer vaccines, and adoptive cell therapies in recent years. Chimeric antigen receptor (CAR) T cells have shown great promise in the treatment of haematological cancers but research towards creating effective CAR T cells against solid cancers including EOC is continuing.

Epithelial ovarian cancer is regarded as immunogenic, as immune cells active against the tumour are identified in the tumour tissue, ascites and blood [32,33]. However, significant immune suppressive responses exist that involve regulatory T cells, inflammatory cytokines and myeloid derived suppressor cells (MDSCs) in the tumour microenvironment. Expression of PD-L1 on tumour cells and monocytes likely contribute to this immune suppression [32,33]. In-vivo studies have also shown a swift response to CAR T cell therapy targeting the epidermal growth factor family of receptor tyrosine kinases (ErbBs) but the tumours regrew soon after the therapy had ceased. Newer generations of CAR T cells are tasked with overcoming immune suppressive elements of tumours, improving entry of these cells to the tumour and increasing their life span within the tumours.

In-vitro and in-vivo experimental studies have shown that EOC is susceptible to immune checkpoint inhibitors such as anti-PD-1 or PD-L1 antibodies [34,35]. Addition of PD-1 antibody to in-vitro co-cultures of unstimulated T cells, with or without carboplatin, showed increased in T cell activation and tumour cell death [35]. An animal model of ovarian cancer using immune deficient mice has shown reduced tumour burden with the addition of a PD-1 inhibitor to standard chemotherapy [36]. In a murine ovarian tumour model, dual blockade of PD-1 and LAG-3 has shown enhanced T cell effector function, reduced tumour growth, increased numbers of CD8+ T cells, and reduction in the frequency of Tregs and MDSCs in the tumour microenvironment [37]. However, these results have not been replicated in clinical trials. Studies of the use of immune checkpoint inhibitors in first treatment or in the recurrent setting have not shown any benefit from anti PD-1 or PD-L1 antibodies. Large phase II trial of patients with recurrent or persistent EOC have shown modest response to PD-L1 inhibitor pembrolizumab (phase II KEYNOTE-100 study) with objective response of around 8% and with median PFS just over 2 months [38].

A randomised phase III clinical trial combining a PD-1 inhibitor avelumab, with or without chemotherapy (pegylated liposomal doxorubicin) in platinum resistant or refractory EOC patients showed no significant improvement in PFS or OS versus chemotherapy alone (JAVELIN ovarian 200 trial) [39].

The combination of anti-PD-1 and VEGF-A blockade increases anti-tumour effect in patients with high expression of VEGF, as compared with those treated with a monotherapy [40]. However, the severe side effects of this combination therapy need to be fully evaluated. A clinical trial of PD-1 inhibitor, durvalumab, in combination with endothelial growth factor receptor inhibitor, cediranib, has shown high incidence of drug-associated adverse events [41].

Poly-adenosine-di-phosphate ribose polymerase inhibitors are thought to improve the response of HRD positive EOC to immunotherapy through the generation of a higher mutation burden, which elevates the level of neoantigen expression. The stimulator of interferon genes pathway is activated by DNA damage and neoantigen expression and plays a role in innate immunity [42]. PD-L1 inhibitors have been shown to strengthen the anti-tumour activity of PARPis by improving anti-tumour immune responses [43], and have shown modest clinical activity in recurrent EOC [44]. In the phase I/II TOPACIO trial, combination therapy with niraparib and pembrolizumab was evaluated for the treatment of platinum-resistant EOC. In the cohort with $BRCA1/2^{mut}$, objective response rate and disease control rate were 45% and 73%, respectively [45].

## OTHER NOVEL AGENTS

Fully understanding the molecular make up of EOC and the knowledge that different pathological subtypes may respond to different treatments is beginning to influence care. For example, low-grade serous ovarian cancers (<10% of all serous ovarian cancers) behave differently to high-grade serous cancer and are relatively chemotherapy resistant. They are characterised by high oestrogen and progesterone receptor expression (which can be targeted with endocrine treatment) and alterations in the MAP kinase cellular pathway. Trametinib, a MEK inhibitor, has demonstrated an improvement in PFS and response rate compared with standard of care chemotherapy in low-grade serous cancers [46]. Further trials with combination treatments are underway.

Many other potential targets have been investigated in EOC (for example, targeting p53, DNA repair or the cell cycle). Many trials now recruit patients based on the molecular markers and multiple agents are being investigated alone or in combination.

## CONCLUSION

Surgery and platinum-based chemotherapy continue to form the backbone of treatment for ovarian cancer. The addition of targeted treatments, particularly PARP inhibitors, are now transforming care and patient outcomes. Further developments will rely on increasing knowledge of ovarian cancer biology and optimally designed clinical trials.

## REFERENCES

1. Sung H, Ferlay J, Siegel RL, et al. Global Cancer Statistics 2020: GLOBOCAN Estimates of Incidence and Mortality Worldwide for 36 Cancers in 185 Countries. Cancer J Clini 2021; 71:209–249.
2. Covens A, Carey M, Bryson P, et al. Systematic review of first-line chemotherapy for newly diagnosed postoperative patients with stage II, III, or IV epithelial ovarian cancer. Gynecol Oncol 2002; 85:71–80.
3. Ledermann JA, Drew Y, Kristeleit RS. Homologous recombination deficiency and ovarian cancer. Eur J Can 2016; 60:49–58.
4. Alsop K, Fereday S, Meldrum C, et al. BRCA mutation frequency and patterns of treatment response in BRCA mutation-positive women with ovarian cancer: a report from the Australian Ovarian Cancer Study Group. J Clin Oncol 2012; 30:2654–2663.
5. Silver DP, Livingston DM. Mechanisms of BRCA1 tumor suppression. Can Discov 2012; 2:679–684.
6. CGARN. Integrated genomic analyses of ovarian carcinoma. Nature 2011;474:609-615.
7. Kuroki L, Guntupalli SR. Treatment of epithelial ovarian cancer. BMJ (Clin Res Ed) 2020; 371:m3773.
8. Santoiemma PP, Powell DJ Jr. Tumor infiltrating lymphocytes in ovarian cancer. Can Biol Ther 2015; 16:807–820.
9. Chelariu-Raicu A, Coleman RL, Sood AK. Anti-Angiogenesis Therapy in Ovarian Cancer: Which Patient is It Most Likely to Benefit? Oncol 2019: 33.
10. Pujade-Lauraine E, Hilpert F, Weber B, et al. Bevacizumab combined with chemotherapy for platinum-resistant recurrent ovarian cancer: The AURELIA open-label randomized phase III trial. J Clin Oncol 2014; 32;1302–1308.
11. Aghajanian C, Blank SV, Goff BA, et al. OCEANS: a randomized, double-blind, placebo-controlled phase III trial of chemotherapy with or without bevacizumab in patients with platinum-sensitive recurrent epithelial ovarian, primary peritoneal, or fallopian tube cancer. J Clin Oncol 2012; 30:2039–2045.

12. Coleman RL, Brady MF, Herzog TJ, et al. Bevacizumab and paclitaxel-carboplatin chemotherapy and secondary cytoreduction in recurrent, platinum-sensitive ovarian cancer (NRG Oncology/Gynecologic Oncology Group study GOG-0213): a multicentre, open-label, randomised, phase 3 trial. Lancet Oncol 2017; 18:779–791.

13. Daniele G, Raspagliesi F, Scambia G, et al. Bevacizumab, carboplatin, and paclitaxel in the first line treatment of advanced ovarian cancer patients: the phase IV MITO-16A/MaNGO-OV2A study. Int J Gynecol Can 2021; 31:875.

14. Burger RA, Brady MF, Bookman MA, et al. Incorporation of bevacizumab in the primary treatment of ovarian cancer. New Engl J Med 2011; 365:2473–2483.

15. Oza AM, Cook AD, Pfisterer J, et al. Standard chemotherapy with or without bevacizumab for women with newly diagnosed ovarian cancer (ICON7): overall survival results of a phase 3 randomised trial. Lancet Oncol 2015; 16:928–936.

16. https://www.england.nhs.uk/publication/national-cancer-drugs-fund-list/ [Last Accessed May 2022].

17. Vergote I, du Bois A, Floquet A, et al. Overall survival results of AGO-OVAR16: A phase 3 study of maintenance pazopanib versus placebo in women who have not progressed after first-line chemotherapy for advanced ovarian cancer. Gynecol Oncol 2019; 155:186–191.

18. du Bois A, Kristensen G, Ray-Coquard I, et al. Standard first-line chemotherapy with or without nintedanib for advanced ovarian cancer (AGO-OVAR 12): a randomised, double-blind, placebo-controlled phase 3 trial. Lancet Oncol 2016; 17:78–89.

19. Monk BJ, Poveda A, Vergote I, et al. Anti-angiopoietin therapy with trebananib for recurrent ovarian cancer (TRINOVA-1): a randomised, multicentre, double-blind, placebo-controlled phase 3 trial. Lancet Oncol 2014; 15:799–808.

20. Ledermann JA, Embleton-Thirsk AC, Perren TJ, et al. Cediranib in patients with relapsed platinum-sensitive ovarian cancer (ICON6): a randomised, double-blind, placebo-controlled phase 3 trial. Lancet 2016; 387:1066–1074.

21. Ray-Coquard I, Pautier P, Pignata S, et al. Olaparib plus Bevacizumab as First-Line Maintenance in Ovarian Cancer. N Engl J Med 2019; 381:2416–2428.

22. NICE. (2016). Olaparib for maintenance treatment of relapsed, platinum-sensitive, BRCA mutation-positive ovarian, fallopian tube and peritoneal cancer after response to second-line or subsequent platinum-based chemotherapy [TA381]. [online] Available from: https://www.nice.org.uk/guidance/ta381/chapter/1-Recommendations [Last Accessed May, 2022].

23. Pujade-Lauraine E, Ledermann JA, Selle F, et al. Olaparib tablets as maintenance therapy in patients with platinum-sensitive, relapsed ovarian cancer and a BRCA1/2 mutation (SOLO2/ENGOT-Ov21): a double-blind, randomised, placebo-controlled, phase 3 trial. Lancet Oncol 2017; 18:1274–1284.

24. Poveda A, Floquet A, Ledermann JA, et al. Olaparib tablets as maintenance therapy in patients with platinum-sensitive relapsed ovarian cancer and a BRCA1/2 mutation (SOLO2/ENGOT-Ov21): a final analysis of a double-blind, randomised, placebo-controlled, phase 3 trial. Lancet Oncol 2021; 22:620–631.

25. NICE. (2021). Olaparib for maintenance treatment of relapsed platinum-sensitive ovarian, fallopian tube or peritoneal cancer. Technology appraisal guidance [TA620]. [online] Available from: https://www.nice.org.uk/guidance/ta620/chapter/1-Recommendations [Last Accessed May, 2022].

26. Mirza MR, Monk BJ, Herrstedt J, et al. Niraparib Maintenance Therapy in Platinum-Sensitive, Recurrent Ovarian Cancer. N Engl J Med 2016; 375:2154–2164.

27. Coleman RL, Oza AM, Lorusso D, et al. Rucaparib maintenance treatment for recurrent ovarian carcinoma after response to platinum therapy (ARIEL3): a randomised, double-blind, placebo-controlled, phase 3 trial. Lancet 2017; 390:1949–1961.

28. Ison G, Howie LJ, Amiri-Kordestani L, et al. FDA Approval Summary: Niraparib for the Maintenance Treatment of Patients with Recurrent Ovarian Cancer in Response to Platinum-Based Chemotherapy. Clin Cancer Res 2018; 24:4066–4071.

29. NICE. (2021). Olaparib plus bevacizumab for maintenance treatment of advanced ovarian, fallopian tube or primary peritoneal cancer. [online] Available from: https://www.nice.org.uk/guidance/ta693 [Last Accessed May, 2022].

30. Moore K, Colombo N, Scambia G, et al. Maintenance Olaparib in Patients with Newly Diagnosed Advanced Ovarian Cancer. N Engl J Med 2018; 379:2495–2505.

31. González-Martín A, Pothuri B, Vergote I, et al. Niraparib in Patients with Newly Diagnosed Advanced Ovarian Cancer. N Engl J Med 2019; 381:2391–2402.

32. Chatterjee J, ai W, Aziz NHA, et al. Clinical Use of Programmed Cell Death-1 and Its Ligand Expression as Discriminatory and Predictive Markers in Ovarian Cancer. Clin Cancer Res 2017; 23:3453–3460.

33. Maine CJ, Aziz NH, Chatterjee J, et al. Programmed death ligand-1 over-expression correlates with malignancy and contributes to immune regulation in ovarian cancer. Cancer Immunol Immunother 2014; 63:215–224.

34. Wahba J, et al. Determining a mechanism of synergistic immuno-chemotherapy in ovarian cancer. Eur J Can. 2016; 61:S217–S218.

35. Natoli M, Bonito N, Robinson JD, et al. Human ovarian cancer intrinsic mechanisms regulate lymphocyte activation in response to immune checkpoint blockade. Cancer Immunol Immunother 2020; 69:1391–1401.

36. Wahba J, Natoli M, Whilding LM, et al. Chemotherapy-induced apoptosis, autophagy and cell cycle arrest are key drivers of synergy in chemo-immunotherapy of epithelial ovarian cancer. Cancer Immunol Immunother 2018; 67:1753–1765.

37. Huang RY, Francois A, McGray AJR, et al. Compensatory upregulation of PD-1, LAG-3, and CTLA-4 limits the efficacy of single-agent checkpoint blockade in metastatic ovarian cancer. Oncoimmunol 2017; 6:e1249561.

38. Matulonis UA, Shapira-Frommer R, Santin AD, et al. Antitumor activity and safety of pembrolizumab in patients with advanced recurrent ovarian cancer: results from the phase II KEYNOTE-100 study. Ann Oncol 2019; 30:1080–1087.

39. Pujade-Lauraine E, Fujiwara K, Ledermann JA, et al. Avelumab alone or in combination with chemotherapy versus chemotherapy alone in platinum-resistant or platinum-refractory ovarian cancer (JAVELIN Ovarian 200): an open-label, three-arm, randomised, phase 3 study. Lancet Oncol 2021; 22:1034–1046.

40. Wallin JJ, Bendell JC, Funke R, et al. Atezolizumab in combination with bevacizumab enhances antigen-specific T-cell migration in metastatic renal cell carcinoma. Nat Commun 2016; 7:12624.

41. Lee JM, Cimino-Mathews A, Peer CJ, et al. Safety and Clinical Activity of the Programmed Death-Ligand 1 Inhibitor Durvalumab in Combination With Poly (ADP-Ribose) Polymerase Inhibitor Olaparib or Vascular Endothelial Growth Factor Receptor 1-3 Inhibitor Cediranib in Women's Cancers: A Dose-Escalation, Phase I Study. J Clin Oncol 2017; 35:2193–2202.

42. Barber GN. STING: infection, inflammation and cancer. Nat Rev Immunol 2015; 15:760–770.

43. Jiao S, Xia W, Yamaguchi H, et al. PARP Inhibitor Upregulates PD-L1 Expression and Enhances Cancer-. Associated Immunosuppression. Clin Cancer Res 2017; 23:3711–3720.

44. Lampert EJ, Zimmer A, Padget M, et al. Combination of PARP Inhibitor Olaparib, and PD-L1 Inhibitor Durvalumab, in Recurrent Ovarian Cancer: a Proof-of-Concept Phase II Study. Clin Cancer Res 2020; 26:4268–4279.

45. Konstantinopoulos PA, Waggoner SE, Vidal GA, et al. TOPACIO/Keynote-162 (NCT02657889): A phase 1/2 study of niraparib + pembrolizumab in patients (pts) with advanced triple-negative breast cancer or recurrent ovarian cancer (ROC)—Results from ROC cohort. J Clin Oncol 2018; 36:106.

46. Gershenson DM, Gourley C, Paul J. MEK Inhibitors for the Treatment of Low-Grade Serous Ovarian Cancer: Expanding Therapeutic Options for a Rare Ovarian Cancer Subtype. J Clin Oncol 2020; 38:3731–3734.

# Chapter 17

# Epithelial ovarian cancer: Comprehensive approach for precision medicine

*Ikuo Konishi*

## INTRODUCTION

Ovarian cancer is the second most common cause of death from gynaecologic cancer in women around the world. According to the World Health Organization (WHO) Globocan 2020, it is estimated that 313,959 new cases and 207,252 deaths occurred in all over the world [1]. The incident rate varies from 4.4 to 10.7, average 6.6, and is still increasing in Asian countries including Japan [2]. Prognosis of ovarian cancer patients remains poor, because the majority of patients with ovarian cancer are diagnosed at advanced stages with peritoneal dissemination. Of those diagnosed with International Federation of Gynaecology and Obstetrics (FIGO) stage III or IV, >70% will have a recurrence within the first 5 years, and recurrent ovarian cancer remains an almost uniformly fatal disease [3]. Over the past several decades, however, there have been significant advancements in the genomic analyses on the biological diversity of ovarian cancer, and in the translational researches for the innovative development of ovarian cancer treatment [4]. Novel targeted drugs have been developed and improved dramatically the survival of advanced cancer patients. The new WHO classification of epithelial ovarian cancer in 2020 defines the main five histological types, such as high-grade serous carcinoma (HGSC), low-grade serous carcinoma (LGSC), endometrioid carcinoma, clear cell carcinoma, and mucinous carcinoma. Rare types are malignant Brenner tumour, mesonephric-like carcinoma, undifferentiated and dedifferentiated carcinoma, and carcinosarcoma [5]. Clinicopathologic and molecular studies have demonstrated that the histogenetic origin and the biological behaviour are clearly different among the histological types [6] (**Figure 17.1**), and therefore, individualised approach has become possible for the detection, diagnosis, and treatment of each type of ovarian cancer [7]. Moreover, precision medicine using the comprehensive genomic analyses has recently been making a breakthrough for ideal personalisation of treatment for each patient [4,7]. In this chapter, therefore, the current status on the proceedings toward precision medicine in the management of ovarian cancer has been thoroughly reviewed, and the future perspective is presented.

**Ikuo Konishi** MD, PhD, Professor Emeritus and the 9th Professor at Department of Gynecology and Obstetrics of Kyoto University, National Hospital Organization, Kyoto Medical Center 1-1 Fukakusa Mukaihata-cho, Fushimi-ku, Kyoto, Japan
Email: konishi@kuhp.kyoto-u.ac.jp

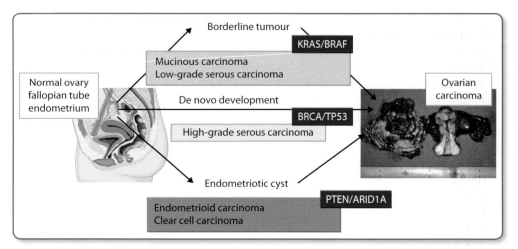

**Figure 17.1** Diversity in development of epithelial ovarian cancer. Ovarian cancer is a heterogeneous group of disease with different clinical and molecular scenarios.

# MODERN ERA OF PRECISION MEDICINE

## Philosophy of physician and patient

Physicians know a priori that there should be one best treatment for the patient, and have earnestly been seeking it among the various available modalities. Because physicians also are aware of the heterogeneity of disease among patients, even after the same clinical diagnosis is made, they try to shed light on the specific nature of the disease for a particular patient, using clinical history, physical examination, laboratory tests, histopathology, and imaging. Collecting all these data, we discuss about the patient at a clinical conference, finally decide the most appropriate treatment plan for this specific patient, and then explain it to the patient and the family. Under such conditions, both the physician and the patient reach a consensus. All of them seem to be happy under such an ideal doctor-patient relationship.

## Era of epidemiology-based medicine

Since the 1980s, however, the term 'evidence-based' has been introduced in clinical decision making. In 1987, David Eddy first used 'evidence-based', and the term 'evidence-based medicine (EBM)' was introduced in medical education [8]. Since 1990, a big wave of EBM has become popular in order to do clinical practice more objectively by application of population-based data to individual patient care [9]. Thus, EBM based on clinical epidemiology was gradually established as a scientific approach for medical practice and decision making. Then, EBM further developed by classifying evidence levels, and now the strongest recommendation is based on data obtained by randomised controlled trials (RCTs), meta-analyses, and systematic reviews [10]. EBM claims that decision making should not be based on a clinician's opinion or expert belief, but on the scientific evidence. Many physicians have been involved in RCTs to seek the necessary scientific evidence, and such great efforts have resulted in success for establishment of novel treatments as standard ones. Thus, we have to continue our efforts to establish the scientific evidence that will be adopted in clinical guidelines and used for daily decision making in clinical practice.

Nevertheless, there have been many critical opinions against EBM expressed to date [11]. Similarly, designed RCTs frequently disagree with one another, and cohort studies with better quality often disagree with those from RCTs. Clinically, important details may be hidden, because EBM does not integrate non-statistical forms of medical information such as professional experience and patient-specific factors. Most importantly, it has been recognised that the usefulness of applying EBM to individual patients is limited [11,12]. Patients are individuals, not groups. Because EBM is based on applying principles of clinical epidemiology to individual patient care, it carries with it many of the assumptions of epidemiological strategy. Individual circumstances and values are varied, and patients respond in their own unique way to a therapy that was not predicted from data by RCTs. This is a limitation of clinical guidelines based on EBM. For individual patients, therefore, our clinical medicine must resolve disagreements between general rules, empirical data, theories, principles, and patient values. In this setting, recent development of personalised medicine using genome analyses appears to overcome the limitations of an EBM approach for clinical decision making [4].

## New era of genomics-based medicine

Advances in clinical oncology and novel drug discoveries are playing the major leadership roles in personalised medicine. The final goal of medicine is increasing patient specificity so that the right treatment is given to the right patient at the right time [4]. Accumulating evidence has clearly demonstrated the heterogeneity between tumours among patients and even in the same patients. In the 21st century, the advancement of comprehensive genomic analyses using next-generation sequencing (NGS) and gene expression profiling using DNA microarray along with bioinformatics reveals the diversity of genome, epigenome, and expression profiles of cancer. If the driver oncogene and the main signalling pathway are identified, the molecular-targeted drug is effective due to the 'oncogene addiction' of cancer cells. One example is EML4-ALK lung cancer. In 2007, Hiroyuki Mano and his colleagues identified the fusion oncogene EML4-ALK in a subset of non-small-cell lung cancer with poor prognosis, and then showed that an ALK kinase inhibitor such as crizotinib dramatically improved the survival of patients [13]. RCT was not necessary for approval of the drug in a short period of time by FDA in 2011. Direction of personalised medicine is now expanding to 'precision medicine'. The NIH in the United States defines precision medicine as an emerging approach for disease treatment and prevention that takes into account individual variability in genes, environment, and lifestyle for each person. It is in contrast to a 'one-size-fits-all' approach, in which disease treatment and prevention strategies are developed for the average person. Thus, all of us are coming into an ideal world for healthcare as well as for better doctor-patient relationship.

In the real world of clinical practice in medical oncology, the selection of drug for breast or lung cancer has already been decided, being based on the genomic characteristics of tumour of the patient. In the field of the management for ovarian cancer, however, we are still struggling due to various difficulties. Since most cases of ovarian cancer lack the strong driver oncogene, genomic analysis by NGS does not work for identification of appropriate therapy. The most important prognostic factor in patients with advanced ovarian cancer is peritoneal dissemination, but its pathogenesis and therapeutic strategy for cure of disease have not yet been determined. Nevertheless, we can see dawn of precision management of ovarian cancer patients, since tremendous efforts have been made by physicians, medical staffs, researchers, and patients, in order to clarify the genomic landscape of ovarian cancer, elucidate the molecular mechanisms of peritoneal dissemination, and also develop the novel treatment modalities.

## OVARIAN CANCER AS DISEASE OF HETEROGENEITY

### Natural history of development and screening of ovarian cancer

Epithelial ovarian cancer is the leading cause of death among female genital malignancies in developed countries. This is due to the difficulty of early detection of ovarian cancer, since more than half of patients present with advanced disease of FIGO stage III or IV. In order to improve the prognosis of ovarian cancer patients, trials for its early detection in postmenopausal women have been conducted using either serum tumour marker CA125 or transvaginal ultrasonography (TVUS) [14]. CA125 (MUC16) is a high molecular weight trans-membrane mucin, and has generally been employed as a useful tumour marker for preoperative assessment of adnexal mass, as well as for monitoring the course of ovarian cancer patients. Although ovarian cancer screening programs using CA125 were tried, the survival benefit has not been reported. CA125 is not always raised in early stage disease and can be elevated in various benign conditions. Currently, only CA125 testing is not recommended in the general population [14]. A recent proteomics study showed that longitudinal use of multiple markers such as HE4, CHI3L1, PEBP4, and AGR2, in addition to CA125, may improve the sensitivity and specificity for early detection of ovarian cancer up to 1 year before diagnosis [15]. In the future, liquid biopsy of novel biomarkers such as circulating cell-free DNAs, extracellular vesicles (EVs), and microRNA may explore the new world for early detection of the silent killers [16,17].

Transvaginal ultrasonography (TVUS) is commonly used in daily clinical practice for visualisation of the solid part suggesting malignancy in the cystic ovarian tumours, and has been expected as an important tool for ovarian cancer screening. Several, single arm prospective studies reported the benefit of TVUS, resulting in an increased detection rate of early stage cancers with better outcome of patients [18,19]. However, RCTs using TVUS with CA125 in Shizuoka, Japan [20], and in PLCO study from United States [21,22] did not show a significant advantage of the screening for early detection or survival benefit. In our detailed analysis of the results of PLCO study, however, the possible benefit of annual screening for earlier detection and decrease of mortality rate was observed [23]. All gynaecologists expected the promising results from the recent and largest RCT, UKCTOCS trial in the United Kingdom [24]. Among a total of 202,562 women, 50,625 (25.0%) were randomised to multimodal, CA125 followed by TVUS screening (MMS), 50,623 (25.0%) to only TVUS screening (USS), and the remaining 101,314 (50.0%) to no screening. At a median follow-up of 16.3 years, 2,055 women were diagnosed as tubal or ovarian cancer, and 522 (1.0%) from MMS group, 517 (1.0%) from USS group, and 1,016 (1.0%) from no screening group. Overall incidence of stage I or II disease was 39.2% higher (95% CI 16.1–66.9) in MMS than in no screening, whereas the difference of stage III or IV was only 10.2% lower (95% CI −21.3–2.4). Among 1,206 women who died of disease, 296 (0.6%) from MMS, 291 (0.6%) from USS, and 619 (0.6%) from no screening. Thus, there was no significant reduction of death in MMS ($p = 0.58$) or USS ($p = 0.36$) compared with no screening. Accumulating evidences clearly indicate that screening program by CA125 and/or TVUS in the general population does not decrease the mortality rate of ovarian cancer. Interestingly, however, among invasive ovarian cancers found in UKCTOCS study, the rate of aggressive cancers including HGSC was 78.6% (1,416/1,802) that is much higher than in Asian countries including Japan [23]. Therefore, there may be different effects of the screening programs among different races due to varied incidence of aggressive types of ovarian cancer.

Until the end of 20th century, natural history of ovarian cancer development had been unclear, since the tumours arise in the abdominal cavity and patients present already having the definite invasive carcinoma. Clinically, evident precursors were not known for epithelial ovarian cancer. In 2003, in order to verify this issue, we retrospectively collected data from the ovarian cancer patients, whose clinical and TVUS findings 12 months or fewer prior to the diagnosis by laparotomy were available. This clinicopathological analysis disclosed the diversity of natural history of cancer development among the histological types [25]. Strikingly, in patients with HGSC, there had been no apparent abnormalities in the adnexal regions 2–12 months prior to the diagnosis, but laparotomy showed all cases to have advanced stage of tumour (**Figure 17.2**). Thus, HGSC seems to develop suddenly from the normal-appearing ovary, and therefore, it is impossible to detect HGSC at earlier stages. This is consistent with a recent concept of histogenetic origin of HGSC as the fallopian tube. In cases of LGSC, however, they had been followed up for benign-appearing cysts, and the tumour was discovered at stage I when the solid lesion appeared in the cyst. Most endometrioid and clear cell carcinomas were also detected at early stages by TVUS due to the appearance of solid components during the follow-up for ovarian endometriotic cyst (**Figure 17.3**). Thus, the periodic follow-up using TVUS for ovarian endometriotic cyst or benign-appearing cyst every 6 months is useful for early detection of LGSC, endometrioid, and clear cell carcinomas. Such heterogeneity of ovarian cancer development is consistent with different results of the screening programs by TVUS among different countries. Currently, ovarian cancer screening using CA125 or TVUS has not been recommended in the general population [22–24], because it is not effective for early detection or decrease in mortality rate of the most common histological type, HGSC. However, a possible benefit of annual check-up using TVUS is the early detection of indolent types of ovarian cancer.

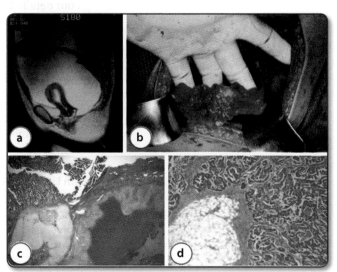

**Figure 17.2** Natural course of de novo development in high-grade serous carcinoma (HGSC). A 34-year-old, infertile woman had been receiving ovulation-induction therapy, and her ovaries were normal-appearing by TVUS. Suddenly, (a) massive ascites developed, and (b) laparotomy revealed peritoneal carcinomatosis. (c) Histological examination revealed HGCS on the ovarian surface and (d) its metastatic lesions in the omentum.

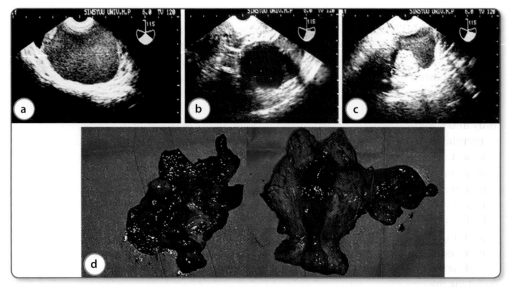

**Figure 17.3** Natural course of development in ovarian endometrioid carcinoma (OEC), arising in endometriotic cyst. (a) A 39-year-old woman had been followed with TVUS every 6 months for her endometriotic cyst, which showed the typical 'fine sands-like appearance' due to intracystic bleeding from endometriosis. (b) One and half years later, endometriosis became inactive and the cystic fluid appeared 'translucent' in TVUS. (c) After 6 months, the solid portion developed in the cyst, (d) and the surgery revealed OEC at stage IA.

Thus, accumulated evidence indicates that ovarian cancer is a heterogeneous group of disease with different clinical and molecular scenarios [4,26] (**Figure 17.1**). Robert J. Kurman and his colleagues classified ovarian cancer into the two groups designated as type I and type II [27]. Type I tumours include LGSC, endometrioid carcinoma, clear cell carcinoma, and mucinous carcinoma, which develop in a stepwise fashion from the precursors, such as ovarian borderline tumour or endometriotic cyst. They are detected at earlier stages, and characterised by gene mutations including KRAS, BRAF, HER2, CTNNB1, PTEN, PIK3CA, and ARID1A. On the other hand, type II tumours comprise of HGSC and undifferentiated carcinoma, which appears to develop de novo from normal-appearing ovary, being found at advanced stages, and associated with poor prognosis. These tumours are chromosomally highly unstable, harbour TP53 mutations, and in approximately 50%, they exhibit homologous recombination deficiency (HRD) including germline and somatic mutations of *BRCA* genes. Thus, the concept of dualistic model of ovarian carcinogenesis is essential for the feasibility of screening and early detection of cancer, as well as for the precision management of cancer in each patient [28].

## Precision diagnosis of ovarian cancer

Clinical conference before surgery or other therapies is very important for deciding on the best management for the patient. All medical staff, not only gynaecologists but also radiologists and pathologists if possible, should gather and discuss the precise diagnosis, possible treatment modalities, and the operative procedure. In case of adnexal mass, the preoperative assessment is especially important, because the clinical diagnosis is not pathological but presumable. However, precise prediction of histological types and malignancy is feasible preoperatively, using the combination of imaging modalities, such as US and MRI, with the levels of serum tumour markers such as CA125, CA19-9, CEA, AFP, and SCC. Tumours with mainly solid and partly cystic lesions with extremely elevated CA125 levels strongly suggest HGSC. They are usually associated with peritoneal disseminations which could be often identified by CT and MRI. Monocystic tumour with solid mural nodule with various sizes suggests either endometrioid or clear cell carcinoma. CA125 levels are slightly elevated. Solid part of the tumour is positive for colour-Doppler study in US, and enhanced by contrast media in MRI, and such findings are useful for differential diagnosis from benign endometriotic cyst. Multi-lobular cystic tumour with the solid part, along with elevated CA19-9 levels, suggests mucinous carcinoma. Non-epithelial tumours such as sex-cord stromal tumours and germ cell tumours show the characteristic symptoms, imaging findings, and specific tumour markers, and therefore, precise diagnosis can be made preoperatively.

Differential diagnosis between primary and metastatic ovarian tumours is important for the precision management of the patient. If the gastrointestinal primary is suspected, the occult blood reaction of faeces should be tested, followed by endoscopic examination of upper and lower intestinal tracts. Abdominal CT is useful for the detection of primary hepatobiliary and pancreatic lesions. Krukenberg tumour especially from gastric cancer shows typical clinical features, such as bilateral, large, spheroid, and totally solid tumours (**Figure 17.4**), which is not infrequently accompanied by hormone production. Generally, the elevated tumour marker is CEA, rather than CA125. These findings strongly suggest typical metastatic tumour, and physicians should immediately look for the primary lesion using various modalities. Metastatic carcinoma from the colon frequently mimics primary ovarian mucinous carcinoma (OMC) [29], and therefore, the precise differential diagnosis will be described in the section on 'Ovarian mucinous carcinoma'.

## Precision prevention of ovarian cancer

Epidemiologically, the risk factors for development of epithelial ovarian cancer are family history of breast and ovarian cancer, infertility, and hormone-replacement therapy. On the other hand, multi-parity, breastfeeding, tubal ligation, and oral contraceptives use are protective for cancer development [2,5,6]. The risk increases with increasing number

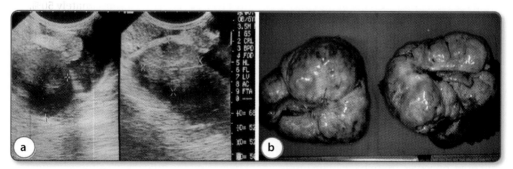

**Figure 17.4** Krukenberg tumour of the ovary, metastasised from gastric cancer. Clinically, (a) typical feature of Krukenberg tumour, such as bilateral, large, spheroid, and completely solid ovarian tumours, is shown in US and (b) macroscopic findings.

of ovulatory cycles in the lifetime (HR 1.92; 95% CI 1.60–2.30) [30]. This is consistent with the classic hypothesis of 'incessant ovulation theory' by Mahmoud F. Fathalla [31]. Gonadotropin hypothesis has been proposed for ovarian carcinogenesis; however, the current consensus is that infertility treatment does not increase the risk independently of other factors [32]. Among the histological types, there are heterogeneous associations of risk factors [30,33]. Lifetime ovulatory cycles increased the risk of serous, endometrioid, and clear cell, but not mucinous carcinomas [30]. Although parity is a protective factor for all histological types, oral contraceptives use is not in the case of mucinous carcinoma [33]. Interestingly, smoking is associated with an increased risk of mucinous, but a decreased risk of clear cell carcinoma [33]. Such heterogeneity in the risk factors also represents the different aetiology of each histological type of ovarian cancer.

In order to reduce the mortality rate, recent attention has focussed on familial ovarian cancer. Since *BRCA1* and *BRCA2* genes were discovered as the cause of hereditary breast and ovarian cancer (HBOC), genetic counselling, and testing for BRCA1/2 has been available in cancer centres. Almost all of ovarian cancers in the BRCA family are histologically HGCS, and 10–15% of sporadic HGCS harbour germline BRCA1/2 mutations. Since the frequency of the presence of BRCA1/2 mutation is higher than expected from the family history of cancer patients, genetic counselling and testing for BRCA1/2 is recommended for all patients with epithelial ovarian cancer [34]. Accumulating data indicate that BRCA1 mutations increase ovarian/fallopian tube cancer risk (40–60%) with an average patient age of 50–53 years, whereas the risk for BRCA2 mutations is lower (11–35%) with slightly higher age of 55–58 years [35,36]. A recent prospective analysis showed that the estimated cumulative risks for breast and ovarian cancer by the age of 70 years for BRCA1 carriers were 60% and 59%, respectively. For BRCA2 carriers, they were 55% and 16.5%, respectively [37]. Thus, BRCA1/2 mutation carriers have a higher risk for both breast and ovarian cancer, and therefore, they need more intensive surveillance and intervention by chemoprevention or prophylactic surgery. Since a reasonable screening method has not been available for ovarian cancer, risk-reducing salpingo-oophorectomy (RRSO) is an important tool for prevention.

The NCCN Guidelines 2020 recommend RRSO for women with BRCA1/2 mutation, typically between ages 35 and 40 years for BRCA1, and between ages 45 and 50 years for BRCA2, after completion of childbearing [38]. In a meta-analysis, RRSO was associated with a significant reduction in the risk of BRCA-associated ovarian or tubal cancer (HR 0.21; 95% CI 0.12–0.39) [39]. In a prospective study of 2,482 women with BRCA1/2 mutations, RRSO is associated with lower all-cause mortality (10% vs. 3%; HR 0.40; 95% CI 0.26–0.61), breast cancer-specific mortality (6% vs. 2%; HR 0.44; 95% CI 0.12–0.76), and ovarian cancer-specific mortality (3% vs. 0.4%; HR 0.21; 95% CI 0.06–0.80) [40]. RRSO has been reported to incidentally detect an occult HGSC, such as ovarian, tubal, and peritoneal cancer, in 4.5–9% of the cases. The precursor of HGSC, serous tubal intraepithelial carcinoma (STIC), was discovered in the fimbria or distal side of the tube in 5–8% of the cases [35,41]. Since the histogenetic origin of serous ovarian and peritoneal cancer has been regarded as the fallopian tube in most cases, only salpingectomy may serve as an alternative method for prevention. Recently, in case of hysterectomy for benign gynaecologic diseases, bilateral salpingectomy is frequently adopted for the possible reduction of future ovarian cancer. Till now, however, there have been limited data regarding the efficacy of salpingectomy for reducing the risk of ovarian cancer [42].

# CLINICAL, PATHOLOGIC, AND GENOMIC LANDSCAPE OF OVARIAN CANCER

## High-grade serous carcinoma

High-grade serous carcinoma (HGSC) is the most common type of epithelial ovarian cancer, and accounts for >50% of ovarian carcinomas. HGCS most often occurs in the sixth and seventh decades, and the mean age is 63 years [5,6]. Nearly all patients present with tumour of advanced stages, FIGO stage III or IV, with peritoneal dissemination. Primary debulking surgery (PDS) followed by the standard chemotherapy with taxane/platinum is effective in >80% of patients, with complete remission of disease after the first-line treatment. However, most patients at advanced stages will have recurrence and eventually die due to peritoneal carcinomatosis exhibiting chemoresistance, and 5-year survival rate of optimally debulked patients is approximately 50%.

Clinically, the tumours are often bilateral and show solid and papillary growth. Preoperative examination of the tumour shows the imaging features of mostly solid tumour intermingled with irregularly cystic lesions (**Figure 17.5**). Serum CA125 levels are extremely elevated to usually >200 U/mL, frequently exceed 1,000 U/mL, whereas serum CA19-9 and CEA levels are within normal limits (**Figure 17.6**). This is in contrast to benign serous cystadenoma, which shows a simple cystic tumour without solid portion and normal CA125 levels (**Figure 17.7**). Serous borderline tumours (SBT) present with unilateral, sometimes bilateral, monocystic tumour with many small solid nodules, each of which is usually <2 cm in size (**Figure 17.8**). CA125 levels are normal or slightly elevated to usually <200 U/mL.

Histologically, the tumour cells exhibit papillary, labyrinthine with slit-like spaces, glandular, or solid architecture (**Figure 17.9**). Nuclei are large and highly atypical with high-mitotic activity, whereas the cytoplasm is scant. Necrosis is common. Immunohistochemically, they are characterised by positivity for WT1, PX8, and CK7, but negative for CK20 [5]. As almost all of HGCSs harbour TP53 mutation or deletion, they show either overexpression or completely negative ('null') for p53 protein. Recently, a subset of HGCS which had been classified as undifferentiated, endometrioid, and transitional cell carcinoma are included in HGSC, which is designated as 'solid, endometrioid, transitional (SET) variant of HGSC' (**Figure 17.10**), since they share the same clinical and immunohistochemical features such as WT1 and p53 positivity. SET tumours tend to occur in women at younger ages or with BRCA germline mutation, and have a better prognosis [5].

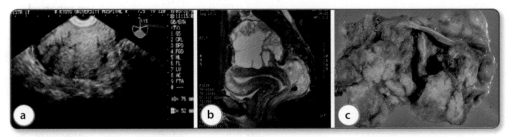

**Figure 17.5** High-grade serous carcinoma (HGSC). Typical clinical feature of HGSC is mostly solid tumour intermingled with irregularly cystic lesions, as shown in (a) US, (b) T2-weighted MRI, and (c) macroscopic findings.

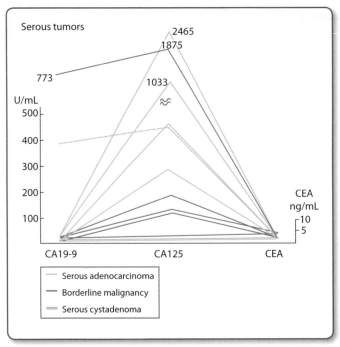

**Figure 17.6** Serum tumour marker, CA19-9, CA125, and CEA, levels in ovarian serous tumours. Serum CA125 levels are extremely elevated to usually > 200 U/mL, frequently exceeds 1,000 U/mL in HGSC, slightly elevated in serous borderline tumours (SBT), and not elevated in benign serous cystadenoma.

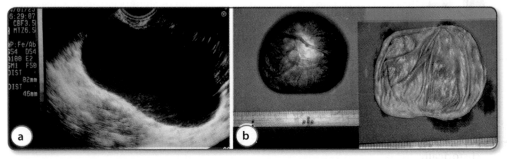

**Figure 17.7** Ovarian serous cystadenoma. Typical clinical feature of benign serous cystadenoma is a simple, unilocular cystic tumour without solid portion, as shown in (a) US and (b) macroscopic findings.

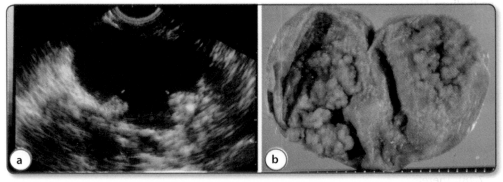

**Figure 17.8** Serous borderline tumour (SBT). Typical clinical feature of SBT is unilateral, sometimes bilateral, monocystic tumour with many small solid nodules, each size of which usually less than 2 cm in size, as shown in (a) US and (b) macroscopic findings.

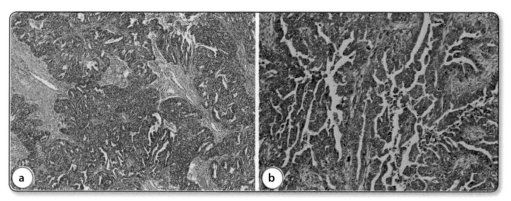

**Figure 17.9** Histopathology of HGSC. Cancer cells of HGSC exhibit papillary, (a and b) labyrinthine with slit-like spaces, glandular, or solid architecture. Nuclei are large and highly atypical with high-mitotic activity.

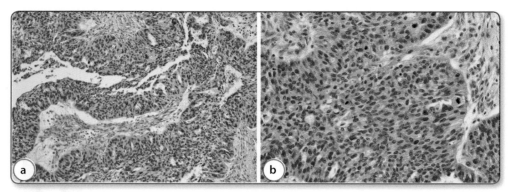

**Figure 17.10** Histopathology of 'SET variant' of HGSC. A 46-year-old woman with germline BRCA1 mutation underwent surgery for ovarian cancer, stage IIIC. Histopathology shows typical SET variant of HGSC, which resembles the feature of (a) endometrioid or (b) transitional carcinoma.

Historically, the cell origin of epithelial ovarian cancer has been proposed by Robert E. Scully that it originates in the ovarian surface epithelium (OSE), and growing toward the various direction of Müllerian metaplasia such as tubal, endometrial, and endocervical epithelium. However, thorough examination of the fallopian tubes removed for prevention of ovarian cancer in BRCA-mutated women disclosed the presence of precursor lesion mainly in the tubal fimbria that is STIC with TP53 mutation [43,44] (**Figure 17.11**). In addition, further studies by immunohistochemistry revealed the epithelial foci of p53 overexpression without cellular atypia and proliferative activities. Such foci are designated as 'p53 signature', and considered to be the earliest event of carcinogenesis. Clonal expansion and genomic evolution from 'p53 signature' to STIC, and to invasive HGSC of ovarian and peritoneal lesions have been demonstrated using whole-genome analysis of the micro-dissected cells from each lesion [45,46]. Reconstructed phylogenic trees in the same patients indicate the sequential accumulation of genomic alterations [45,46], and clonal evolution with heterogeneous blanching to sub-clones during the progression [47,48]. Therefore, HGSC is currently thought to be originated from the secretory cells in the distal portion of fallopian tube, and less commonly from the OSE or its inclusion cysts of the ovary. Strikingly, STICs showed the same allelic imbalances as those in the ovarian and

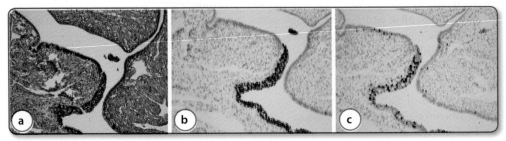

**Figure 17.11** Serous tubal intraepithelial carcinoma (STIC). Histopathologic features of STIC are (a) stratification of tubal epithelial cells, (b) overexpression of p53 protein, and (c) increased proliferative activity in Ki-67 immunostainings.

tubal carcinomas, and the time interval between STIC and ovarian cancer is estimated to be 6.5 years [45,46]. In addition, genomic analyses of incidentally found tubal lesions such as 'p53 signatures', dormant STICs, and proliferative STICs from women without ovarian cancer suggest the long latent period of time at least two decades during 'p53 signature' and dormant STICs [46]. However, the time for spreading from STIC to ovary or other peritoneal sites is estimated to be short, <2 years [45,48].

In 2011, The Cancer Genome Atlas (TCGA) Research Network reported comprehensive genomic and epigenetic changes in >300 cases of HGSC, and also showed various patterns of gene expression profile [49]. Of the HGSC cases analysed, germline mutation of BRCA1 was found in 8%, and that of BRCA2 was 6%. For somatic mutations, nearly all cases harboured mutations in TP53 (96%). Pathological review of the TP53-negative cases and their re-classification revealed that all HGSC cases have a TP53 abnormality including a case of homozygous deletion. Thus, TP53 mutation is the universal phenomenon as the genomic features of HGSC. In contrast, the frequency of somatic mutations other than TP53 is <5% i.e. NF1 (4%), BRCA1 (3%), BRCA2 (3%), CDK12 (3%), and RB1 (2%). Thus, TCGA study confirmed that mutation of driver oncogene is extremely rare in the prototype of epithelial ovarian cancer HGSC, and therefore, targeted drugs against driver oncogenes such as EGFR, HER2, KRAS, and BRAF are usually not effective for HGSC.

Emerging importance is the aberrations of the homologous recombination (HR) pathway genes [26], including BRCA1 germline mutation (8%), BRCA1 somatic mutation (3%), BRCA2 germline mutation (6%), BRCA2 somatic mutation (3%), BRCA1 promoter methylation (10%), CDK12 mutations (3%), and other HR gene mutations such as FA genes, RAD genes and DNA damage response genes (5.5%), and RAD51C promoter methylation (2%). Thus, approximately 40% of HGSCs are designated as 'HR deficient'. In addition, PTEN inactivation (6%) is one of the mechanisms of RAD51, and overexpression and amplification of EMSY (7%) inhibits BRCA2 function. These cases are considered as 'possibly HR deficient'. Accordingly, approximately 50% of HGSC cases are characterised by HRD. Eventually, widespread copy number alterations characteristically occur in HGSC. TCGA analysis identified eight regional copy number gains and 22 losses [49]. Among focal amplifications observed in 63 regions, the most common amplification for CCNE1, MYC, and MECOM were detected in >20% of cases. Homozygous deletions of the region encoding tumour suppressor genes, such as PTEN, RB1, and NF1, were also detected. Extensive copy number abnormalities are consistent with the early loss of TP53 along with intrinsic or acquired HRD, both of which cause the defect in DNA repair. Such genetic characteristics cause the unstable genome, loss of tumour suppressor genes, and aberrant chromosomes, all of which drive clonal evolution and expansion during the progression. This is the essential nature of HGSC as aggressive cancer showing frequent metastasis via peritoneal dissemination.

Since HGSC lack actionable driver mutations, which are usually present in breast and lung cancers, Michel J. Birrer said that another strategy 'targeting the untargetable' is needed for novel therapy of ovarian cancer [50]. In this sense, recent development of poly-(ADP-ribose) polymerase (PARP) inhibitor is a breakthrough as the evolutional treatment for HGSC [51]. Basically, HRD exhibits the extreme platinum sensitivity of this tumour, since platinum-DNA adducts lead to DNA breaks, resulting in double-strand breaks. Such breaks are repaired using HR pathway, but if HRD is present, those will be repaired using another repair system of single-strand DNA breaks, which depend on the PARP complex. Inhibition of this alternative repair pathway by PARP inhibitors results in the ultimate death of cancer cells with HRD, which has been designated as 'synthetic lethality'. Actually, PARP inhibitors in combination with platinum-based chemotherapy have been shown to be very effective in tumours with HRD, and the survival of the patients has been dramatically improved, as described in 'TARGETED THERAPIES' section. However, HGSC cancer cells maintain the genomic instability, evolve, and escape from 'synthetic lethality'. Therefore, we should proceed further to overcome the resistance to PARP inhibitors.

With regard to mRNA expression profile, TCGA analyses revealed the four subtypes of HGSC, i.e. 'immunoreactive', 'differentiated', 'proliferative', and 'mesenchymal' [49]. 'Immunoreactive' subtype is characterised by expression of T-cell chemokine ligands (CXCL10 and CXCL11) and the receptor (CXCR3). 'Differentiated' subtype shows high expression of ovarian tumour (MUC16 and MUC1) and tubal markers (SLP1), whereas 'proliferative' subtype exhibits increased expression of transcription factors (HMGA2 and SOX11) and proliferation markers (MCM2 and PCNA). 'Mesenchymal' subtype is characterised by high expression of the genes of HOX and stromal component (FAP, ANGPTL2, and ANGPTL1). Importantly, subsequent studies reported the significant differences in the survival of patients among the subtypes [52,53]. Patients with 'immunoreactive' subtype showed the best survival, then 'differentiated', followed by 'proliferative', and 'mesenchymal' the worst. Importantly, patients with 'mesenchymal' subtype accounting for 23% of all cases had a median survival of 23 months with platinum-resistant rate of 63%, in contrast to those with other subtypes showing a median survival of 46 months and platinum-resistant rate of 23% [52].

Our analysis on the histopathological features along with the mRNA expression profile of HGSC patients has revealed that 'differentiated' subtype in TCGA is histologically well-differentiated grade 1 carcinoma showing papilloglandular pattern (PG), and 'proliferative' is poorly differentiated grade 3 carcinoma with solid and proliferative pattern (SP). Thus, they represent the conventional histological grades. In contrast, 'mesenchymal' is associated with dense desmoplastic stroma showing mesenchymal transition pattern (MT), and 'immunoreactive' is characterised by histological pattern of immune reactive (IR), where many lymphocytes are surrounding the cancer nest [54] (**Figure 17.12**). Therefore, the latter two represent mainly the total gene expressions of cancer tissues including those from the microenvironment. Thus, our histopathological study confirmed again the prognostic significance of histological grade, and also disclosed that tumour microenvironment is more important for the patient prognosis. Using the light microscopy for pathological classification the four subtypes (PG, SP, MT, and IR), it becomes easier

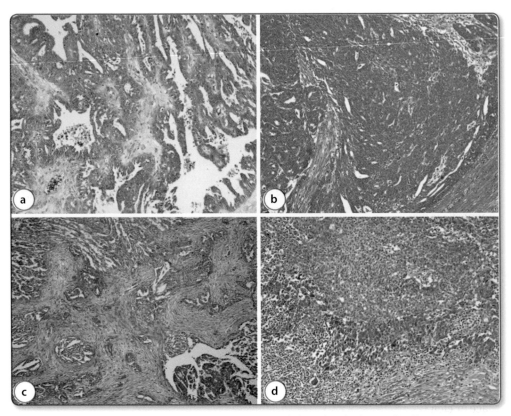

**Figure 17.12** Molecular four subtypes of HGSC in TCGA. Histopathological study along with mRNA expression profile in HGSC shows that 'differentiated' subtype in TCGA is well-differentiated grade 1 carcinoma showing (a) papilloglandular pattern (PG), and (b) 'proliferative' is poorly differentiated grade 3 carcinoma with solid and proliferative pattern (SP). 'Mesenchymal' is associated with dense desmoplastic stroma showing (c) mesenchymal transition pattern (MT), and 'immunoreactive' is characterised by histological pattern of immune reactive (IR), (d) where many lymphocytes are surrounding the cancer nest.

to predict the patient prognosis in clinical practice. Imaging with MRI and CT for the characteristic patterns of tumour growth is also useful for the preoperative assessment on the histological subtypes [55].

Expression profile subtyping of HGSC implicates the future direction of precision management of ovarian cancer. Specialised treatment is needed for patients with 'mesenchymal' or MT subtype, which shows chemoresistance with the worst survival of patients. In 2013, JGOG 3,016 study in Japan demonstrated that a dose-dense paclitaxel and carboplatin (TC) chemotherapy containing high-dose weekly-given paclitaxel significantly improved the progression-free survival (PFS) and overall survival (OS) of advanced cancer patients, compared with the standard TC chemotherapy every 3 weeks [56]. Then, our sub-analysis (JGOG 3016A1) on the histological findings of HGSC patients showed that dose-dense TC regimen had significantly improved PFS of the patients with MT subtype [57]. Regarding the efficacy of anti-VEGF antibody, bevacizumab, HGSC patients with 'proliferative' subtype obtained the greatest and significant benefit in PFS, and those with 'mesenchymal' subtype did a non-significant improvement [58]. Therefore, in the era of precision medicine, gene expression profiling of HGSC might play an important role in the selection of chemotherapeutic regimen and/or in the indication of targeted drugs.

## Low-grade serous carcinoma

Low-grade serous carcinoma accounts for approximately 5% of all epithelial ovarian cancer. Patients with LGSC present over a wide range of age, median 43 years, >10 years younger than those with HGSC [5]. LGSC shows a more indolent clinical course than HGSC [59]. Since LGSC develops from the precursor lesion such as SBT especially showing micro-papillary pattern (**Figure 17.13**), it may be detected at early stages during the follow-up of ovarian cystic lesion [25]. Unexpectedly, however, more than half of patients with LGSC are found at advanced stages, and the long-term survival is poor. This is because LGSC is resistant to taxane/platinum chemotherapy, and the complete cytoreduction is the only prognostic indicator. When the patients have the extra-ovarian diseases, median PFS and OS are 28 and 100 months, respectively [5]. In clinical practice, therefore, it is very much important to pathologically make a differential diagnosis between LGSC and HGSC before starting treatment, especially considering neoadjuvant chemotherapy (NAC) for advanced diseases. Even if NAC is considered as an appropriate therapy due to high-volume disease, laparoscopic examination with the biopsy of the disseminated tissues is essential. If the biopsy reveals the pathological diagnosis as LGSC, physicians should re-consider the primary surgery for the patient.

Macroscopically, LGSC is often bilateral and exhibits papillary growth. Calcification is frequent in ovarian and extra-ovarian lesions, and therefore the tumour may be incidentally detected by abdominal X-ray. Microscopically, LGSC exhibits a variety of patterns, such as small nests, glands, papillae, or micro-papillae, all of which are often surrounded by a clear space or cleft (**Figure 17.13**). Large papillae may invade stroma being surrounded by clear spaces, and are designated as 'inverted macro-papillae' [5]. The tumour cells tend to be uniformly rounded with scant cytoplasm. The nuclei exhibit mild atypia, and mitotic count is low. Necrosis is very rare, and psammoma bodies are often present. When numerous psammoma bodies exist, such tumours have been called as 'psammomacarcinoma'. The

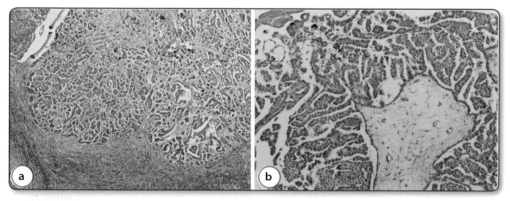

**Figure 17.13** Low-grade serous carcinoma (LGSC). A 27-year-old woman with bilateral ovarian tumours at stage IIIC underwent surgery. (a) Histopathology shows typical LGSC, such as small nests, glands, and micro-papillae, surrounded by a clear space or cleft. (b) This tumour is accompanied by adjacent lesions with SBT with micro-papillary pattern.

tumours are frequently associated with a co-existing SBT. Immunohistochemically, the tumour cells are positive for CK7, PAX8, ER, and WT1. Typically, p53 exhibits wild-type immunoreactivity.

Typical gene mutations of LGSC are KRAS and BRAF, and their occurrence is mutually exclusive [26,60]. The frequency of these mutations has been reported as 15.4–54.5% (mean 24.2%) for KRAS and 0–32% (mean 7.8%) for BRAF. In contrast, TP53 mutation is absent in LGSC. Such molecular features are common to those of SBT, which has been considered as the precursor for LGSC. NRAS mutation was also reported to be present in 3.6–22% (mean 8.3%). Whole-genome sequencing of 19 cases of LGCS showed that, in addition to KRAS, BRAF, and NRAS, somatic mutations are present in USP9X and EIFAX, both of which are linked to the regulation of mTOR pathway [60]. Recent comprehensive genomic analyses on 71 cases of LGSC disclosed, in addition to the mutations of RAS/RAF pathway genes in 47%, the presence of putative novel driver mutations, such as USP9X (27%), MACF1 (11%), ARID1A (9%), NF2 (4%), DOT1L (6%), and ASH1L (4%) [61].

Targeted therapy directed to the pathway of driver gene might be feasible in LGSC. A phase II GOG trial of a MEK inhibitor, selumetinib, in 52 patients with recurrent LGSC showed that the overall response rate (ORR) as 15.4% (CR 1, PR 7; 8/52) and disease control rate (DCR) as 80.8% (SD 65.4%; 34/52). The median PFS was 11 months, and the toxicities were acceptable [62]. A patient with recurrent LGSC with KRAS mutation experienced a dramatic clinical response to MEK inhibitor, binimetinib [63]. A recent RCT for binimetinib versus physician's choice chemotherapy (PCC) in a total of 303 patients with recurrent LGSC showed a meaningful difference between binimetinib and PCC in ORR (16% vs. 13%), and median OS (25.3 months vs. 20.8 months) [64]. In addition, KRAS mutation was significantly associated with response to binimetinib (OR 3.4; 95% CI 1.53–7.66; $p$ = 0.003), and also with prolonged PFS (17.7 months in KRAS mutant vs. 10.8 months in KRAS wild-type; $p$ = 0.006). In addition, a woman of metastatic LGSC with BRAF mutation has responded completely to the treatment with combined BRAF and MEK inhibitors [65]. These studies might recommend us the use of MEK inhibitors for recurrent LGSC patients [66]. In the era of precision medicine, therefore, whole-genome sequencing has encouraged us to identify the driver oncogene and try the matched targeted drug for the patient with recurrent or metastatic LGSC.

LGSC is known to express the estrogen and progesterone receptors (ER and PgR), as a recent systematic review and meta-analysis showed that the expression of ER is observed in 80.7% (95% CI 72.2–89.1%) and that of PgR in 54.4% (95% CI 44.3–64.4%), suggesting those to be the target of hormonal therapy [67]. A patient with ER-positive LGSC underwent optimal debulking surgery and received adjuvant chemotherapy with liposomal doxorubicin and carboplatin, but the recurrent tumour rapidly enlarged. After the initiation of aromatase inhibitor, letrozole, the patient showed a prolonged PR for 34 months [68]. In a retrospective study on 27 cases with advanced LGSC who underwent primary cytoreductive surgery followed by hormonal monotherapy using letrozole (55.5%) or anastrozole (37.1%), 3-year PFS and OS were 79.0% and 92.6%, respectively. After a median follow-up of 41 months, only six patients had a recurrence and two patients died of the disease [69]. A prospective PARAGON trial using anastrozole in 36 patients with recurrent or metastatic, ER-positive LGSC demonstrated the response rate as PR in 14%, SD in 50%, and PD in 36%. Median PFS was 11.1 months, and the clinical benefit at 6 months was obtained in 61% [70]. Thus, hormonal monotherapy using aromatase inhibitor would be an appropriate choice as the first-line adjuvant treatment for LGSC with ER expression.

## Ovarian endometrioid carcinoma

Ovarian endometrioid carcinoma (OEC) accounts for approximately 10% of epithelial ovarian cancer [5]. The frequency of OEC had been reported as 15–20%, but many high-grade OEC cases are currently classified as 'SET variant' of HGSC, and therefore, its incidence has decreased. The mean patient age is 55 years, and this tumour occurs also in the setting of Lynch syndrome. In approximately one quarter of patients, OEC is associated with co-existence of endometrial endometrioid carcinoma (EEC) or hyperplasia [5]. Most tumours (85–90%) are associated with endometriosis, arising mainly in ovarian endometriotic cyst and rarely in extra-ovarian endometriosis [71]. Smaller number of OEC arises in the benign or borderline endometrioid adenofibromas. Regarding the FIGO stage, if applying the recent criteria of pathological diagnosis of OEC, most of patients are at stage I or II, and the percentage of stage III or IV is reported as <3%. Since OEC has been considered to respond well to the standard taxane/platinum chemotherapy, the molecular targeted drugs specific for OEC have not received attention.

Clinically, OEC is usually unilateral and large, mean size of 11 cm in diameter, with a smooth surface (**Figure 17.14**). The cut section shows a tumour having both cystic and solid portions, with frequent haemorrhage and necrosis. Typical OEC arising in endometriotic cyst represents the polypoid fragile nodule protruding into the lumen of old blood-filled or brownish-serous fluid or squamous debris-containing cyst (**Figures 17.3** and **17.14**). There is no specific pattern of the imaging features in OEC, but the solid part tends to be relatively

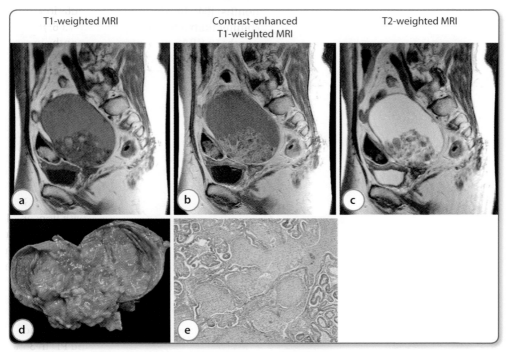

**Figure 17.14** Ovarian endometrioid carcinoma (OEC). A 54-year-old woman underwent surgery for ovarian unilocular, cystic tumour with solid part. (a) MRI findings of T1- weighted, (b) contrast-enhanced T1- weighted, and (c) T2- weighted images show the (d) contrast-enhancement in the solid part, (e) which is histologically OEC with prominent squamous metaplasia.

large and irregular in shape, compared with that of ovarian clear cell carcinoma (OCCC), and is positive with colour-Doppler US and enhanced by contrast media in MRI (**Figure 17.15**). Clinical follow-up of endometriotic cyst every 6 months using TVUS is usually able to detect the cancer at early stages. TVUS for young women complaining of abdominal pain shows the typical 'fine sands-like appearance' of the cystic fluid due to bleeding from active endometriosis. Malignant change is rare in such active phase of endometriosis. With advancing age, however, endometriosis becomes inactive and the cystic fluid becomes 'translucent' in TVUS. Malignant change tends to occur in such cases (**Figure 17.3**). Thus, physicians should pay more attention to the perimenopausal women with endometriosis.

Microscopically, OEC resembles the feature of grade 1-2 EEC, which typically shows a confluent back-to-back or cribriform arrangement of glands (**Figure 17.16**). The glands are composed of endometrial-like cuboidal cells with smooth luminal borders. Villoglandular or papillary growth pattern also occurs. OEC arising in adenofibroma shows the co-existence of fibromatous stroma (**Figure 17.16**). The tumours with solid growth >50% are classified as grade 3 OEC, but recently they are frequently classified as HGSC after immunohistochemical analysis. Squamous metaplasia commonly exists, and mucinous differentiation may be observed. Immunohistochemically, OECs are negative for WT1 and Napsin 1, and most cases exhibit the reactivity for wild-type p53 [5]. The tumours

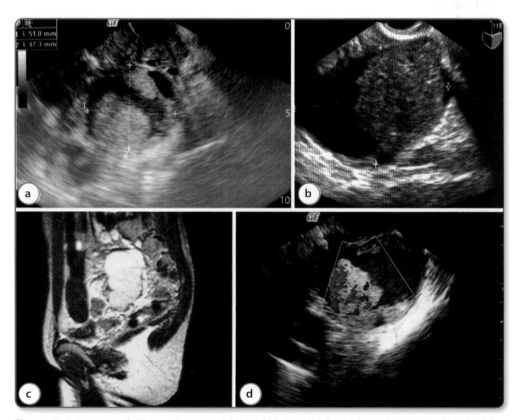

**Figure 17.15** Imaging with US and MRI in typical OEC. In OEC, (a and b) the solid part shows relatively large and irregular shaped tumour in US, which is (c) enhanced by contrast media in MRI, and (d) positive with colour-Doppler US.

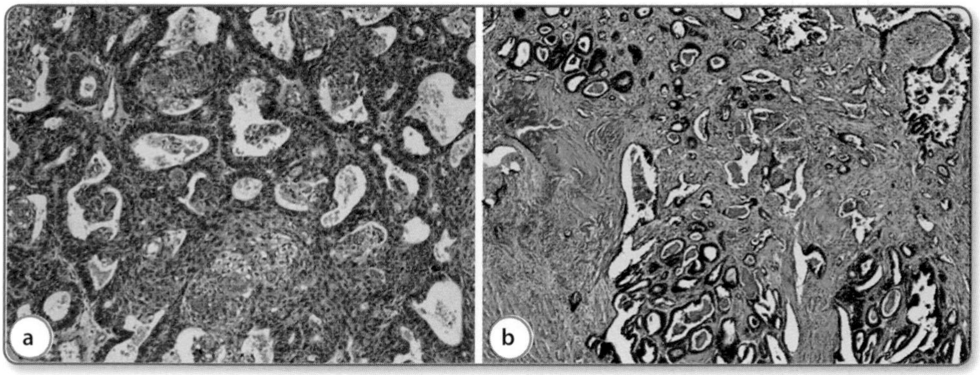

**Figure 17.16** Histopathology of OEC. Histopathology of OEC resembles the feature of grade 1–2 endometrial endometrioid carcinoma (EEC), (a) confluent back-to-back or cribriform arrangement of glands. Squamous metaplasia is frequently observed. Another type, (b) OEC arising in adenofibroma shows the co-existence of fibromatous stroma.

with high-grade endometrioid features with WT1-positivity and p53-abnormality should be classified as HGSC. Typical OEC are positive for ER, PgR, PAX8, CK7, and vimentin. Clinically, although OEC frequently expresses ER, the estrogen-dependent growth like breast cancer has not been demonstrated, and hormonal therapy is not indicated. Differential diagnosis between OEC and OCCC is made by immunohistochemistry for Napsin A and HNF1β, both of which are positive in OCCC but not in OEC.

Endometriosis-related ovarian cancers are OEC or OCCC, but each shows different modes of carcinogenesis, as Masaki Mandai hypothesised that OEC develops under unopposed estrogen environment like EEC, whereas OCCC arises in the condition of oxidative stress in the ovarian endometriotic cyst [71]. Actually, molecular alterations of OEC resemble those of EEC [6,26,72], as the common abnormalities are Wnt/β-catenin signalling pathway (CTNNB1 mutations 30–50%), PIK3/PTEN pathway (PIK3CA 15–40%; PTEN 20%), MAPK pathway (KRAS 12–33%), and SWI/SNF complex (ARID1A 30%). Deficiency of mismatch repair in OEC is reported to be lower than EEC, and microsatellite instability (MSI) has been observed in 13–20%. The molecular four subtypes of endometrial cancers by TCGA can be applied to OEC, and the frequency is 3% POLE (ultra-mutated), 19% MSI (hypermutated), 17% copy-number-high (serous-like), and 61% copy-number-low (endometrioid) [72]. Since an immune checkpoint inhibitor, anti-PD-1 antibody, is indicated for solid tumours with MSI-high, substantial number of OEC cases could be the target of immunotherapy. Whole genome sequencing analysis of OEC along with patients survival showed that patients with CTNNB1 mutation were detected at early stages and showed good prognosis [73]. In OEC cases with co-existence of EEC, although the concept of 'independent primary' was generally accepted by pathologic features of each tumour, recent genomic studies have demonstrated the clonal relationship between the two lesions, suggesting that endometrial cancer cells are transported via reflux through the fallopian tube and implanted to the ovary [74]. Interestingly, a recent phylogenic genome analysis elegantly demonstrated the clonal expansion and evolution from normal endometrium with gene mutation, to endometriotic cyst, and eventually to endometriosis-associated ovarian cancer such as OEC and OCCC [75,76].

## Ovarian clear cell carcinoma

Ovarian clear cell carcinoma represents approximately 10–12% of epithelial ovarian cancers in North America and Europe, whereas it shows a higher prevalence in Asian women, and especially in Japan it occurs in 25% of all ovarian cancers [5]. OCCC has been known to arise frequently in ovarian endometriotic cysts [71]. Since OCCC is associated with reduced response to taxane/platinum chemotherapy, patients with advanced disease show poor prognosis [77,78]. The mean age of patients is 50–53 years, and clinically it is the most common neoplasm to be associated with venous thromboembolism and paraneoplastic hypercalcaemia. Sometimes, cerebral infarction precedes the detection of ovarian cancer, being designated as 'Trousseau syndrome'. Although >50% cases of OCCC present at stage I, they are finally staged as IC after the tumour rupture due to severe adhesions of endometriosis.

Clinically, OCCC is typically unilateral, with a mean size of 13 cm, and the cut surface shows unilocular cystic tumour with solid nodules protruding toward the lumen (**Figure 17.17**), although OCCC less frequently shows the completely solid tumour, which represents another type arising in the adenofibromatous background. Preoperative check-up with various imaging modalities shows that the typical feature of OCCC is a relatively large, cystic tumour with ball-like solid nodule in the wall (**Figure 17.18**). On MRI, solid part is enhanced with contrast media, and frequently the necrotic layer covers the surface of solid nodule, which represents the hypoxic portion of the tumour (**Figure 17.19**). In clinical practice, ovarian endometriotic cysts are diagnosed using TVUS as benign, if they have the cystic wall without solid portions associated with the cystic fluid showing the 'fine sands-like appearance' due to intracystic haemorrhage. However, intracystic bleeding or presence of clots and tissue debris mimics the solid portion suggestive of malignancy (**Figure 17.20**). In such case, colour-Doppler TVUS or contrast-enhanced MRI is very useful for differential diagnosis (**Figures 17.18** and **17.19**). During pregnancy, however, decidual change of the ectopic endometrium in the cystic wall results in the production of many small solid nodules mimicking malignancy, which show the positivity in colour-Doppler US (**Figure 17.21**). Therefore, one should be careful about over-diagnosis and over-treatment of decidualised benign endometriotic cyst during pregnancy.

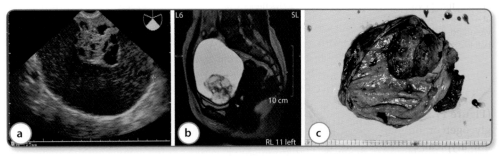

**Figure 17.17** Ovarian clear cell carcinoma (OCCC). Typical clinical feature of OCCC is a large, unilateral, monocystic tumour with ball-like solid nodule protruding toward the lumen, as shown in (a) US, (b) T2-weighted MRI, and (c) macroscopic findings. A 48-year-old woman had been treated with endocrine therapy. During the follow-up with TVUS every 6 months, the solid portion appeared and gradually increased in size. Laparotomy showed stage IA OCCC.

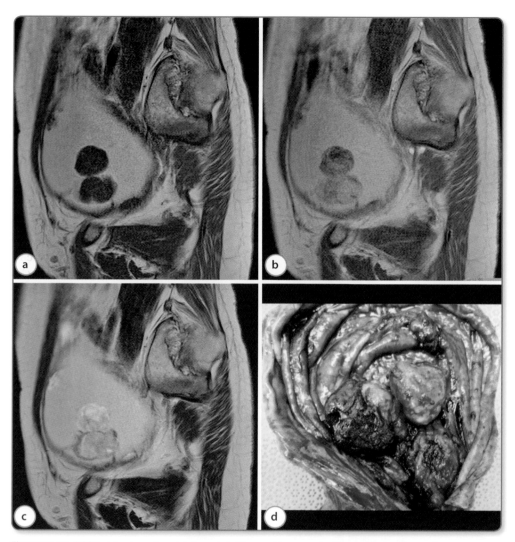

**Figure 17.18** OCCC arising in endometriotic cyst. A 48-year-old woman had been followed for ovarian endometriotic cyst since the age of 27 years. Her dysmenorrhea disappeared at 46 years and menopause occurred at 47 years, but the cyst increased in size and the solid part appeared at 48 years of age. MRI findings of (A) T1-weighted, (B) contrast-enhanced T1-weighted, and (C) T2-weighted images show the contrast-enhancement in the ball-like solid part. Laparotomy showed stage IC1 OCCC.

Microscopically, OCCC displays tubulocystic, papillary, and solid architecture (**Figure 17.22**), being composed of the polygonal cells with clear cytoplasm containing glycogen or 'hobnail' cells with scant cytoplasm (**Figure 17.23**). Nuclei are enlarged and atypical, but the mitotic figures are rare. Stromal hyalinisation is common, and eosinophilic hyaline globules are often present. OCCC arising in adenofibroma is accompanied by the fibromatous stroma (**Figure 17.23**). Immunohistochemically, the tumour cells are typically positive for HNF1β, histological marker of this neoplasm, and also show positivity for PAX8 and Napsin A. On the other hand, they are usually negative

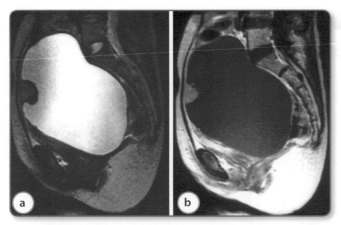

**Figure 17.19** Contrast-enhanced MRI in OCCC. Typical MRI findings of OCCC are large cystic tumour with ball-like solid nodule, as shown in (a) T2-weighted MRI. Contrast-enhancement shows (b) the necrotic layer covering the surface of solid nodule, which represents the hypoxic portion of the tumour.

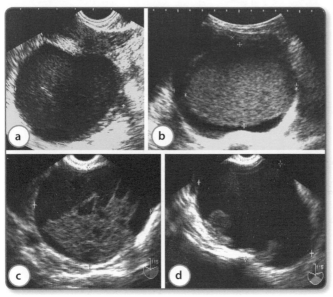

**Figure 17.20** US images of ovarian endometriotic cyst mimicking malignancy. Typical features in US for ovarian endometriotic cysts are the cystic wall without solid portions and the cystic fluid showing (a and b) 'fine sands-like appearance'. However, (c) intracystic bleeding or (d) presence of clots and tissue debris mimics the solid portion suggestive of malignancy. In such case, colour-Doppler TVUS or contrast-enhanced MRI is useful for differential diagnosis.

for WT1, ER, and PgR, which are used for differential diagnosis from HGSC [5]. Abnormal immunoreactivity for p53 is rare.

Pathogenesis of OCCC arising in ovarian endometriotic cyst has been addressed by our hypothesis that the oxidative stress from free-iron of menstrual blood accumulating in the cystic fluid causes the DNA damage, resulting in the cancer development [79]. Then, we identified the specific expression profile pattern of OCCC ('OCCC signature'), characterised by continuous upregulation of glucose metabolism genes and oxidative stress-related genes, such as HNF1β, SOD2, hypoxia-inducible factor-1 alpha (HIF-1α), interleukin-6 (IL-6), and STAT3, via epigenetic mechanism [80]. Among them, HNF1β signalling pathway plays a central role in the stress tolerance and altered glucose metabolism. Metabolome analyses demonstrated that up-regulated HNF1β expression enhances anaerobic glucose metabolism ('Warburg effect'), which is involved in the development of chemoresistance [81]. Accordingly, the tumour cells have survived via epigenetic and

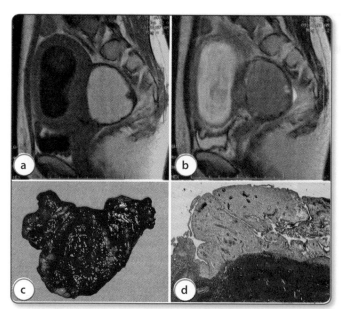

**Figure 17.21** Decidualised endometriotic cyst during pregnancy. During pregnancy, ovarian endometriotic cyst may show the presence of small, solid-like nodules in the cyst wall, as shown in (a) T1-weighted and (b) T2-weighted MRI images. Resection of the cyst revealed that (c) it is not neoplasm but (d) the decidualised ectopic endometrium.

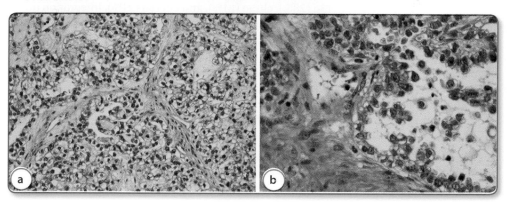

**Figure 17.22** Histopathology of OCCC. Cancer cells of OCCC display tubulocystic, papillary, and solid architecture, being composed of the (a) polygonal cells with clear cytoplasm containing glycogen or (b) 'hobnail' cells with scant cytoplasm. Mitotic figures are rare.

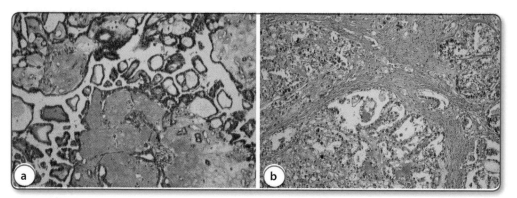

**Figure 17.23** Histopathology of OCCC. In OCCC, (a) stromal hyalinisation is common and eosinophilic hyaline globules are often present. (b) Another type OCCC arising in adenofibroma is accompanied by the fibromatous stroma.

genetic evolution under the stressful environment of the endometriotic cyst, and acquired platinum resistance. Since knockdown of HNF1β decreased the intracellular level of glutathione and increased the sensitivity of cisplatin, the characteristic glucose metabolism due to upregulation of HNF1β pathway will be the possible target of OCCC. In addition, renal clear cell carcinomas also show the similar expression profile as 'OCCC signature', suggesting the effectiveness of a multi-kinase inhibitor, sorafenib, in patients with OCCC [82]. Clinical benefit from sorafenib was actually reported in the patients with recurrent OCCC [83].

Trial of identification of the OCCC-specific gene alteration resulted in the discovery of ARID1A encoding BAF250a [84,85]. ARID1A is one of the members of SWI/SNF chromatin re-modelling complex, which alters the position of nucleosomes along DNA and functions as a tumour suppressor. Our genomic and immunohistochemical analyses on all members of SWI/SNF complex in OCCC disclosed that loss of expression of not only ARID1A but also other members is associated with faster growth and nuclear atypia. The patients with loss of at least one member of SWI/SNF complex showed significantly more advanced stages and shorter PFS and OS [86]. Our whole exome sequencing of 39 cases of OCCC showed the somatic mutation of ARID1A (62%), PIK3CA (51%), MLL3 (15%), KRAS (10%), ARID1B (10%), PPP2R1A (10%), PIK3R1 (8%), and PTEN (5%). Copy number variation analysis identified frequent amplification in chr8q (64%), chr20q (54%), and chr17q (46%), as well as deletion in chr19p (41%), chr13q (28%), chr9q (21%), and chr18q (21%). Integration of the analyses showed that important aberrant pathways are KRAS/PIK3CA (82%), MYC/retinoblastoma (75%), in addition to the chromatin re-modelling complex switch (85%) [87]. Thus, these pathways could be the therapeutic target for OCCC in the era of precision medicine [88]. Actually, the 'OCCC gene signature' is correlated with the expression profile of the responders to immune checkpoint inhibitor, nivolumab [89]. Regarding cytotoxic chemotherapy, although the regimen with irinotecan and cisplatin (CPT-P) received attention as the specific regimen for OCCC [90], JGOG3017/GCIG trial for CPT-P versus TC chemotherapy did not show a significant difference in PFS and OS [91].

## Ovarian mucinous carcinoma

Ovarian mucinous tumours present with an absolutely unilateral, very large, sometimes >30 cm in diameter, multi-loculated cystic tumour with a smooth surface. In the US and MRI, multi-lobular tumour with simple and thin septa suggests benign cystadenoma (**Figure 17.24**), whereas that having a collection of numerous micro-cysts suggests mucinous borderline tumour (MBT) (**Figure 17.25**). The presence of a definite solid part in the large multi-loculated tumour suggests carcinoma (**Figure 17.26**). Serum tumour marker of ovarian mucinous tumours is not CA125, but CA19-9, which is frequently elevated in both carcinomas and MBTs, but not in benign cystadenomas (**Figure 17.27**). Primary OMC is uncommon, and comprises only 2–3% of epithelial ovarian cancers [5,92]. This is because many metastatic mucinous carcinomas from the gastrointestinal tract had been misdiagnosed as ovarian primary [29]. Krukenberg tumours can easily be diagnosed for their typical macroscopic and imaging features (**Figure 17.4**). In contrast, metastatic tumours especially from colon cancer frequently show the multi-lobular cystic tumour mimicking the ovarian primary. Generally, however, compared with the smooth-surfaced tumour in the ovarian primary (**Figures 17.28** and **17.29**), metastatic tumours tend to be bilateral, smaller in size, usually <20 cm, and show the characteristic nodular configuration of the tumour surface (**Figures 17.30** to **17.32**), solid part with necrosis is evident within the tumour. Patients present with the gastrointestinal signs including faecal occult blood and elevated serum tumour marker CEA levels (**Figure 17.33**). Ovarian multi-cystic tumour with extremely elevated CEA levels, rather than CA125, indicates the metastatic tumour is mainly from colon cancer. Thus, preoperative clinical and laboratory examinations using endoscopy and CT usually find the primary lesions such as stomach, colon, pancreas, biliary tract, breast, or others. Important exception is an appendiceal primary. Malignant or low-malignant tumours of the appendix frequently metastasise to the ovary, which mimics the primary OMC or MBT. Pseudomyxoma peritonei is caused by appendiceal lesions in almost all cases, and even if ovarian tumours are present, they are metastatic ones. Therefore, if ovarian 'mucinous carcinomas' are found by frozen sections at laparotomy, surgeons should search for the possible primary tumours in the gastrointestinal tracts, and perform appendectomy even if it is normal in size.

Usually, primary OMC presents as FIGO stage I, unilateral, large tumour with the size of >20 cm. Cut section shows a multi-lobular, cystic, and mucus-containing tumour with solid parts. Microscopically, the carcinomas are accompanied by the adjacent, borderline,

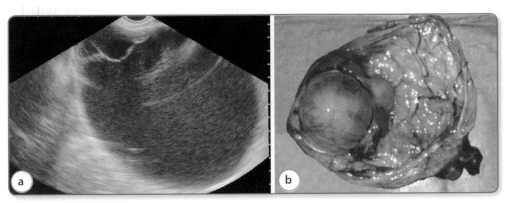

**Figure 17.24** Ovarian mucinous cystadenoma. Ovarian mucinous tumours show unilateral, very large, multiloculated cystic tumour with the smooth surface. In benign mucinous cystadenoma, the tumour is a multi-lobular tumour with simple and thin septa, and no solid portions, as shown in (a) US and (b) macroscopic findings.

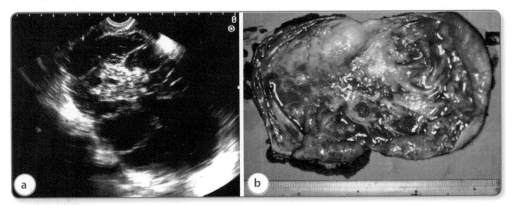

**Figure 17.25** Mucinous borderline tumour (MBT). In MBT, the tumour is unilateral, very large, multi-loculated cystic tumour with the smooth surface, frequently accompanied by the collection of numerous micro-cysts, not solid, as shown in (a) US and (b) macroscopic findings.

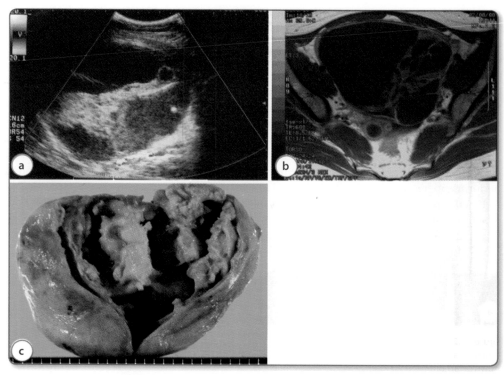

**Figure 17.26** Ovarian mucinous carcinoma (OMC). Among ovarian mucinous tumours with the feature of unilateral, very large, multi-lobulated cystic tumour, the presence of definite solid part in (a) US, (b) contrast-enhanced T1-weighted MRI, and (c) macroscopic findings, suggests the malignancy.

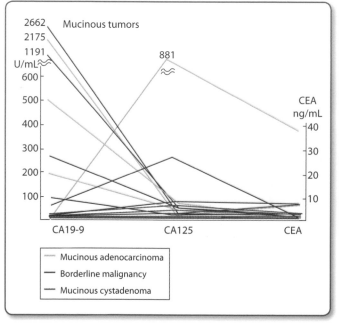

**Figure 17.27** Serum tumour marker, CA19-9, CA125, and CEA, levels in ovarian mucinous tumours. Tumour marker of ovarian mucinous tumours is not CA125, but CA19-9, which is frequently elevated in both OMC and MBTs, but not in benign mucinous cystadenomas.

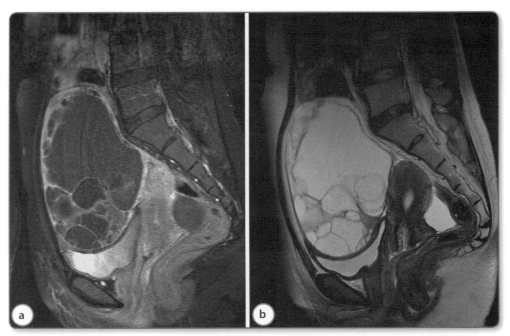

**Figure 17.28** Differential diagnosis: Typical MRI finding in primary OMC. Primary OMC presents usually with stage IA, unilateral, very large, with size of >20 cm, multi-lobular, cystic tumour with the solid part. Such findings are shown in (a) contrast-enhanced T1-weighted and (b) T2-weighted MRI images.

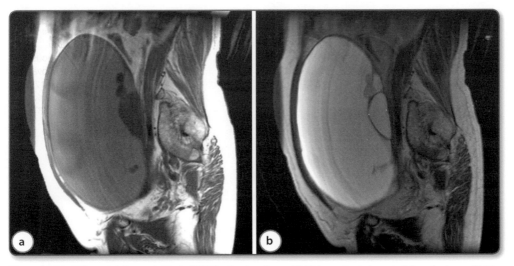

**Figure 17.29** Differential diagnosis: Typical MRI finding in primary OMC. Important characteristics of primary OMC are absolute unilaterality and the smooth surface of the multi-lobulated cystic tumour.

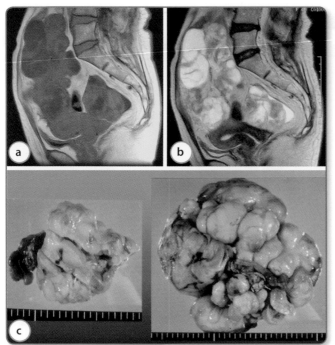

**Figure 17.30** Differential diagnosis: Typical MRI finding in metastatic ovarian cancer (colon cancer). In contrast to primary ovarian mucinous tumours, metastatic tumours frequently show the bilaterality and the characteristic nodularity of the tumour surface, as shown in (a) T1-weighted and (b) T2-weighted MRI, and (c) macroscopic findings.

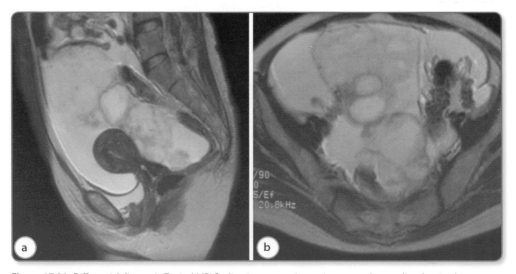

**Figure 17.31** Differential diagnosis: Typical MRI finding in metastatic ovarian cancer (appendiceal cancer). Bilaterality and nodularity of the surface are shown in (a) T1-weighted and (b) T2-weighted MRI images.

or benign-like lesions (**Figure 17.33**). Thus, OMC have been considered to develop from MBT via adenoma-carcinoma sequence [93], and therefore, surgical intervention of MBT is important for the prevention of OMC development. In MBT, when the carcinomatous epithelium is present without invasion, the tumour is designated as MBT with

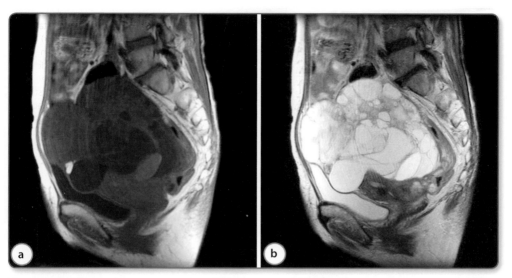

**Figure 17.32** Differential diagnosis: Typical MRI finding in metastatic ovarian cancer (pancreatic cancer). Metastatic tumour from the pancreatic carcinoma mimics primary OMC in both macroscopic and microscopic features. However, it is noticeable that the surface of the ovarian tumour is very nodular, as shown in (a) T1-weighted and (b) T2-weighted MRI images.

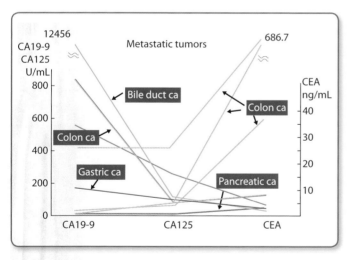

**Figure 17.33** Serum tumour marker, CA19-9, CA125, and CEA, levels in metastatic ovarian tumours. It is very important for differential diagnosis that CA125 is not so high, but CA19-9 or CEA is extremely elevated in metastatic tumours. ca, cancer.

intraepithelial carcinoma (**Figure 17.34**). If the carcinomatous lesion with desmoplastic stroma is small <5 mm in size, the tumour is diagnosed as MBT with micro-invasive carcinoma. In OMC, carcinomas show mainly the expansile/confluent (**Figure 17.35**) and rarely infiltrative/destructive pattern of growth. The patients with the latter infiltrative growth have been reported to show worse prognosis. The tumour cells resemble those of intestinal, gastric, and pyloric glands. When the cells resemble the endocervical cells with the mixture of various müllerian-type epithelial cells, the tumour should be classified as endometrioid carcinoma, because 'seromucinous carcinoma' category has been deleted

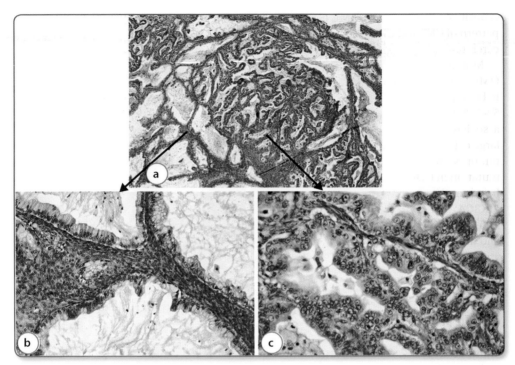

**Figure 17.34** Histopathology of MBT with intra-epithelial carcinoma. OMC develop from MBT via adenoma-carcinoma sequence, and therefore, tumours frequently consist of both (a) malignant and borderline lesions. (b) MBT of mainly borderline lesions with (c) the carcinomatous epithelium without invasion is classified as 'MBT with intraepithelial carcinoma'.

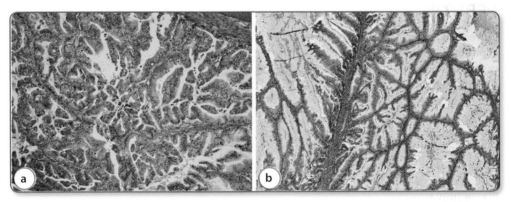

**Figure 17.35** Histopathology of OMC. In most cases of OMC, cancer cells are (a) gastrointestinal type cells, and show the expansile and (b) confluent pattern of growth.

from the new WHO classification [5]. Generally, prognosis of patients with OMC is favourable. Rarely, some patients experience peritoneal recurrence, and the tumour will not respond to the standard taxane/platinum chemotherapy. Immunohistochemically, the tumour cells are diffusely positive for CK7 and variably positive for CK20 and PAX8. CA19-9 is typically positive, whereas CA125, WT1, Napsin A, ER, and PR are negative. P53 is positive in some part of OMC cases, in contrast to p53-negative in MBT [5]. Staining pattern of CK7 and CK20 is useful for differential diagnosis between OMC and metastatic carcinoma.

Mutations of KRAS, BRAF, and CDKN2A have been well known to be often present in OMC as well as in MBT, and therefore, RAS/RAF and p16/INK4A pathways are thought to be important in the early carcinogenesis [93]. In contrast, TP53 mutation is present in 50–70% of OMC but in lower percentage in MBT, and is considered as a late event, being associated with genomic instability [26]. A recent whole-genome sequencing study in a large cohort of >500 cases of mucinous tumours including OMC and benign/borderline tumours showed that the most frequent genetic event in OMC is copy number loss or mutation in CDKN2A (76%), followed by KRAS (64%) and TP53 (64%) mutations [94]. Importantly, amplification of ERBB2 was seen in 26%, and mutations of RNF43, BRAF, PIK3CA, and ARID1A were present in 8–12% of OMC cases. In contrast, OMC patients with HRD or mismatch repair deficiency are very rare. Analyses of the tumour grade of OMC and metastatic OMC cases showed that TP53 mutation along with copy number alterations are key drivers for tumour progression. Mutation patterns of OMC were clearly different from those of colorectal, appendiceal, and pancreatic carcinomas, suggesting that OMC has primary ovarian origin. The potential targets of OMC are RNF43, ERBB2, and RAS/RAF, and their inhibitors could be the candidates of a drug for a patient with recurrent OMC after the gene panel testing of the tumour [95]. Actually, of the two patients with recurrent OMC with overexpression and amplification of ERBB2, the tumour in one patient responded dramatically to trastuzumab in combination with conventional chemotherapy [96]. Thus, in the era of precision medicine, whole-genome sequencing or gene panel testing might be useful in recurrent OMC in the search for a driver oncogene and matched targeted drug.

# CLINICAL, PATHOLOGIC, AND MOLECULAR ASPECTS OF PERITONEAL DISSEMINATION

More than 50% of patients with epithelial ovarian cancer present with advanced diseases at either stage III or IV. Since the most important factor for poor prognosis of ovarian cancer is peritoneal dissemination, novel development of precision treatment targeting the disease process is mandatory, being based on the complete elucidation of its clinical, pathological, and molecular aspects. In 1889, Stephan Paget proposed the 'seed' and 'soil' theory, and since then, pathogenesis of peritoneal dissemination has been discussed with the biological interactions among cancer cells, peritoneal mesothelial cells, endothelial cells, immune cells, and cancer-associated fibroblasts (CAFs) under the specific microenvironment [97]. In this metastasis, cancer cells appear to behave in the same way as human embryos implant to extrauterine sites in ectopic pregnancy, or as the endometrial tissues implant to the peritoneal cavity in endometriosis.

Interestingly, genomic alterations specific for the peritoneal dissemination have not been identified, even in the era of whole-genome sequencing. However, the epigenetic evolution of cancer cells may play a pivotal role in the disease process, and the gene expression profiling may also disclose the specific tumour microenvironment. Further clinical and basic research is needed to clarify the pathogenesis of peritoneal dissemination, in order to find the true target for novel treatment. In addition, recent attention has focussed on the clonal evolution of ovarian cancer cells as well as the acquisition of cancer stem cell (CSC)-like properties in the tumour microenvironment.

Thus, peritoneal dissemination of ovarian cancer cells has been discussed in reference to the key words such as clonal evolution, epigenetics, CSC, and tumour microenvironment. Based on the results from analyses for the peritoneal dissemination, appropriate strategies for surgery, cytotoxic chemotherapy, and molecular-targeted therapies should be established. Until now, data have accumulated mainly on the HGSC cancer cell, and therefore, the description below is on treating the peritoneal dissemination of HGSC.

## Biology of peritoneal dissemination and microenvironment

Peritoneal dissemination is a unique metastatic process, which consists of detachment of cancer cells from the primary lesion, floating in the ascitic fluid, attachment to the peritoneal mesothelium, invasion into the sub-mesothelial space, along with immune evasion and re-modelling of the tumour microenvironment including angiogenesis (**Figure 17.36**). After the cell proliferation and colonisation in the metastatic sites, cancer cells show frequent epithelio-mesenchymal transition (EMT) along with desmoplastic reaction of the surrounding stroma. From the first metastatic lesions, ovarian cancer cells metastasise again to other peritoneal or retroperitoneal sites. Thus, the peritoneal dissemination of ovarian cancer cells is a dynamic process in the peritoneal cavity, and pathologically, ovarian cancer cells show different faces according to the above sequential steps of the metastasis. Essentially, metastasis of cancer cells is the strategy for cell survival, most of which is an escape from the stressful condition. Thus, the metastasis represents various aspects of crosstalk between cancer cells and their microenvironment, such as escape from microenvironment, adaptation to microenvironment, and rearrangement of microenvironment.

### Detachment of cancer cells and hypoxia

The first step of peritoneal dissemination of HGSC is detachment of cancer cells from the primary lesion in either the fallopian tube or ovary. HGSC cells are characterised as having high proliferative activity, and tend to form papillary or solid tumours. Cancer cells at the tip of papillary or solid lesions, being away from the blood supply, are exposed to hypoxia, so that these cells show an increased expression of HIF-1$\alpha$ [98]. Interestingly, we discovered first that the cancer cells under hypoxia are associated with loss of expression of E-cadherin (**Figure 17.37**), which is the most important intercellular adhesion molecule

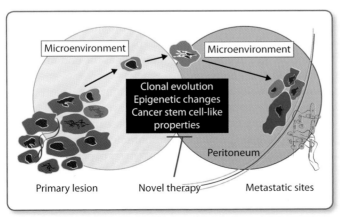

**Figure 17.36** Peritoneal dissemination of ovarian cancer cells. Peritoneal dissemination is the unique metastatic process, characterised by the biological interactions between cancer cells and other cells under the specific microenvironment. HGSC cancer cells clonally evolve with epigenetic changes and acquire cancer stem cell (CSC)-like properties in the metastasis, which will be targeted by novel treatments.

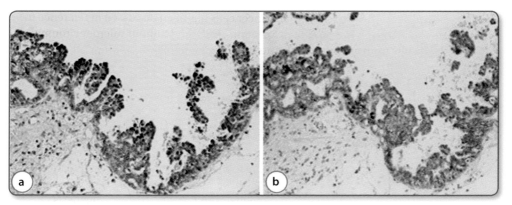

**Figure 17.37** Expression of HIF-1α with loss of E-cadherin expression in HGSC cancer cells. HGSC cancer cells at the tip of papillary lesion are exposed to hypoxia and (a) express HIF-1α, (b) being associated with loss of E-cadherin expression, and detach from the primary lesion.

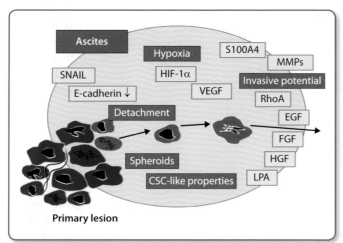

**Figure 17.38** Detachment of ovarian cancer cells in peritoneal dissemination. HGSC cancer cells under hypoxia detach from the primary lesion, and initiate the hypoxia-responsive signalling of target genes, such as VEGF and S100A4, which are involved in ascites formation and migration of cancer cells.

of epithelial cells, as well as the determinant molecule for cancer progression [99]. Hypoxic environment in vitro has been demonstrated to attenuate the expression of E-cadherin via upregulation of the transcription factor SNAIL, along with the increase in cell motility and invasive capacity. Thus, hypoxia plays an important role in the acceleration of detachment of ovarian cancer cells from the primary lesion into the peritoneal cavity (**Figure 17.38**) [98]. Loss of E-cadherin expression is usually coupled with the expression of N-cadherin, being referred as the phenomenon of 'cadherin-switch' of cancer cells [99].

Under hypoxia, ovarian cancer cells start the process of peritoneal dissemination with the formation of spheroids. Actually, many spheroids can be pathologically identified as floating in the tubal fluid in the vicinity of STIC (**Figure 17.39**), or in the ascites close to the greater omentum (**Figure 17.40**). Since spheroid formation is one of characteristic features of CSCs in vitro [100], ovarian cancer cells starting dissemination might have already acquired the CSC-like properties. In earlier studies on ovarian CSC-like cells, cancer-initiating cells have been isolated from the ascitic cancer cells in patients with HGSC [101].

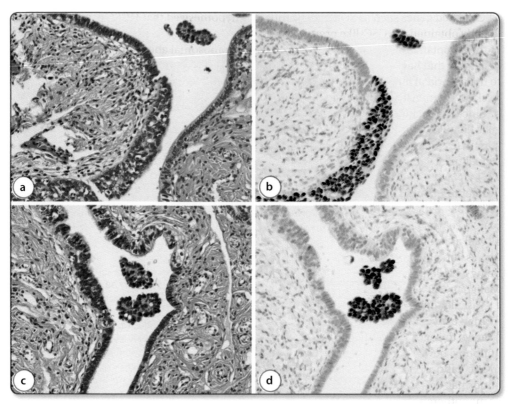

**Figure 17.39** Spheroids in the vicinity of STIC, floating in the tubal fluid. HGSC cancer cells start the peritoneal dissemination with the formation of spheroids from STIC, as shown in (a) HE section and (b) p53 immunostaining. Spheroids are floating in the tubal fluid, as shown in (c) HE section and (d) p53 immunostaining.

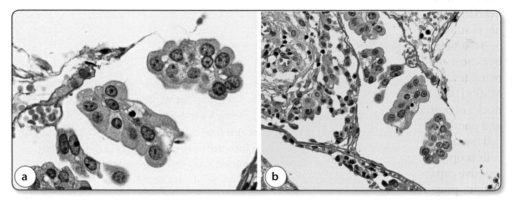

**Figure 17.40** Spheroids in the ascites approaching the greater omentum. Spheroids of HGSC cancer cells are (a) floating in the ascitic fluid, and (b) attach to the mesothelial cells of the omentum.

Since hypoxia has been implicated as a driver in the maintenance of niches for CSCs in various cancers [102], it is of particular interest that ovarian cancer spheroids are placed in the hypoxic condition from the beginning. Hypoxia promotes the acquisition of CSC-like state through the increased expression of CSC markers like CD133 and CD44, along with

CSC-related genes such as SOX2 [103]. Thus, it is hypothesised that HGSC cancer cells have already obtained the CSC-like properties during the period of the precursor of HGSC, STIC in the fallopian tube. This is consistent with the chromosomal aberrations due to genomic instability that have reportedly been present in STIC [46,47], possibly due to DNA damages to the fimbria of fallopian tubes under high levels of reactive oxygen species (ROS) from the backflow of menstrual blood.

Since the ascitic fluids contain half the soluble oxygen as blood [102], ovarian cancer cells floating in the ascites continue to be exposed to hypoxia (**Figure 17.38**). Hypoxia stimulates the expression of HIF-1$\alpha$, initiating the hypoxia-responsive downstream signalling of various target genes, such as GLUT-1, PDK-1, VEGF, S100A4, CXCR4, OCT4, NANOG, SOX2, and Notch, which are crucial for regulating glucose metabolism, proliferation, migration, inflammation, angiogenesis, and self-renewal of various cancer cells [103]. Especially in peritoneal dissemination, VEGF produced by ovarian cancer cells plays a central role in the increased vascular permeability resulting in ascites accumulation as well as neovascularisation in the metastatic sites. In 1997, we first reported that elevated expression of VEGF in epithelial ovarian cancer is an important poor prognostic factor, being correlated with advancing stage of disease in patients with ovarian cancer [104]. Malignant ascites contain high levels of VEGF.

Vascular endothelial growth factor is a key player for the peritoneal dissemination of ovarian cancer, and therefore, targeted therapy with anti-VEGF antibody is an important strategy to control the malignant behaviour of ovarian cancer cells [105]. Anti-VEGF antibody, bevacizumab, is a recombinant humanised monoclonal IgG antibody that binds to circulating VEGF, normalises tumour vessels that are structurally and functionally abnormal, and enhances the effects of chemotherapy. After phase II trials for bevacizumab as monotherapy showing the favourable response rates of 16–21%, all of phase III trials with chemotherapy plus bevacizumab and maintenance with bevacizumab showed a significantly longer PFS in patients with primary and recurrent ovarian cancer. Since then, bevacizumab has been commonly prescribed for patients with advanced ovarian cancer in both the first-line and the second-line treatments [106]. Recently, however, it is known that ovarian cancer cells acquire the resistance to bevacizumab via various mechanisms, and a novel strategy to overcome the resistance is mandatory.

S100A4 (metastasin) is a small Ca-binding protein of the S100 family, and is secreted by cancer cells in the form of EVs, which stimulate angiogenesis and invasiveness, up-regulates matrix metalloproteinases (MMPs), and down-regulates tissue inhibitors of MMPs [107]. We demonstrated that an increased expression of S100A4 protein in the nuclei of ovarian cancer cells is significantly associated with peritoneal dissemination and poor prognosis of patients [108]. Ovarian cancer cells secrete S100A4 and express the cell membrane receptor RAGE for S100A4. Transcription of *S100A4* gene in HGSC cancer cells is up-regulated by hypoxic conditions, and is associated with EMT and increased invasive capacity in vitro, suggesting its pivotal role as autocrine/paracrine factor for tumour progression. Interestingly, we also found that elevated expression of S100A4 protein is correlated with hypomethylation of *S100A4* gene in ovarian cancer cases. In addition, chronic hypoxia in vitro is shown to induce the hypomethylation of CpG sites in the first intron of *S100A4* gene, resulting in the constitutive overexpression of S100A4 [109]. Thus, the epigenetic mechanism is working in ovarian cancer cells for adaptation to the hypoxic microenvironment. Recently, epigenetic reprogramming has been implicated in the dynamic transformation of cancer cells, such as determination of metastatic phenotype, clonal evolution process, or acquisition of CSC-like properties [110].

Recently, high levels of serum S100A4 transcripts have been identified in patients with various cancer, being associated with tumour progression and poor prognosis [111–114]. EVs released by cancer cells have been implicated in cell-to-cell signal mediators like the language of cancer cells, and therefore, S100A4 could be the novel therapeutic target for various cancers [115]. Intracellular signalling of S100A4 is transferred via RhoA, one of RAS-like small GTP-binding proteins, which mediates the autocrine/paracrine stimulation of not only S100A4 but also EGF, FGF, HGF, and lysophosphatidic acid (LPA). Increased expression of RhoA has been reported in the disseminated lesions as compared with that in the primary lesion [116]. Treatment with Rho inhibitors or Rho kinase inhibitors suppresses the S100A4-stimulated invasion of ovarian cancer cells in vitro. Statins have been known to inhibit the signal transduction of RhoA, via inhibition of mevalonate pathway, and is shown to suppress the peritoneal dissemination of ovarian cancer cells in mouse model [117]. Thus, statins have recently received attention as a promising drug for the suppression of peritoneal dissemination of ovarian cancer [118]. Epidemiologically, a population-based cohort study from Canada reported that postdiagnosis use of statins is associated with better ovarian cancer survival in the full cohort (HR 0.76; 95% CI 0.64–0.89) and among women with HGSC (HR 0.80; 95% CI 0.67–0.96) [119]. Recently, similar results have also been obtained from Australian national data [120].

## Attachment of cancer cells and inflammation

The second step of peritoneal dissemination is the approach of ovarian cancer cell spheroids to the peritoneal mesothelium (**Figure 17.40**), followed by attachment and arrangement of the microenvironment to facilitate invasion and colonisation (**Figure 17.41**). Clinically, reddish change of the peritoneal surface is frequently seen at laparotomy in patients with ovarian cancer, and its pathological examination reveals the presence of inflammation with extensive angiogenesis mimicking the granulation tissue of wound healing (**Figure 17.42**). Cell to cell communication between ovarian cancer cells and peritoneal mesothelial cells has thoroughly been investigated [121,122]. Ovarian cancer cells produce various molecules such as HGF, transforming growth factor-beta (TGF-β), and interleukin-1beta (IL-1β), and induce the transformation of normal mesothelial cells into the mesenchymal-like mesothelial cells, which promote the adhesion of cancer cells on the peritoneum, as well as enhance vascular permeability and angiogenesis via VEGF production [122].

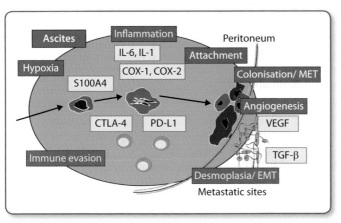

**Figure 17.41** Tumour microenvironment of the metastatic sites in peritoneal dissemination. HGSC cancer cells attach to the peritoneal surface, invade, colonise, and metastasise again, under various microenvironments of immune evasion, inflammation, and epithelio-mesenchymal transition (EMT).

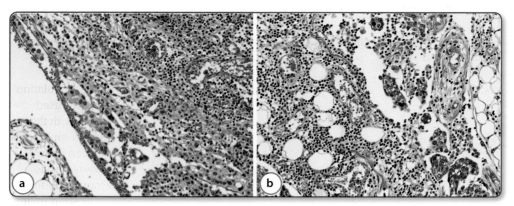

**Figure 17.42** Inflammatory microenvironment in the attachment phase of peritoneal dissemination. Histopathology of attachment and sub-mesothelial invasion shows the presence of inflammation (a) with extensive angiogenesis mimicking the granulation tissue of wound healing, (b) with extensive infiltration of lymphatic cells.

Malignant ascites of advanced ovarian cancer have been reported to contain elevated levels of various cytokines, such as tumour necrosis factor-alpha (TNF-$\alpha$), IL-6, IL-8, and LPA, all of which can be involved in the inflammatory change and disruption of the integrity of peritoneal surface [123]. Pro-inflammatory prostaglandins are known to be important in the physiological process of reproduction, and expression of the enzymes COX-1 and COX-2 catalysing the production of prostaglandins from arachidonic acid is reportedly increased in ovarian cancer [124]. Thus, various cytokines and prostaglandins might be involved in acute and chronic inflammatory responses in the peritoneal dissemination.

Such inflammatory microenvironment of the peritoneal cavity may be appropriate for the implantation of ovarian cancer spheroids [121–123]. This phenomenon seems to be analogous to the pathogenesis of endometriosis, in which the transplantation of endometrial tissues occurs under inflammatory conditions with high levels of cytokines. Port-site recurrence frequently occurs after laparoscopic surgery for ovarian cancer, suggesting an important role of inflammation in the implantation of cancer cells in the wound. In peritoneal dissemination, it is likely that ovarian cancer cells change the microenvironment of the peritoneal surface into the inflammatory condition, in which cancer cells are able to implant and survive easily. Therefore, inflammatory reaction in the attachment phase of peritoneal dissemination might be one of several appropriate targets for preventing the metastasis of ovarian cancer, and anti-inflammatory drugs like aspirin have received attention. Interestingly, a large cohort study reported that, compared with never users, the current and postdiagnosis use of either aspirin (HR 0.68; 95% CI 0.52–0.89) or non-aspirin non-steroidal anti-inflammatory drugs (NSAIDs) (HR 0.67; 95% CI 0.51–0.87) is associated with improved ovarian cancer-specific survival [125]. This study gives a great impact to the future management of ovarian cancer, and clinical trials are needed to test the possible benefit of anti-inflammatory medications combined with standard chemotherapy.

## Colonisation and epithelio-mesenchymal transition

The third step is the colonisation and proliferation of ovarian cancer cells at the disseminated sites of peritoneum under the normoxic condition after obtaining an appropriate blood supply (**Figure 17.43**). A reverse, mesenchymal-epithelial transition

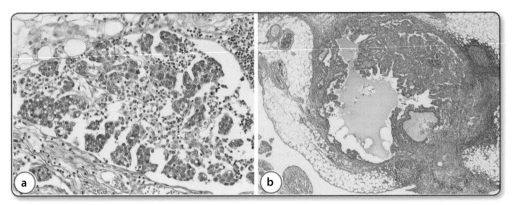

**Figure 17.43** Colonisation of ovarian cancer cells in the metastatic sites. Colonisation and proliferation of HGSC cancer cells start at (a) the disseminated sites, and under the normoxic condition, cancer cells show (b) less-invasive features resembling those in the primary lesions.

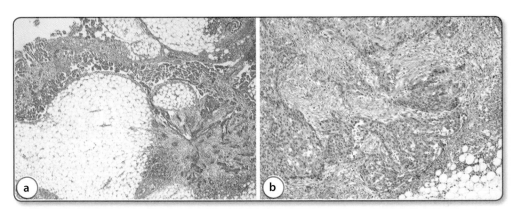

**Figure 17.44** Epithelio-mesenchymal transition (EMT) at metastatic sites. HGSC cancer cells exhibit high proliferative activity, and (a) the tumour microenvironment becomes hypoxic again. Ovarian cancer cells re-start the invasion and migration into the surrounding stroma, being associated with desmoplastic reaction, and show (b) the typical feature of EMT.

(MET) occurs in such lesions, as the expression of E-cadherin is reportedly increased in the ovarian cancer cells at metastatic sites [126]. Here, ovarian cancer cells may show the pathologically less-invasive features resembling those in the primary lesions of HGSC (**Figure 17.43**). In most cases of HGSC, however, cancer cells have an extremely high-proliferative activity, and the tumour microenvironment becomes hypoxic again. Then, ovarian cancer cells restart the invasion and migration into the surrounding stroma, being associated with desmoplastic reaction (**Figure 17.44**). The stroma consists of CAFs, immune cells, endothelial cells, and the extracellular matrix. Neovascularisation is again observed. Here, ovarian cancer cells exhibit the typical features of EMT, which is characterised by the transformation into spindle-like shape of cancer cell with eosinophilic cytoplasm containing many cytoskeletons for enhanced migratory capacity (**Figure 17.45**). Both cancer cells and CAFs secrete MMPs re-modelling the tumour microenvironment. Eventually, an edematous microenvironment appears and increases the intercellular

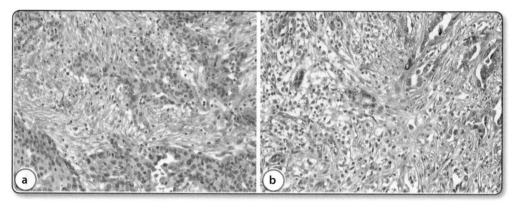

**Figure 17.45** HGSC cancer cells in EMT with cancer-associated fibroblasts (CAF). (a) EMT is characterised by transformation into spindle-like shape of cancer cell with eosinophilic cytoplasm for enhanced migratory capacity. (b) Spindle-shaped cancer cells are intermingled with CAF, immune cells, and endothelial cells in EMT.

communications using exosomes among cancer cells, stromal cells, and immune cells, resulting in the enhancement of motility of cancer cells. Such features of ovarian cancer toward EMT associated with the stromal desmoplasia are more frequently observed in the metastasis to the greater omentum, being clinically called as 'omental cake'. Adipocytes in the omentum may also contribute to the behaviour of ovarian cancer cells via production of various adipokines [127,128].

Deregulation of TGF-β signalling plays an important role in ovarian carcinogenesis [129]. Our microarray analysis comparing the gene expressions between the ovarian and omental tumours identified the activation of TGF-β pathway in the omental metastasis [130]. Expression of TGF-β signalling molecules, such as TGF-β receptor type 2 and phosphorylated SMAD2, is increased in the omental metastases. This is consistent with the finding that, among a variety of cytokines and growth factors, TGF-β signalling plays a fundamental role in EMT, metastasis, and stemness [131]. Hypoxia also regulates CSC-associated genes and induces EMT via TGF-β signalling pathways. Since the desmoplastic stroma with CAFs serves as the convenient niche for CSCs, EMT might be essential for the survival of ovarian CSC-like cells. In the histopathology of HGSC, EMT with desmoplastic stroma is most frequently seen in the 'mesenchymal' or MT subtype [49,54], which consists of the mixture of epithelial-like cells in the centre and mesenchymal-like cells in the invading front (**Figure 17.45**). Such hybrid phenotype is known to display increased CSC-like properties accompanied by enhanced resistance to anticancer drugs [103,131]. This is consistent with the chemoresistant nature of 'mesenchymal' or MT subtype in HGSC [49]. Accordingly, ovarian CSCs-like cells with EMT as well as the desmoplastic micro-environment should be targeted adequately by novel treatments in order to overcome the chemoresistance. In mouse model of peritoneal dissemination of ovarian cancer, treatment with inhibitor for TGF-β signalling pathway was effective for better survival [130], and now, various anti-TGF-β drugs are under clinical trials [132].

## Immune environment of peritoneal dissemination

Immune environment plays a crucial role in the progression of ovarian cancer cells [133]. Cancer cells having various gene mutations express cancer-specific antigens, which are recognised by the host immune cells, resulting in the immunoreactions to eradicate the cancer cells. However, cancer cells express molecules on the cell surface or produce various cytokines in order to escape from the host immune mechanisms. Among them, the immune checkpoint molecules such as CTLA-4 and PD-1/PD-L1 (ligand of PD-1) have recently received much attention in the modern era of immunotherapy with immune checkpoint inhibitors [134]. In addition, various immune cells are recruited under the inflammatory environment of peritoneal dissemination, and may support the acquisition of CSC-like properties as well as the progression of ovarian cancer cells [135].

Immune cells include macrophages, dendritic cells (DCs), neutrophils, mast cells, lymphocytes, and myeloid-derived suppressor cells (MDSCs). Macrophages residing in tumours are called tumour-associated macrophages (TAMs), and frequently detected in ovarian cancer tissues and in malignant ascites. TAMs present two main phenotypes i.e. the anti-tumour M1 macrophages and pro-tumour M2 macrophages. Strikingly, almost all TAMs in the primary lesions and ascites of ovarian cancer patients are M2 macrophages [135,136]. M2 macrophages are activated by direct contact with ovarian cancer cells, and secrete IL-6 and IL-10, resulting in an activation of signal transducer and activator of transcription 3 (STAT3) which play an important role in tumour progression and chemoresistance of ovarian cancer cells [137]. M2 macrophages have also been reported to inhibit the proliferation of T lymphocytes, accelerate the immunosuppression by T regulatory (Treg) cells, and express the ligand receptors for CTLA-4 and PD-1. M2 macrophages also play an important role in the tissue repair, re-modelling of the extracellular matrix, and angiogenesis [136]. This is consistent with the pathological features of the inflammatory peritoneal surface in the peritoneal dissemination of ovarian cancer. DCs capture endogenous or exogenous antigens, process them, and present the antigenic peptides to CD4+ and CD8+ T cells, via major histocompatibility complex class II (MHC II) and MHC I molecules, respectively. Thus, DCs play key roles in the anti-tumour host immune system. In ovarian cancer patients, dysfunction of DCs has been reported to occur in the immune-modulating microenvironment such as IL-6, IL-10, and VEGF, tumour-derived EVs, activation of STAT3, and the abnormal intracellular lipid accumulation [135,137].

Actual function of lymphocytes existing within the tumour tissues remains undetermined, but these cells are termed as tumour-infiltrating lymphocytes (TILs), consisting of B cells and T cells such as CD4+, CD+8 T cells, and Treg cells. In HGSC, the presence of CD+8 T cells has been reported to correlate with better survival of patients [138,139]. Among the four molecular subtypes of HGSC, the best prognosis has been reported in the patients with 'immunoreactive' or IR subtype [52,53], which shows pathological features of the prominent infiltration of immune cells [54]. On the other hand, the infiltration of Treg cells indicates the poor clinical outcomes of ovarian cancer patients [140]. Treg cells regulate the immune response via several mechanisms, such as secreting immunosuppressive molecules like IL-10 and TGF-β, modulating the maturation of DCs, and inhibiting the effector lymphocytes via the expression of CTLA-4. Recently, MDSCs have received attention as a key player for the immunosuppression in cancer [141]. MDSCs are a heterogenic population of immature myeloid cells that differ in morphology and function from terminally differentiated mature myeloid cells such as macrophages, DCs, or neutrophils. MDSCs also include myeloid cells at various stages of differentiation that expand from bone marrow into peripheral organs, including the tumour microenvironment, and co-express the myeloid surface marker GR-1 and CD11b [135]. MDSCs promote tumour progression via various mechanisms, such as immune suppression by targeting effector

T cells, activation of Treg cells, generation of oxidative stress, and facilitation of angiogenesis. Our analysis on advanced ovarian cancer found that the expression of VEGF inhibits the tumour immunity, recruiting MDSCs via GM-CSF expression. In addition, MDSC infiltration is enhanced in patients showing resistance to anti-VEGF therapy [142]. Thus, anti-VEGF therapy might induce the tumour hypoxia and GM-CSF expression, resulting in the recruitment of MDSCs and inhibition of the tumour immunity. Accumulating evidence suggests that MDSCs increase the stemness of ovarian CSC-like cells via various signalling pathways [143,144].

The mechanism of 'escape from the host immune' in cancer has recently been disclosed [105,134]. An immune reaction to antigens including cancer cells is initiated with antigen recognition by DCs (cognitive phase). DCs migrate to lymph nodes and present the antigens to T cells, which recognise the cancer cells and become activated. At the same time, a second signal is sent via interaction of specific molecules known as immune checkpoint molecules i.e. B7, CD28, and CTLA-4. When the interaction between B7 and CD28 occurs, active immunity is initiated. If the interaction between B7 and CTLA-4 is stronger, the response is inhibited. Such pro- or anti-immune mechanism also occurs when T cells recognise the target (effector phase). If the interaction between PD-1 on T cells and PD-L1 (ligand of PD-1) on target cells is stronger, the immunologic attack will be attenuated. Cancer cells that frequently express either CTLA-4 or PD-L1, escape the attack by T cells. Therefore, immunotherapy using anti-CTLA-4 antibodies for the cognitive phase or anti-PD-L1/ PD-1 antibodies for the effector phase is a novel therapy with immune checkpoint inhibitors [134]. We first showed the efficacy of monotherapy with anti-PD-1 antibody, nivolumab, for patients with platinum-resistant recurrence of ovarian cancer, and 2 of the 20 patients showed CR and survived >5 years [145]. Thus, clinical trials with immune checkpoint inhibitors have opened a new window for ovarian cancer treatment. However, the ORR in the monotherapy with immune checkpoint inhibitor is relatively low in ovarian cancer patients, and the various combinations with other targeted drugs are under clinical trials.

## Cancer stem cell-like cells in ovarian cancer

### Evolution of cancer stem cell-like cells in ovarian cancer

Various aspects of the tumour microenvironment in peritoneal dissemination, such as hypoxia, inflammation, EMT with desmoplastic stroma, and immune environment, are discussed with reference to the niches for CSCs [102,103]. It has been proposed that the recurrence and reduced efficacy of chemotherapy are caused by the presence of CSCs in the niches. The existence of CSCs in ovarian cancer tissues has not yet been confirmed. However, the natural course of advanced ovarian cancer with peritoneal dissemination, such as apparent regression after cytotoxic chemotherapy, recurrence in most patients, and progression with chemoresistance, strongly suggests intratumoural heterogeneity, consisting of both quiescent CSC-like cells with chemoresistance and actively proliferating non-CSC-like cells responding to chemotherapy [146]. Thus, the clinical course of advanced ovarian cancer fits well the CSC concept.

Cancer stem cells have been defined as a 'cellular population within a tumour which exhibits the capacity of self-renewal and causes the heterogeneous lineages of cancer cells that comprise the tumour tissue' [102, 103]. CSCs constitute a small population of tumour cells with enhanced metastatic capacity and with strong resistance to anticancer therapies.

Biological characteristics of CSCs have been reported as ability of repair of DNA damage, immunosuppressive phenotype, metabolic reprogramming, resistance to oxidative stress, and capability to expel anticancer agents. Interestingly, however, specific morphological features of CSC have not been described. Also, the genomic alterations specific for acquiring the biologic characteristics of CSC have not been identified, as previous trials with whole-exome sequencing of CSC showed the same genetic alterations with non-CSC cells [147]. Thus, the nature of CSC has been implicated only by the changes of expression of various genes including upregulation of CSC markers, epigenetic alteration of genes, and the interaction with the specific microenvironment named as 'niche'. Nevertheless, the presence of CSC-like cells in ovarian cancer, mainly of HGSC, has strongly been suggested by successful isolation of a single tumourigenic clone among a mixed population of cells derived from the ascites of a patient with advanced ovarian cancer [101]. Ovarian cancer-initiating cells with self-renewing capacity and positivity for CSC markers have been cloned from ovarian cancer tissues [102]. These CSC-like cells have been examined by flow cytometry and are enriched in the side population (SP), being able to efflux the Hoechst33342 dye by the cell transporters [148]. Thus, SP cells have been considered as having CSC-like properties.

There have been several hypothetical models about the lineage relationship between CSCs and non-CSCs [103]. The classic hierarchical model suggests that cancers are hierarchically organised in the same manner as normal tissues, and CSCs share similar molecular properties to normal stem cells. In the fallopian tubes or ovary, normal stem cells have been theorised to exist in the transformation zone between the fimbria and the peritoneal mesothelium or in the hilar region of ovarian surface. Tumours may have a hierarchical structure with tumourigenic CSCs at the top which generate the differentiated non-CSCs, which form most of the tumour mass and is highly sensitive to chemotherapy. In contrast, CSCs remain quiescent and resistant to chemotherapy targeting fast-proliferating cells. In this model, CSCs have been considered as phenotypically stable. In contrast, another plasticity model proposes that cancer cells can switch between CSC-like state and differentiated non-CSC state, so that non-tumourigenic cancer cells can de-differentiate to acquire CSC-like properties [103]. CSC-like phenotype is flexible, and the specific tumour microenvironment may play an important role in the dynamic process. Chemotherapy has also been shown to give selective pressure, resulting in the enrichment of CSC possibly due to the plasticity. Actually, phenotypic heterogeneity has been reported to be present in cancer-initiating cells from patients with HGSC [149]. In case of ovarian cancer, therefore, the plasticity model may fit the nature of CSC-like cells.

The third theory for CSC is the clonal evolution model, in which cancer cells can evolve during the development and progression, and finally acquire the CSC-like properties as the result of clonal evolution. HGSC is a representative of tumour with genomic instability due to loss of DNA repair function, and accumulated evidence indicates that various different clones evolve in the peritoneal dissemination [45–47]. After various kinds of chemotherapy, ovarian cancer cells recur with different clinical, pathological, and molecular features, being presumably based on the biological characteristics of HGSCs. Therefore, we hypothesised that, during the development and progression of HGSC, loss of various key genes due to the genomic instability contributes to the acquisition of CSC-like properties. In order to address this hypothesis, a study of functional genomics screen using a shRNA library targeting 15,000 genes was conducted in ovarian cancer cells, and then, the six novel genes, *MSL3*, *ZNF691*, *VPS45*, *ITGB3BP*, *TLE2*, and *ZNF498*, have been identified [150].

The suppression of each gene markedly increases the proportion of SP cells, which exhibit the capacity for spheroid formation, single cell clonogenicity, in vivo tumourigenicity, chemoresistance, along with activation of Hedgehog pathway. VPS45 and ITGB3BP have been known as tumour suppressor, and TLE2 is a corepressor of Wnt-β catenin pathway. Clinicopathologically, loss of expression of MSL3, ZNF691, and VPS45 has reportedly been correlated with poor prognosis of ovarian cancer patients. This may be consistent with the clonal evolution of CSC-like cells in ovarian cancer. HGSC cells show extensive genetic alterations including loss of the responsible genes even in the early carcinogenic phase of STIC, and may already have acquired CSC-like properties. During peritoneal dissemination and under various anti-cancer therapies, the genome of HGSC cells continuously changes. In addition, epigenetic reprogramming for adaptation of new environment may also play an important role in the subsequent evolution of CSC-like cells [109,110,151,152]. In ovarian cancer, therefore, CSC-like properties may be different among patients or according to the different phases of clonal evolution.

## Cancer stem cell-like cells and chemoresistance

Several markers for CSCs, such as CD133, ALDH, CD44, CD117, and CD 326, have been identified in ovarian cancer [102,103,146]. CD133, a trans-membrane glycoprotein, is the most common CSCs marker as expressed in the tumour-initiating cells of various cancers, being involved in stem cell maintenance and expansion. In ovarian cancer, CD133 is important in tumour initiation, self-renewal, and chemoresistance, however, the expression of CD133 is heterogeneous and may represent the plasticity of CSCs-like cells [151]. ALDH is an enzyme implicated in detoxification and efflux of chemotherapeutic drugs, and has been reported in ovarian cancer to play a key role in spheroid formation, self-renewal, and high proliferative and differentiation capacities. CD44 is a receptor for the extracellular matrix components that enable CSCs to sense environmental changes, and may be involved in EMT. CD44 has also been associated with spheroid formation, self-renewal, maintenance of CSC-like properties, and chemoresistance [103]. CD117 is a receptor of tyrosine kinase, c-Kit, activated by binding to its ligand, stem cell factor, which activates cell-signalling cascades for cell proliferation, apoptosis, adhesion, and differentiation. CD326 is a trans-membrane glycoprotein, EpCAM, expressed in various cancers, and was isolated using an in vivo limiting dilution assay in ovarian cancer [146]. Clinicopathologic studies of ovarian cancer patients showed that CD133 overexpression is significantly correlated with FIGO stage and tumour grade. Overexpression of ALDH, CD44, or CD117 is reportedly associated with poor survival of ovarian cancer patients. Expression of CD326 is increased in ovarian cancer tissues after chemotherapy, and is more frequently observed in platinum-resistant diseases [153].

Clinically, one of the most important issues for the management of ovarian cancer is chemoresistance, being caused by various mechanisms such as the enhancement of DNA damage response and repair, increased drug efflux via the transporters, ability of detoxification for drugs, increased adaptation to stressful conditions such as hypoxia and low nutrients, and attaining quiescence with activation of survival pathways [102,103]. These mechanisms work in ovarian CSC-like cells via their intrinsic machineries, as all of the CSC marker molecules such as CD133, ALDH, CD44, CD117, and CD326 have been reported to play pivotal roles in chemoresistance. In addition, signals from the niches in the tumour microenvironment have also been implicated in chemoresistance [102]. Hypoxia stimulates HIF-1α to initiate hypoxia-responsive signalling and maintain cancer cells in a quiescent state, shielding them from drugs targeting proliferating cells. Under inflammatory conditions, various cytokines and growth factors also contribute to the chemoresistance of ovarian CSC-like cells [123,135]. Especially, autocrine production of IL-6 from ovarian cancer cells makes them resistant to cisplatin and paclitaxel via decreased proteolytic cleavage of caspase-3 [154]. Production of IL-6 is associated with increased expression of multidrug resistant genes MDR1 and GSTπ, and antiapoptotic genes Bcl-2 and Bcl-xl, suggesting that IL-6 promotes drug resistance by increasing drug efflux and reducing apoptosis. COX-2 has also been associated with chemoresistance, as primary ovarian cancer refractory to platinum-based chemotherapy contained many COX-2 positive cancer cells [123]. Increased expression of TGF-β in the recurrent ovarian cancer has been implicated in chemoresistance, since the inhibition of TGF-β signalling reverses the sensitivity to cisplatin in the chemoresistant cancer cells. TGF-β signalling regulates ovarian CSC-like cells via modulation of tissue trans-glutaminase 2, which plays an important role in EMT and stemness. Dynamic EMT state showing epithelial/ mesenchymal hybrid phenotype in cancer represents the plasticity of CSC-like cells, and is correlated with increased stemness and chemoresistance [103,131]. In our clinical experience about the effect of NAC, patients with HGSC with 'mesenchymal' or MT subtype show the least response to the treatment with taxane and platinum. Thus, ovarian CSC-like cells in the strongest niche of EMT should be the target of novel therapy in ovarian cancer management.

## Novel treatment targeting ovarian CSC-like cells

Most patients with advanced ovarian cancer develop recurrence acquiring chemoresistance. This is presumably caused by the presence of CSC-like cells which cannot completely be eradicated by cytoreductive surgery with first-line cytotoxic chemotherapy. The small subpopulation of CSC-like cells forms again the tumour bulk population, which appears as recurrent tumour. Therefore, treatment strategy in the era of precision medicine should focus on the occult presence of ovarian CSC-like cells. The ultimate goal of cancer treatment is complete eradication of cancer including CSC-like cells, and therefore, novel development of various drugs targeting ovarian CSC-like cells as well as their niches is urgently needed.

Several drugs for targeting ovarian CSC-like cells and their niches have been under consideration or clinical trial [103,155,156]. Molecules targeting the CSC markers such as CD44, CD117, or ADLH have been unsuccessful due to safety issues, since most of the drugs target stemness factors that are shared with normal stem cells. Various therapies targeting the signalling pathways in ovarian CSC-like cells, such as Notch, Wnt, and Hedgehog, might be possible, and the combinations of the conventional chemotherapy with the drugs i.e. RO4929097, MK-0752, and enoticumab for Notch signal, sonidegib, and vismodegib for Hedgehog signal, ipafricept for Wnt signal, have been under clinical trial. IL-6 plays an important role in the inflammatory environment of ovarian CSC-like cells. Siltuximab, an anti-IL-6 antibody, sensitises the paclitaxel-resistant ovarian cancer cells, but did not show the benefit in vivo. Tocilizumab, a monoclonal antibody blocking IL-6R, may be promising, since ovarian cancer patients who received the highest dose of tocilizumab showed longer OS. TGF-β signalling plays a central role in EMT and chemoresistance of ovarian CSC-like cells, and therefore, inhibition of TGF-β signalling could be valuable. Small molecule inhibitors, such as LY2109761 and LY3157299, targeting the TGF-β signalling pathways have been under clinical trial for patients with various cancers including ovarian cancer. Anti-EpCAM antibody, catumaxomab, has been tried in patients with peritoneal carcinomatosis. Until now, however, drugs targeting ovarian CSC-like cells and their niches have not yet been approved for clinical practice.

At present, the definite tool for complete eradication of ovarian CSC-like cells is surgery, and therefore, reconsideration of operative procedures is necessary for patients with advanced ovarian cancer. Surgery for peritoneal dissemination needs a personalised approach. In case of low-volume disease, complete resection with macroscopic no residual tumour (R0 surgery) may be feasible, when the additional operations can be appropriately performed in addition to the standard surgery. In case of high-volume disease, however, primary surgical approach is very difficult and it may be better to choose NAC followed by interval debulking surgery (IDS). In most patients with HGCS, NAC is effective and 'apparently complete surgery' will become feasible in IDS. However, surgeons cannot identify the presence of residual CSC-like cells under the normal-appearing peritoneal surface after NAC. Thus, 'apparently complete surgery' at IDS is not enough for complete eradication of all CSC-like cells. This important issue will be discussed in the section on 'Precision surgery for advanced ovarian cancer'.

# SURGERY FOR OVARIAN CANCER

## Precision surgery for early ovarian cancer

The standard treatment of epithelial ovarian cancer is optimal staging, PDS, followed by postoperative taxane/platinum chemotherapy [3,157]. Although the completeness of surgery is the most important prognostic factor for ovarian cancer patients, precision surgery should be highly individualised for the patient according to her desires such as preservation of fertility and quality of life (QOL), as well as the biological characteristics of the tumour. Since the prognosis of patients with ovarian cancer at early stages (FIGO stage I and II) is generally favourable, fertility-preserving surgery can be considered for young women.

### Fertility-sparing surgery for early ovarian cancer

Fertility-sparing surgery (FSS) has been considered for young women with ovarian cancer at early stage and with low-grade histology, who strongly desire child-bearing. Recently, this issue has become more important with advancing age of marriage and pregnancy in women. For the surgical procedure, unilateral salpingo-oophorectomy with partial omentectomy has been employed. Biopsy from the contralateral, normal-appearing ovary, and systematic lymphadenectomy can be omitted, considering the maintenance of fertility [157]. However, thorough surgical staging procedures including cytological sampling from various sites, biopsies from the suspected lesions, and lymph node sampling are needed to confirm the early stage of disease, because, approximately 30% of patients with the tumour apparently confined to the ovary have been upstaged after the complete surgery. According to a systematic review of literature on FSS from 2000 to 2020 [158], recurrence occurred in 9.1% (62/622) of patients with grade 1–2 carcinoma, and in 25.6% (32/125) with grade 3 carcinoma including OCCC ($p < 0.001$). Death rate was 8.8% (219/2,489) in grade 1–2 carcinomas, which is significantly lower compared to 30% (213/711) in grade 3 carcinoma ($p < 0.001$).

FSS had been usually employed in apparently stage I carcinoma with favourable histological features, that is, serous, endometrioid, or mucinous carcinoma with grade 1–2 histology. There is controversy with regards to FSS for OCCC, which is classified as grade 3, but frequently develops in young women who desire fertility preservation [159].

Our multicentre, retrospective JCOG study on a total of 211 stage I (stage IA 126 and IC 85) patients was performed in order to re-consider the indication of FSS for various histological types including OCCC [160]. Five-year OS and recurrence-free survival (RFS) were 100% and 97.8% for stage IA and favourable histology, 100% and 100% for stage IA OCCC, 100% and 33.3% for stage IA and non-clear grade 3, 96.9% and 92.1% for stage IC and favourable histology, 93.3% and 66.0% for stage IC OCCC, and 66.7% and 66.7% for stage IC and non-clear grade 3. Regarding reproductive outcome, 53.6% (45/84) of patients who were nulliparous at FSS and married at the time of investigation gave birth to 56 healthy children. This study has confirmed that FSS is a safe treatment for stage IA patients with grade 1–2, non-clear cell histology, and even in stage IC, prognosis is favourable after FSS followed by adjuvant chemotherapy. Interestingly, we showed that patients with OCCC at stage IA having favourable prognosis could be candidates for FSS, whereas the patients with OCCC at stage IC tended to recur, even if they were designated as IC due to the surgical rupture of tumour (stage IC1). Thus, severe adhesion of endometriosis has an impact as prognostic indicator. A recent review on FSS on a total 60 patients with OCCC showed that 16.6% of patients had recurrence, but there was no difference in survival and recurrence rates among patients who underwent FSS and those who had radical surgery. The total clinical pregnancy rate was 32% with 24% live birth rate in 12 patients [161]. In the era of precision medicine, these data should be explained to the patients who desire to undergo FSS.

## Systematic lymphadenectomy in early ovarian cancer

Benefit of systematic lymphadenectomy for ovarian cancer at early stages has been controversial. The frequency of lymph node metastasis is reported as 5–13% of ovarian cancers in which the tumour is apparently confined to the ovary. Pelvic nodes are affected in 5–14%, and para-aortic nodes in 4–12% [157]. Therefore, systematic pelvic and para-aortic lymphadenectomy is usually needed for accurate staging. In a retrospective study on a total of 6,686 women with clinical stage I ovarian cancer (pT1), lymphadenectomy improved significantly the 5-year disease-specific survival of all patients [162]. In contrast, a RCT on systematic lymphadenectomy versus lymph node sampling in 268 patients with pT1 and pT2 ovarian cancer showed that lymphadenectomy did not significantly influence PFS and OS of patients [163]; for systematic lymphadenectomy and sampling, 5-year PFS was 78.3% and 71.3% ($p = 0.166$), and 5-year OS was 84.2% and 81.3% ($p = 0.513$), respectively, although lymphadenectomy detected a higher proportion of patients with metastatic lymph nodes (22% vs. 9%; $p = 0.007$). Nevertheless, a recent systematic review and meta-analysis showed that lymphadenectomy is associated with improved OS (HR 0.75; 95% CI 0.68–0.82) [164]. A multicentre, retrospective cohort study reported an improvement of 5-year disease-free survival of patients at early stages [165]. Generally, the prognosis of patients with lymph node metastases only is better than that with peritoneal dissemination, and new FIGO stage classification for such cases has been revised from stage IIIC to stage IIIA1. Thus, resection of metastatic nodes is very important not only in the accurate staging, but also in the prognosis and QOL in pT1 patients, since adjuvant chemotherapy is indicated if positive, and can be omitted if negative [157]. In the era of precision medicine, therefore, individualised treatment is possible according to the systematic lymphadenectomy in patients with early stage ovarian cancer.

## Minimally invasive surgery for ovarian cancer

Role of minimally invasive surgery (MIS) in gynaecologic oncology has been continually expanding, and today, advanced laparoscopic and robotic-assisted laparoscopic techniques are commonly used to treat endometrial cancers. For patients with ovarian cancer, gynaecologic surgeons traditionally hesitate to perform laparoscopic procedures due to the concern about adequacy for staging, the possibility of tumour spillage, and the risk of port-site metastasis, and therefore, the standard surgical approach has been open laparotomy [157]. Now, laparoscopic evaluation has been adopted for assessment on the feasibility of PDS to no visible disease, and assessment of the peritoneal lesions for patients in complete remission after the primary treatment. Especially, diagnostic laparoscopy triaging patients to either performing PDS immediately or giving NAC first is important as a standard approach for patients with advanced disease [166].

Recently, however, MIS with usual or robotic laparoscopy has been attempted for treatment of selected patients with both early and advanced diseases of ovarian cancer. Review of six retrospective studies on early ovarian cancer showed that there was no difference in upstaging rate, PFS, and OS, between open laparotomy and MIS [167]. The controversial issues in early stage disease have been discussed on intraoperative tumour rupture/spillage and port-site metastasis [168], and various modalities preventing them have been developed and used. The major concern is oncologic outcome of patients who underwent MIS. A recent systematic review and meta-analysis of 19 observational studies on a total of 7,213 patients, open 4,982 and MIS 2,285, showed no significant differences in OS at 3 and 5 years between the two groups, in not only early stage but also advanced stage subgroups [169]. Recently, MIS has also been tried in the secondary surgery for patients with recurrent tumour, and sometimes, successful complete cytoreduction was reported. So far, MIS is not currently recommended as standard for tumour debulking surgery. In the near future, however, MIS would be considered as the precision surgery for a group of selected patients.

## Precision surgery for advanced ovarian cancer

The end-point of surgery should be the complete extirpation of cancer cells with a safe margin. Nevertheless, we have been talking about ovarian cancer surgery using the term 'optimal debulking'. We should confirm again that the final goal of surgery is not 'optimal' but 'complete'.

### Primary debulking surgery

The standard surgical strategy for patients with advanced ovarian cancer is primary debulking surgery (PDS), including the removal of intraperitoneal disseminations and metastases as completely as possible [157]. Rationale of the debulking is that it is technically feasible, since typically ovarian cancer is confined within the peritoneal borders, and usually does not invade deep into abdominal organs. Bulky tumour contains necrotic and hypoxic areas which contain cancer cells resistant to chemotherapy, and theoretically, debulking surgery will change the microenvironment where cancer cells become chemosensitive. In 1975, C Thomas Griffiths reported that survival of advanced ovarian cancer improved as the size of residual tumour decreased [170]. Then, based on the review of two GOG studies in 1992, the term 'optimal cytoreduction' was introduced and defined as a residual tumour <2 cm [171]. Finally, a largest trial GOG182 ($n = 4,312$) showed that median PFS and OS of stage III+IV patients were 29 and 68 months in no residual tumour, 16 and 44 months in residual tumour $\leq 1$ cm, and 13 and 30 months in residual tumour > 1 cm. Since then, the size of a residual tumour up to 1 cm has commonly been used as the definition of 'optimal cytoreduction', and that >1 cm as 'suboptimal' [172]. In all of data on survival, however, the group of patients who underwent complete extirpation to no residual tumour (R0) shows the best survival. Currently, according to the advancement of surgical technologies, the goal of debulking surgery appears to have evolved to that of complete gross resection of all visible diseases, R0 surgery [173,174], which may result in the successful eradication of all CSC-like cancer cells.

Thus, in PDS of advanced ovarian cancer, gynaecologic oncologists by themselves or in collaboration with intestinal and hepato-biliary surgeons have been trying to do R0 surgery. In addition to the standard procedures such as bilateral salpingo-oophorectomy and total hysterectomy, and omentectomy, additional operations should be performed for various peritoneal tumours. En bloc resection of the primary tumour with stripping of the peritoneum of lateral wall and vesicouterine fossa can be performed easily (**Figure 17.46**). The extent of omentectomy either complete or partial depends on the degree of tumour involvement (**Figure 17.47**). If the tumour invasion in the cul-de-sac peritoneum is severe, co-resection of the tumour with recto-sigmoid colon, followed by colorectal anastomosis is reasonable. Resection of small and large intestines, followed by reconstruction, will be done, if the number of anastomosis is small. Recently, upper abdominal surgery has also become a standard procedure. Disseminations on the liver and the diaphragm can be resected using careful surgical techniques (**Figures 17.48** and **17.49**). Splenectomy is considered as the tumour dissemination frequently occurs in this area. Eventually, the complete removal of peritoneal tumours is often feasible in low-volume disease. However, in case of high-volume disease especially with disseminations on the small intestines and the mesentery, it may not be possible to perform complete R0 surgery in PDS.

## Neoadjuvant chemotherapy and interval debulking surgery

It might be reasonable to give chemotherapy first if PDS is anticipated to result in suboptimal outcomes even after maximal cytoreduction. Thus, neoadjuvant chemotherapy (NAC) followed by interval debulking surgery (IDS) was tried for patients with high-volume disease, and in many cases, optimal or complete cytoreduction was feasible in IDS. Then, prospective RCTs were conducted to compare PDS and NAC+IDS in patients with advanced ovarian cancer. Two early studies, EORTC and CHORUS, demonstrated NAC+IDS are not inferior to PDS in regard to PFS and OS of patients [175]. In addition, rate of severe postoperative complications and deaths is lower in NAC+IDS. Since then, NAC+IDS has received enthusiastic attention as an alternative standard treatment for advanced disease, but has also encountered many critiques [176]. Maximal effort for cytoreduction was poor in these RCTs, as operation time was too short and complete or optimal surgery rate in PDS group was very low. However, the third RCT of SCORPION demonstrated clearly that, under the maximal effort of cytoreduction in both arms, PFS and OS are equivalent between PDS and NAC+IDS, and that postoperative complication rate is significantly lower in NAC+IDS [177]. In this study, patients were ideally recruited using laparoscopic assessment of tumour burden. The fourth RCT in Japan, JCOG0602, also showed the superiority of NAC+IDS in terms of postoperative complication, although non-inferiority of NAC+IDS to PDS was not confirmed [178].

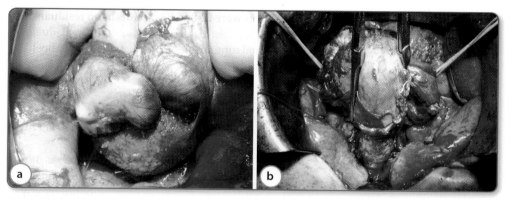

**Figure 17.46** En bloc resection in primary debulking surgery (PDS). (a) In patients with advanced ovarian cancer with peritoneal dissemination, (b) en bloc resection of the primary tumour with stripping of the peritoneum of lateral wall and vesicouterine fossa is performed.

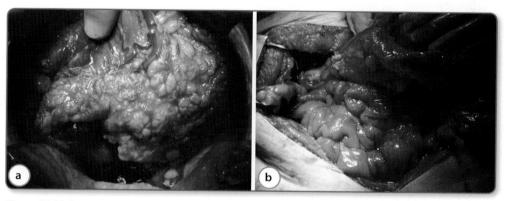

**Figure 17.47** Omentectomy in PDS. The greater omentum frequently show (a) 'omental cake', and in such case, (b) complete omentectomy is performed.

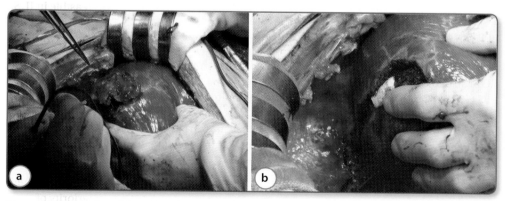

**Figure 17.48** Resection of disseminated tumour on the surface of liver. (A) Disseminations on the liver are resected using careful surgical techniques, followed by (B) appropriate haemostasis.

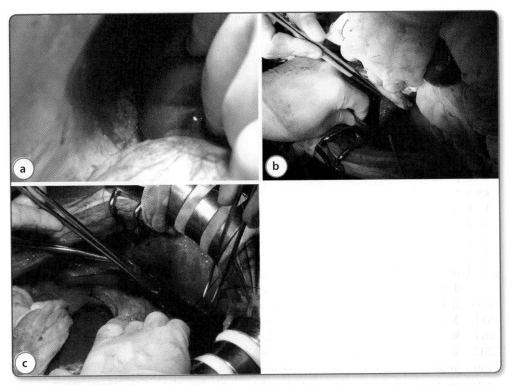

**Figure 17.49** Resection of disseminated tumour on the diaphragm. When the dissemination on (a) the diaphragm is present, (b) peritoneal stripping or resection of tumour with the diaphragm wall, (c) followed by the repair suture, is performed.

A systematic review and meta-analysis of 17 studies comprising 3,759 patients showed that, compared to NAC+IDS group, patients in PDS group were significantly more likely to have a grade ≥3 morbidity with an overall rate of 21.2% compared to 8.8% (95% CI 1.9–4.0; $p < 0.0001$), and were more likely to die within 30 days of surgery (OR 6.1; 95% CI 2.1–17.6; $p = 0.0008$) [179]. Although NAC+IDS was associated with significantly increased optimal and complete cytoreduction rates (OR 1.9; 95% CI 1.3–2.9; $p = 0.001$; and OR 2.2; 95% CI 1.5–3.3; $p = 0.0001$, respectively), NAC+IDS did not confer any additional survival benefit (OR 1.0; $p = 0.76$). A recent review and meta-analysis from Cochrane Database for RCTs also found little or no difference with regard to OS (HR 0.95; 95% CI 0.84–1.07) or PFS (HR 0.97; 95% CI 0.87–1.07) [180]. During or after these RCTs, the rate of NAC use for advanced ovarian cancer has dramatically increased from 8.6% to 22.6% between 2004 and 2013, and from 17.6% to 45.1% between 2006 and 2016 in the United States [181]. Such increase is also occurring in Japan, as the nationwide data on the primary treatment of advanced cancer showed double increase of NAC+IDS from 2002 to 2015. Thus, NAC+IDS has become a choice of treatment for patients with advanced ovarian cancer in the world.

A controversy about PDS versus NAC+IDS is the possible inferiority of NAC+IDS in the long-term survival of patients. A large-scale retrospective study using National Cancer Database in the United States from 2004 to 2015 showed that, comparing PDS ($n = 26,717$)

and NAC+IDS ($n$ = 9,885), the survival was significantly better in PDS group than NAC+IDS ($p < 0.001$). Patients who underwent PDS-R0 (no macroscopic residual tumour) showed the best median survival (62.6 months, 95% CI 60.5–64.5), and those with IDS-R1 (macroscopic residual tumour) showed the worst median survival (29.5 months, 95% CI 28.4–31.9). The survival curve of PDS-R1 overlaps that of IDS-R0 (median survival 38.9 vs. 41.8 months, respectively, HR 0.93; 95% CI 0.87–1.0) [182]. Other reports showed similar outcomes [183,184]. Although various causes for the difference in the survival between PDS and NAC+IDS groups have been considered, the most important point is that 'R0 in IDS' is essentially different from R0 in PDS. Actually, microscopic residual cancer cells are found in 25% of 'normal-appearing peritoneum' after NAC [185]. A prospective pathologic study on the presence of residual tumour after NAC in the sites having initially disseminated tumour > 1 cm in diameter revealed that the rate of occult cancer cells identified was 71.4% in the rectosigmoid colon, 70.3% in the transverse mesentery, 68.3% in the greater omentum, 61.9% in the right diaphragm, 61.1% in the paracolic gutters, and in 56.6% in the vesicouterine fossa [186]. Thus, cancer cells still remain under the normal-appearing peritoneum very frequently after NAC, and gynaecologic surgeons should consider the possibility of occult presence of tumour at IDS.

Another concern is that NAC may facilitate chemoresistance. A study on the response to re-treatment with platinum-based chemotherapy in patients who had undergone either PDS or NAC+IDS showed that platinum-resistance occurred in 55% after PDS and in 89% after NAC+IDS ($p < 0.001$) [187]. These findings may be consistent with the presence of CSC-like cells and the possible increase in stemness after NAC. Various causes, such as interruption of chemotherapy for IDS, unrecognised residual cancer cells at IDS, increased number of CSC-like cells, and NAC-induced gene alterations, may possibly contribute to the chemoresistance in patients treated with NAC+IDS [188]. The timing of IDS after NAC might be important for suppressing the chemoresistance of tumour cells, and we are awaiting the results of the on-going trial [189]. What can we do now? At present, we have to make an effort to perform 'true R0 surgery' i.e. maximal effort to resect all of the tumour including the occult ones, as much as we can.

In NCCN guidelines, therefore, NAC+IDS is not yet the standard treatment for advanced ovarian cancer, and is recommended for situations such as confirmed poor surgical candidate or low likelihood of optimal cytoreduction. The ideal treatment for patient is PDS resulting in no macroscopic residual disease. However, if severe postoperative complication occurs, patient survival will be compromised due to delay of adjuvant chemotherapy. The risk of death within 90 days is high after aggressive PDS for frail patients, and an appropriate triage is needed [190]. Therefore, NAC+IDS might be the best treatment for patients with high-risk complications or with high-volume tumour. Decision of either PDS or NAC should be determined by several factors such as tumour burden, tumour sites, and the capability of the group of surgeons, in addition to the condition of patient. Considering various methods for the prediction of completeness of surgery [188], it is reasonable to use laparoscopy for either PDS OR NAC. (**Figure 17.50**). Laparoscopic parameters proposed for the prediction of surgical outcome are stomach infiltration, diaphragmatic carcinomatosis, peritoneal carcinomatosis, omental caking, mesenteric retraction, bowel infiltration, and superficial liver metastases [191]. At the triaging laparoscopy, it is important to record the sites of disseminated nodules. Then, at IDS after NAC, it is essential to make an effort to perform 'true R0 surgery', which treats not only the macroscopic tumours but also 'normal-appearing peritoneum' having the occult cancer cells.

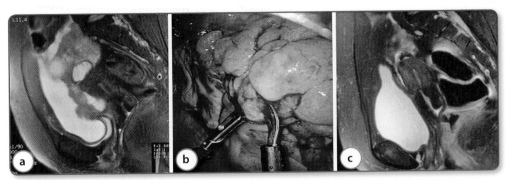

**Figure 17.50** Laparoscopy before neoadjuvant chemotherapy (NAC). (a) In advanced ovarian cancer with high-volume disease, laparoscopy is essential for identifying the location of peritoneal disseminations, and (b) for histopathologic confirmation of diagnosis with biopsy. In most cases, (c) NAC is very much effective and the interval-debulking surgery (IDS) is performed.

## Toward precision surgery: Imaging occult cancer cells

In the era of precision medicine, several strategies using new technologies have been conducted to achieve 'true R0 surgery'. The most promising one is the fluorescence image-guided surgery (FIGS). This technology has the capability to provide the surgeon with real-time feedback and may optimise the precision surgery. FIGS has been performed with untargeted dyes, such as indocyanine green (ICG) or with contrast agents targeting the specific molecule on the cancer cells. Since ICG has commonly been employed in the detection of sentinel lymph node of gynaecologic cancers, it seems reasonable to expand to cytoreductive surgery for peritoneal carcinomatosis. A recent systematic review on 71 patients including 26 ovarian cancer patients and 353 peritoneal nodules reported that sensitivity varied from 72.4% to 100%, specificity from 54.2% to 100% [192]. In case of advanced ovarian cancer, however, peritoneal scars after NAC had little affinity for ICG, and it may be difficult to identify occult cancer under the peritoneum using ICG only.

In this sense, the use of target molecule in FIGS has received enthusiastic attention. The putative targeted molecules are folate receptor alpha (FRα), HER2, CD24, and GnRH receptors [193]. Among them, FRα-targeting FIGS contrast agents have been improved to OTL38, which is a folate analogue conjugated to a NIR fluorescent dye, named as pafolacianine sodium, binding FRα in cancer cells [194]. Near-infrared fluorescent (NIRF) imaging was used to visualise target lesions, and 44 patients were evaluated for safety, and 225 lesions from 29 patients were evaluated for efficacy [195]. Sensitivity was 85.93% and PPV was 88.14%. In 48.3% (14/29) of patients, at least one additional lesion was detected by OTL38 alone. Recently, the same authors reported the results of a phase III randomised trial for OTL38 in 150 patients. In 33% of patients, NIRF imaging with OTL38 revealed additional lesions that had not been planned for resection and not identified by normal white light and palpation ($p < 0.001$). The tumour-found rate was 39.7% in patients who received IDS. R0 resection was obtained in 62.4% of patients [196]. Thus, NIRF imaging with OTL38 is very much promising for the detection of occult cancer cells even in IDS after NAC, and is expected to be commonly used in the era of precision medicine.

Another approach is photodynamic diagnosis (PDD) and therapy (PDT) modalities that use photosensitisers for fluorescence detection or photochemical treatment of cancer for peritoneal carcinomatosis [197]. In patients with ovarian cancer, PDD has been tried using a photosensitiser 5-aminolevulinic acid, reporting a sensitivity of 95% and specificity of 100% for peritoneal dissemination of ovarian cancer with accurate detection of micro-metastases [197]. However, chemotherapy prior to PDD increases the false positive detection rates due to inflammatory responses. For PDT, clinical trials were performed between 1990 and 2006, using intravenous porfimer sodium, a first-generation photosensitiser. However, there have been no new trial results published since 2012. This is due to a lack of tumour specificity of the photosensitiser, resulting in severe adverse events such as capillary leak syndrome characterised by fluid redistribution and hypovolemia, gastrointestinal perforation, and anastomotic leakages. Thus, targeted PDT and PDD have currently been under preclinical testing in order to increase the specificity [198].

## Systematic lymphadenectomy in PDS or IDS

The role of systematic lymphadenectomy in patients with advanced ovarian cancer has been controversial [164]. Early retrospective studies reported its benefit for better survival of patients. Two RCTs to compare systematic lymphadenectomy versus resection of bulky nodes only showed that systematic lymphadenectomy improved PFS but not OS in patients with optimally debulked disease, and a higher rate of lymph node metastasis in this group of patients [199,200]. Since the strongest prognostic factor in advanced ovarian cancer is the presence and size of residual tumour after cytoreductive surgery, systematic lymphadenectomy has not usually been performed in patients who had residual tumours in PDS. Controversial issue was whether lymphadenectomy should be done or not for patients who underwent R0 surgery. Strikingly, a recent RCT on 647 patients with advanced ovarian cancer (LION), to compare systematic lymphadenectomy ($n$ = 323) or no lymphadenectomy ($n$ = 324) in R0 surgery [199], clearly demonstrated that PFS and OS were similar in both groups, although positive nodes were detected in 55.7% of patients having lymphadenectomy. In addition, serious postoperative complication is higher in the lymphadenectomy group. Even in R0 surgery at IDS, systematic lymphadenectomy did not improve the survival and QOL of patients [201,202], except in one study from France [203].

Thus, patients with advanced ovarian cancer who underwent macroscopically complete resection do not benefit from systematic lymphadenectomy. As seen in the revision of FIGO staging, lymph node metastasis has decreased significantly in value as the prognostic factor for patients with advanced ovarian cancer. In conclusion, systematic lymphadenectomy is not indicated for patients with advanced ovarian cancer irrespective of the presence or absence of residual tumour after debulking surgery for the peritoneal cavity.

## Precision surgery for recurrent ovarian cancer

Initial multimodal treatment combined with cytoreductive surgery and taxane/platinum chemotherapy is effective in most patients with advanced ovarian cancer, leading to a period of disease remission. Afterwards, however, approximately half of the patients relapse within 2 years and >70% relapse within 5 years. The current treatment guidelines are as follows. Since recurrence usually means incurable disease, the goal of treatment for recurrence is not the cure of disease but the prolongation of survival and/or improvement of QOL, including the relief of cancer-related symptoms. However, as physicians, we have to consider first the possibility of cure because the recurrent condition is extremely varied among patients. Therefore, the treatment for recurrence should be individualised according to the condition of patient and the nature of recurrent tumour, such as histological type, location sites, number, and biological characteristics. In this sense, secondary debulking surgery (SDS) for recurrent ovarian cancer is a possible choice of treatment.

In order to eradicate CSC-like cells of ovarian cancer, surgery is the only tool for treatment. Therefore, the possibility of surgical approach should always be considered first in both primary and recurrent settings. If the recurrent tumour is localised in the lymph nodes, retroperitoneal space, or in the pelvic peritoneum, the possibility of its complete extirpation as well as cure of disease is highly expected. In our experience at Kyoto University Hospital from 2000 to 2015, among a total of 142 patients with recurrent ovarian cancer from all stages, the survival of the selected 38 patients who could fortunately undergo the secondary surgery was significantly better than that in the remaining 104 patients who received chemotherapy only (median OS 134.6 vs. 43.3 months; $p < 0.0001$). Generally, however, if the recurrent tumours are distributed in various sites of whole peritoneal cavity or when the tumour progression is rapid, complete extirpation is difficult, and the prognosis of such patients is very poor. Thus, physicians usually hesitate to do surgery in the recurrent setting. Recently, however, SDS for platinum-sensitive recurrence has been under strong debate and its significance is controversial.

The first RCT for SDS (GOG 213) in women with platinum-sensitive recurrent ovarian cancer was conducted from 2007 to 2011 [204]. A total of 485 patients underwent randomisation, 240 to secondary cytoreduction before chemotherapy and 245 to chemotherapy alone. R0 surgery was achieved in 67% of the patients in the surgery group. Platinum-based chemotherapy with bevacizumab followed by bevacizumab maintenance was administered to 84% of the patients overall and was equally distributed between the two groups. Median PFS was longer in the surgery group than in the no-surgery group, although the difference was not significant. It was striking that HR for death in the surgery versus the no-surgery group was 1.29 (95% CI 0.97–1.72; $p = 0.08$), which corresponded to a median OS of 50.6 months and 64.7 months, respectively. In contrast, the results of AGO DESKTOP III/ENGOT trial showed distinct results favouring SDS at the ASCO Annual Meeting 2017 [205]. In this study, patients were eligible only if they cleared AGO-score for prediction of complete cytoreduction i.e. good performance status, <500 mL of ascites, and complete cytoreduction at the primary surgery [206]. Platinum-sensitive 407 patients were randomised to either chemotherapy alone or surgery plus chemotherapy, being performed in the period before the use of bevacizumab. Median PFS was 14 months in the chemotherapy alone and 19.6 months in the surgery plus chemotherapy (HR 0.66; 95% CI 0.52–0.83; $p < 0.001$). Since the prognosis of patients for the surgery group who could not undergo R0 surgery was poorer than those who received chemotherapy alone, the prediction of complete surgery such as using AGO-score is essential in clinical practice.

Another criterion for the prediction of R0 surgery in SDS is the Tian model (**Table 17.1**) [207]. In a retrospective analysis on 52 platinum-sensitive, recurrent patients between 2004 and 2016, being classified as low-risk in Tian model as complete resection anticipated, 22 of the 52 underwent SDS whereas the remaining 30 received chemotherapy alone [208]. The rate of complete resection of SDS was 73% (16/22). The SDS group had significantly longer PFS (HR 0.45; 95% CI 0.22–0.91; $p = 0.027$) and OS (HR 0.28; 95% CI 0.11–0.72; $p = 0.008$) than the chemotherapy group. A recent meta-analysis of the three RCTs ($n = 1,250$) reported that SDS is associated with significantly better PFS improvement than systemic therapy alone (95% CI 0.61–0.78; $p < 0.001$), and the benefit was greater for R0 surgery subpopulation (HR 0.56; 95% CI 0.48–0.66; $p < 0.001$) [209]. Accordingly, in case of platinum-sensitive recurrence, SDS is one of the important strategies for better survival of patients, but complete R0 surgery should be guaranteed. Selection of truly

**Table 17.1 Tian's risk model for secondary cytoreductive surgery**

| Impact factor | Scoring* | | | | | |
|---|---|---|---|---|---|---|
| | 0 | 0.8 | 1.5 | 1.8 | 2.4 | 3.0 |
| FIGO stage | I/II | III/IV | | | | |
| Residual disease at primary surgery | No | | Yes | | | |
| DFI (mo) | ≥16 | | | | <16 | |
| PS at recurrence | 0–1 | | | | 2–3 | |
| CA125 at recurrence | ≤105 | | | >105 | | |
| Ascites at recurrence | Absent | | | | | Present |

*≤4.7 is categorised as low-risk and >4.7 as high-risk.
CA125, cancer antigen 125; DFI, disease-free interval; FIGO, International Federation of Gynaecology and Obstetrics;
PS, performance status

suitable patients for surgery is an essential requirement [210]. To do so, AGO-score or Tian model is a beneficial tool for the prediction of its feasibility. In the era of precision surgery, SDS should be considered as an important tool for eradicating CSC-like cells and better survival of the patient.

# CYTOTOXIC CHEMOTHERAPY

In the modern management of ovarian cancer, cytotoxic chemotherapy has been playing an indispensable role to improve the survival and QOL in patients especially with advanced stage of disease. Appropriate combination of surgery and the standard taxane/platinum chemotherapy still occupies the central part in the treatment of ovarian cancer [3]. Recently, however, epoch-making development of molecular targeted drugs such as anti-VEGF antibody and PARP inhibitors has opened new avenues of treatment for ovarian cancer patients [105], and currently, these drugs are also included in the standard treatment in combination with the cytotoxic chemotherapy [3,7]. The current status of such drugs is described in the section on 'TARGETED THERAPIES'.

The important milestone in development of cytotoxic chemotherapy was the introduction of cisplatin in 1976, and since then, platinum-based chemotherapy has been the mainstay in the treatment for ovarian cancer. Since paclitaxel was introduced in 1993, the combination double chemotherapy with taxane and platinum was developed [211]. Through international RCTs, intravenous administration of paclitaxel and carboplatin (TC) every 3 weeks for six cycles has been the gold standard, for more than two decades both in adjuvant and neoadjuvant settings [212]. In case of intolerance to paclitaxel, another taxane docetaxel has been used. The combination of paclitaxel and carboplatin appears to play complementary roles to cover most ovarian cancer patients, since the expression signature patterns of cancer for the sensitivity to each drug are completely different to each other [213].

## Chemotherapy for early ovarian cancer

For early stage diseases, the need for adjuvant chemotherapy has been the issue of strong debate. Several prospective studies demonstrated that the prognosis of patients with stage IA or IB, histologically grade 1 or 2, ovarian cancer who underwent accurate surgical staging was extremely favourable without adjuvant chemotherapy [214,215]. In 2003, however, two RCTs, ACTION and ICON1, which compared the adjuvant chemotherapy versus observation in patients with early ovarian cancer, reported that adjuvant chemotherapy significantly improved both RFS and OS, although the improvement was not significant in optimally staged patients [216,217]. A meta-analysis including five RCTs involving 1,277 women with early stage diseases indicated better PFS and OS in women who underwent adjuvant platinum-based chemotherapy than those who did not [218]. Especially, women who were suboptimally staged or had high-risk disease received the greatest benefit from adjuvant chemotherapy. On the other hand, its benefit for women who underwent optimal staging and had low-risk disease remains uncertain. Accordingly, it has been generally accepted that adjuvant chemotherapy can be omitted in patients with stage IA or IB, grade 1 tumours, who underwent complete surgical staging [211].

## Chemotherapy for advanced ovarian cancer

More than 50% of patients with epithelial ovarian cancer present with advanced diseases of either stage III or IV. Since the most important factor for poor prognosis of epithelial ovarian cancer is peritoneal dissemination, all of the treatment modalities have been focussing on the control of peritoneal disease. Although >80% of patients respond well to first-line standard chemotherapy with intravenous TC regimen every 3 weeks for six cycles, approximately 70% of patients experience recurrence. Therefore, additional treatments to TC have enthusiastically been tried, but the third cytotoxic drug such as gemcitabine, liposomal doxorubicin, or topotecan, in addition to TC, could not improve the survival of patients. Currently, however, instead of cytotoxic drug, targeted drugs such as anti-VEGF antibody and PARP inhibitors have been incorporated mainly as the maintenance therapy combined with platinum-based chemotherapy [3,7].

With regard to the possible modification of TC regimen, dose-dense TC treatment has received much attention. In 2013, JGOG3016 study reported that dose-dense TC significantly improved both PFS and OS of advanced ovarian cancer patients [56]. In dose-dense TC regimen, carboplatin AUC 6 was given in the same way as the conventional regimen. However, paclitaxel 80 mg/m$^2$ is given weekly on days 1, 8, and 15, in contrast to 180 mg/m$^2$ on day 1 in the conventional one. Thus, the total dose of paclitaxel is increased. Of the 631 patients, 312 underwent dose-dense regimen, whereas 319 underwent conventional regimen. Median follow-up was 76.8 months. Median PFS was significantly longer 28.2 months in the dose-dense group than 17.5 months in the conventional group (HR 0.76; 95% CI 0.62–0.91; $p = 0.0037$). Median OS was 100.5 months versus 62.2 months, respectively (HR 0.79; 95% CI 0.63–0.99; $p = 0.039$). This report has given a striking influence to the standard TC regimen, but subsequent trials of both GOG262 and ICON8 with concurrent use of bevacizumab did not replicate the benefits of dose-dense TC [219,220]. This may be due to the additional use of bevacizumab or ethnic differences [221].

## Intraperitoneal chemotherapy

Another important issue of controversy is intraperitoneal chemotherapy (IP). Theoretically, intravenous administration is suitable for the treatment of peritoneal dissemination of ovarian cancer, since prolonged exposure to higher local concentrations of the drugs is achieved by IP for the tumours on the peritoneal surface. Early three RCTs using intraperitoneal administration of cisplatin showed the survival benefit for optimally debulked patients with stage III ovarian cancer [222]. In 2006, the NCI of the United States issued a clinical alert supporting the use of IP chemotherapy. However, IP may show higher toxicity, and is sometimes associated with complications with an implanted subcutaneous port and catheter system. Successful implementation of IP requires education and experience for development as standard of care. Thus, a less toxic, more feasible outpatient regimen was needed, and trials of IP administration of carboplatin have been conducted. Although OV21 study showed some improvement in PD rate at 9 months, 24.5% in IP arm versus 38.6% in control ($p = 0.065$), this study did not proceed to phase III study [223]. In a large-scale RCT (GOG252), a total of 1,560 patients were randomised to either IV carboplatin, or IP carboplatin, or IP cisplatin, in combination with paclitaxel [224]. All participants received bevacizumab, and median follow-up was 84.8 months. Median PFS was 24.9 months in IV carboplatin, 27.4 months in IP carboplatin, and 26.2 months in IP cisplatin. Median OS was 75.5, 78.9, and 72.9 months, respectively. There were no statistical differences in both PFS and OS between the IV regimen and either of the IP regimens. Thus, in the new era of bevacizumab use, the benefit of IP seems to have disappeared, and at present, one RCT for IP carboplatin is awaiting survival data. Recent attention has moved to the combination of IP with hyperthermic therapy.

## Hyperthermic intraperitoneal chemotherapy

Since the prognosis of patients with various cancers having peritoneal dissemination is generally poor, hyperthermic therapy has been tried for colon, gastric, and ovarian cancers. The rationale of hyperthermic intraperitoneal chemotherapy (HIPEC) is to eradicate all microscopic disease with higher local concentrations of cytotoxic drugs further potentiated with heat. Application of HIPEC to ovarian cancer may be advantageous, because HIPEC is a single treatment delivered at the time of cytoreductive surgery. Technologies for performing HIPEC have been described in details [225]. Following complete cytoreductive surgery, HIPEC is usually performed using an open platform. After the tentative closing of skin, the abdomen is warmed with hyperthermic saline to 42–43°C. Once the target temperature is reached, chemotherapy is infused into the circuit and perfused for 30–90 minutes with simultaneous vigorous manual agitation of abdomen. After perfusion is completed, the heated chemotherapy solution is drained, an additional wash is performed, and the final reconstruction is performed or ostomies constructed.

Since 2005, several case series and case-control studies established the feasibility and safety of HIPEC in ovarian cancer patients. In 2018, a striking report appeared [226]. A multicentre phase III RCT, analysing 245 patients with poor prognosis stage III ovarian cancer patients who underwent NAC, demonstrated that the IDS plus HIPEC had advantage in both PFS and OS. After a median follow-up of 4.7 years, median PFS was 10.7 in IDS without HIPEC and 14.2 months in IDS plus HIPEC (HR 0.66; 95% CI 0.50–0.87; $p = 0.003$). Median OS was 33.9 and 45.7 months, respectively (HR 0.67; 95% CI 0.48–0.94; $p = 0.02$). The adverse events are abdominal pain, infection, ileus, and thromboembolic events, but the incidence was not significantly increased in HIPEC [227]. Currently, HIPEC has also been applied to patients with recurrent ovarian cancer [228]. Thus, HIPEC has received enthusiastic attention as a promising strategy to obtain better survival in patients with advanced or recurrent ovarian cancer. The standardisation for giving HIPEC safely for patients with ovarian cancer is mandatory. Although it is possible that CSC-like cells with their niche in the peritoneal dissemination may also be resistant to hyperthermia, a recent study with in vivo mouse model reported a promising effect of HIPEC on ovarian CSC-like cells [229].

## Chemotherapy for recurrent ovarian cancer

There have been excellent advancements in the treatment for patients with recurrent ovarian cancer i.e. reconsideration and challenge for SDS, choice of chemotherapeutic regimen depending on the platinum-free interval (PFI), development of novel targeted drugs such as anti-VEGF antibody and PARP inhibitors, whole-genome sequencing for the search of matched drug, as well as the improvement of best supportive care [230,231]. Thus, the treatment of choice for recurrence is essential for the survival and better QOL of patients. SDS is indicated in selected patients who could undergo complete R0 surgery. In the modern era of novel developments of targeted drugs, however, most patients tend to have systemic therapy with the combination of cytotoxic and targeted drugs. Historically, recurrence has been classified into three categories according to chemosensitivity [230,231]. Effectiveness of the second-line therapy depends on the time period of PFS between the completion of the first-line therapy and the occurrence of recurrent tumour, and currently PFI is the most reliable predictor. Thus, recurrence with PFI under 6 months is designated as 'platinum-resistant', PFI within 6–12 months as 'partially platinum-sensitive', and PFI over 12 months as 'fully platinum-sensitive'.

The current standard regimen for platinum-sensitive recurrence is the carboplatin-containing combination, such as carboplatin with either paclitaxel, pegylated liposomal doxorubicin (PLD), gemcitabine, or topoisomerase inhibitors such as topotecan and irinotecan, since such combination has shown better results than carboplatin alone. Thus, one of the above combinations has been selected most frequently for platinum-sensitive recurrence. Recently, however, bevacizumab has been added to the doublet chemotherapy, since significant improvement of PFS was shown in patients with platinum-sensitive recurrence [232]. Other important drugs are PARP inhibitors which have drastically improved PFS of patients with platinum-sensitive recurrence. The use of PARP inhibitors was first approved as monotherapy for maintenance after platinum-based chemotherapy only in patients with BRCA-mutation [233], but soon expanded to all patients with platinum-sensitive recurrence [234]. Considering the clinical evidence, sequencing the treatment with platinum-based chemotherapy, PARP inhibitor, and bevacizumab would be scheduled for platinum-sensitive recurrence [235].

Patients with platinum-resistant disease had been considered as incurable, and the aim of treatment was believed to be only palliation. In clinical practice, patients usually receive non-platinum single-agent chemotherapy, which shows some activity and lower toxicity than combination chemotherapy [230]. Recently, however, the benefit of addition of bevacizumab to single-agent chemotherapy has been demonstrated in patients with platinum-resistant recurrence [236]. Use of a PARP inhibitor may also be considered, although most patients with platinum-resistant recurrence are HRD-negative [234]. Efficacy of the immune checkpoint inhibitors is so far limited [237], however, our trial with nivolumab showed the dual response in 2 of the 20 patients [145]. Targeted drugs against driver oncogene might be indicated in type I ovarian cancers [66]. In the era of precision medicine, therefore, physicians should search for new strategies for the improvement of survival, for the maintenance of QOL and an excellent end-of-life care [238]. Indication and the use of novel targeted drugs for patients with recurrent ovarian cancer will be discussed in the following section.

# TARGETED THERAPIES

The drugs targeting the signalling pathways of cancer cells are classified into two categories. One is the monoclonal antibody that does not penetrate the cell membranes but binds with the ligands and receptors of the specific growth factors. Another is the low molecular organic compound that can enter the cytoplasm and act on targets such as tyrosine kinases and DNA repair machineries [105]. In the 21st century, there have been dramatic developments in ovarian cancer treatment targeting various intercellular and intracellular signalling pathways, especially anti-angiogenesis, anti-DVA repair, and anti-immune evasion in cancer cells.

## Anti-angiogenesis therapies

Angiogenesis, the formation of new blood and lymphatic vessels from existing vasculature, is a crucial process involved in solid tumour growth and progression. VEGF secreted from the cancer cells plays a central role in angiogenic signals, stimulating endothelial cell migration, endothelial cell proliferation, and microvessel formation. Anti-VEGF antibody, bevacizumab, is a recombinant humanised monoclonal IgG antibody that binds to circulating VEGF and prevents it from binding to its receptors. Bevacizumab was expected to be effective in ovarian cancer, since VEGF plays a central role in the peritoneal dissemination and angiogenesis [104]. Adverse events are hypertension, proteinuria, and serious gastrointestinal toxicities such as perforation and fistula.

The two phase III trials, GOG218, and ICON7, for newly diagnosed advanced or high-risk ovarian cancer demonstrated that TC chemotherapy plus bevacizumab and maintenance with bevacizumab showed a significantly longer PFS for 2–4 months, but not in OS [239,240]. Strikingly, in the final analysis of ICON7, benefit of bevacizumab was seen in patients with higher risk of recurrence (stage III with $\geq$ 2 cm residual disease and stage IV), as median OS was 39.7 months versus 30.2 months (HR 0.78; 95% CI 0.63–0.97) [241]. Also in the final analysis of GOG 218, median OS in stage IV patients was 42.8 months in bevacizumab versus 32.6 months in placebo (HR 0.75; 95% CI 0.59–0.95) [242]. For the patients with recurrence, both of the phase III trials, OCEANS and AURELIA, also showed significant improvement in PFS, but not in OS, in the chemotherapy plus bevacizumab group. In the OCEANS for platinum-sensitive recurrence, median PFS was 12.4 months in the bevacizumab versus 8.4 months in the control (HR 0.484; 95% CI 0.388–0.605; $p < 0.0001$) and ORR was 78.5% versus 57.4%, respectively ($p < 0.0001$) [232]. In the AURELIA for platinum-resistant recurrence, median PFS was 6.7 months with bevacizumab versus 3.4 months without (HR 0.48; 95% CI 0.38–0.60; $p < 0.001$), and ORR was 27.3% versus 11.8%, respectively ($p = 0001$) [236]. Following these studies, bevacizumab is commonly employed as a standard of care in both primary and recurrent settings.

In the era of precision medicine, predictive biomarkers for the sensitivity to bevacizumab have been under exploration. In GOG218 study, BRCA1/2 and other HRD mutations were not predictive of bevacizumab activity. Among molecular subtypes of HGSC, addition of bevacizumab is significantly more effective in 'proliferative' followed by 'mesenchymal' subtypes [58]. Sub-analysis of ICON7 comparing serum samples between five responders and five non-responders to bevacizumab, followed by validation in independent cohort of 115 patients, showed that candidate biomarkers are mesothelin, fms-like tyrosine kinase-4 (FLT4), and α1-acid glycoprotein (AGP). A combination of the three markers with CA125 may be useful for the prediction of response to bevacizumab [243].

As antiangiogenic drugs, multi-kinase inhibitors that inhibit various tyrosine kinase signallings including VEGF pathway, such as pazopanib, nintedanib, and cediranib, have been tried in ovarian cancer patients. Trials with pazopanib and nintedanib showed an improvement in median PFS; for pazopanib benefit of 5.6 months (HR 0.77; 95% CI 0.64–0.91; $p = 0.0021$) and for nintedanib 1.4 months (HR 0.84; 95% CI 0.72–0.98; $p = 0.024$), respectively [244,245]. HR for PFS in these studies was similar to that of bevacizumab. However, final analysis of both trials did not show the benefit of OS [246,247], and none of the oral tyrosine kinase inhibitors has been submitted for licensing for ovarian cancer treatment. Cediranib is an oral VEGF receptor and c-Kit inhibitor having anti-tumour activity in various recurrent cancers, and has been shown to be effective in platinum-sensitive recurrence in ICON6 trial. After a median follow-up of 25.6 months, strong evidence of an effect of concurrent plus maintenance cediranib on PFS was observed (HR 0.56; 95% CI 0.44–0.72; $p < 0.0001$). In this final survival analysis, there was a 7.4 months difference but not significant in median survival (HR 0.86; 95% CI 0.67–1.11; $p = 0.24$) [248]. Recently, the possibility of synergy combining cediranib with PARP inhibitor has received attention, and the clinical trial ICON9 is ongoing.

## Poly-(ADP-ribose) polymerase inhibitors

PARP inhibitor maintenance therapy is the latest breakthrough in the management of not only recurrent ovarian cancer but also newly diagnosed advanced cancer. PARP is a key enzyme involved in the repair of single-strand DNA breaks, which is the major complementary DNA repair pathway in cancer cells with HRD. PARP inhibitors block this back-up pathway, thereby leading to cell death referred as 'synthetic lethality' [249]. Since HRD exists in approximately 50% of HGSC due to BRCA germline mutation, BRCA somatic mutation, BRCA methylation, and epigenetic loss of other factors in the HR pathway, many patients with advanced ovarian cancer mainly of HGSC are sensitive to PARP inhibitors. For the prediction of sensitivity to PARP inhibitors, functional HRD status is examined using the companion diagnostics such as Myriad MyChoice test, in addition to the genetic analysis for BRCA mutations. If the companion test is positive, the tumours are designated as 'HRD-positive', and otherwise 'HRD-negative'.

From 2012 to 2017, trials evaluating PARP inhibitors, such as olaparib, niraparib, and rucaparib, showed a dramatic benefit for survival in patients with platinum-sensitive recurrent ovarian cancer [233,250–252]. In 2018, the results of SOLO-1 trial for newly diagnosed advanced ovarian cancer led to approval of olaparib as the first-line maintenance therapy in patients with germline BRCA1/2 mutation, establishing a new standard of care [253]. In 2019, the three phase III trials, evaluating the first-line use of PARP inhibitors beyond BRCA1/2 mutations, showed a significant improvement of PFS; in PRIMA trial for niraparib, in PAOLA-1 for olaparib plus bevacizumab, and in VELIA for veliparib with concurrent chemotherapy and maintenance [254–256]. These results led to the recent approval of maintenance niraparib irrespective of biomarker status, and olaparib in combination with bevacizumab in HRD-positive advanced ovarian cancer [257]. Thus, PARP inhibitors have been incorporated as the standard first-line treatment for advanced ovarian cancer. Benefit from PARP inhibitors is strongest in women with HRD-positive/BRCA-mutated, modest in those who had HRD-positive/BRCA-wild-type, but the least in those with HRD-negative tumours. Thus, the assessment of HRD status of cancer is essential for the prediction of efficacy. Physicians are asked by the patient, 'what is the best option of treatment for me?' To answer the question, we have to know the HRD status of tumour in the patient, either BRCA-mutated, HRD-positive, or HRD-negative, using the molecular tests for predictive biomarkers [258].

Recent recommendations on the use of PARP inhibitors for newly diagnosed advanced ovarian cancer have been proposed in ESMO Open-Cancer Horizons round table discussions [259]. In patients with BRCA-mutated tumours, based on the data of improvement of PFS, the incorporation of PARP inhibitor switch maintenance in the first-line setting should be the standard of care for all patients with BRCA1/2 mutation-associated newly diagnosed advanced ovarian cancer. In patients with HRD-positive tumours, there is a significant and clinically meaningful benefit of adding PARP inhibitor maintenance therapy, alone or in combination with bevacizumab, following response to platinum-based chemotherapy. Molecular tests for HRD are better guides for the use of PARP inhibitors. With regard to the duration of therapy, after the first-line platinum-based chemotherapy, PARP inhibitors should be maintained for at least 2 years for olaparib and 3 years for niraparib to cover the period of maximum risk of recurrence.

Controversial issue is the indication of PARP inhibitors for patients with HRD-negative tumours. Patients with HR-negative cancer have the worst prognosis, and the results for this group were different among the three RCTs of first-line PARP inhibitors [254–256]. The PRIMA trial reported a statistically significant improvement in PFS with niraparib versus placebo (HR 0.68; 95% CI 0.49–0.94) in the HRD-negative subgroup. Median PFS was relatively short as 8.1 months versus 5.4 months, respectively, which could be explained by the high-risk population [254]. The PAOLA-1 trial did not show any benefit of adding olaparib to bevacizumab compared with bevacizumab alone in the HRD-negative subgroup (HR 1.00; 95% CI 0.75–1.35). Median PFS was 16.6 months versus 16.2 months, respectively [255]. In the VELIA trial, there was no significant improvement in PFS (HR 0.81; 95% CI 0.6–1.09), with a median PFS of 15.0 months in veliparib versus 11.5 months in control [256]. In summary, only niraparib can be considered as the maintenance therapy options in patients with HRD-negative cancer. Patients with histological subtypes other than HGSC should not routinely be considered for PARP inhibitor maintenance therapy. Decisions will be individualised, considering the licensed indication and HRD testing.

Common adverse events include anaemia, fatigue, and nausea. Drug-specific ones are thrombocytopenia and hypertension for niraparib. Such adverse events could be usually managed with dose reductions and interruptions, while definitive discontinuations should be reserved for severe situations. Studies have focused on the development of acute myeloid leucemia (AML) or myelodysplastic syndrome (MDS), the incidence of which have been reported as <2% in the first-line and 8% in the second-line use of the drug. Thus, appropriate counselling and surveillance are needed. Patients deemed to be at potential risk or with a history of hematological disease of AML or MDS should not receive PARP inhibitors [259].

There are several resistance mechanisms to PARP inhibitors, such as the phenomenon of secondary reverse mutations in BRCA gene during recurrence leading to loss of HRD. The unmet need is the treatment for the patients with HRD-negative ovarian cancers which are deemed also to be chemoresistant. Therefore, there is emergence of several trials investigating the role of adding other agents such as immune checkpoint inhibitors, as combination therapy with PARP inhibitors in order to either modify the HRD status or the tumour immune microenvironment.

## Novel Immunotherapy

Historically, various kinds of immunotherapy have been tried for patients with ovarian cancer, and most of them were not successful [260]. Tumour-specific antigens have been considered as the promising targets of novel immunotherapy using monoclonal antibody or antibody-drug conjugate [261]. CA125 (MU16) is the most common tumour marker of ovarian cancer, and a RCT with anti-CA125 mouse monoclonal antibody, oregovomab, was conducted as consolidation treatment in patients with advanced cancer, resulting in no significant improvement in the time to relapse [262]. A recent MIMOSA trial with murine monoclonal anti-idiotypic antibody that functionally imitates CA-125, abagovomab, as maintenance therapy, did not prolong PFS and OS in patients with advanced cancer [263].

Folate receptor alpha has been reportedly overexpressed in 80–90% of ovarian cancer, but is only minimally expressed in normal tissues, suggesting FRα as a promising target. FRα expression induces drug resistance by enhancing the antiapoptotic capacity of tumour cells. Recent trial with anti-FRα monoclonal antibody, farletuzumab, in combination with taxane/platinum chemotherapy, did not show the survival benefit in platinum-sensitive recurrent patients. However, mirvetuximab soravtansine (MIRV) under clinical trial is interesting. This is an antibody-drug conjugate comprising a FRα-binding antibody, cleavable linker, and the maytansinoid DM4, a potent tubulin-targeting agent. A phase III study FORWARD I comparing MIRV and PCC in patients with platinum-resistant ovarian cancer was conducted in a total of 366 patients [264]. Although the benefit of PFS did not reach statistical significance, all secondary end-points showed the superior outcomes of MIRV in FRα-high population, such as improved ORR (24% vs. 10%) and CA125 responses (53% vs. 25%). In a report presented at ASCO Annual Meeting 2021, treatment with MIRV in combination with bevacizumab resulted in the ORR of 47% and median duration of response of 9.7 months, suggesting a promising role of MIRV in recurrent ovarian cancer.

In 2018, Tasuku Honjo and James P Allison received the Nobel Prize in Physiology or Medicine for their discoveries of immune checkpoint molecules, such as PD-1 and CTLA-4, respectively. These molecules play pivotal roles in the 'escape from the host immune' mechanisms in cancer [265]. Cancer cells frequently express either PD-L1 or CTLA-4, reduce the immune attack by host T cells, and therefore, immunotherapy using anti-PD-1, PD-L1, and CTLA-4 antibody is a novel targeted therapy against the immune checkpoint signals. Currently, treatment with such drugs has been incorporated in the standard treatment of various cancers [260,265]. This is the paradigm shift of the 21st century in cancer therapy, since the effect of these drugs is durable, and if response is obtained, patients with advanced cancer will have unprecedented long-term survival [260,266].

In 2010, we conducted the first clinical trial using anti-PD-1 antibody, nivolumab, in a total of 20 patents with platinum-resistant, recurrent ovarian cancer [145]. The ORR was 15% with CR 2 and PR 1, and DCR was 45% with SD six patients. Interestingly, the response was durable, as two patients with CR showed no evidence of disease 5 years after the treatment. Trial of KEYNOTE-028 with another PD-1 antibody, pembrolizumab, included 26 patients with recurrent ovarian cancer, and showed ORR of 11.5% with one CR and two PR patients. The duration of response was >6 months [267]. Treatment with anti-PD-L1 antibody, avelumab, was found to be associated with ORR of 9.6% among 125 patients with platinum-resistant patients [268]. Another PD-L1 antibody, atezolizumab, also demonstrated a response in 2 of the 8 heavily pretreated patients [269]. The largest trial as monotherapy for ovarian cancer is the KEYNOTE-100 trial [270], in which 376 patients with recurrent ovarian cancer were treated with pembrolizumab every 3 weeks, showed ORR to be <10% and median PFS 2.1 months. In summary for recurrent ovarian cancer, unfortunately, the efficacy of immune checkpoint inhibitors as monotherapy is limited, although the effect is durable when the response is obtained. In current clinical practice, only pembrolizumab can be used for patients with recurrent ovarian cancer, if the tumour is shown to be MSI-high by the companion diagnostics. Considerable number of patients with endometriosis-related ovarian cancer such as OEC and OCCC show positivity for MSI. Thus, the indication of pembrolizumab should be searched for in patients with recurrent ovarian cancer.

Regarding the possibility of dual block, a phase II trial of nivolumab alone versus nivolumab plus anti-CTLA-4 antibody, ipilimumab, was tried in a total of 100 patients with recurrent ovarian cancer [271]. ORR was 12.2% in nivolumab versus 31.4% in nivolumab plus ipilimumab (OR 3.28; $p = 0.034$), but the toxicity increased in the combination. Accumulating evidence suggests that the key factor for the response to immune checkpoint inhibitors is high tumour mutational burden (TMB) or MSI-high, as well as the gene expression profile (GEP) for T-cell-inflamed microenvironment. Most patients with HGSC show low TMB and low GEP, and might be responsible for the resistance to immune checkpoint inhibitors. As it is hypothesised that chemotherapy promotes antigen release and enhances tumour-specific T-cell activation, combination of immune checkpoint inhibitors with chemotherapy has been tried. In JAVELIN 200 trial, 566 patients with platinum-resistant recurrent patients were randomised to either avelumab alone, avelumab plus PLD, or PLD alone. However, addition of avelumab did not significantly prolong either PFS or OS [272].

Combination of immune checkpoint inhibitors with antiangiogenic drugs has also been under clinical trials. In a phase II trial with nivolumab plus bevacizumab on 38 patients with recurrent ovarian cancer [273], the ORR was 40.0% (95% CI 19.1–64.0%) in platinum-sensitive, and 16.7% (95% CI 3.6–41.4%) in platinum-resistant participants. Median PFS was 8.1 months (95% CI 6.3–14.7). For newly diagnosed advanced ovarian cancer patients, the IMagyn050/GOG 3015/ENGOT OV-39/trial was conducted from 2017 to 2019 [274]. A total of 1,301 patients with FIGO stage III or IV who had either PDS with macroscopic residual disease or NAC+IDS, and received standard TC chemotherapy and bevacizumab followed by maintenance bevacizumab, were randomised to either atezolizumab or placebo given during chemotherapy and in the maintenance phase. The median PFS for atezolizumab and placebo was 19.5 months versus 18.4 months, respectively (HR 0.92; 95% CI 0.79–1.07; $p = 0.28$). In the PD-L1-positive population, 20.8 months versus 18.5 months (HR 0.80; 95% CI 0.65–0.99; $p = 0.038$). The current evidence does not support the universal use of immune checkpoint inhibitors in newly diagnosed ovarian cancer.

Thus, although various trials with immune checkpoint inhibitors as monotherapy or combination with chemotherapy have enthusiastically been conducted for ovarian cancer patients, they have not yet demonstrated a significant benefit for survival. Nevertheless, long-term responders have been observed in all the trials, indicating that better biomarkers for patient selection are needed. Gene signatures predicting the response to nivolumab have recently been reported [89]. More importantly, we need a strategy to convert cold tumours into inflamed ones responding to anti-PD-1/ PD-L1 therapy. Thus, attention is focused now on the possibility of combination of immune checkpoint inhibitors with PARP inhibitors. In a single-arm phases I and II trial (TOPACIO/KEYNOTE-162) for combination of pembrolizumab with niraparib in a total of 62 patients with platinum-resistant recurrent ovarian cancer, ORR was 18% (90% CI 11–29%), with a DCR of 65% (90% CI 54–75%), including 3 CR, 8 PR, and 28 SD [275]. Currently, there are four international, on-going RCTs involving >5,000 patients with newly diagnosed advanced ovarian cancer, investigating the combination of PD-1/PD-L1 inhibitors with PARP inhibitors.

## NEXT-GENERATION SEQUENCING AND MATCHED THERAPY

In the era of precision medicine, personalised therapy for each patient is the attractive challenge, with a great impact on the management of ovarian cancer [4,105]. Every day, physicians are faced with the patient with recurrent ovarian cancer who is enthusiastically seeking a better treatment, and therefore, physicians have to discuss the currently accumulated evidence including the genomic features of recurrent cancer using NGS for possible alternative treatment specialised to the patient. Genome profiling for the formalin-fixed, paraffin-embedded tumour tissues, using the NGS panel, such as FoundationOne CDx, NCC Oncopanel, Ion AmpliSeq Cancer Hotspot Panel, PleSSision-160 Panel, TruSight Tumour 170 Panel, or others, followed by the tumour boards by specialists, has been available now in the central and local cancer centres in many countries. Continuous development and cost reduction of NGS technologies enhance the chance of its application for various cancers. At present, the discovery rate of matched therapy is relatively low in ovarian cancers, due to lack of strong driver gene in the type II ovarian cancers. In case of type I ovarian cancers, however, it is essential to search the potential target, since they frequently have mutated driver oncogenes.

In the real world data, actionable gene alterations have been identified in >80% of the cases examined, but the frequency of identification of druggable gene variants varied from 6% to 77% of the cases [276–281]. In a series at Vienna Medical University, among 44 patients with recurrent ovarian cancer patients, 38 (86%) had at least one mutation, and in 31 (77%) patients, targeted treatment such as everolimus, cetuximab, sunitinib, aromatase inhibitor, or immune checkpoint inhibitor was possible. A total of 12 (39%) of the 31 patients received the recommended therapy, and the clinical benefit was obtained in 42% [276]. A prospective molecular profiling program of genome-matched therapy for type I ovarian cancer at University Toronto Cancer Centre demonstrated that 35 (64%) of the 55 patients had at least one mutations, and among them, 14 patients with KRAS/NRAS mutations were treated with MEK inhibitor and there were seven PR, seven SD, and one PD [280]. In an earlier RCT for precision medicine SHIVA trial for various cancers, treatment with matched targeted agents based on the actionable molecular alterations did not improve PFS in heavily pre-treated patients, compared with treatment by PCC [282]. Nevertheless, incorporation of NGS into the treatment of ovarian cancer will be an essential strategy for seeking personalised therapy for the patient, especially in type I ovarian cancers. For type II ovarian cancers, genetic testing for BRCA mutations as well as molecular testing for HRD is most important for the personalised use of PARP inhibitors, and these tests are usually included in the panel tests. Thus, in the era of precision medicine, gene panel testing by NGS is becoming the essential tool for searching the most appropriate treatment for the patient.

More recently, liquid biopsy examining the gene profiling of circulating cell-free DNA samples has been tried in ovarian cancer patients. Development of a blood-based assay to survey the genomic landscape of human tumours and its dynamic evolution provides considerable clinical opportunities to optimise therapeutic regimens [283]. Currently, several gene panel tests for liquid biopsy such as Guardant360 CDx and FoundationOne

Liquid CDx are available for solid tumours. Although the length of circulating tumour DNA fragment is short, the NGS technologies making it feasible to monitor the most important genomic features of HGSC, such as TP53 and BRCA mutations as well as chromosomal aberrations. Recently, liquid biopsy has been expanded to the examination of EVs and microRNAs, both of which represent the tumour microenvironment and may be useful for characterising the tumour [284,285]. The potential roles of microRNA in ovarian cancer as factors for poor prognostic or prediction of chemosensitivity have been enthusiastically analysed, and a recent meta-analysis reported that the 12 microRNAs (miR-9, miR-21, miR-100, miR-141, miR-145, miR-200a, miR-200b, miR-200c, miR-203, miR-205, miR-214, and miR-429) should be included in future studies for validation [286].

Currently, the usefulness of liquid biopsy for the detection of genomic alterations using NGS in patients with ovarian cancer is still limited. A series at Wakayama University Hospital, the comprehensive mutational profile was examined in 51 pre-treated ovarian cancer patients, and 48 (94%) showed one or more somatic mutations. Higher concentration of cell-free DNA was significantly correlated with worse PFS of patients [287]. At University of California San Diego, a total of 105 patients with gynaecologic cancer underwent cell-free DNA testing, and 79 (75.2%) showed ≥1 alteration in the liquid samples. Of the 50 ovarian cancer patients, genomic alterations found were TP53 (64.0%), PIK3CA (18.0%), KRAS (16.0%), BRAF (16.0%), MYC (12.0%), MET (12.0%), CDK6 (12.0%), CCNE1 (10.0%), and EGFR (10.0%). Of the 105 patients, OS was compared between the matched treatment with cell-free DNA analysis ($n = 33$) and the treatment by PCC ($n = 22$). Matched treatment was an independent prognostic factor for the better OS in multivariate analysis (HR 0.34; 95% CI 0.16–0.75) [288]. Due to the genomic instability, ovarian cancers especially of HGSC will change their genomes in the clonal evolution during the tumour progression. Since the liquid biopsy is useful for the detection of clonal changes of cancer under various treatments with cytotoxic and targeted drugs, the blood-based analysis would be the mainstay for monitoring the patients surviving with recurrent ovarian cancer.

# FUTURE PERSPECTIVE FOR PRECISION MEDICINE

With the recent development of targeted drugs along with the improvement of cytoreductive surgery, we are now in the corner of real advancement of management for patients with advanced and recurrent ovarian cancer. In the coming decades, patients will benefit from further achievement of success in the clinical trials for new drugs and novel treatment modalities. Furthermore, we are coming into the new era of precision medicine, where treatment and prevention of disease takes into account individual variability in genes, environment, and lifestyle for each person. The final goal is increasing patient specificity so that the right treatment is given to the right patient at the right time. Various data act as predictive biomarkers to select a specific therapy, and also to indicate accurate risk assessment, monitoring, and predicting resistance and tolerability to a treatment regimen for each patient. Therefore, each surgical procedure and each anti-cancer drug will be directed to the specific location of CSC-like tumour cells, and to the specific signalling of cancer cells under the particular tumour microenvironment, because they are continuously evolving with genomic and epigenomic changes. Accordingly, we must consider now the two-dimensional map model of the cancer genomic profiling, which shows both the diversity in carcinogenesis (X-axis) and the diversity of evolution in progression (Y-axis) (**Figure 17.51**). The place of each patient will be identified on the map via comprehensive

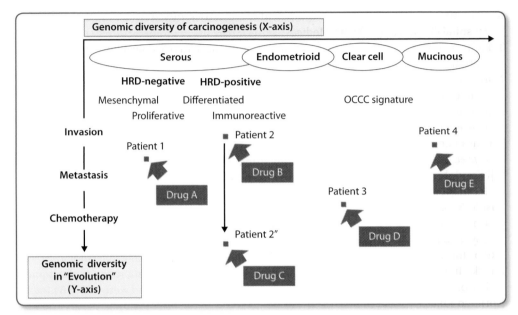

**Figure 17.51** Two-dimension model of cancer genome for precision medicine. Two-dimensional map model of the cancer genomic profiling, both the diversity in carcinogenesis (X-axis) and the diversity of evolution in progression (Y-axis) are considered. The place of each patient will be identified on the map, and the right treatment is given to the right patient at the right time in the future precision medicine.

genomic profiling, and each treatment will be given at an appropriate timing in the near future. Further research is necessary to advance precision medicine for better survival and QOL in each patient with ovarian cancer.

## CONFLICTS OF INTEREST

I declare no conflict of interest.

## ACKNOWLEDGEMENTS

I sincerely appreciate my collaborators for their tremendous efforts for our clinical, basic, and translational researches for the patients with ovarian cancer.

Masaki Mandai, MD, PhD. The 10th Professor and Chairman, Department of Gynecology and Obstetrics, Kyoto University Graduate School of Medicine, Kyoto Japan.

Junzo Hamanishi, MD, PhD. Associate Professor, Department of Gynecology and Obstetrics, Kyoto University Graduate School of Medicine, Kyoto, Japan.

Ken Yamaguchi, MD, PhD. Associate Professor, Department of Gynecology and Obstetrics, Kyoto University Graduate School of Medicine, Kyoto Japan.

Masafumi Koshiyama, MD, PhD. Professor, Department of Human Nursing, The University of Shiga Prefecture, Hikone, Japan.

Hideki Kuroda, MD, PhD. Department of Palliative Care, Kyoto Baptist Hospital, Kyoto, Japan.

Kaoru Abiko, MD, PhD. Director, Department of Obstetrics and Gynecology, National Hospital Organization, Kyoto Medical Center, Kyoto, Japan.

Takuma Hayashi, PhD. Director, Gynecologic Cancer Research, Clinical Research Center, National Hospital Organization, Kyoto Medical Center, Kyoto, Japan.

Noriomi Matsumura, MD, PhD. Professor and Chairman, Department of Obstetrics and Gynecology, Kindai University Faculty of Medicine, Osaka, Japan.

Ayako Suzuki, MD. Associate Professor, Department of Obstetrics and Gynecology, Kindai University Faculty of Medicine, Osaka, Japan.

Tsukasa Baba, MD, PhD. Professor and Chairman, Department of Obstetrics and Gynecology, Iwate Medical University School of Medicine, Morioka, Japan.

Eiji Kondoh, MD, PhD. Professor and Chairman, Department of Obstetrics and Gynecology, Kumamoto University Faculty of Life Sciences, Kumamoto, Japan.

Toshio Nikaido, PhD. Professor and Chairman, Department of Regenerative Medicine, University of Toyama Graduate School of Medicine and Pharmaceutical Sciences, Toyama, Japan.

Akiko Horiuchi, MD, PhD, Director, Horiuchi Ladies Clinic, Matsumoto, Japan.

Kazuko Itoh, MD, PhD, Director, Department of Obstetrics and Gynecology, Ina Central Hospital, Ina, Japan

Norihiko Kikuchi, MD, PhD. Associate Professor, Department of Obstetrics and Gynecology, Shinshu University School of Medicine, Matsumoto, Japan.

Ryusuke Murakami, MD, PhD. Director, Department of Gynecology, Shiga General Hospital, Moriyama, Japan.

I deeply thank my teachers for their enthusiastic education for my career in gynecology and obstetrics.

Toshio Nishimura, MD, PhD. The 5th Professor and Chairman, Department of Gynecology and Obstetrics, Kyoto University Graduate School of Medicine, Kyoto Japan.

Masahiko Ukita, MD, PhD. Director, Department of Obstetrics and Gynecology, Kurashiki Central Hospital, Kurashiki, Japan.

Takahide Mori, MD, PhD. The 7th Professor and Chairman, Department of Gynecology and Obstetrics, Kyoto University Graduate School of Medicine, Kyoto Japan.

Shingo Fujii, MD, PhD. The 8th Professor and Chairman, Department of Gynecology and Obstetrics, Kyoto University Graduate School of Medicine, Kyoto Japan.

Finally, I am also grateful to Ms Nikita Chauhan for her kind and professional assistance for publication of this chapter.

# REFERENCES

1. WHO. (2020). Ovary. Cancer incidence and mortality statistics worldwide and by region. [online] Available from: https://gco.iarc.fr/today/home [Last accessed May, 2022].
2. Nomura H, Iwasa N, Yoshihara T, et al. Epidemiology and etiology of ovarian cancer. In: Katabuchi H (Ed). Frontiers in Ovarian Cancer Science. Singapore: Springer; 2017. pp. 1–13.
3. Kurnit KC, Fleming GF, Ernst Lengyel E. Updates and new options in advanced epithelial ovarian cancer treatment. Obstet Gynecol 2021; 137:108–121.
4. Konishi I. Toward precision medicine in gynecology and obstetrics. In: Konishi I (Ed). Precision Medicine in Gynecology and Obstetrics. Singapore: Springer; 2017. pp. 1–8.
5. WHO. Tumours of the ovary. Female Genital Tumours. WHO Classification of Tumours, 5th edition. Lyon: IARC; 2020. pp. 31–167.
6. Seidman JD, Ronnett BM, Shih IM, et al. Epithelial tumors of the ovary. In: Kurman RJ, Ellenson LH, Ronnett BM (Eds). Blaustein's Pathology of the Female Genital Tract, 7th edition. Switzerland: Springer; 2019. pp. 841–966.

7.    Lheureux S, Braunstein M, Oza AM. Epithelial ovarian cancer: Evolution of management in the era of precision medicine. CA Cancer J Clin 2019; 69:280–304.

8.    Eddy DM. Clinical decision making: From theory to practice. Practice policies - What are they?. JAMA 1990; 263:877–878.

9.    Evidence-Based Medicine Working Group. Evidence-based medicine: A new approach to teaching the practice of medicine. JAMA 1992; 268:2420–2425.

10.   Farmer A. Medical practice guidelines: Lessons from the United States. BMJ 1993; 307:313–317.

11.   Cohen AM, Starvi PZ, Hersh WR. A categorization and analysis of the criticisms of Evidence-Based Medicine. Int J Med Inform 2004; 73:35–43.

12.   Kenny NP. Does good science make good medicine? Incorporating evidence into practice is complicated by the fact that clinical practice is as much as art as science. CMAJ 1997; 157:33–36.

13.   Soda M, Choi YL, Enomoto M, et al. Identification of the transforming EML4-ALK fusion gene in non-small-cell lung cancer. Nature 2007; 448:561–566.

14.   Kobayashi H. Screening and prevention of ovarian cancer. In: Katabuchi H (Ed). Frontiers in Ovarian Cancer Science. Singapore: Springer; 2017. pp. 57–81.

15.   Whitwell HJ, Worthington J, Blyuss O, et al. Improved early detection of ovarian cancer using longitudinal multimarker models. Br J Cancer 2020; 122:847–856

16.   Yokoi A, Matsuzaki J, Yamamoto Y, et al. Integrated extracellular microRNA profiling for ovarian cancer screening.  Nat Commun 2018; 9:4319.

17.   Feeney L, Harley IJ, McCluggage WG, et al. Liquid biopsy in ovarian cancer: Catching the silent killer before it strikes. World J Clin Oncol 2020; 11:868–889.

18.   Sato S, Yokoyama Y, Sakamoto T, et al. Usefulness of mass screening for ovarian carcinoma using transvaginal ultrasonography.  Cancer 2000; 89:582–588.

19.   van Nagell JR Jr, Miller RW, DeSimone CP, et al. Long-term survival of women with epithelial ovarian cancer detected by ultrasonographic screening. Obstet Gynecol 2011; 118:1212–1221.

20.   Kobayashi H, Yamada Y, Sado T, et al. A randomized study of screening for ovarian cancer: A multicenter study in Japan. Int J Gynecol Cancer 2008; 18:414–420.

21.   Buys SS, Partridge E, Black A, et al. Effect of screening on ovarian cancer mortality: The prostate, lung, colorectal and ovarian (PLCO) cancer screening randomized controlled trial. JAMA 2011; 305:2295–2303.

22.   Pinsky PF, Yu K, Kramer BS, et al. Extended mortality results for ovarian cancer screening in the PLCO trial with median 15 years follow-up. Gynecol Oncol 2016; 143:270–275.

23.   Koshiyama M, Matsumura N, Konishi I. Clinical efficacy of ovarian cancer screening. J Cancer 2016; 7:1311–1316.

24.   Menon U, Gentry-Maharaj A, Burnell M, et al. Ovarian cancer population screening and mortality after long-term follow-up in the UK Collaborative Trial of Ovarian Cancer Screening (UKCTOCS): A randomised controlled trial. Lancet 2021; 397:2182–2193.

25.   Horiuchi A, Itoh K, Shimizu M, et al. Toward understanding the natural history of ovarian carcinoma development: A clinicopathological approach. Gynecol Oncol 2003; 88:309–317.

26.   Romero I, Leskelä S, Mies BP, et al. Morphological and molecular heterogeneity of epithelial ovarian cancer: Therapeutic implications. EJC Suppl 2020; 15:1–15.

27.   Shih IeM, Kurman RJ. Ovarian tumorigenesis: A proposed model based on morphological and molecular genetic analysis. Am J Pathol 2004; 164:1511–1518

28.   Koshiyama M, Matsumura N, Konishi I. Recent concepts of ovarian carcinogenesis: Type I and type II. Biomed Res Int 2014; 934261.

29.   Seidman JD, Kurman RJ, Ronnett BM. Primary and metastatic mucinous adenocarcinomas in the ovaries: Incidence in routine practice with a new approach to improve intraoperative diagnosis. Am J Surg Pathol 2003; 27:985–993.

30.   Trabert B, Tworoger SS, O'Brien KM, et al. The risk of ovarian cancer increases with an increase in the lifetime number of ovulatory cycles: An analysis from the Ovarian Cancer Cohort Consortium (OC3). Cancer Res 2020; 80:1210–1218.

31.   Fathalla MF. Incessant ovulation: A factor in ovarian neoplasia? Lancet 1971; 2:163.

32.   Konishi I. Gonadotropins and ovarian carcinogenesis: A new era of basic research and its clinical implications. Int J Gynecol Cancer 2006; 16:16–22.

33.   Wentzensen N, Poole EM, Trabert B, et al. Ovarian cancer risk factors by histologic subtype: An analysis from the Ovarian Cancer Cohort Consortium. J Clin Oncol 2016; 34:2888–2898.

34.   Konstantinopoulos PA, Norquist B, Lacchetti C, et al. Germline and somatic tumor testing in epithelial ovarian cancer: ASCO Guideline. J Clin Oncol 2020; 38:1222–1245.

35. Reyes MC, Crum CP, van Diest PJ. BRCA1/2-associated hereditary breast and ovarian cancer syndrome. Female Genital Tumours. WHO Classification of Tumours, 5th edition. Lyon: IARC; 2020. pp. 544–545.

36. Sekine M, Enomoto T. Hereditary ovarian cancer. In: Katabuchi H (Ed). Frontiers in Ovarian Cancer Science. Singapore: Springer; 2017. pp. 15–35.

37. Mavaddat N, Peock S, Frost D, et al. Cancer risks for BRCA1 and BRCA2 mutation carriers: Results from prospective analysis of EMBRACE. J Natl Cancer Inst 2013 ;105:812–822.

38. Daly MB, Pal T, Berry MP, et al. Genetic/familial high-risk assessment: Breast, ovarian, and pancreatic. In: NCCN Clinical Practice Guidelines in Oncology (NCCN Guidelines). 2020, Version 2.2021. J Natl Compr Canc Netw 2021;19:77–102.

39. Finch PM, Lubinski J, Møller P, et al. Impact of oophorectomy on cancer incidence and mortality in women with a BRCA1 or BRCA2 mutation. J Clin Oncol 2014; 32:1547–1553.

40. Domchek SM, Friebel TM, Singer CF, et al. Association of risk-reducing surgery in BRCA1 or BRCA2 mutation carriers with cancer risk and mortality. JAMA 2010; 304:967–975.

41. Powell CB, Chen LM, McLennan J, et al. Risk-reducing salpingo-oophorectomy (RRSO) in BRCA mutation carriers: Experience with a consecutive series of 111 patients using a standardized surgical-pathological protocol. Int J Gynecol Cancer 2011; 21:846–851.

42. Kotsopoulos J, Narod SA. Prophylactic salpingectomy for the prevention of ovarian cancer: Who should we target? Int J Cancer 2020; 147:1245–1251.

43. Kindelberger DW, Lee Y, Miron A, et al. Intraepithelial carcinoma of the fimbria and pelvic serous carcinoma: Evidence for a causal relationship. Am J Surg Pathol 2007; 31:161–169.

44. Kurman RJ, Shih IM. The origin and pathogenesis of epithelial ovarian cancer: A proposed unifying theory. Am J Surg Pathol 2010; 34:433–443.

45. Labidi-Galy SI, Papp E, Hallberg D, et al. High grade serous ovarian carcinomas originate in the fallopian tube. Nat Commun 2017; 8:1093.

46. Wu RC, Wang P, Lin SF, et al. Genomic landscape and evolutionary trajectories of ovarian cancer precursor lesions. J Pathol 2019; 248:41–50.

47. Masoodi T, Siraj S, Siraj AK, et al. Genetic heterogeneity and evolutionary history of high-grade ovarian carcinoma and matched distant metastases. Br J Cancer 2020; 122:1219–1230.

48. Chien J, Neums L, Powell AFLA, et al. Genetic evidence for early peritoneal spreading in pelvic high-grade serous cancer. Front Oncol 2018; 8:58.

49. Cancer Genome Atlas Research Network. Integrated genomic analyses of ovarian carcinoma. Nature 2011; 474:609–615.

50. Birrer MJ. Ovarian cancer: Targeting the untargetable. Am Soc Clin Oncol Educ Book 2014;13-5.

51. Curtin NJ. The development of rucaparib/rubraca: A story of the synergy between science and serendipity. Cancers (Basel) 2020; 12:564.

52. Verhaak RG, Tamayo P, Yang JY, et al. Prognostically relevant gene signatures of high-grade serous ovarian carcinoma. J Clin Invest 2013; 123:517–525.

53. Konecny GE, Wang C, Hamidi H, et al. Prognostic and therapeutic relevance of molecular subtypes in high-grade serous ovarian cancer. J Natl Cancer Inst 2014; 106:dju249.

54. Murakami R, Matsumura N, Mandai M, et al. Establishment of a novel histopathological classification of high-grade serous ovarian carcinoma correlated with prognostically distinct gene expression subtypes. Am J Pathol 2016; 186:1103–1113.

55. Ohsuga T, Yamaguchi K, Kido A, et al. Distinct preoperative clinical features predict four histopathological subtypes of high-grade serous carcinoma of the ovary, fallopian tube, and peritoneum. BMC Cancer 2017; 17:580.

56. Katsumata N, Yasuda M, Isonishi S, et al. Long-term results of dose-dense paclitaxel and carboplatin versus conventional paclitaxel and carboplatin for treatment of advanced epithelial ovarian, fallopian tube, or primary peritoneal cancer (JGOG 3016): A randomised, controlled, open-label trial. Lancet Oncol 2013; 14:1020–1026.

57. Murakami R, Matsumura N, Michimae H, et al. The mesenchymal transition subtype more responsive to dose dense taxane chemotherapy combined with carboplatin than to conventional taxane and carboplatin chemotherapy in high grade serous ovarian carcinoma: A survey of Japanese Gynecologic Oncology Group study (JGOG3016A1). Gynecol Oncol 2019; 153:312–319.

58. Kommoss S, Winterhoff B, Oberg AL, et al. Bevacizumab may differentially improve ovarian cancer outcome in patients with proliferative and mesenchymal molecular subtypes. Clin Cancer Res 2017; 23:3794–3801.

59. Slomovitz B, Gourley C, Carey MS, et al. Low-grade serous ovarian cancer: State of the science. Gynecol Oncol. 2020; 156:715–725.
60. Hunter SM, Anglesio MS, Ryland GL, et al. Molecular profiling of low grade serous ovarian tumours identifies novel candidate driver genes. Oncotarget 2015; 6:37663–37677.
61. Cheasley D, Nigam A, Zethoven M, et al. Genomic analysis of low-grade serous ovarian carcinoma to identify key drivers and therapeutic vulnerabilities. J Pathol 2021; 253:41–54.
62. Farley J, Brady WE, Vathipadiekal V, et al. Selumetinib in women with recurrent low-grade serous carcinoma of the ovary or peritoneum: An open-label, single-arm, phase 2 study. Lancet Oncol 2013; 14:134–140.
63. Han C, Bellone S, Zammataro L, et al. Binimetinib (MEK162) in recurrent low-grade serous ovarian cancer resistant to chemotherapy and hormonal treatment. Gynecol Oncol Rep 2018; 25:41–44.
64. Monk BJ, Grisham RN, Banerjee S, et al. MILO/ENGOT-ov11: Binimetinib versus physician's choice chemotherapy in recurrent or persistent low-grade serous carcinomas of the ovary, fallopian tube, or primary peritoneum. J Clin Oncol 2020; 38:3753–3762.
65. Tholander B, Koliadi A, Botling J, et al. Complete response with combined BRAF and MEK inhibition in BRAF mutated advanced low-grade serous ovarian carcinoma. Ups J Med Sci 2020; 125:325–329.
66. Gershenson DM, Gourley C, Paul J. MEK Inhibitors for the treatment of low-grade serous ovarian cancer: Expanding therapeutic options for a rare ovarian cancer subtype. J Clin Oncol 2020; 38:3731–3734.
67. Voutsadakis IA. A systematic review and meta-analysis of hormone receptor expression in low-grade serous ovarian carcinoma. Eur J Obstet Gynecol Reprod Biol 2021; 256:172–178.
68. Watson CH, Secord AA. Durable response to hormonal therapy in a patient with rapidly progressive low-grade serous ovarian cancer: A case report. Gynecol Oncol Rep 2020; 33:100598.
69. Fader AN, Bergstrom J, Jernigan A, et al. Primary cytoreductive surgery and adjuvant hormonal monotherapy in women with advanced low-grade serous ovarian carcinoma: Reducing overtreatment without compromising survival? Gynecol Oncol 2017; 147:85–91.
70. Tang M, O'Connell RL, Amant F, et al. PARAGON: A Phase II study of anastrozole in patients with estrogen receptor-positive recurrent/metastatic low-grade ovarian cancers and serous borderline ovarian tumors. Gynecol Oncol 2019; 154:531–538.
71. Mandai M, Yamaguchi K, Matsumura N, et al. Ovarian cancer in endometriosis: Molecular biology, pathology, and clinical management. Int J Clin Oncol 2009; 14:383–391.
72. Cybulska P, Paula ADC, Tseng J, et al. Molecular profiling and molecular classification of endometrioid ovarian carcinomas. Gynecol Oncol 2019; 154:516–523.
73. Hollis RL, Thomson JP, Stanley B, et al. Molecular stratification of endometrioid ovarian carcinoma predicts clinical outcome. Nat Commun 2020; 11:4995.
74. Schultheis AM, Ng CKY, De Filippo MR, et al. Massively parallel sequencing-based clonality analysis of synchronous endometrioid endometrial and ovarian carcinomas. J Natl Cancer Inst 2016; 108:djv427.
75. Suda K, Nakaoka H, Yoshihara K, et al. Clonal expansion and diversification of cancer-associated mutations in endometriosis and normal endometrium. Cell Rep 2018; 24:1777–1789.
76. Yachida N, Yoshihara K, Yamaguchi M, et al. How does endometriosis lead to ovarian cancer? The molecular mechanism of endometriosis-associated ovarian cancer development. Cancers (Basel) 2021; 13:1439.
77. Sugiyama T, Kamura T, Kigawa J, et al. Clinical characteristics of clear cell carcinoma of the ovary. Cancer 2000; 88:2584–2589.
78. Okamoto A, Glasspool RM, Mabuchi S, et al. Gynecologic Cancer InterGroup (GCIG) consensus review for clear cell carcinoma of the ovary. Int J Gynecol Cancer 2014; 24:S20–25.
79. Mandai M, Matsumura N, Baba T, et al. Ovarian clear cell carcinoma as a stress-responsive cancer: Influence of the microenvironment on the carcinogenesis and cancer phenotype. Cancer Lett 2011; 310:129–133.
80. Yamaguchi K, Mandai M, Oura T, et al. Identification of an ovarian clear cell carcinoma gene signature that reflects inherent disease biology and the carcinogenic processes. Oncogene 2010; 29:1741–1752.
81. Mandai M, Amano Y, Yamaguchi K, et al. Ovarian clear cell carcinoma meets metabolism; HNF-1beta confers survival benefits through the Warburg effect and ROS reduction. Oncotarget 2015; 6:30704–30714.
82. Matsumura N, Mandai M, Okamoto T, et al. Sorafenib efficacy in ovarian clear cell carcinoma revealed by transcriptome profiling. Cancer Sci 2010; 101:2658–2563.
83. Koshiyama M, Matsumura N, Baba T, et al. Two cases of recurrent ovarian clear cell carcinoma treated with sorafenib. Cancer Biol Ther 2014; 15:22–25.

84. Jones S, Wang TL, Shih IeM, et al. Frequent mutations of chromatin remodeling gene ARID1A in ovarian clear cell carcinoma. Science 2010; 330:228–231.

85. Wiegand KC, Shah SP, Al-Agha OM, et al. ARID1A mutations in endometriosis-associated ovarian carcinomas. N Engl J Med 2010; 363:1532–1543.

86. Abou-Taleb H, Yamaguchi K, Matsumura N, et al. Comprehensive assessment of the expression of the SWI/SNF complex defines two distinct prognostic subtypes of ovarian clear cell carcinoma. Oncotarget 2016; 7:54758–54770.

87. Murakami R, Matsumura N, Brown JB, et al. Exome sequencing landscape analysis in ovarian clear cell carcinoma shed light on key chromosomal regions and mutation gene networks. Am J Pathol 2017; 187:2246–2258.

88. Takahashi K, Takenaka M, Okamoto A, et al. Treatment strategies for ARID1A-deficient ovarian clear cell carcinoma. Cancers (Basel) 2021; 13:1769.

89. Murakami R, Hamanishi J, Brown JB, et al. Combination of gene set signatures correlates with response to nivolumab in platinum-resistant ovarian cancer. Sci Rep 2021; 11:11427.

90. Takano M, Sugiyama T, Yaegashi N, et al. Progression-free survival and overall survival of patients with clear cell carcinoma of the ovary treated with paclitaxel-carboplatin or irinotecan-cisplatin: Retrospective analysis. Int J Clin Oncol 2007; 12:256–260.

91. Sugiyama T, Okamoto A, Enomoto T, et al.Randomized phase III trial of irinotecan plus cisplatin compared with paclitaxel plus carboplatin as first-line chemotherapy for ovarian clear cell Ccarcinoma: JGOG3017/GCIG trial. J Clin Oncol 2016; 34:2881–2887.

92. Ricci F, Affatato R, Carrassa L, et al. Recent insights into mucinous ovarian carcinoma. Int J Mol Sci 2018;19:1569.

93. Mandai M, Konishi I, Kuroda H, et al. Heterogeneous distribution of K-ras-mutated epithelia in mucinous ovarian tumors with special reference to histopathology. Hum Pathol 1998; 29:34–40.

94. Cheasley D, Wakefield MJ, Ryland GL, et al. The molecular origin and taxonomy of mucinous ovarian carcinoma. Nat Commun 2019; 10:3935.

95. Gorringe KL, Cheasley D, Wakefield MJ, et al. Therapeutic options for mucinous ovarian carcinoma. Gynecol Oncol 2020; 156:552–560.

96. McAlpine JN, Wiegand KC, Vang R, et al. HER2 overexpression and amplification is present in a subset of ovarian mucinous carcinomas and can be targeted with trastuzumab therapy. BMC Cancer 2009; 9:433.

97. Mikuła-Pietrasik J, Uruski P, Tykarski A, et al. The peritoneal 'soil' for a cancerous 'seed': A comprehensive review of the pathogenesis of intraperitoneal cancer metastases. Cell Mol Life Sci 2018; 75:509–525.

98. Imai T, Horiuchi A, Wang C, et al. Hypoxia attenuates the expression of E-cadherin via up-regulation of SNAIL in ovarian carcinoma cells. Am J Pathol 2003; 163:1437–1447.

99. Rosso M, Majem B, Devis L, et al. E-cadherin: A determinant molecule associated with ovarian cancer progression, dissemination and aggressiveness. PLoS One 2017; 12:e0184439.

100. Liao J, Qian F, Tchabo N, et al. Ovarian cancer spheroid cells with stem cell-like properties contribute to tumor generation, metastasis and chemotherapy resistance through hypoxia-resistant metabolism. PLoS ONE 2014; 9:e84941.

101. Zhang S, Balch C, Chan MW, et al. Identification and characterization of ovarian cancer-initiating cells from primary human tumors. Cancer Res 2008; 68:4311–4320.

102. Jain S, Annett SL, Morgan MP, et al. The cancer stem cell niche in ovarian cancer and its impact on immune surveillance. Int J Mol Sci 2021; 22:4091.

103. Terraneo N, Jacob F, Dubrovska A, et al. Novel therapeutic strategies for ovarian cancer stem cells. Front Oncol 2020; 10:319.

104. Yamamoto S, Konishi I, Mandai M, et al. Expression of vascular endothelial growth factor (VEGF) in epithelial ovarian neoplasms: Correlation with clinicopathology and patient survival, and analysis of serum VEGF levels. Br J Cancer 1997; 76:1221–1227.

105. Basu P, Mukhopadhyay A, Konishi I. Targeted therapy for gynecologic cancers: Toward the era of precision medicine. Int J Gynaecol Obstet 2018; 143:131–136.

106. Liu S, Kasherman L, Fazelzad R, et al. The use of bevacizumab in the modern era of targeted therapy for ovarian cancer: A systematic review and meta-analysis. Gynecol Oncol 2021; 161:601–612.

107. Fei F, Qu J, Zhang M, et al. S100A4 in cancer progression and metastasis: A systematic review. Oncotarget 2017; 8:73219–73239.

108. Kikuchi N, Horiuchi A, Osada R, et al. Nuclear expression of S100A4 is associated with aggressive behavior of epithelial ovarian carcinoma: an important autocrine/paracrine factor in tumor progression. Cancer Sci 2006; 97:1061–1069.

109. Horiuchi A, Hayashi T, Kikuchi N, et al. Hypoxia upregulates ovarian cancer invasiveness via the binding of HIF-1α to a hypoxia-induced, methylation-free hypoxia response element of S100A4 gene. Int J Cancer 2012; 131:1755–1767.

110. Chatterjee A, Rodger EJ, Eccles MR. Epigenetic drivers of tumourigenesis and cancer metastasis. Semin Cancer Biol 2018; 51:149–159.

111. Link T, Kuhlmann JD, Kobelt D, et al. Clinical relevance of circulating MACC1 and S100A4 transcripts for ovarian cancer. Mol Oncol 2019; 13:1268–1279.

112. Alanazi B, Munje CR, Rastogi N, et al. Integrated nuclear proteomics and transcriptomics identifies S100A4 as a therapeutic target in acute myeloid leukemia. Leukemia 2020; 34:427–440.

113. Ganaie AA, Mansini AP, Hussain T, et al. Anti-S100A4 antibody therapy is efficient in treating aggressive prostate cancer and reversing immunosuppression: Serum and biopsy S100A4 as a clinical predictor. Mol Cancer Ther 2020; 19:2598–2611.

114. Sun H, Wang C, Hu B, et al. Exosomal S100A4 derived from highly metastatic hepatocellular carcinoma cells promotes metastasis by activating STAT3. Signal Transduct Target Ther 2021; 6:187.

115. Bresnick AR. S100 proteins as therapeutic targets. Biophys Rev 2018; 10:1617–1629.

116. Horiuchi A, Imai T, Wang C, et al. Up-regulation of small GTPases, RhoA and RhoC, is associated with tumor progression in ovarian carcinoma. Lab Invest 2003; 83:861–870.

117. Horiuchi A, Kikuchi N, Osada R, et al. Overexpression of RhoA enhances peritoneal dissemination: RhoA suppression with lovastatin may be useful for ovarian cancer. Cancer Sci 2008; 99:2532–2539.

118. Kobayashi Y, Kashima H, Rahmanto YS, et al. Drug repositioning of mevalonate pathway inhibitors as antitumor agents for ovarian cancer. Oncotarget 2017; 8:72147–72156.

119. Hanley GE, Kaur P, Berchuck A, et al. Cardiovascular medications and survival in people with ovarian cancer: A population-based cohort study from British Columbia, Canada. Gynecol Oncol 2021; S0090–8258(21)00427-3.

120. Feng JL, Dixon-Suen SC, Jordan SJ,. Statin use and survival among women with ovarian cancer: An Australian national data-linkage study. Br J Cancer 2021; 125:766–771.

121. van Baal JOAM, van Noorden CJF, Nieuwland R, et al. Development of peritoneal carcinomatosis in epithelial ovarian cancer: A review. J Histochem Cytochem 2018; 66:67–83.

122. Mogi K, Yoshihara M, Iyoshi S, et al. Ovarian cancer-associated mesothelial cells: Transdifferentiation to minions of cancer and orchestrate developing peritoneal dissemination. Cancers (Basel) 2021; 13:1352.

123. Savant SS, Sriramkumar S, O'Hagan HM. The role of inflammation and inflammatory mediators in the development, progression, metastasis, and chemoresistance of epithelial ovarian cancer. Cancers (Basel) 2018; 10:251.

124. Beeghly-Fadiel A, Wilson AJ, Keene S, et al. Differential cyclooxygenase expression levels and survival associations in type I and type II ovarian tumors. J Ovarian Res 2018; 11:17.

125. Merritt MA, Rice MS, Barnard ME, et al. Pre-diagnosis and post-diagnosis use of common analgesics and ovarian cancer prognosis (NHS/NHSII): a cohort study. Lancet Oncol 2018; 19:1107–1116.

126. Imai T, Horiuchi A, Shiozawa T, et al. Elevated expression of E-cadherin and alpha-, beta-, and gamma-catenins in metastatic lesions compared with primary epithelial ovarian carcinomas. Hum Pathol 2004; 35:1469–1476.

127. Nieman KM, Kenny HA, Penicka CV, et al. Adipocytes promote ovarian cancer metastasis and provide energy for rapid tumor growth. Nat Med 2011; 17:1498–1503.

128. Motohara T, Masuda K, Morotti M, et al. An evolving story of the metastatic voyage of ovarian cancer cells: Cellular and molecular orchestration of the adipose-rich metastatic microenvironment. Oncogene 2019; 38:2885–2898.

129. Matsumura N, Huang Z, Mori S, et al. Epigenetic suppression of the TGF-beta pathway revealed by transcriptome profiling in ovarian cancer. Genome Res 2011; 21:74–82.

130. Yamamura S, Matsumura N, Manda M, et al. The activated transforming growth factor-beta signaling pathway in peritoneal metastases is a potential therapeutic target in ovarian cancer. Int J Cancer 2012; 130:20–28.

131. Deshmukh AP, Vasaikar SV, Tomczak K, et al. Identification of EMT signaling cross-talk and gene regulatory networks by single-cell RNA sequencing. Proc Natl Acad Sci USA 2021; 118:e2102050118.

132. Roane BM, Arend RC, Birrer MJ. Review: Targeting the transforming growth factor-beta pathway in ovarian cancer. Cancers (Basel) 2019; 11:668.

133. Salas-Benito D, Vercher E, Conde E, et al. Inflammation and immunity in ovarian cancer. EJC Suppl 2020; 15:56–66.

134. Hamanishi J, Mandai M, Konishi I. Immune checkpoint inhibition in ovarian cancer. Int Immunol 2016; 28:339–348.

135. Yang Y, Yang Y, Yang J, et al. Tumor microenvironment in ovarian cancer: Function and therapeutic strategy. Front Cell Dev Biol 2020; 8:758.

136. Noy R, Pollard JW. Tumor-associated macrophages: From mechanisms to therapy. Immunity 2014; 41:49–61.

137. Takaishi K, Komohara Y, Tashiro H, et al. Involvement of M2-polarized macrophages in the ascites from advanced epithelial ovarian carcinoma in tumor progression via Stat3 activation. Cancer Sci 2010; 101:2128–2136.

138. Hamanishi J, Mandai M, Iwasaki M, et al. Programmed cell death 1 ligand 1 and tumor-infiltrating CD8+ T lymphocytes are prognostic factors of human ovarian cancer. Proc Natl Acad Sci USA 2007; 104:3360–3365.

139. Goode EL, Block MS, Kalli KR, et al. Dose-response association of CD8+ tumor-infiltrating lymphocytes and survival time in high-grade serous ovarian cancer. JAMA Oncol 2017; 3:e173290.

140. Curiel TJ, Coukos G, Zou L, et al. Specific recruitment of regulatory T cells in ovarian carcinoma fosters immune privilege and predicts reduced survival. Nat Med 2004; 10:942–949.

141. Mabuchi S, Sasano T, Komura N, et al. Targeting myeloid-derived suppressor cells in ovarian cancer. Cells 2021; 10:329.

142. Horikawa N, Abiko K, Matsumura N, et al. Anti-VEGF therapy resistance in ovarian cancer is caused by GM-CSF-induced myeloid-derived suppressor cell recruitment. British Journal of Cancer 2020; 122:778–788.

143. Komura N, Mabuchi S, Shimura K, et al. The role of myeloid-derived suppressor cells in increasing cancer stem-like cells and promoting PD-L1 expression in epithelial ovarian cancer. Cancer Immunol Immunother 2020; 69:2477–2499.

144. Taki M, Abiko K, Baba T, et al. Snail promotes ovarian cancer progression by recruiting myeloid-derived suppressor cells via CXCR2 ligand upregulation. Nat Commun 2018; 9:1685.

145. Hamanishi J, Mandai M, Ikeda T, et al. Safety and antitumor activity of anti-PD-1 antibody, nivolumab, in patients with platinum-resistant ovarian cancer. J Clin Oncol 2015; 33:4015–4022.

146. Motohara T, Katabuchi H. Ovarian cancer stemness: Biological and clinical implications for metastasis and chemotherapy resistance. Cancers (Basel) 2019; 11:907.

147. Mazzoldi EL, Pastò A, Pilotto G, et al. Comparison of the genomic profile of cancer stem cells and their non-stem counterpart: The case of ovarian cancer. J Clin Med 2020; 9:368.

148. Szotek PP, Pieretti-Vanmarcke R, Masiakos PT, et al. Ovarian cancer side population defines cells with stem cell-like characteristics and mullerian inhibiting substance responsiveness. Proc Natl Acad Sci USA 2006; 103:11154–11159.

149. Stewart JM, Shaw PA, Gedye C, et al. Phenotypic heterogeneity and instability of human ovarian tumor-initiating cells. Proc Natl Acad Sci U S A 2011; 108:6468–6473.

150. Yamanoi K, Baba T, Abiko K, et al. Acquisition of a side population fraction augments malignant phenotype in ovarian cancer. Sci Rep 2019; 9:14215.

151. Baba T, Convery PA, Matsumura N, at al. Epigenetic regulation of CD133 and tumorigenicity of CD133+ ovarian cancer cells. Oncogene 2009; 28:209–218.

152. Ciriello G, Magnani L. The many faces of cancer evolution. iScience 2021; 24:102403.

153. Tao Y, Li H, Huang R, et al. Clinicopathological and prognostic significance of cancer stem cell markers in ovarian cancer patients: Evidence from 52 studies. Cell Physiol Biochem 2018; 46:1716–1726.

154. Wang Y, Niu XL, Qu Y, et al. Autocrine production of interleukin-6 confers cisplatin and paclitaxel resistance in ovarian cancer cells. Cancer Lett 2010; 295:110–123.

155. Dzobo K, Senthebane DA, Ganz C, et al. Advances in therapeutic targeting of cancer stem cells within the tumor microenvironment: An updated review. Cells 2020; 9:1896.

156. Muñoz-Galván S, Carnero A. Targeting cancer stem cells to overcome therapy resistance in ovarian cancer. Cells 2020; 9:1402.

157. Mikami M. Primary surgical treatment of epithelial ovarian cancer. In: Katabuchi H (ed). Frontiers in Ovarian Cancer Science. Singapore: Springer: 2017. pp. 191–205.

158. Schuurman T, Zilver S, Samuels S, et al. Fertility-sparing surgery in gynecologic cancer: A systematic review. Cancers (Basel) 2021; 13:1008.

159. Kajiyama H, Shibata K, Suzuki S, et al. Is there any possibility of fertility-sparing surgery in patients with clear-cell carcinoma of the ovary? Gynecol Oncol 2008; 111:523–526.

160. Satoh T, Hatae M, Watanabe Y, et al. Outcomes of fertility-sparing surgery for stage I epithelial ovarian cancer: A proposal for patient selection. J Clin Oncol 2010; 28:1727–1732.

161. Prodromidou A, Theofanakis C, Thomakos N, et al. Fertility sparing surgery for early-stage clear cell carcinoma of the ovary: A systematic review and analysis of obstetric outcomes. Eur J Surg Oncol 2021; 47:1286–1291.

162. Chan JK, Munro EG, Cheung MK, et al. Association of lymphadenectomy and survival in stage I ovarian cancer patients. Obstet Gynecol 2007; 109:12–19.

163. Maggioni A, Benedetti Panici P, Dell'Anna T, et al. Randomised study of systematic lymphadenectomy in patients with epithelial ovarian cancer macroscopically confined to the pelvis. Br J Cancer 2006; 95:699–704.

164. Chiyoda T, Sakurai M, Satoh T, et al. Lymphadenectomy for primary ovarian cancer: A systematic review and meta-analysis. J Gynecol Oncol 2020; 31:e67.

165. Bizzarri N, du Bois A, Fruscio R, et al. Is there any therapeutic role of pelvic and para-aortic lymphadenectomy in apparent early stage epithelial ovarian cancer? Gynecol Oncol 2021; 160:56–63.

166. Koirala P, Moon AS, Chuang L. Clinical utility of preoperative assessment in ovarian cancer cytoreduction. Diagnostics (Basel) 2020; 10:568.

167. Kong Q, Wei H, Zhang J, et al. Comparison of the survival outcomes of laparoscopy versus laparotomy in treatment of early-stage ovarian cancer: A systematic review and meta-analysis. J Ovarian Res 2021; 14:45.

168. Tantitamit T, Lee CL. Is it the time for laparoscopic management of early-stage ovarian malignancies? Gynecol Minim Invasive Ther 2018; 7:93–103.

169. Jochum F, Vermel M, Faller E, et al. Three and five-year mortality in ovarian cancer after minimally invasive compared to open surgery: A systematic review and meta-analysis. J Clin Med 2020; 9:2507.

170. Griffiths CT. Surgical resection of tumor bulk in the primary treatment of ovarian carcinoma. Natl Cancer Inst Monogr 1975; 42:101–104.

171. Hoskins WJ, Bundy BN, Thigpen JT, et al. The influence of cytoreductive surgery on recurrence-free interval and survival in small-volume stage III epithelial ovarian cancer: A Gynecologic Oncology Group study. Gynecol Oncol 1992; 47:159–166.

172. Bookman MA, Brady MF, McGuire WP, et al. Evaluation of new platinum-based treatment regimens in advanced-stage ovarian cancer: A phase III trial of the Gynecologic Cancer Intergroup. J Clin Oncol 2009; 27:1419–1425.

173. Tseng JH, Cowan RA, Zhou Q, et al. Continuous improvement in primary debulking surgery for advanced ovarian cancer: Do increased complete gross resection rates independently lead to increased progression-free and overall survival? Gynecol Oncol 2018; 151:24–31.

174. Nishikimi K, Tate S, Matsuoka A, et al. Aggressive surgery could overcome the extent of initial peritoneal dissemination for advanced ovarian, fallopian tube, and peritoneal carcinoma. Sci Rep 2020; 10:21307.

175. Vergote I, Coens C, Nankivell M, et al. Neoadjuvant chemotherapy versus debulking surgery in advanced tubo-ovarian cancers: Pooled analysis of individual patient data from the EORTC 55971 and CHORUS trials. Lancet Oncol 2018; 19:1680–1687.

176. Fotopoulou C, Sehouli J, Aletti G, et al. Value of neoadjuvant chemotherapy for newly diagnosed advanced ovarian cancer: A European perspective. J Clin Oncol 2017; 35:587–590.

177. Fagotti A, Ferrandina MG, Vizzielli G, et al. Randomized trial of primary debulking surgery versus neoadjuvant chemotherapy for advanced epithelial ovarian cancer (SCORPION-NCT01461850). Int J Gynecol Cancer 2020; 30:1657–1664.

178. Onda T, Satoh T, Ogawa G, et al. Comparison of survival between primary debulking surgery and neoadjuvant chemotherapy for stage III/IV ovarian, tubal and peritoneal cancers in phase III randomised trial. Eur J Cancer 2020;130:114–125.

179. Bartels HC, Rogers AC, McSharry V, et al. A meta-analysis of morbidity and mortality in primary cytoreductive surgery compared to neoadjuvant chemotherapy in advanced ovarian malignancy. Gynecol Oncol 2019; 154:622–630.

180. Coleridge SL, Bryant A, Kehoe S, et al. Chemotherapy versus surgery for initial treatment in advanced ovarian epithelial cancer. Cochrane Database Syst Rev 2021; 2:CD005343.

181. Knisely AT, St Clair CM, Hou JY, et al. Trends in primary treatment and median survival among women with advanced-stage epithelial ovarian cancer in the US from 2004 to 2016. JAMA Netw Open 2020; 3:e2017517.

182. Lyons YA, Reyes HD, Mcdonald ME, et al. Interval debulking surgery is not worth the wait: A National Cancer Database study comparing primary cytoreductive surgery versus neoadjuvant chemotherapy. Int J Gynecol Cancer 2020; 30:845–852.

183. Kim SR, Kotsopoulos J, Sun P, et al. The impacts of neoadjuvant chemotherapy and of cytoreductive surgery on 10-year survival from advanced ovarian cancer. Int J Gynaecol Obstet 2021; 153:417–423.

184. Matsuo K, Matsuzaki S, Nusbaum DJ, et al. Possible candidate population for neoadjuvant chemotherapy in women with advanced ovarian cancer. Gynecol Oncol 2021; 160:32–39.

185. Bhatt A, Bakrin N, Kammar P, et al. Distribution of residual disease in the peritoneum following neoadjuvant chemotherapy in advanced epithelial ovarian cancer and its potential therapeutic implications. Eur J Surg Oncol 2021; 47:181–187.

186. Tate S, Nishikimi K, Kato K, et al. Microscopic diseases remain in initial disseminated sites after neoadjuvant chemotherapy for stage III/IV ovarian, tubal, and primary peritoneal cancer. J Gynecol Oncol 2020; 31:e34.

187. Rauh-Hain JA, Nitschmann CC, Worley MJ Jr, et al. Platinum resistance after neoadjuvant chemotherapy compared to primary surgery in patients with advanced epithelial ovarian carcinoma. Gynecol Oncol 2013; 129:63–68.

188. Patel A, Iyer P, Matsuzaki S, et al. Emerging trends in neoadjuvant chemotherapy for ovarian cancer. Cancers (Basel) 2021; 13:626.

189. Reuss A, du Bois A, Harter P, et al. TRUST: Trial of radical upfront surgical therapy in advanced ovarian cancer (ENGOT ov33/AGO-OVAR OP7). Int J Gynecol Cancer 2019; 29:1327–1331.

190. Narasimhulu DM, Thannickal A, Kumar A, et al. Appropriate triage allows aggressive primary debulking surgery with rates of morbidity and mortality comparable to interval surgery after chemotherapy. Gynecol Oncol 2021; 160:681–687.

191. Fagotti A, Vizzielli G, De Iaco P, et al. A multicentric trial (Olympia-MITO 13) on the accuracy of laparoscopy to assess peritoneal spread in ovarian cancer. Am J Obstet Gynecol 2013; 209:462.e1–462.

192. Baiocchi GL, Gheza F, Molfino S, et al. Indocyanine green fluorescence-guided intraoperative detection of peritoneal carcinomatosis: Systematic review. BMC Surg 2020; 20:158.

193. de Jong JM, Hoogendam JP, Braat AJAT, et al. The feasibility of folate receptor alpha- and HER2-targeted intraoperative fluorescence-guided cytoreductive surgery in women with epithelial ovarian cancer: A systematic review. Gynecol Oncol 2021:S0090–8258(21)00423–6.

194. Hoogstins CE, Tummers QR, Gaarenstroom KN, et al. A novel tumor-specific agent for intraoperative near-infrared fluorescence imaging: A translational study in healthy volunteers and patients with ovarian cancer. Clin Cancer Res 2016; 22:2929–2938.

195. Randall LM, Wenham RM, Low PS, et al. A phase II, multicenter, open-label trial of OTL38 injection for the intra-operative imaging of folate receptor-alpha positive ovarian cancer. Gynecol Oncol 2019; 155:63–68.

196. Tanyi JL, Chon HS, Morgan MAl, et al. Phase 3, randomized, single-dose, open-label study to investigate the safety and efficacy of pafolacianine sodium injection (OTL38) for intraoperative imaging of folate receptor positive ovarian cancer. J Clin Oncol 2021; 15:5503–5503.

197. Liu Y, Endo Y, Fujita T, et al. Cytoreductive surgery under aminolevulinic acid-mediated photodynamic diagnosis plus hyperthermic intraperitoneal chemotherapy in patients with peritoneal carcinomatosis from ovarian cancer and primary peritoneal carcinoma: Results of a phase I trial. Ann Surg Oncol 2014; 21:4256–4262.

198. Xu S, Bulin AL, Hurbin A, et al. Photodynamic diagnosis and therapy for peritoneal carcinomatosis: Emerging perspectives. Cancers (Basel) 2020; 12:2491.

199. Harter P, Sehouli J, Lorusso D, et al. A randomized trial of lymphadenectomy in patients with advanced ovarian neoplasms. N Engl J Med 2019; 380:822–832.

200. Panici PB, Maggioni A, Hacker N, et al. Systematic aortic and pelvic lymphadenectomy versus resection of bulky nodes only in optimally debulked advanced ovarian cancer: A randomized clinical trial. J Natl Cancer Inst 2005; 97:560–506.

201. Lai Y, Peng H, Tong C. Role of lymphadenectomy during interval debulking surgery performed after neoadjuvant chemotherapy in patients with advanced ovarian cancer. Front Oncol 2021; 11:646135.

202. Seidler S, Koual M, Achen G, et al. Clinical impact of lymphadenectomy after neoadjuvant chemotherapy in advanced epithelial ovarian cancer: A review of available data. J Clin Med 2021; 10:334.

203. Bund V, Lecointre L, Velten M, et al. Impact of lymphadenectomy on survival of patients with serous advanced ovarian cancer after neoadjuvant chemotherapy: A French national multicenter study (FRANCOGYN). J Clin Med 2020; 9:2427.

204. Coleman RL, Spirtos NM, Enserro D, et al. Secondary surgical cytoreduction for recurrent ovarian cancer. N Engl J Med 2019; 381:1929–1939.

205. Du Bois A, Vergote I, Ferron G, et al. Randomized controlled phase III study evaluating the impact of secondary cytoreductive surgery in recurrent ovarian cancer: AGO DESKTOP III/ENGOT ov20. J Clin Oncol 2017; 35:5501.

206. Harter P, Sehouli J, Reuss A, et al. Prospective validation study of a predictive score for operability of recurrent ovarian cancer: The Multicenter Intergroup Study DESKTOP II. Int J Gynecol Cancer 2011; 21:289–95.

207. Tian WJ, Chi DS, Sehouli J, et al. A risk model for secondary cytoreductive surgery in recurrent ovarian cancer: An evidence-based proposal for patient selection. Ann Surg Oncol 2012; 19:597–604.
208. So M, Miyamoto T, Murakami R, et al. The efficacy of secondary cytoreductive surgery for recurrent ovarian, tubal, or peritoneal cancer in Tian-model low-risk patients. J Gynecol Oncol 2019; 30:e100.
209. Marchetti C, Fagotti A, Tombolini V, et al. The role of secondary cytoreductive surgery in recurrent ovarian cancer: A systematic review and meta-analysis. Ann Surg Oncol 2021; 28:3258–3263.
210. Capozzi VA, Rosati A, Turco LC, et al. Surgery vs. chemotherapy for ovarian cancer recurrence: what is the best treatment option. Gland Surg 2020; 9:1112–1117
211. Nagase S, Ohta T, Seino M. Primary chemotherapy and targeted molecular therapy of epithelial ovarian cancer. In: Katabuchi H (Ed). Frontiers in Ovarian Cancer Science.Singapore; Springer; 2017. pp. 207–224.
212. Ozols RF, Bundy BN, Greer BE, et al. Phase III trial of carboplatin and paclitaxel compared with cisplatin and paclitaxel in patients with optimally resected stage III ovarian cancer: a Gynecologic Oncology Group study. J Clin Oncol 2003; 21:3194–3200.
213. Murakami R, Matsumura N, Brown JB, et al.Prediction of taxane and platinum sensitivity in ovarian cancer based on gene expression profiles. Gynecol Oncol 2016; 141:49–56.
214. Young RC, Walton LA, Ellenberg SS, et al. Adjuvant therapy in stage I and stage II epithelial ovarian cancer. Results of two prospective randomized trials. N Engl J Med 1990; 322:1021–1027.
215. Monga M, Carmichael JA, Shelley WE, et al. Surgery without adjuvant chemotherapy for early epithelial ovarian carcinoma after comprehensive surgical staging. Gynecol Oncol 1991; 43:195–197.
216. Trimbos JB, Vergote I, Bolis G, et al. Impact of adjuvant chemotherapy and surgical staging in early-stage ovarian carcinoma: European Organisation for Research and Treatment of Cancer-Adjuvant ChemoTherapy in Ovarian Neoplasm trial. J Natl Cancer Inst 2003; 95:113–125.
217. Colombo N, Guthrie D, Chiari S, et al. International Collaborative Ovarian Neoplasm trial 1: A randomized trial of adjuvant chemotherapy in women with early-stage ovarian cancer. J Natl Cancer Inst 2003; 95:125–132.
218. Lawrie TA, Winter-Roach BA, Heus P, et al. Adjuvant (post-surgery) chemotherapy for early stage epithelial ovarian cancer. Cochrane Database Syst Rev 2015; 12:CD004706.
219. Chan JK, Brady MF, Penson RT, et al. Weekly vs. every-3-week paclitaxel and carboplatin for ovarian cancer. N Engl J Med 2016; 374:738–748.
220. Clamp AR, James EC, McNeish IA, et al. Weekly dose-dense chemotherapy in first-line epithelial ovarian, fallopian tube, or primary peritoneal carcinoma treatment (ICON8): Primary progression free survival analysis results from a GCIG phase 3 randomised controlled trial. Lancet 2019; 394:2084–2095.
221. Pirolli R, de Alencar VTL, Estati FL, et al. Comparison of dose-dense vs. 3-weekly paclitaxel and carboplatin in the first-line treatment of ovarian cancer in a propensity score-matched cohort. BMC Cancer 2021; 21:525.
222. Fujiwara K, Hasegawa K, Nagao S. Landscape of systemic therapy for ovarian cancer in 2019: Primary therapy. Cancer 2019; 125:4582–4586.
223. Provencher DM, Gallagher CJ, Parulekar WR, at al. OV21/PETROC: a randomized Gynecologic Cancer Intergroup phase II study of intraperitoneal versus intravenous chemotherapy following neoadjuvant chemotherapy and optimal debulking surgery in epithelial ovarian cancer. Ann Oncol 2018; 29:431–438.
224. Walker JL, Brady MF, Wenzel L, et al. Randomized trial of intravenous versus intraperitoneal chemotherapy plus bevacizumab in advanced ovarian carcinoma: An NRG Oncology/Gynecologic Oncology Group study. J Clin Oncol 2019; 37:1380–1390.
225. Riggs MJ, Pandalai PK, Kim J, et al. Hyperthermic intraperitoneal chemotherapy in ovarian cancer. Diagnostics (Basel) 2020; 10:43.
226. van Driel WJ, Koole SN, Sikorska K, et al. Hyperthermic intraperitoneal chemotherapy in ovarian cancer. N Engl J Med 2018; 378:230–240.
227. Zhang G, Zhu Y, Liu C, et al. The prognosis impact of hyperthermic intraperitoneal chemotherapy (HIPEC) plus cytoreductive surgery (CRS) in advanced ovarian cancer: The meta-analysis. J Ovarian Res 2019;12:33.
228. Cianci S, Riemma G, Ronsini C, et al. Hyperthermic intraperitoneal chemotherapy (HIPEC) for ovarian cancer recurrence: Systematic review and meta-analysis. Gland Surg 2020; 9:1140–1148.
229. Wu CC, Hsu YT, Chang CL. Hyperthermic intraperitoneal chemotherapy enhances antitumor effects on ovarian cancer through immune-mediated cancer stem cell targeting. Int J Hyperthermia 2021; 38:1013–1022.
230. Yanazume S, Kobayashi H. Treatment of recurrent epithelial ovarian cancer. In: Katabuchi H (ed). Frontiers in Ovarian Cancer Science. Singapore: Springer; 2017. pp. 243–265.

231. Pignata S, Pisano C, Di Napoli M, et al. Treatment of recurrent epithelial ovarian cancer. Cancer 2019; 125:4609–4615.

232. Aghajanian C, Blank SV, Goff BA, et al. OCEANS: A randomized, double-blind, placebo-controlled phase III trial of chemotherapy with or without bevacizumab in patients with platinum-sensitive recurrent epithelial ovarian, primary peritoneal, or fallopian tube cancer. J Clin Oncol 2012; 30:2039–2045.

233. Pujade-Lauraine E, Ledermann JA, Selle F, et al. Olaparib tablets as maintenance therapy in patients with platinum-sensitive, relapsed ovarian cancer and a BRCA1/2 mutation (SOLO2/ENGOT-Ov21): A double-blind, randomised, placebo-controlled, phase 3 trial. Lancet Oncol 2017; 18:1274–1284.

234. Elyashiv O, Wong YNS, Ledermann JA. Frontline maintenance treatment for ovarian cancer. Curr Oncol Rep 2021; 23:97.

235. Pignata S, Cecere SC. How to sequence treatment in relapsed ovarian cancer. Future Oncol 2021; 17:1–8.

236. Pujade-Lauraine E, Hilpert F, Weber B, et al. Bevacizumab combined with chemotherapy for platinum-resistant recurrent ovarian cancer: The AURELIA open-label randomized phase III trial. J Clin Oncol 2014; 32:1302–1308.

237. Indini A, Nigro O, Lengyel CG, et al. Immune-checkpoint inhibitors in platinum-resistant ovarian cancer. Cancers (Basel) 2021; 13:1663.

238. Friedlander ML. Do all patient with recurrent ovarian cancer need systemic therapy? Cancer 2019; 125:4602–4608.

239. Burger RA, Brady MF, Bookman MA, et al. Incorporation of bevacizumab in the primary treatment of ovarian cancer. N Engl J Med 2011;365:2473–2483.

240. Perren TJ, Swart AM, Pfisterer J, et al. A phase 3 trial of bevacizumab in ovarian cancer. N Engl J Med. 2011;365:2484–2496.

241. Oza AM, Cook AD, Pfisterer J, et al. Standard chemotherapy with or without bevacizumab for women with newly diagnosed ovarian cancer (ICON7): Overall survival results of a phase 3 randomised trial. Lancet Oncol. 2015; 16:928–936.

242. Tewari KS, Burger RA, Enserro D, et al. Final overall survival of a randomized trial of bevacizumab for primary treatment of ovarian cancer. J Clin Oncol 2019; 37:2317–2328.

243. Collinson F, Hutchinson M, Craven RA, et al. Predicting response to bevacizumab in ovarian cancer: A panel of potential biomarkers informing treatment selection. Clin Cancer Res 2013; 19:5227–5239.

244. du Bois A, Floquet A, Kim JW, et al. Incorporation of pazopanib in maintenance therapy of ovarian cancer. J Clin Oncol 2014; 32:3374–3382.

245. du Bois A, Kristensen G, Ray-Coquard I, et al. Standard first-line chemotherapy with or without nintedanib for advanced ovarian cancer (AGO-OVAR 12): A randomised, double-blind, placebo-controlled phase 3 trial. Lancet Oncol 2016; 17:78–89.

246. Vergote I, du Bois A, Floquet A, et al. Overall survival results of AGO-OVAR16: A phase 3 study of maintenance pazopanib versus placebo in women who have not progressed after first-line chemotherapy for advanced ovarian cancer. Gynecol Oncol 2019; 155:186–191.

247. Ray-Coquard I, Cibula D, Mirza MR, et al. Final results from GCIG/ENGOT/AGO-OVAR 12: A randomised placebo-controlled phase III trial of nintedanib combined with chemotherapy for newly diagnosed advanced ovarian cancer. Int J Cancer 2020; 146:439–448.

248. Ledermann JA, Embleton-Thirsk AC, Perren TJ, et al. Cediranib in addition to chemotherapy for women with relapsed platinum-sensitive ovarian cancer (ICON6): Overall survival results of a phase III randomised trial. ESMO Open 2021; 6:100043.

249. Farmer H, McCabe N, Lord CJ, et al. Targeting the DNA repair defect in BRCA mutant cells as a therapeutic strategy. Nature 2005; 434:917–921.

250. Ledermann J, Harter P, Gourley C, et al. Olaparib maintenance therapy in platinum-sensitive relapsed ovarian cancer. N Engl J Med 2012; 366:1382–1392.

251. Mirza MR, Monk BJ, Herrstedt J, et al. Niraparib maintenance therapy in platinum-sensitive, recurrent ovarian cancer. N Engl J Med 2016; 375:2154–2164.

252. Coleman RL, Oza AM, Lorusso D, et al. ARIEL3 investigators Rucaparib maintenance treatment for recurrent ovarian carcinoma after response to platinum therapy (ARIEL3): A randomised, double-blind, placebo-controlled, phase 3 trial. Lancet 2017; 390:1949–1961.

253. Moore K, Colombo N, Scambia G, et al. Maintenance olaparib in patients with newly diagnosed advanced ovarian cancer. N Engl J Med 2018; 379:2495–2505.

254. Gonzalez-Martin A, Pothuri B, Vergote I, et al. Niraparib in patients with newly diagnosed advanced ovarian cancer. N Eng J Med 2019; 381:2391–2402.

255. Ray-Coquard I, Pautier P, Pignata S, et al. Olaparib plus bevacizumab as first-line maintenance in ovarian cancer. N Engl J Med 2019; 381:2416–2428.
256. Coleman RL, Fleming GF, Brady MF, et al. Veliparib with first-line chemotherapy and as maintenance therapy in ovarian cancer. N Engl J Med 2019; 381:2403–2415.
257. Arora S, Balasubramaniam S, Zhang H, et al. FDA approval summary: Olaparib monotherapy or in combination with bevacizumab for the maintenance treatment of patients with advanced ovarian cancer. Oncologist 2020; 26:e164–e172.
258. Miller RE, Leary A, Scott CL, et al. ESMO recommendations on predictive biomarker testing for homologous recombination deficiency and PARP inhibitor benefit in ovarian cancer. Ann Oncol 2020; 31:1606–1622.
259. Banerjee S, Gonzalez-Martin A, Harter P, et al. First-line PARP inhibitors in ovarian cancer: Summary of an ESMO Open - Cancer Horizons round-table discussion. ESMO Open. 2020; 5:e001110.
260. Mandai M, Hamanishi J, Abiko K, et al. Immunotherapy for gynecologic cancer. In: Konishi I, ed. Precision Medicine in Gynecology and Obstetrics. Singapore: Springer; 2017. pp. 69–85.
261. Hartnett EG, Knight J, Radolec M, et al. Immunotherapy advances for epithelial ovarian cancer. Cancers (Basel) 2020; 12:3733.
262. Berek JS, Taylor PT, Gordon A, et al. Randomized, placebo-controlled study of oregovomab for consolidation of clinical remission in patients with advanced ovarian cancer. J Clin Oncol 2004; 22:3507–3516.
263. Sabbatini P, Harter P, Scambia G, et al. Abagovomab as maintenance therapy in patients with epithelial ovarian cancer: A phase III trial of the AGO OVAR, COGI, GINECO, and GEICO-the MIMOSA study. J Clin Oncol 2013; 31:1554–1561.
264. Moore KN, Oza AM, Colombo N, et al. Phase III, randomized trial of mirvetuximab soravtansine versus chemotherapy in patients with platinum-resistant ovarian cancer: primary analysis of FORWARD I. Ann Oncol 2021; 32:757–765.
265. Chamoto K, Hatae R, Honjo T. Current issues and perspectives in PD-1 blockade cancer immunotherapy. Int J Clin Oncol 2020; 25:790–800.
266. González-Martín A, Sánchez-Lorenzo L. Immunotherapy with checkpoint inhibitors in patients with ovarian cancer: Still promising? Cancer 2019; 125:4616–4622.
267. Varga A, Piha-Paul S, Ott PA, et al. Pembrolizumab in patients with programmed death ligand 1-positive advanced ovarian cancer: Analysis of KEYNOTE-028. Gynecol Oncol 2019; 152:243–250.
268. Disis ML, Taylor MH, Kelly K, et al. Efficacy and safety of avelumab for patients with recurrent or refractory ovarian cancer: Phase 1b results from the JAVELIN solid tumor trial. JAMA Oncol 2019; 5:393–401.
269. Liu JF, Gordon M, Veneris J, et al. Safety, clinical activity and biomarker assessments of atezolizumab from a Phase I study in advanced/recurrent ovarian and uterine cancers. Gynecol Oncol 2019; 154:314–322.
270. Matulonis UA, Shapira-Frommer R, Santin AD, et al. Antitumor activity and safety of pembrolizumab in patients with advanced recurrent ovarian cancer: Results from the phase II KEYNOTE-100 study. Ann Oncol 2019; 30:1080–1087.
271. Zamarin D, Burger RA, Sill MW, et al. Randomized phase II trial of nivolumab versus nivolumab and ipilimumab for recurrent or persistent ovarian cancer: An NRG Oncology study. J Clin Oncol 2020; 38:1814–1823.
272. Pujade-Lauraine E, Fujiwara K, Ledermann JA, et al. Avelumab alone or in combination with chemotherapy versus chemotherapy alone in platinum-resistant or platinum-refractory ovarian cancer (JAVELIN Ovarian 200): An open-label, three-arm, randomised, phase 3 study. Lancet Oncol 2021; 22:1034–1046.
273. Liu JF, Herold C, Gray KP, et al. Assessment of combined nivolumab and bevacizumab in relapsed ovarian cancer: A phase 2 clinical trial. JAMA Oncol 2019; 5:1731–1738.
274. Moore KN, Bookman M, Sehouli J, et al. Atezolizumab, bevacizumab, and chemotherapy for newly diagnosed stage III or IV ovarian cancer: Placebo-controlled randomized phase III trial (IMagyn050/GOG 3015/ENGOT-OV39). J Clin Oncol 2021; 39:1842–1855.
275. Konstantinopoulos PA, Waggoner S, Vidal GA, et al. Single-arm phases 1 and 2 trial of niraparib in combination with pembrolizumab in patients with recurrent platinum-resistant ovarian carcinoma. JAMA Oncol 2019; 5:1141–1149.
276. Aust S, Schwameis R, Gagic T, et al. Precision medicine tumor boards: Clinical applicability of personalized treatment concepts in ovarian cancer. Cancers (Basel) 2020; 12:548.
277. Saotome K, Chiyoda T, Aimono E, et al. Clinical implications of next-generation sequencing-based panel tests for malignant ovarian tumors. Cancer Med 2020; 9:7407–7417.

278. Lee YJ, Kim D, Kim HS, et al. Integrating a next generation sequencing panel into clinical practice in ovarian cancer. Yonsei Med J 2019; 60:914–923.
279. Varnier R, Le Saux O, Chabaud S, et al. Actionable molecular alterations in advanced gynaecologic malignancies: Updated results from the ProfiLER programme. Eur J Cancer 2019; 118:156–165.
280. Spreafico A, Oza AM, Clarke BA, et al. Genotype-matched treatment for patients with advanced type I epithelial ovarian cancer (EOC). Gynecol Oncol 2017; 144:250–255.
281. Gunderson CC, Rowland MR, Wright DL, et al. Initiation of a formalized precision medicine program in gynecologic oncology. Gynecol Oncol 2016; 141:24–28.
282. Le Tourneau C, Delord JP, Gonçalves A, et al. Molecularly targeted therapy based on tumour molecular profiling versus conventional therapy for advanced cancer (SHIVA): A multicentre, open-label, proof-of-concept, randomised, controlled phase 2 trial. Lancet Oncol 2015; 16:1324–1334.
283. Paracchini L, D'Incalci M, Marchini S. Liquid biopsy in the clinical management of high-grade serous epithelial ovarian cancer: Current use and future opportunities. Cancers (Basel) 2021; 13:2386.
284. Chang L, Ni J, Zhu Y, et al. Liquid biopsy in ovarian cancer: Recent advances in circulating extracellular vesicle detection for early diagnosis and monitoring progression. Theranostics 2019; 9:4130–4140.
285. Shimizu A, Sawada K, Kimura T. Pathophysiological role and potential therapeutic exploitation of exosomes in ovarian cancer. Cells 2020; 9:814.
286. Ferreira P, Roela RA, Lopez RVM, et al. The prognostic role of microRNA in epithelial ovarian cancer: A systematic review of literature with an overall survival meta-analysis. Oncotarget 2020; 11:1085–1095.
287. Noguchi T, Iwahashi N, Sakai K, et al. Comprehensive gene mutation profiling of circulating tumor DNA in ovarian cancer: Its pathological and prognostic impact. Cancers (Basel) 2020; 12:3382.
288. Charo LM, Eskander RN, Okamura R, et al. Clinical implications of plasma circulating tumor DNA in gynecologic cancer patients. Mol Oncol 2021; 15:67–79.